SPORTS SCIENCE HANDBOOK

The Essential Guide to Kinesiology, Sport and Exercise Science

Volume 2: I–Z

by

Simon P. R. Jenkins

Published in Great Britain by
MULTI-SCIENCE PUBLISHING CO. LTD
5 Wates Way, Brentwood, Essex CM15 9TB, UK

© 2005 Simon P.R. Jenkins

ISBN 0906522 37 4

Contents

To my late father, Gilbert Ivor Jenkins

Foreword

The trend in professions relating to sport and exercise, including physical education, has been to move from general issues towards more specialized concerns with respect to the scientific knowledge available. Scientific technology has advanced to the stage that human movement can be analyzed using three-dimensional high-speed digital video analysis and athletic potential can be determined using biochemical analysis.

Much of what students learn has a strong interrelationship that requires a common base of theoretical knowledge and practical application. Terminology is often a barrier in the study of human movement, especially in the scientific disciplines. Dr. Jenkins' *Sports Science Handbook* brings a clear focus of how Kinesiology, Sport & Exercise Science, Physical Education, and Health interrelate and provides a framework of commonality in which to discuss key concepts. It is an impressive collection of diligently researched and useful references.

I believe that this book will become highly regarded in the USA, as well as many other nations, and it will be heavily used as an authoritative reference book. It is a must for every university library; for departments related to health, physical education and sports science; and especially for professors and students in these fields.

DANNY R. MIELKE, Ed.D.; M.P.H.; C.H.E.S.
Professor, Eastern Oregon University

Preface

As a boy, growing up in the UK, my dreams included playing rugby for Wales and winning the British Open golf championship. I didn't fulfill those dreams, but I did become a good all-round sportsman. I was obsessed with playing sport, but eventually my motivation turned to finding out why I was unable to emulate my heroes. It was the urge to understand the processes involved in skill acquisition, performance enhancement and injury prevention that drove me to study sports science, and to pursue it as my vocation. Having completed my undergraduate degree, I was inspired by my father's book, *Oil Economist's Handbook*, to produce a similar book for sports science.

When the first edition of *Sports Science Handbook* was published, I was in the midst of my doctoral studies at the University of Oxford, with a thesis entitled, "Conscious and Unconscious Control in Highly Learned Motor Actions." My research was carried out on the PGA European Tour, at the same time as I worked as a caddie. My theoretical, empirical and experiential insights made me realize why I was never going to win the British Open.

After completing my doctoral work in 1994, I became a lecturer in sports science at St. Mary's University College, specializing in psychology and also teaching courses in research methods and statistics. At the University of Surrey (Guildford), an opportunity arose to lead the development of a new sports science program designed specifically for part-time adult learners. At Surrey, I learned much from colleagues, such as Dr. Joe Millward in nutritional science, and Nicky Gilbert in dietetics, who contributed to my courses. Subsequently, at the University of Wales (Swansea), I led the development of a new sports science degree for full-time students. My understanding of chemistry was enhanced through developing a course on exercise metabolism with Dr. Tony Wellington. Basic knowledge in chemistry is important for being able to gain a thorough understanding of many questions in exercise science. I also led the development of a state-of-the-art motion analysis laboratory, and gained new perspectives on biomechanics by working with colleagues in physics and engineering. By 2001, I had delivered or developed courses in most of the subdisciplines related to sports science.

Between 1997 and 2001, I was also an Associate Coach for the English Golf Union, working in the Winter Coaching Program for Potential Boy Internationals in the South Region. I worked with the professional golf teachers, Steve Rolley and Gary Smith, providing education and training on fitness, diet and psychology. Most of the boys dreamed of winning the British Open, and my corpus of knowledge from sports science, as well as my research on golf, should increase the probability that at least one of these boys will fulfill that dream.

Having worked in the USA since 2002, I am currently working as a Visiting Lecturer at Pepperdine University. Two of the coaches at Pepperdine are Dr. Marv Dunphy, who was Head Coach of the gold-medal winning USA Volleyball team at the 1988 Olympic Games; and Paul Westphal, who was a successful NBA coach after a stellar career as a player with the

University of Southern California and the Boston Celtics. During one of his coaching classes in 2004, which I sat in on, Dunphy conducted an interview with Westphal, who was asked whether it was more important for one of his players to get a degree or to be drafted for the NBA. Westphal replied, "There's a politically correct answer, but I'm not going to give it. I want to see the young man succeed and fulfill his dreams." For some student-athletes, making a good college team and getting a degree is the fulfillment of a dream; an end in itself. For other student-athletes, college is a stepping-stone for, say, becoming an NBA player or an Olympian.

Consider the case of Matt Leinart, who was quarterback of national football champions University of Southern California in 2005 and also the recipient of the Heisman Trophy. Rather than enter the 2005 NFL Draft, with the prospect of making millions of dollars, Leinart decided to stay at the University of Southern California for his final year of eligibility, which would also allow him to achieve the final 18 credits required for his sociology degree. Leinart said he thought his decision "made a statement to college football – maybe to student-athletes about school being more important" than money (*Los Angeles Times*, 15 January 2005).

My involvement in providing education and training for NCAA Division I athletes has largely been through teaching a health and life skills course, based on the NCAA program, "Challenging Athletes' Minds for Personal Success" (CHAMPS). Objectives of the CHAMPS program include: supporting the efforts of every student-athlete toward intellectual development and graduation; using athletics as a preparation for success in life; respecting diversity; and enabling student-athletes to make meaningful contributions to their communities.

Following my experience in adapted physical education at Eastern Oregon University and also in golf coaching for the Special Olympics, I was inspired to develop an adapted physical activity program at Pepperdine. This program provides opportunity for persons with developmental disabilities, such as Down syndrome, to participate in golf and aquatics. The life skills of many students from my CHAMPS classes at Pepperdine have enabled the Adapted Physical Activity program to be a success.

The major addition of information on disabilities and health for this edition of the *Sports Science Handbook* reflects my work in this area over the last four years. The desire to understand the relevant psychology and physiology was driven by the practical experience. Consider these words from the reflective journal of a student on the Adapted Aquatics Program at Eastern Oregon University:

"I worked with a girl who has autism, cerebral palsy, and a Dandy-Walker cyst. I never knew that an individual could have so many disorders. She walks around school with a walker, and according to the aide, she maneuvers it very well. She also controls her upper body better than most people with cerebral palsy, and she does not drool. As I learned from talking to the aide, my girl feeds herself and she also lets people know what she wants by using cue cards. She is also very capable of maneuvering herself in her wheelchair, as I found out when she raced us, while we were on scooters. Although my girl has all these disorders and handicaps, she is a very unique and wonderful person. All the days she is in a good mood, she is a blast. She smiles and laughs a lot. She even grunts a little. In the pool, she is usually very active and cooperative and seems to be having fun. On the days she is not in a very good mood, you just try to make it fun. Working with my girl was exciting, memorable and fulfilling."

Using the Book

A feature of the *Sports Science Handbook* is that the language used in scientific journals is maintained as much as possible, in order to gain an understanding of terminology and concepts. Development of the book has been driven by a 'top-down' approach in which overviews of important areas are compiled, before detail is added. Many entries provide a concise and comprehensive coverage of a particular subject matter. Within these entries, some scientific terms are highlighted in bold and are defined. Most of the scientific terms that are not highlighted in bold are defined in a separate entry, but the author has avoided use of a signifier (such as an asterisk) for highlighting the terms that are defined in a separate entry. No hard and fast rules were used to determine where scientific terms are defined, but an attempt has been made to make the book user-friendly. The book is largely a 'review of authoritative reviews;' thus to avoid unnecessary cluttering of the text, citations in the text are minimized. Instead, a bibliography is provided at the end of the entry and further bibliographies attached to cross-referenced terms or to entries for relevant subdisciplines. There is also a general bibliography, which includes textbooks that were used extensively by the author when compiling this latest edition of the *Sports Science Handbook*.

The *Sports Science Handbook* provides concise and up-to-date overviews of subject matter and clarifies confusing issues. It can be used, for example, to distinguish: ability vs. skill; cellulite vs. stretch marks; cholesterol vs. lipoprotein; convulsion vs. seizure; creep vs. stress relaxation; force vs. work; hypnosis vs. meditation; learning disability vs. mental retardation; medial tibial stress syndrome vs. shin splints; negative reinforcement vs. punishment; power vs. strength; reflex vs. stereotypy; stretch reflex vs. stretch-shortening cycle; and torque vs. torsion.

The book can be used as a source of reference for introductory or foundation courses that are concerned with: (i) the nature and scope of kinesiology and its various professional applications; (ii) key concepts and terminology within the subdisciplines; (iii) the historical and philosophical foundations of the field; and (iv) the use of historical knowledge to understand current issues, controversies and future directions.

Readership

The book will be useful to students throughout their academic career as a handbook for work on essays, projects, laboratory reports, exam revision, and thesis ideas. Teachers in high

Foreword

The trend in professions relating to sport and exercise, including physical education, has been to move from general issues towards more specialized concerns with respect to the scientific knowledge available. Scientific technology has advanced to the stage that human movement can be analyzed using three-dimensional high-speed digital video analysis and athletic potential can be determined using biochemical analysis.

Much of what students learn has a strong interrelationship that requires a common base of theoretical knowledge and practical application. Terminology is often a barrier in the study of human movement, especially in the scientific disciplines. Dr. Jenkins' *Sports Science Handbook* brings a clear focus of how Kinesiology, Sport & Exercise Science, Physical Education, and Health interrelate and provides a framework of commonality in which to discuss key concepts. It is an impressive collection of diligently researched and useful references.

I believe that this book will become highly regarded in the USA, as well as many other nations, and it will be heavily used as an authoritative reference book. It is a must for every university library; for departments related to health, physical education and sports science; and especially for professors and students in these fields.

DANNY R. MIELKE, Ed.D.; M.P.H.; C.H.E.S.
Professor, Eastern Oregon University

Acknowledgements

To Dr. Danny Mielke, who provided me with the initial opportunity to work in the USA as a sabbatical replacement, Assistant Professor in the Department of Physical Education and Health at Eastern Oregon University in La Grande for the academic year 2001-2002; and to whom I am indebted for mentoring and inspiration in many aspects of sport, physical education, and health in the USA. It is most appropriate that Dr. Mielke has kindly written the foreword for this edition of the *Sports Science Handbook*.

To Dr. Peggy Anderson, also of the Department of Physical Education and Health at Eastern Oregon University, for facilitating my work in the Adapted Aquatics Program with Mr. Bill Durand of the Union-Baker School District, before she took leave for her sabbatical year. Working in this program has been the most rewarding experience of my career. I am grateful to Mr. Durand for enabling me to learn so much from his expertise in adapted physical education; and to the PE students at Eastern Oregon University, who were so devoted to their work. To Dr. Caroline Vos Strache, who brought me to Pepperdine University in Malibu for 2002–2003 as her sabbatical replacement to coordinate the major in Physical Education.

To Dr. Doug Swartzendruber, who made me welcome for an extended period of employment as a Visiting Lecturer in the Natural Science Division at Pepperdine and who supported my efforts to develop an adapted physical activity program for persons with developmental disabilities.

To Mike Anderson, my colleague in Physical Education at Pepperdine, for making my life easy when it came to matters of academic administration.

To Kimberlee Rodriguez of the Athletics Department at Pepperdine, for our many discussions about the lives of student-athletes and for encouraging students to take my classes.

To my students at Pepperdine University, who read and provided comments on entries that were being prepared for this edition, especially Morgan Matthies and Joey Parker; and, specifically, to students in my History & Philosophy class, whose feedback convinced me to embed the chronology items in the main part of the book rather than in a separate section: Nelson Caraballo, Jasmine Clarendon, Amber Coffman, Teiosha George, Amber Heydel, Terrance Johnson, Marvin Lea, Glen McGowan, Derek Mills, Leslie Pacheco, Ali Pavoni, Maytal Shvartz, and Ashley Swanson.

To my publisher, Bill Hughes, for his confidence in the vision of this book for the US market.

To my family and friends for continual support and encouragement; and especially to my wife, Chrys, who provided limitless patience, as well as guidance and assistance on editing; and spurred me to write a preface explaining why the book is a vocational project.

Introduction

Kinesiology

The *Sports Science Handbook* has now adopted a subtitle that includes the term 'kinesiology,' which can be defined as the study of movement or, more generally, the study of physical activity (Newell, 1990). In 1993, the American Academy of Physical Education (AAPE) changed its name to the American Academy of Kinesiology and Physical Education (AAKPE).

While the term 'kinesiology' has become accepted in higher education, the term 'physical education' is the correct name for the teaching of exercise and sport activities (and related theoretical knowledge) in elementary and high schools, because it has long been understood by society (Spirduso, 1990).

The American Academy of Kinesiology and Physical Education (AAKPE) provides information about doctoral programs that focus on the study of physical activity. Based on a survey of programs at 61 doctoral institutions (69 departments) by the AAKPE, the most frequently used terms in departmental titles are: kinesiology (22), exercise and/or sport(s) science(s) (21), health (14), physical education (6) and human performance (5). The widespread use of the term 'kinesiology' is shown also by the fact that eight of the eleven "Big Ten" Schools in the USA now have a department (or division) with 'kinesiology' in its name. None of these schools has a department with 'physical education' in its name, but the Department of Kinesiology at the University of Indiana is in the School of Health, Physical Education & Recreation. The term 'sport & exercise science,' or simply 'exercise science,' is now often used by departments that embrace contexts other than sport, especially those concerned with health. Only one of the "Big Ten" schools (University of Iowa) has 'exercise science' in the name of a department, but three other schools have named programs or majors at undergraduate level in 'exercise science.' The University of Michigan defines the scope of its major in 'movement science' as being biomechanics, physiology and motor control, but the University of Wisconsin-Madison uses a broader definition of 'movement science' and also has a major in 'exercise science.' The Exercise Science option at Wisconsin-Madison prepares students for graduate study in exercise physiology, cardiac rehabilitation, sport psychology, or biomechanics; whereas the Movement Science option prepares students for graduate study in motor behavior, motor control/learning, motor development, sport psychology, or biomechanics. What the University of Wisconsin-Madison calls 'movement science' is called 'exercise science' at the University of Indiana (Bloomington) and the University of Iowa. Ohio State University uses 'exercise science' to refer to the field of health-related fitness (fitness evaluation/exercise prescription), but Penn State University calls this 'movement science.'

The chronology of name changes at Michigan State University, one of the "Big Ten" schools, is a good reflection of historical trends and the fact that 'kinesiology' is perhaps the best 'catch-all' term for university departments to use in their name: Department of Physical Culture and Athletics (1899); Department of Physical Training (1916); Department of Physical Education (1921); Department of Physical Education, Health and Recreation (1944); Department of Health, Physical Education and Recreation (1954); Department of Health and Physical Education (1981); School of Health Education, Counseling Psychology and Human Performance (1985); Department of Physical Education and Exercise Science (1990); and Department of Kinesiology (1998).

Physical Education as an Academic Discipline

Central to historical accounts of the development of kinesiology from physical education are the University of California, Berkeley and the University of California, Los Angeles (UCLA). In the early 1940s, the Executive Committee of the College of Letters and Science at the University of California (Berkeley) completed a review of the physical education department and concluded that its curriculum was lacking in academic content. As a result, the physical education department proposed a new major that met the College's criteria for academic standards. Elsewhere, physical education continued to be regarded as an area of teaching rather than an academic discipline. Many physical educators argued that academic theory, empirical research and scholarship are of little use to those engaged in the practice of teaching children and youths in schools.

In the early 1960s, James Conant studied the education of the nation's teachers and recommended that graduate programs in physical education be abolished due to lack of academic credibility. In 1962, the Fisher Bill was passed in the state of California. It created a single-subject teaching credential that limited a teacher to a specific subject field. Physical education was identified as a nonacademic area, but it could be classified as an academic area if certain criteria were met. Following the Fisher Bill and Conant's report, physical education departments in universities and colleges underwent academic reform.

In the 1950s, the Physical Education Department at the University of California, Los Angeles (UCLA) offered one of the finest teacher preparation programs in the USA (Smith, 1999). The first research facility, the Human Performance Laboratory, was dedicated in 1958. With the establishment of California's Master Plan for Higher Education in 1960, most teacher preparation programs for University of California undergraduates were discontinued. Consequently, the School of Applied Arts at UCLA was disestablished. The Physical Education Department was transferred to the Life Science Division in the College of Letters and Science, and the tenured faculty members designed new educational programs in the science of human movement. A revised physical education major, involving primarily one of three allied fields of study – physiology, psychology or sociology – was approved in 1962. This major became a model for adoption by other universities, especially after the State Board of Education approved it in 1965 as being equivalent to that of an academic subject-matter major. Camille Brown, a professor of physical education at UCLA, was described by *Quest* as "an accomplished conceptual synthesizer who works in the areas of human movement theory and physical education curriculum." The Kinesiology Department at UCLA was established in 1972 and was the first of its kind in the USA. In 1990, however, the Kinesiology Department at UCLA became the Physiological Science Department, when it was decided to decrease the scope of the department's research and education programs and focus primarily on physiology.

The American Alliance for Health, Physical Education, and Recreation (AAHPER) formed a panel in 1963 to address the professional preparation of physical education teachers and it publicly refuted the views of James Conant. In 1964, Franklin M. Henry spoke at the annual meeting of the National College Physical Education Association for Men (NCPEAM) on: "Physical Education – An Academic Discipline." Henry proposed that physical education must not only become a credible academic discipline, but also it must preside over the profession (practice) of physical education. Henry defined an academic discipline as an organized body of knowledge that is theoretical and scholarly, without any requirement of practical application, as distinguished from technical and professional knowledge (Henry, 1978).

In the history of physical education, a distinction is made between 'education of the physical' and 'education through the physical.' Charles McCloy was a champion of 'education of the physical,' in which the purpose of physical activity is to develop the physical body. Jesse F. Williams advocated 'education through the physical,' in which the purpose of sport and physical education is to build character. Following Franklin M. Henry's address in 1964, there was a shift away from both 'education of the physical' and 'education through the physical' towards a disciplinary-oriented approach in higher education.

Subdisciplines

For three years in the mid 1960s, the "Big Ten" directors met to discuss "The Body of Knowledge in Physical Education." Five subdisciplines were covered at all three meetings: history/philosophy of sport; exercise physiology, motor learning/sport psychology; biomechanics; and sport sociology. These subdisciplines represented much of what, at the time, was considered to be the body of knowledge for "the study of human movement (Thomas, 1990). By 1980, all the leading graduate programs in kinesiology across the USA were based on a subdisciplinary model (Swanson and Massengale, 1997).

Interdisciplinary and Cross-disciplinary

The subdisciplines have typically maintained their interdisciplinary connections (e.g. exercise physiology to physiology and biochemistry), but they have not sufficiently developed the cross-disciplinary connections (e.g. exercise physiology to biomechanics to psychology) that would broaden the impact of knowledge and research (Newell, 1990; Sharp, 2003). An example of an attempt to promote the cross-disciplinary approach can be found in the Department of Kinesiology at University of Illinois (Urbana-Champaign). The academic programs are organized around five clusters of core concepts related to the study of human movement: (i) Biodynamics of Physical Activity ("the study of work output, energy, and efficiency of movements as it relates to the nature of exercise stress, the mechanics of human movement, and fitness throughout the human lifespan"); (ii) Social Science of Physical Activity ("the study of the antecedents and consequences of involvement in physical activity and sport as well as the impact that physical activity and sport have upon individuals, society and culture"); (iii) Coordination, Control and Skill ("the study of the mechanisms and processes involved in the acquisition and performance of human motor skills"); (iv) Pedagogical Kinesiology ("the study of the organizational and instructional concepts essential for the efficient and effective conduct of physical activity programs, particularly those that relate to physical education and sport contexts"); and (v) Therapeutic Kinesiology ("the study of movement as a therapeutic vehicle for health and wellness, particularly the prevention and rehabilitation of injury, disease or movement dysfunction").

References

American Academy of Kinesiology and Physical Education. AAKPE Doctoral Program Information. 3 June 2004. Http://www.aakpe.org/

Brown, C. (1967). The structure of knowledge of physical education. *Quest* (monograph IX), 53-67.

Conant, J. (1963). *The education of American teachers*. New York: McGraw-Hill.

Department of Kinesiology (2000). College of Applied Life Studies. University of Illinois at Urbana-Champaign. Http://www.kines.uiuc.edu/overview

Dunn, J.M. (2001). Honoring the past – embracing the future. *Quest* 53(4), 495-506.

Estes, S.G. and Mechikoff, R.A. (1999). *Knowing Human Movement*. San Francisco, CA: Benjamin Cummings

Henry, F. (1964). Physical education as an academic discipline. *Journal of Health, Physical Education, and Recreation* 35(7), 32-33, 69.

Henry, F. (1978). *The academic discipline of physical education*. *Quest* 29, 13-29.

McCloy, C.H. (1940). *Philosophical basis for physical education*. New York: F.S. Crofts & Co.

Newell, K.M. (1990). Physical education in higher education: Chaos out of order. *Quest* 42(3), 227-242.

Newell, K.M. (1990). Physical activity, knowledge types, and degree programs. *Quest* 42(3), 243-268.

Newell, K. (1990). Kinesiology: The label for the study of physical activity in higher education. *Quest* 42(3), 269-278.

Sharp, R.L. (2003). Doctoral education: The mixture perspective. *Quest* 55, 82-85.

Smith, J.L. (1999). University of California: In Memoriam. Donald Thomas Handy, Kinesiology: Los Angeles. Http://dynaweb.oac.cdlib.org:8088/dynaweb/uchist/public/inmemoriam/inmemoriam1999/@Generi c..._

Swanson, R.A. and Massengale, J.D. (1997). Exercise and sport science in 20th century America. In: Massengale, J.D. and Swanson, R.A. (eds). *The history of exercise and sport science*. pp1-14. Champaign, IL: Human Kinetics.

Spirduso, W.W. (1990). Commentary: The Newell epic – A case for academic sanity. *Quest* 42, 297-304.

Thomas, J.R. (1990). The body of knowledge: A common core. In: Corbin, C.B. and Eckert, H.M. (eds). *The evolving undergraduate major*. pp5-12. Champaign, IL: Human Kinetics.

Williams, J.F. (1930). Education through the physical. *Journal of Higher Education* 1, 279-282.

Wrynn, A. (2003). Contesting the canon: Understanding the history of the evolving discipline of kinesiology. *Quest* 55(3), 244-256.

Zeigler, E.F. and McCristal, K.J. (1967). A history of the Big Ten Body-of-Knowledge Project in physical education. *Quest* 9, 79-84.

Survey of the eleven "Big Ten" Schools, December 2004

Department of Exercise Science. University of Iowa. Http://uiowa.edu/~exsci

Department of Health and Kinesiology. Purdue University. Http://www.sla.purdue.edu/academic/hk

Department of Kinesiology. College of Applied Life Studies. University of Illinois at Urbana-Champaign. Http://www.kines.uiuc.edu/

Department of Kinesiology. College of Education. Michigan State University. Http://edweb6.educ.msu.edu/kin.

Department of Kinesiology. College of Health and Human Development. Penn State University. Http://www.hhdev.psu.edu/kines/

Department of Kinesiology. School of Education. University of Wisconsin-Madison. Http://www.education.wisc.edu/kinesiology

Department of Kinesiology. School of Health, Physical Education and Recreation. Indiana University (Bloomington). Http://www.indiana.edu/~kines/

Division of Kinesiology. University of Michigan. Http://www.kines.umich.edu

Division of Kinesiology. College of Education and Human Development. University of Minnesota. Http://education.umn.edu/Kin

School of Physical Activity and Educational Services. College of Education. Ohio State University. Http://www.coe.ohio-state.edu/paes

Department of Physical Therapy & Human Movement Sciences. Feinberg School of Medicine. Northwestern University. Http://www.nupt.northwestern.edu

General Bibliography

American College of Sports Medicine (2001). *ACSM's resource manual for Guidelines for exercise testing & prescription*. 4th ed. Philadelphia, PA: Lippincott Williams & Wilkins.

Anderson, M.K., Hall, S.J. and Martin, M. (2004). *Foundations of athletic training: Prevention, assessment and management*. 3rd ed. Philadelphia, PA: Lippincott, Williams and Wilkins.

Anshel, M.II. (2003). *Sport psychology: From theory to practice*. 4th ed. San Francisco: Benjamin Cummings.

Antonio, J. and Stout, J.R. (2001). *Sports supplements*. Philadelphia, PA: Lippincott Williams & Wilkins.

Brown, S.P. (2000). *Introduction to exercise science*. Philadelphia, PA: Lippincott Williams & Wilkins.

Coakley, J. (2004). *Sports in society. Issues and controversies*. 8th ed. Boston, MA: McGraw-Hill.

Cox, R.H. (2002). *Sport psychology: Concepts and applications*. 5th ed. Boston, MA: McGraw-Hill.

Eitzen, D.S. and Sage, G.H. (2003). *Sociology of North American sport*. 7th ed. Boston, MA: McGraw-Hill.

Enoka, R.M. (2002). *Neuromechanics of human movement*. 3rd ed. Champaign, IL: Human Kinetics.

Gallahue, D.L. and Ozmun, J.C. (2002). *Understanding motor development. Infants, children, adolescents, adults*. 5th ed. New York, NY: McGraw-Hill.

Germann, W.J. and Stanfield, C.L. (2001). *Principles of human physiology*. San Francisco, CA: Benjamin Cummings.

Gill, D.L. (2000). *Psychological dynamics of sport and exercise*. 2nd ed. Champaign, IL: Human Kinetics.

Guyton, A.C. and Hall, J.E. (2000). *Textbook of medical physiology*. 10th ed. Philadelphia, PA: W.B. Saunders Co.

Hall, S.J. (2003). *Basic biomechanics*. 4th ed. Boston, MA: WCB McGraw Hill.

Hamill, J. and Knutzen, K.M. (2003). *Biomechanical basis of human movement*. 2nd ed. Philadelphia, PA: Lippincott Williams & Wilkins.

Hamilton, N. and Luttgens, K. (2002). *Kinesiology. Scientific basis of human motion*. 10th ed. Madison, WI: Brown & Benchmark.

Harries, M. et al. (1998). *Oxford textbook of sports medicine*. 2nd ed. Oxford: Oxford University Press.

Haywood, K.M. and Getchell, N. (2004). *Life span motor development*. 4th ed. Champaign, IL: Human Kinetics.

Horn, T. (2002, ed). *Advances in sport psychology*. 2nd ed. Champaign, IL: Human Kinetics.

Housh, T.J. and Housh, D.J. (2000, eds). *Introduction to exercise science*. Boston, MA: Allyn and Bacon.

Houston, M.E (2001). *Biochemistry primer for exercise science*. 2nd ed. Champaign, IL: Human Kinetics.

Insel, P., Turner, R.E. and Ross, D. (2004). *Nutrition*. 2nd ed. Sudbury, MA: Jones and Bartlett.

Irvin, R., Iversen, D. and Roy, S. (1998). *Sports medicine. Prevention, assessment, management and rehabilitation of athletic injuries*. 2nd ed. Boston, MA: Allyn & Bacon.

Kamen, G. (2001). *Foundations of Exercise Science*. Philadelphia, PA: Lippincott, Williams and Wilkins.

Kreighbaum, E. and Barthels, K.M. (1996). *Biomechanics: A qualitative approach*. 4th ed. Needham Heights, MA: Allyn and Bacon.

Leonard, W. (1998). *Sociological perspectives of sport*. 5th ed. San Francisco, CA: Benjamin Cummings.

Levangie, P.K. and Norkin, C.C. (2001). *Joint structure and function: A comprehensive analysis*. 3rd ed. Philadelphia, PA: F.A. Davis Company.

Le Veau, B.F. (1992). *Williams and Lissner's biomechanics of human motion*. 3rd ed. Philadelphia, PA: W.B. Saunders.

Marieb, E.N. (2002). *Anatomy and physiology*. San Francisco, CA: Benjamin Cummings.

Mathews, C.K., Van Holde, K.E. and Ahern, K. (2000). *Biochemistry*. 3rd ed. San Francisco, CA: Benjamin/Cummings.

McArdle, W.D, Katch, F.I. and Katch, V.L. (2004). *Exercise physiology. Energy, nutrition, and human performance*. 5th ed. Philadelphia, PA: Lippincott Williams & Wilkins.

Mechikoff, R.A. and Estes, S.G. (2002). *A history and philosophy of sport and physical education. From ancient civilization to the modern world*. 3rd ed Boston, MA: McGraw-Hill.

Nieman, D.C. (2003). *Exercise testing and prescription*. 5th ed. Boston, MA: McGraw-Hill.

Payne, V.G. and Isaacs, L.D. (2005). *Human motor development. A lifespan approach*. 6th ed. Boston, MA: McGraw-Hill.

Plowman, S.A. and Smith, D.L. (2003). *Exercise physiology for health, fitness and performance*. 2nd ed. San Francisco, CA: Benjamin Cummings.

Polidoro, J.R. (2000). *Sport and physical activity in the modern world*. San Francisco, CA: Benjamin Cummings.

Powers, S.K. and Dodd, S.L. (2003). *Total fitness and wellness*. 3rd ed. San Francisco, CA: Benjamin Cummings.

Powers, S.K. and Howley, E.T. (2004). *Exercise physiology. Theory and application to fitness and performance*. 5th ed. Boston, MA: McGraw-Hill.

Rasch, P.J. (1989). *Kinesiology and applied anatomy*. 7th ed. Philadelphia, PA: Lea & Febiger.

Robergs, R.A. and Roberts, S.O. (2000). *Fundamental principles of exercise physiology*. Boston, MA: McGraw-Hill.

Rose, D.J. (1997). *A multilevel approach to the study of motor control and learning*. San Francisco, CA: Benjamin Cummings.

Safran, M.R., McKeag, D.B. and Van Camp, S.P. (1998). *Manual of sports medicine*. Philadelphia, PA: Lippincot-Raven.

Schmidt, R.A. and Wrisberg, C.A. (2004). *Motor learning and performance*. 3rd ed. Champaign, IL: Human Kinetics.

Schmidt, R.A. and Lee, T.D. (1999). *Motor control and learning. A behavioral emphasis*. 3rd ed. Champaign, IL: Human Kinetics.

Sherill, C. (2004). *Adapted physical activity, recreation, and sport: Crossdisciplinary and lifespan*. 6th ed. Boston, MA: McGraw-Hill.

Sherry, E. and Wilson, S. (1998). *Oxford handbook of sports medicine*. 2nd ed. New York: Oxford University Press.

Siedentop, D. (2004). *Introduction to physical education, fitness and sport*. 5th ed. Boston, MA: McGraw-Hill.

Silva, J.M. and Stevens, D.E. (2002, eds). *Psychological foundations of sport*. Boston, MA: Allyn & Bacon.

Stryer, L, Berg, J. and Tymoczko, J. (2002). *Biochemistry*. 5th ed. New York: W.H. Freeman.

Swanson, R.A. and Spears, B. (1995). *History of sport and physical education in the United States*. 4th ed. Boston, MA: WCB/McGraw-Hill.

Tortora, G.J. and Grabowski, S.R. (2003). *Principles of anatomy and physiology*. 10th ed. New York: John Wiley and Sons.

Vander, A., Sherman, J. and Luciano, D. (2001). *Human physiology. The mechanisms of body function*. 8th edition. Boston, MA: McGraw-Hill.

Van Raalte, J.L. and Brewer, B.W. (1996). *Exploring sport and exercise psychology*. Washington, DC: American Psychology Association.

Wann, D.L. (1997). *Sports psychology*. Upper Saddle River, NJ: Prentice Hall.

Williams, J.M. (2001, ed). *Applied sport psychology: Personal growth to peak performance*. 4th ed. Boston, MA: McGraw-Hill.

Wilmore, J.H. and Costill, D.L. (2004). *Physiology of sport and exercise*. 3rd ed. Champaign, IL: Human Kinetics.

Winnick, J.P. (2000, ed). *Adapted physical education and sport*. 3rd ed. Champaign, IL: Human Kinetics.

Wuest, D.A. and Buecher, C.A. (2003). *Foundations of physical education, exercise science, and sport*. 14th ed. Boston, MA: McGraw-Hill.

I

IDEOLOGY In order to understand the social significance of sport, it is necessary to understand the values within which sports are embedded. Values get transmitted and reproduced by sports even if those values are contradictory. The values possessed by a person depend on the concepts that person possesses and, in turn, on the ideology acquired by that person. The most well-known uses of the term ideology are those noted by Williams (1976, 1977) as being inspired by the work of Karl Marx, in which it has been used in three ways: i) a system of beliefs characteristic of a particular class or group; ii) a system of illusory beliefs or false ideas that can be contrasted with true or scientific knowledge; and iii) the general process of the production of meanings and ideas.

Ideology is concerned with the creation as well as the diffusion of meaning. Dominant ideology produces cultural continuity, but there is always the potential for the development of oppositional ideas that can overthrow the dominant ones and lead to cultural change. Guttman's (1978) characteristics of modern sports provide a guide to what dominant sport values are. Tomlinson (1999) argues that dominant values are not unproblematically dominant, however. Sports cultures are full of contradictions: e.g. individualism defies collective responsibility; spontaneity defies routinization; play defies the development of work effort; and participation can defy the urge to win. Williams (1963) used the term 'cultural fiction' to refer to dissociation between cultural values and observed behavior. An example of a cultural fiction in sport is amateurism.

See also CHARACTER BUILDING; OLYMPIC IDEOLOGY; VALUES.

Bibliography

Guttmann, A. (1978). *From ritual to record*. New York: Columbia University Press.

Sage, G.H. (1998). *Power and ideology in American sport: A critical perspective*. 2nd ed. Champaign, IL: Human Kinetics.

Tomlinson, A. (1999). *The game's up: Essays in the cultural analysis of sport, leisure and popular culture*. Aldershot, England: Ashgate Publishing Ltd.

Williams, R. (1963). *American Society - A sociological interpretation*. 2nd ed. London: Alfred A Knopf.

Williams, R. (1976). *Keywords: A vocabulary of culture and society*. London: Fontana.

Williams, R. (1977). *Marxism and Literature*. Oxford: Oxford University Press.

IDIOPATHIC Of, or pertaining to, a disease without recognizable cause.

ILIAC ARTERY See under ARTERIAL ENDOFIBROSIS.

ILIAC CREST See under HIP POINTER.

ILIOCRISTALE An anatomical landmark that is the most lateral point on the iliac crest (crista iliaca).

ILIOINGUINAL NERVE See under HIP JOINT, NERVES.

ILIOPSOAS BURSITIS See under HIP JOINT, BURSITIS.

ILIOSPINALE An anatomical landmark that is the inferior aspect of the tip of the anterior superior iliac spine. The designated landmark is the undersurface of the tip of the anterior superior iliac spine, not the most frontally curved aspect. It is the origin of the *sartorius* muscle, thus slight movement of the thigh enables identification of the muscle and then the landmark.

ILIOTIBIAL BAND Iliotibial tract. It is a thick band of connective tissue that extends down the outside of the thigh from the iliac crest of the pelvis, over the knee to its attachment on the lateral condyle of the tibia (**Gerdy's tubercle**) and lateral proximal fibular head. It attaches to the pelvis via the *tensor fasciae latae* and *gluteus maximus*. The primary function of the iliotibial band is to provide static stability to the lateral aspect of the knee. Avulsion injuries may occur at Gerdy's tubercle.

See also HIP JOINT, BURSITIS.

ILIOTIBIAL BAND SYNDROME 'Runner's knee.' An extra-articular cause of snapping-hip syndrome in which there is excessive friction between the iliotibial band and the lateral femoral epicondylar eminence. It is a common overuse injury in runners and cyclists.

In knee flexion greater than 30 degrees, the iliotibial band lies on, or posterior to, the lateral femoral epicondyle. When the knee is in an extended position, the iliotibial band is anterior to it. Flexion and extension of the knee under stress can therefore produce irritation and inflammation within the iliotibial band, the underlying bursa and the periosteum of the lateral femoral epicondyle.

Iliotibial band syndrome may be caused by training errors, such as a sudden increase in distance or excessive downhill running. Intrinsic risk factors include a prominent lateral epicondyle, forefoot pronation, a tight iliotibial band, excessive genu varus and leg length discrepancy. In the UK, iliotibial band syndrome occurs more commonly in the right knee because the roads are cambered such that the right leg is the 'downhill' leg when running into the face of the traffic (i.e. the right side of the road).

IMAGERY The process of forming images. An image is a cognitive (mental) representation, reproduction or reconstruction of sensations or perceptions. Sensory stimulation is not necessary for the formation of an image. For sports skills, vision and kinesthesis are the most important modalities for imagery. A distinction has been made between internal and external imagery. **External imagery** involves a person viewing himself/herself from the perspective of an external observer (as if watching a video recording). **Internal imagery** involves the person imaging from his/her own perspective. Research attempting to show internal imaginal rehearsal is 'better' than external imaginal rehearsal, or vice-versa, is probably fruitless. It is possible, however, that one perspective may be better suited to certain aspects of task performance and to certain individuals. There is both anecdotal and experimental evidence that negative imagery inhibits athletic performance.

Gould and Damarjian (1996) suggest the following guidelines for the effective use of imagery: practice imagery regularly; use all the senses to enhance the vividness of imagery; practice controlling images; use both internal and external perspectives; combine imagery with relaxation; develop coping strategies through imagery; use imagery in practice as well as competition; use video- and audio-tapes to enhance imagery skills; use triggers or cues to facilitate the quality of imagery; emphasize dynamic imagery focusing on kinesthetic feel of the movements; imagine in real time; and keep a diary to record monitor evaluate progress.

See also HYPNOSIS; MAGNETIC RESONANCE IMAGING; MENTAL PRACTICE.

Bibliography

Gould, D. and Damarjian, N. (1996). Imagery training for peak performance. In Van Raalte, J.L. and Brewer, B.W. (eds). *Exploring sport and exercise psychology*. pp25-50. Washington, DC: American Psychological Association.

Howe, B.L. (1991). Imagery and sport performance. *Sports Medicine* 11(1), 1-5.

Sheikh, A.A. and Korner, E.R. (1994, eds). *Imagery in sports and physical performance*. Amityville, NY: Baywood Publishing Company.

IMMOBILIZATION The process of holding a joint or bone in place with a splint, cast or brace. This is done to prevent an injured area from moving while it heals. There is the possibility of decreased circulation if a cast, splint, or brace fits too tightly.

Casts are generally used for immobilization of a broken bone. Use of **splints** include: to immobilize a dislocated joint while it heals; for finger injuries, such as fractures or baseball finger; to immobilize an injured arm or leg immediately after an injury. **Slings** are often used to support the arm after a fracture or other injury. They are generally used along with a cast or splint, but are sometimes used alone as a means of immobilization. **Braces** are used to support, align or hold a body part in the correct position. A **collar** is generally used for neck injuries. A soft collar can relieve pain by restricting movement of the head and neck. It also transfers some of the weight of the head from the neck to the chest. A stiff collar is generally used to support the neck when there has been a fracture in one of the bones of the neck. **Traction** involves using a method for applying tension to correct the alignment of two structures (such as two bones) and hold them in the correct position. Skin traction is a combination of a splint and traction that is applied to the arms or legs by strips of adhesive tape placed over the skin of the arm or leg.

Prolonged bed rest can result in sores on the skin (**decubitus ulcers**), skin infection, buildup of fluid in the lungs or an infection in the lungs (pneumonia) and urinary infection. Prolonged bed rest can also cause diminished capacity of the heart, decreased plasma and blood volumes, and impaired control of blood vessels. The hypovolemia and diminished vasomotor tone caused by prolonged bed rest may cause orthostatic hypotension. The initial stimulus for acclimatization to bed rest appears to be a greatly decreased hydrostatic pressure within the cardiovascular system that involves shift of blood from the lower extremities into the upper body, increase in central venous pressure and diuresis.

Muscle strength declines rapidly during limb immobilization, because of a decrease in muscle size and a decrease in tension per unit of muscle cross-sectional area. Muscle fatigability also increases rapidly after immobilization.

If a muscle is fixed in a lengthened position, sarcomeres are added; if the muscle is in a shortened position, sarcomeres are lost and there is decreased glycogen, ADP, creatine phosphate and creatine. It will not result in muscle atrophy if it involves significant muscle stretch. For example, immobilization of an ankle that is fully plantar flexed results in substantial atrophy of the plantar flexors while immobilization in full dorsal flexion results in much less atrophy or even hypertrophy in some cases.

See also NEUROMUSCULAR ELECTRICAL STIMULATION.

Bibliography

Booth, F.W. (1987). Physiologic and biochemical effects of immobilization on muscle. *Clinical Orthopedics* 219, 15-20.

Lieber, R.L. (2002). *Skeletal muscle structure, function, and plasticity. The Physiological basis of rehabilitation*. 2nd ed. Philadelphia, PA: Lippincott Williams & Wilkins.

IMMUNITY   The ability of the body to resist agents that can cause disease. The **immune system** protects against, recognizes, attacks and destroys foreign substances (**antigens**). It also brings long-term immunity to infectious diseases. **Cells of the immune system** are mainly leukocytes, but also other cells such as liver cells that produce soluble mediators. **Soluble mediators** are produced primarily by immune cells that act either directly on the antigen or indirectly by signaling other immune cells to act or release additional mediators. Soluble mediators include antibodies (immunoglobulins), cytokines, complement proteins, inflammatory mediators and acute phase proteins. **Immune system processes** for dealing with antigens include cytotoxic reactions, apoptosis, lysis, neutralization, opsinization, phagocytosis and chemotaxis.

The immune system can be subdivided into non-specific and specific systems. **The non-specific immune system** is the first line of defense against antigens. It does not have to recognize foreign substances or cells and involves processes associated with both external structures (especially the skin and the respiratory tract) and internal structures (especially natural killer cells, neutrophils and macrophages). When the body's skin is broken, or an internal injury occurs, an inflammatory response develops, which initially is caused by local release of molecules from the damaged tissue. These events lead to increased localized blood flow and migration of phagocytes to the damaged area. Several proteins assist the function of phagocytes, including complement proteins. The **specific immune system** involves the production of cells or antibodies to provide defense against specific antigens. It can be subdivided into humoral and cell-mediated immunity.

Humoral immunity exists within the fluid components of the body such as the blood and is mediated by the B-cell lymphocytes. After exposure to an antigen, B-cell lymphocytes become either plasma cells or memory cells. **Plasma cells** produce antibodies. The antibodies (immunoglobulins) circulate in the blood and lymph, where they bind to bacteria, toxins and free viruses; inactivate them temporarily and facilitate their destruction by phagocytes or complement proteins. **Cell-mediated immunity** is provided by T-cell lymphocytes that directly attack and lyse cells infected by viruses, parasites, cancer cells or grafts. Chemical mediators are then released in order to enhance inflammation and to activate lymphocytes and macrophages.

Possible mechanisms by which exercise may affect immune system include: direct stimulation of immune function; stimulation of the sympathetic nervous system; altered levels of hormones (especially norepinephrine, epinephrine, cortisol, growth hormone, prolactin and thyroxine); increased body temperature; and exercise-induced cell damage (with the release of acute-phase proteins).

At rest, trained individuals have slightly elevated non-specific immunity. Moderate exercise training generally results in leukocytosis (increased number of leucocytes), but has little effect on serum immunoglobulin levels. Following prolonged, intense exercise, the number of lymphocytes in the blood is suppressed, the function of natural killer cells and B-cell lymphocytes is inhibited, and immunoglobulin levels may be worsened. Decreased blood flow during exercise to the spleen could affect the number of circulating lymphocytes. The **Open Window theory** postulates that after prolonged heavy exercise, there is an 'open window' of altered immunity (which may last between 3 and 72 hours) when viruses and bacteria may gain a foothold, increasing the risk of sub-clinical and clinical infection. The risk of upper-respiratory tract infection appears to be especially high during the one or two week period following marathon-type events.

See also AIDS; CANCER; UPPER RESPIRATORY TRACT INFECTION.

Bibliography

Brenner, I.K.M., Shek, P.N. and Shephard, R.J. (1994). Infection in athletes. *Sports Medicine* 17(2), 86-107.

Heath, G.W., Macera, C.A. and Nieman, D.C. (1992). Exercise and upper respiratory tract infections. Is there a relationship? *Sports Medicine* 14(6), 353-365.

Mackinnon, L.T. (1999). *Advances in exercise immunology*. Champaign, IL: Human Kinetics.

Nielsen, H.B. (2003). Lymphocyte responses to maximal exercise: A physiological perspective. *Sports Medicine* 33(11), 853-867.

Nieman, D.C. and Nehlsen-Cannarella, S.L. (1991). The effects of acute and chronic exercise on immunoglobulins. *Sports Medicine* 11(3), 183-201.

Nieman, D.C. (1997). Exercise immunology: Practical applications. *International Journal of Sports Medicine* 18(1), S91-S100.

Nieman, D.C. and Pedersen, B.K. (1999). Exercise and immune function. Recent developments. *Sports Medicine* 27(2), 73-80.

Pedersen, B.K. and Bruunsgaard, H. (1995). How physical exercise influences the establishment of infections. *Sports Medicine* 19(6), 393-400.

IMMUNOGLOBULINS   Antibodies. These are serum proteins that are synthesized in response to the entry of a foreign substance (antigen) and are capable of binding with the antigen. Plasma cells release immunoglobulins into the circulation. **Immunoglobulins** activate non-specific immune mechanisms to attack the specific antigen and to stimulate complement proteins. Immunoglobulins are produced by B-cell lymphocytes in lymph tissue or by a cell-mediated response from T-cells. There are five different types of immunoglobulin: IgG and IgM neutralize toxins, bacteria and viruses and promote phagocytosis; IgA has a protective function; IgD has unknown function; and IgE is the antibody associated with atopic allergies, such as anaphylaxis.

IMMUNOSUPPRESANT   An agent capable of suppressing immune responses.

IMP   See under AMMONIA; PURINE NUCLEOTIDE CYCLE.

IMPACT   Impulsive force. A collision between two bodies that occurs when relatively large contact forces exist during a very short interval of time.

IMPINGEMENT SYNDROME   In general, an impingement syndrome exists when pressure increases within a confined anatomical space and the enclosed tissues are negatively affected.

See ROTATOR CUFF.

IMPULSE   The product of the magnitude of a force and its time of application. It is the area under a force-time curve. The Standard International units are newton seconds (N.s). The US Customary units are pound force seconds (lbf.s). A large change in an object's state of motion may result from a small force acting for a relatively long time, or from a large force acting for a relatively short time. The **impulse-momentum relationship** states that the change in momentum experienced by a body under the action of a force is equal to the impulse of the resultant force.

INCIDENCE   See under EPIDEMIOLOGY.

INCLUSION BODY MYOSITIS   An inflammatory muscle disease that appears after the age of 50 years and is more common in men than women. It is an autoimmune disorder. Symptoms include weakness of arms, legs and hands, especially thighs, wrists and fingers. It progresses slowly and there is no standard treatment.

Bibliography
Myositis Association. Http://www.myositis.org

INCONTINENCE   See under URINARY INCONTINENCE.

INDIVIDUAL DIFFERENCES   See under PERSONALITY; TRAINING

INERTIA   The resistance offered by a body to a change of its state of rest or motion. An **inertial force (effective force)** is the fictitious (pseudo) force acting on a body as a result of using a non-inertial frame of reference, e.g. centrifugal force in a rotating coordinate system.

An **inertial frame of reference** is a non-accelerating (constant velocity) frame of reference and one in which Newton's laws of motion hold. Consider the act of juggling. The degree of difficulty in juggling balls in a room that is standing still is the same as it is in an autobus that is traveling at constant velocity. A **non-inertial frame of reference** is an accelerating frame of reference and one in which Newton's laws of motion does not hold. A non-inertial frame of reference does not have a constant velocity. The frame could be traveling in a straight line, but be either increasing or decreasing its speed, or it could be traveling along a curved path at a constant speed. The frame could be traveling along a curved path and also increasing or decreasing its speed. Consider a person in an automobile when the brakes are abruptly applied: the person feels that she is being pushed toward the front of the car, but there is no actual force pushing her forward. The automobile is a non-inertial frame of reference, because it is slowing down. The ground is stationary and therefore is an inertial frame of reference. When the brakes are applied the person continues with forward motion relative to the ground in accordance with Newton's 1st law.

D'Alembert's principle states that bodies in motion are considered to be in a state of dynamic equilibrium, with all acting forces resulting in equal and oppositely-directed inertial forces. D'Alembert's principle converts a dynamics problem to a statics problem by introducing a fictitious force equal in magnitude to the product of the mass of the body and its acceleration, and directed opposite to the acceleration. It shows that Newton's 3rd law of motion applies to bodies that are free to move as well as to stationary bodies.

See also MOMENT OF INERTIA; NEWTON'S LAWS.

INTEROCEPTORS   Receptors located in blood vessels, visceral organs, muscles and the nervous system. They provide information about conditions in the internal environment.

INFANT EXERCISE PROGRAMS   The American Academy of Pediatrics recommends that structured infant exercise programs should not be promoted as being therapeutically beneficial for the development of healthy infants, and that parents be encouraged to provide a safe, nurturing, and minimally structured play environment for their infant. In most infant exercise programs, massage techniques, passive exercises and holding an infant in various positions are used. The bones of infants are more susceptible to trauma than those of older children and adults.

Bibliography

American Academy of Pediatrics (1988, 1994). Infant exercise programs. *Pediatrics* 82(5), 800.

INFANT SWIM PROGRAMS Recognition of the swimming reflex, and the belief that it will promote voluntary swimming later in life, has contributed substantially to the popularity of infant swim programs. Benefits of early aquatic experiences include important parent-child learning time, while the child explores and learns new skills in a novel environment. However, children are generally not ready for swimming until their 4th birthday. Prior to this level, longer instructional periods are required due to limitations in neuromuscular capacity. Programs that advocate constant use of flotation do not allow the child to learn the body's inherent floating qualities. Swimming skills (i.e. standard swimming strokes) should be distinguished from water safety skills (i.e. survival flotation, energy conservation 'swimming,' or poolside safety behavior). An estimated 5 to 10 million infants and preschool children participate in formal aquatic instruction programs.

Infant and toddler aquatic programs do not decrease the risk of drowning. In fact, drowning is a leading cause of unintentional injury and death in the pediatric age group. In the USA, drowning rates are highest among children of ages 1 through 2 years. Total submersion should be prohibited so as to avoid hyponatremia. Infants are also at risk of hypothermia.

In swimming pools, most diseases are passed person-to-person, not through the water (chlorine is an effective disinfecting agent). The incidence of ear infection in young children is high due to the short Eustachian tube from the middle ear, which prevents adequate air and fluid exchange during periods of congestion when mucous membranes are swollen.

Bibliography

American Academy of Pediatrics (2000). Swimming programs for infants and toddlers. *Pediatrics* 105(4), 868-870.

Blanksby, B.A. et al. (1995). Children's readiness for learning front crawl swimming. *Australian Journal of Science and Medicine in Sport* 27, 34-37.

INFANT WALKER Baby walker. A device that is designed to support a pre-ambulatory infant, with feet on the floor, and to allow mobility while the infant is learning to walk. It is comprised of a wheeled base, which supports a rigid frame holding a fabric seat with leg openings and usually a plastic tray. Parents give various reasons for using walkers, e.g. to keep the infant quiet and happy, to encourage mobility and promote walking, and to hold the infant during feeding.

Walkers do not help a child learn to walk, but rather delay normal motor and mental development. Infants cannot see their feet in a walker; lack of visual feedback is an impediment to learning. Infant walkers also inhibit the development of balance.

Estimated annual sales of infant walkers in the USA are more than 3 million. Each year a large number of infants suffer severe injuries from infant walkers. In 1999, an estimated 8,800 children younger than 15 months were treated in hospital emergency departments in the USA for injuries associated with infant walkers. 34 infant walker-related deaths were reported from 1973 through 1998. The vast majority of injuries occur from falls down stairs, and head injuries are common. Adult supervision cannot be relied upon to prevent infant walker-related injuries. The American Academy of Pediatrics recommends a ban on the manufacture and sale of mobile infant walkers. If parents insist on using a mobile walker, it is vital that they choose a walker that meets the performance standards of ASTM F977-96 to prevent falls down stairs. Because the safest infant walker is one without wheels, stationary activity centers should be promoted as a safer alternative to mobile walkers.

Bibliography

American Academy of Pediatrics (2001). Injuries

associated with infant walkers. *Pediatrics* 108(3), 790-792.

INFARCTION Infarct. Localized death of tissue caused by obstructed inflow of arterial blood.

INFERIOR Located below another part of the body; nearer the feet than the head.
See also SUPERIOR.

INFERTILITY Diminished or absent capacity to produce offspring. **Sterility** denotes complete inability to produce offspring.
See under TESTOSTERONE.

INFLAMMATION The body's first line of defense against attack such as that imposed by injury or bacterial infection. The five cardinal signs of inflammation are heat, redness, swelling, pain and loss of function. Classic inflammation and repair involves three overlapping phases: acute vascular inflammatory response, repair and regeneration, and remodeling. The first phase starts at the moment of injury and usually lasts 3 to 5 days. It is characterized by edema that accompanies cellular inflammation. It involves the activation of vasoactive mediators, chemical mediators such as histamine, and activation of platelets in the coagulation system. The second phase begins in 48 hours and lasts on average 6 to 8 weeks. It is characterized by exuberant cellular activity together with vascular proliferation leading to the formation of granulation tissue. In the third phase, there is increased organization of extracellular matrix and a more normal biochemical profile. Scar tissue is often formed and this can significantly compromise the biomechanics of the remodeled tissue. Some tissues, e.g. articular cartilage, do not produce a classic inflammatory pattern or response after injury.
See ASPIRIN; CORTICOSTEROIDS; NONSTEROIDAL ANTI-INFLAMMATORY DRUGS.

INFLAMMATORY MEDIATORS Substances that control the development of inflammation; e.g. histamine, platelet activating factor and serotonin; all three of which bring about increased vascular permeability and smooth muscle contraction.

INFRAPATELLAR FAT PAD SYNDROME See HOFFA'S DISEASE.

INGEST To eat or take in through the mouth.

INGUINAL LIGAMENT A fibrous band running from the anterior superior iliac spine to the tubercle of the tibia. See under HERNIA.

INHIBITION i) Prevention of an effector being activated by the action of nerve impulses. ii) The blocking of one physiological or psychological process by another.

INJURY Trauma implies an injury from a mechanical force that is applied external to the involved tissue and results in structural stress in tissue.
Acute injury results rapidly from a macrotraumatic mechanism, and is characterized by an orderly and timely reparative process that results in the sustained restoration of anatomic and functional integrity. **Chronic injury** can begin as microscopic damage to a tissue's structure, and is characterized by failure to proceed through an orderly and timely reparative process, or it may have proceeded through the repair process without establishing sustained anatomic and functional integrity. Chronic injury response may be 'inflammatory dominant' or 'structural-degenerative dominant.' The **inflammatory-dominant response** is typically a response of irritated synovial tissue due to direct trauma, hemobursa, hemarthrosis or associated arthritis. The **structural-degenerative dominant response** is a pattern of connective tissue injury response resulting from failed adaptation to increased exercise demand, most often in combination with a failure of healing and repair. Tissue rupture may result from progressive degeneration. Such a response is most common in tendon.
A distinction can be made between primary and secondary injury. **Primary injury** is an immediate consequence of trauma. Secondary injury may be either an injury that manifests itself some after the initial trauma (e.g. diffuse axonal injury in the brain

may not appear until days after the initial trauma) or an injury that develops as an accommodation to the primary injury (i.e. the 'Dizzy Dean syndrome').

Some authors have criticized the use of nebulous terms such as 'shin splints' and 'Little League elbow' that have minimal clinical or biomechanical utility.

See also CATASTROPHIC INJURY; OVERUSE INJURIES; SPORTS MEDICINE.

Chronology

•1937 • Baseball pitcher Dizzy Dean broke his left big toe, and returned to action too soon. As a consequence of altering his pitching technique to accommodate the pain caused by the toe injury, Dean suffered an injury to his pitching shoulder that effectively finished his career. Dean won less than 20 games the remainder of his career, but gained Hall of Fame status based on his 120-62 record from 1932 – 1936.

Bibliography

Bird, S.R., Black, N. and Newton, P. (1997). *Sports injuries: Causes, diagnoses, treatment and prevention*. Cheltenham: Stanley Thornes.

Bull, R.C. (1999). *Handbook of sports injuries*. St Louis, MI: McGraw-Hill.

Caine, D. et al. (1994). *Epidemiology of sports injuries*. Champaign, IL: Human Kinetics.

Field, L.D. and Savoie, F.H. (1998). Common elbow injuries in sport. *Sports Medicine* 26(3), 193-205.

Fu, F.H. and Stone, D.A. (1994). *Sports injuries. Mechanisms. Prevention. Treatment*. Baltimore: Williams and Wilkins.

Peterson, L. and Renstrom, P. (2001). *Sports injuries - Their prevention and treatment*. 3rd ed. London: Martin Dunitz.

Rettig, A.C. (1998). Elbow, forearm and wrist injuries in the athlete. *Sports Medicine* 25(2), 115-130.

Safran, M.R., McKeag, D.B. and Van Camp, S.P. (1998). *Manual of sports medicine*. Philadelphia, PA: Lippincot-Raven.

Whiting, W.C. and Zernicke, R.F. (1998). *Biomechanics of musculoskeletal injury*. Champaign, IL: Human Kinetics.

INJURY, PSYCHOLOGY OF Emotional recovery from injury is not linear, but cyclical: the balance between distress and coping varies over weeks, days and even within a day. **Distress** includes symptoms such as anxiety, depression, fear, anger and guilt. In addition to distress, there is denial and blame. **Denial** includes feelings of shock and disbelief, avoidance, minimizing and outright failure to accept the severity of injury. Denial may be directed to severity of injury, level of psychological distress, prognosis for recovery, need for surgery or complex rehabilitation and/or impact on athletic career. **Preoccupation with blame** can trigger emotions such as anger, guilt, mistrust and hopelessness. **Determined coping** involves moving beyond passive acceptance and proactively channeling knowledge, skill and energy into emotional recovery. It includes exploration and commitment.

Bibliography

Heil, J. (2000). The injured athlete. In Hanin, Y.L. (ed). *Emotions in sport*. pp245-266. Champaign, IL: Human Kinetics.

INJURY RISK FACTORS Risk factors for injuries in sport can be subdivided into two categories: intrinsic (personal) and extrinsic (environmental). **Intrinsic risk factors** are biological, psychological and social characteristics predisposing a person to an injury such as leg length discrepancy, misalignments, muscular insufficiency, muscular imbalance, hyperflexibility, hypoflexibility, gender differences, growth, aging, obesity, disease and compromised immunity. **Extrinsic risk factors** are related to the type of sports activity, the manner in which it is performed, the environmental conditions and the equipment used. Extrinsic factors include excessive load on the body (e.g. type and speed of movement, number of repetitions, footwear and surface), training errors (e.g. overdistance, fast progression, high intensity, poor technique and fatigue) and environmental stressors (e.g. dark, heat/cold, humidity, altitude and wind).

Bibliography

Caine, D. et al. (1994). *Epidemiology of sports injuries*.

Champaign, IL: Human Kinetics.

Inklaar, H. (1994). Soccer injuries II: Aetiology and prevention. *Sports Medicine* 18(2), 81-93.

Jones, H.H., Cowan, D.N., and Knapik, J.J. (1994). Exercise, training and injuries. *Sports Medicine* 18(3), 202-214.

INNATE   A term used to describe some process or characteristic that is in-born.

See also CONGENITAL; INSTINCT.

INNER EAR   See under EAR.

INNERVATION   Nerve supply.

INOSINE   A nucleoside involved in the formation of purines. It is one of a number of unusual bases found in transfer RNA. Some of the reported metabolic roles of inosine, such as facilitation of ATP synthesis, have been exploited by sellers of dietary supplements containing inosine. There is no scientific data to support the use of inosine supplements as an ergogenic aid.

INOSINE MONOPHOSPHATE   See under AMMONIA.

INOSITOL   Part of cell membrane phospholipids. The body synthesizes inositol from glucose. There are nine forms of inositol, but myo-inositol is the only one involved in human nutrition. Inositol phospholipids, a family of lipids that contain inositol derivatives, are precursors of eicosanoids.

INOTROPIC   Pertaining to the force of muscle contraction; it usually refers to cardiac muscle.

INSERTION   See under MUSCLE ATTACHMENTS.

INSPIRATORY CAPACITY   The maximal volume of gas that can be inspired from the resting- expiratory level.

INSPIRATORY RESERVE VOLUME   The amount of gas that can be inspired from the end-inspiratory position. See also VITAL CAPACITY.

INSTINCT   An inherited invariant behavioral sequence, which is evoked by particular environmental stimuli.

INSTRUMENTAL CONDITIONING   See OPERANT CONDITIONING.

INSULIN   A protein hormone secreted by the beta cells of the **islets of Langerhans**, which are endocrine tissues found in the pancreas. The pancreas regulates glucose metabolism in all body tissues except the brain. It promotes the transport of carbohydrates, fatty acids and amino acids into the cells. Secretion of insulin is controlled by the blood glucose level at the pancreas. An increase in the blood glucose level stimulates insulin secretion. Conversely, a decrease in the blood glucose level causes less insulin to be secreted. An increase in blood amino acid levels also stimulates insulin secretion. **Chronic hyperinsulinemia** (excessive insulin in the blood) could result in serious disorders of carbohydrate and fat metabolism.

Insulin appears to suppress food intake by inhibiting the synthesis of neuropeptide Y, which is a potent stimulator of food intake. A drop in insulin levels activates neuropeptide Y. With the hypothalamus, neuropeptide Y triggers an integrated response that leads to decreased energy expenditure, increased food intake and obesity. Leptin appears to act, at in part, by inhibiting neuropeptide Y synthesis and release in the hypothalamus.

Insulin secretion falls during exercise, but insulin sensitivity increases. In trained individuals, the insulin level does not fall as far during exercise as in the untrained individual. This allows progressively more energy to be derived from free fatty acids.

Insulin has anti-catabolic effects on skeletal muscle protein under certain conditions. With regard to the use of insulin as an ergogenic aid, there is no convincing evidence that chronic increases in circulating insulin enhance muscle mass in individuals who have been undergoing strength training.

Insulin has a sodium-retaining effect on the kidney, augments catecholamine release, increases vascular sensitivity to vasoconstrictor substances, and decreases vascular sensitivity to vasodilator substances. Insulin also increases production of tissue growth factors and facilitates retention of cellular calcium. See also AMYLIN.

INSULIN-LIKE GROWTH FACTORS IGFs. Somatomedins. These are small polypeptides that are secreted by the liver after growth hormone stimulates liver cell DNA to synthesize them. IGFs travel in the blood attached to binding proteins and are released as free hormones to interact with receptors. IGF-1 (somatomedin C) production is stimulated by growth hormone, is released mainly by the liver, but may also be secreted by bone, fat cells, the testes and the heart. It facilitates amino acid and glucose transport, and glycogen synthesis, and it has anabolic effects in bone and cartilage. Responses of IGF-1 to heavy exercise are not clear.

See also GENE THERAPY.

INSULIN RESISTANCE A condition in which body tissues require a greater-than-normal quantity of insulin. It can be considered as decreased effectiveness of insulin to clear blood glucose. Insulin resistance can occur as a result of decreased insulin responsiveness or insulin sensitivity.

Insulin responsiveness is the biological response that is achieved with maximally stimulating levels of insulin. A higher biological response indicates a better insulin responsiveness. Decreased insulin responsiveness is associated with a post-insulin receptor defect.

Insulin sensitivity indicates how well cells to respond to insulin to increase glucose uptake. It is the percentage of maximal biological response elicited by submaximal insulin levels. A higher percentage of biological response for a given sub-maximal insulin level indicates greater insulin sensitivity. Decreased insulin sensitivity is often associated with an insulin receptor defect.

The manifestations of insulin resistance are **hyperinsulinemia** (excess insulin in the blood) and impaired glucose tolerance. **Impaired glucose tolerance** refers to a condition in which the blood glucose level is higher than normal, but not high enough to be classified as diabetic. A **glucose tolerance test** is used to determine how effectively an

individual can remove high levels of glucose from the blood. A concentrated solution of glucose is ingested and the blood glucose is subsequently measured over a period of several hours.

Physical activity has a beneficial effect on insulin sensitivity in normal individuals, as well as those with insulin resistance. Up to 2 hours after exercise, glucose uptake is in part elevated due to insulin-dependent mechanisms. This probably involves a contraction-induced increase in the amount of GLUT-4 associated with the plasma membrane and T-tubules. A single session of exercise can increase insulin sensitivity for at least 16 hours after exercise in both healthy as well as Type-2 diabetic individuals.

Exercise training is associated with increased insulin sensitivity, thus less insulin is needed to handle a given carbohydrate load in order to maintain or improve glucose homeostasis. Exercise training improves insulin sensitivity via increased oxidative enzymes, glucose transporters (e.g. GLUT-4) and capillarity in muscle as well as by decreasing abdominal fat. The improvements in insulin sensitivity with resistance training are similar in magnitude to those achieved with aerobic exercise. The improvements in glucose metabolism after body weight loss and exercise training may in some cases be partially attributed to changes in body composition, including decreases in total and central body fat. Central (abdominal) obesity is much more strongly associated with insulin resistance than is overall obesity. Insulin resistance is also present in individuals with diabetes mellitus, and may develop with aging.

See also METABOLIC SYNDROME.

Bibliography
Borghouts, L.B. and Keizer, H.A. (2000). Exercise and insulin sensitivity: A review. *International Journal of Sports Medicine* 21(1), 1-12.

Chisholm, D.J, Campbell, L.V. and Kraegen, E.W. (1997). Pathogenesis of the insulin resistance syndrome (syndrome X). *Clinical and Experimental Pharmacology and Physiology* 24(9), 782-784.

Ryan, A.S. (2000). Insulin resistance with aging: Effects of diet and exercise. *Sports Medicine* 30(5), 327-346.

INSULIN SENSITIVITY   See under INSULIN RESISTANCE.

INTEGRATION See under MOTOR DEVELOPMENT.

INTERCARPAL JOINTS There are three sets of intercarpal joints: articulations of the first row of carpal bones (scaphoid, semilunar, cuneiform and pisiform), articulations of the second row of carpal bones (trapezium, trapezoid, os magnum and unciform) and articulations of the two rows with each other (mid-carpal joint). These joints are mainly gliding joints.
    See also HAND; WRIST.

INTERDIGITAL NEUROMA   See MORTON'S NEUROMA.

INTERFERONS See under CYTOKINES.

INTERLEUKINS See under CYTOKINES.

INTERPHALANGEAL (FINGER) JOINTS Hinge joints between the phalanges of the fingers. Movements permitted are flexion/extension. The head and base of the phalanges form the articulating surfaces. See HAND; JERSEY FINGER; PROXIMAL INTER-PHALANGEAL JOINTS; TRIGGER FINGER.

INTERPHALANGEAL (TOE) JOINTS   Hinge joints between the phalanges of the foot. The permitted movements are flexion and extension. See FOOT.

INTERSECTION SYNDROME   Pain, swelling and crepitus at the crossover between the first and second extensor compartments of the wrist, where the tendons of the *abductor pollicis longus* and *extensor pollicis brevis* muscles cross the tendons of the *extensor carpi radialis longus* and *extensor carpi radialis brevis* muscles. It is caused by exercise involving repeated and rapid flexion and extension of the wrist, e.g. canoeing.

INTERSTITIAL   Of, pertaining to, or situated in a space between two things. It is often used to refer to 'intercellular.'

INTERSTITIAL FLUID   The water and solute contents of the fluid found between the cells of tissues, but not the plasma in blood and lymph vessels.

INTERTARSAL JOINTS   Gliding joints between the tarsal bones of the foot (talus, calcaneus, navicular, cuboid and cuneiforms). The joints between the 3 cuneiforms, cuboid and 5 metatarsals produce little motion. The **cuneonavicular** joint is a synovial joint formed by the navicular bone and the 3 cuneiforms. The **intercuneiform** and **cuneocuboid** joints are synovial joints continuous with the cuneonavicular joint cavity. See also MIDTARSAL JOINTS.

INTERVAL TRAINING   A form of training that involves periods of exercise interspersed with regular periods of rest or exercise of decreased intensity. It enables more high-intensity exercise to be performed in training. Exercise involving the phosphocreatine system generally has an exercise-to-rest ratio of 1:3, the lactic acid system has a ratio of 1:2 and the oxygen system has a ratio of 1:1. Duration of recovery is generally 30 to 90 seconds, 60 to 240 seconds and 120 to 310 seconds, respectively. Repetitions are typically 25 to 30, 10 to 20 and 3 to 5, respectively. Short aerobic interval training has been shown to prevent glycogen depletion by using lipids compared with continuous exercise performed at the same velocity.
    It has been proposed that that the velocity-at-maximal oxygen uptake might represent an optimal training stimulus for improvements in endurance fitness. If interval sessions are constructed with the goal of allowing the longest possible training time at the velocity-at-maximal oxygen uptake, then each repetition needs to be longer than 60% of the time for which exercise can be sustained at velocity-at-maximal oxygen uptake. Care should be taken in measuring velocity-at-maximal oxygen uptake because of the phenomenon of oxygen drift.
    Fartlek is an unsystematic form of interval training. The performer subjectively determines the peri-

ods of more intensive exercise and rest intervals or periods of decreased intensity of exercise. Fartlek is a Swedish word meaning 'speed play.' It is suitable for exercising over rough and hilly terrain. See also CIRCUIT TRAINING; TRAINING FOR DISTANCE RUNNING.

Chronology
•1930s • Interval training was developed by Hans Reindell, a German cardiologist, who used exercise to improve the fitness of some of his patients.
•1939 • Rudolf Harbig beat the world record for the 800 m by nearly 2 seconds. His record of 1:46.6 lasted until 1955. Harbig was trained by German coach Woldemar Gerschler, a professor at the University of Freiburg, who was the first to systematically apply interval training to elite athletes. Believing that the heart adapted and grew stronger during the interval, Gerschler would not allow the runner to begin the next repetition until their pulse rate had returned to 120 bpm. If this did not occur within 90 seconds of the end of the previous repetition, the workout was deemed to be too difficult and was adjusted. Gerschler divided the year into three training periods, each of which contributed to the racing peak. The year began with four months of cross-country training (7 to 13 miles per day). In the next period quantity intervals (ranging from 10 x 660 yards to 4 x 2 miles) were run at half to three quarters of racing effort. The last period, just prior to the competitive season, involved four months of quality intervals (such as 12 x 200 meters or 4 x 1,000 meters). As the speed of training increased, from cross-country running to quantity intervals to quality intervals, the daily mileage decreased. During the racing season itself, the athlete would run only three to four miles and day and – perhaps twice a week - do short interval sessions (such as 10 x 100 meters).
•1952 • In the Olympics, Emil Zatopek of Czechoslovakia won gold medals in the 5,000 meters, 10,000 meters and Marathon. Zatopek popularized interval training in the 1950s.
•1956 • Gordon Pirie, three years after having been tested and given a new training program by Woldemar Gerschler, ran 5,000 meters in 13:36.8; a new world record.

•1958 • Coach Karl Adam's Ratzeburg Ruderclub eight, astonished the West German rowing establishment by winning the National Championship. Adam employed innovative equipment, including unusually long oars with short, wide blades and short boats. He shattered previously accepted ideas about training in rowing by using heavy weights in the gym and interval training in the water.

Bibliography
Billat, L.V. (2001). Interval training for performance: A scientific and empirical practice. Special recommendations for middle- and long-distance running. Part I: Aerobic interval training. *Sports Medicine* 31(1), 13-31.

Billat, L.V. (2001). Interval training for performance: A scientific and empirical practice. Special recommendations for middle- and long-distance running. Part II: Anaerobic interval training. *Sports Medicine* 31(2), 75-90.

Daniels, J. and Scardina, N. (1984). Interval training and performance. *Sports Medicine* 1, 327-334.

Jones, A.M. and Carter, H. (2000). The effect of endurance training on parameters of aerobic fitness. *Sports Medicine* 29(6), 373-386.

Laursen, P.B. and Jenkins, D.G. (2002). The scientific basis for high-intensity interval training: Optimizing training programmes and maximizing performance in highly-trained endurance athletes. *Sports Medicine* 32(1), 53-73.

INTERVERTEBRAL DISK   See under SPINE.

INTESTINE   See under GASTROINTESTINAL SYSTEM.

INTRA-ABDOMINAL INJURIES   See under APPENDIX; BLADDER; KIDNEY; LIVER; PANCREAS; SPLEEN.

INTRA-ABDOMINAL PRESSURE   Pressure within the abdomen. Intra-abdominal pressure is created by the abdominal muscles, the diaphragm and the muscles of the pelvic floor. It is increased by contraction of these muscles. It can be can be measured with a pressure transducer that is attached to a catheter and inserted into the abdominal cavity through the nasal cavity. The deep abdominal muscles (*transversus abdominis* and *obliquus abdominis internus*), rather than the *rectus abdominis*, are the most important of the abdominal muscles for intra-abdominal pressure, because they are primarily visceral compressors rather than trunk flexors. *Transversus abdominis* is the primary abdominal muscle responsible for generation of intra-abdominal pressure. Its fibers are horizontally oriented, thus it creates compression and an increase in intra-abdominal pressure without an accompanying flexor moment. If the *rectus abdominis* contracts to increase intra-abdominal pressure, it produces a flexion torque that counteracts the anti-flexion effect of intra-abdominal pressure as the diaphragm and pelvic floor spread out. Sit-up type movements, that involve significant work by the *rectus abdominis*, do not usually mimic the coordination between the abdominal muscles that is inherent in the mechanisms that generate intra-abdominal.

Because the intra-abdominal cavity contains mainly liquid and viscous material, it can be considered an incompressible element that can transmit forces from the muscles encasing the cavity to the supporting structures of the trunk. Intra-abdominal pressure and co-contraction of trunk musculature increases the stability of the spinal column. It adds tension to the thoracolumbar fascia, thus increasing the force of the extension moment that the thoracolumbar fascia can generate. Intra-abdominal pressure may decrease the forces required by the *erector spinae* muscles to perform a lift and also the associated compressive and shear forces on the intervertebral disks. Recent research evidence suggests that intra-abdominal pressure decreases compressive force acting on the lumbar spine by 7%. It is thought that the higher the intra-abdominal pressure, the greater the lifting load the spine can support without being injured.

During weightlifting, at the onset of a lift, there is an initial rapid increase in intra-abdominal pressure that may last for less than 0.5 s before decreasing during the remainder of the lift. For intra-abdominal pressure to fully stabilize the spine during heavy weight lifting, it would have to exceed the systolic pressure within the aorta, effectively cutting off the blood flow to the viscera and lower limbs. Regarding breathing during weightlifting, the spine must be stabilized regardless of whether the individual is inhaling or exhaling. In general, breathing should be trained independently of the exertion.

Spine stabilization ('core strength') exercises are directed at improving function by conditioning the muscles around the lumbar spine and increasing intra-abdominal pressure. Many athletic techniques require core stabilization to more effectively transmit forces throughout the body segment chain. Stiffening of the torso is taught for many motor tasks, e.g. when an athlete in a contact sport might experience unexpected loading.

A **weightlifting (back) belt** can be used to increase intra-abdominal pressure during weight lifting. If a lifter trains with a belt, however, the abdominal muscles that contribute to the generation of intra-abdominal pressure may not be strengthened as much as they would in the absence of belt use during training. Neuromuscular control patterns of muscles that generate intra-abdominal pressure may develop differently when a belt is used during training. If a lifter who is accustomed to wearing a belt then attempts lifting without one, he may generate less intra-abdominal pressure than if he had trained regularly without a belt. While weightlifters have traditionally been encouraged to wear a belt for maximal lifts, there is no conclusive evidence that back belts increase the stiffness of the spine, and no proven relationship between this stiffness and the decrease in injury. Weightlifting belts appear to modulate lifting mechanics in some positive ways in some people and in negative ways in others (McGill, 2002). Belts may give people a false sense of security. In the USA, the National Institute for Occupational Safety and Health (NIOSH) does not recommend the use of back belts to prevent low back injuries.

See also VALSALVA MANEUVER.

Bibliography

McGill, S. (2002). *Low back disorders: Evidence-based prevention and rehabilitation*. Champaign, IL: Human Kinetics.

National Institute for Occupational Safety and Health (1994). Workplace use of back belts.

DHHS (NIOSH) Number 94-122. Http://www.cdc.gov/niosh/backbelt.html

Norris, C.M. (1993). Abdominal muscle training in sport. *British Journal of Sports Medicine* 27(1), 19-27.

Norris, C.M. (2000). *Back stability*. Champaign, IL: Human Kinetics.

Perkins, M.S. and Bloswick, D.S. (1995). The use of back belts to increase intra-abdominal pressure as a means of preventing low back injuries: A survey of the literature. *International Journal of Occupational and Environmental Health* 1(4), 326-335.

Reyna, J.R. Jnr et al. (1995). The effect of lumbar belts on isolated lumbar muscle. Strength and dynamic capacity. *Spine* 20(1), 68-73.

Zatsiorsky, V.M. (1995). *Science and practice of strength training*. Champaign, IL: Human Kinetics.

INTRACELLULAR   Located inside one or more cells.

INTRAPULMONARY PRESSURE The pressure within the lungs. It is because intrapulmonary pressure is greater than intrathoracic pressure that the lungs are prevented from collapsing. See under BREATHING.

INTRATHORACIC PRESSURE   The pressure within the thoracic cage.
See under INTRAPULMONARY PRESSURE.

INTRINSIC FACTOR   See under VITAMIN B_{12}.

INTRINSIC MOTIVATION   Participation in an activity 'for its own sake,' without extrinsic rewards such as prizes. Deci's (1975) **Cognitive Evaluation theory** is based on the premise that intrinsically motivated behavior is derived from a person's innate need to feel competent and self-determining. Intentional behavior may be either self-determined or controlled. On the matter of extrinsic rewards, a person's interpretation of the reward (rather than the reward itself) is the critical factor in motivation. A reward has two aspects: controlling and informational. The controlling aspect conflicts with the need for self-determination. When the controlling aspect is high, rewards undermine intrinsic motivation. It is hypothesized that superior performance on complex tasks results from self-determined functioning, whereas superior performance on simple tasks often results when people are given difficult performance standards. Regarding the control aspect, money is more salient than verbal feedback. The informational aspect of a reward affects an individual's feelings of competence. A high informational aspect can provide either positive or negative information. The problem is that rewards tend to be given to a select few. Most rewards have both controlling and informational aspects. Rewards or events that provide positive information enhance perceived competence and intrinsic motivation. On the other hand, negative information about competence detracts from intrinsic motivation. Cognitive Evaluation theory implies that coaches and instructors should minimize the controlling aspects of rewards, use rewards for informational purposes and ensure that all participants have a reasonable chance to earn positive feedback.

Deci and Ryan (2000) proposed four types of extrinsic motivation: external regulation (behaviors that are not self-determined, because they are regulated through external means such as rewards and external constraints); introjected regulation (behaviors that are partly internalized by the person, but that remain non-self-determined because contingencies from external control sources have been internalized without having been endorsed by the individual); identified regulation (behaviors that are performed by choice because the individual judges them as important); and integrated regulation (behaviors that are so integrated in a person's life that they are part of the person's self and value system).

Sport and exercise participants are not simply intrinsically or extrinsically motivated, or even amotivated, but rather have all three types of motivation to various degrees (Vallerand, 2001). Intrinsic and extrinsic motivation and amotivation exist at three levels of generality: the global, contextual and situational levels. Motivation at a given level results from two potential sources: social factors and top-down effects from motivation at the proximal level. The impact of social factors on motivation is mediated by perceptions of competence, autonomy and relatedness. Vallerand postulates that consequences are decreasingly positive from intrinsic motivation to amotivation. Autonomy, competence and relatedness are mediators at all levels of the model.

Pelletier et al. (1995) showed that the more athletes perceived their coaches to be caring and involved, the more they were self-determined in their motivation towards their sport. Coaches can nurture athletes' intrinsic and self-determined extrinsic motivation by being autonomy supportive while providing structure and being involved. Although an autonomy-supportive style has been shown repeatedly to foster athletes' intrinsic and self-determined extrinsic motivation, Western culture still promotes a controlling style of teaching and coaching. An autonomy-supportive style implies that coaches provide opportunities for choices, emphasize task relevance, explain reasons underlying rules and limits, acknowledge athletes' feelings and perspective, give athletes opportunities to take initiatives, provide non-controlling motivational strategies, and prevent ego-involvement in their athletes. Many coaches adopt a controlling interpersonal style because they believe, falsely, that it will bring about better results. Western culture has been highly influenced by the behavioral approach to motivation, which advocates rewards and punishments as the most efficient motivational strategies. Coaches have a tendency to be more controlling with athletes who appear more difficult and non-self-determined in their motivation.

Bibliography

Deci, E.L. (1992). On the nature and functions of motivation theories. *Psychological Science* 3(3), 1992.

Deci, E.L. and Ryan, R.M. (1985). *Intrinsic motivation and self determination in human behavior*. New York: Plenum Press.

Deci, and Ryan, (2000). The 'what' and 'why' of goal pursuits: Human needs and the self-determination of behavior. *Psychological Inquiry* 11, 227-268.

Mageau, G.A. and Vallerand, R.J. (2003). The coach-athlete relationship: A motivational model.

Journal of Sports Sciences 21, 883-904.

Pelletier, L.G. et al. (1995). Toward a new measure of intrinsic motivation, extrinsic motivation, and amotivation in sports: The Sport Motivation Scale (SMS). *Journal of Sport and Exercise Psychology* 17, 35-53.

Vallerand, R.J. (2001). A hierarchical model of intrinsic and extrinsic motivation in sport and exercise. In Roberts, G.C. (2001). *Advances in motivation in sport and exercise*. pp263-319. Champaign, IL: Human Kinetics.

INVERSE STRETCH REFLEX See under GOLGI TENDON ORGANS; STRETCHING.

IN VITRO A term used in the context of scientific experimentation to indicate the occurrence of biological processes in isolation from the whole organism. An *in vitro* experiment is an experiment that is carried out with components isolated from cells.

IN VIVO Within the living organism. An *in vivo* experiment is performed with in tact cells.

IODINE An element, which as a 'trace element' in the human body, is a component of the thyroid hormones and is essential for functioning of the thyroid gland. Much of the iodine in food is in the form of **iodide** (the reduced form) and **iodates** (salts of iodine). In the intestinal tract, iodine is reduced to iodide and absorbed in the small intestine. In the body, inorganic iodide is distributed in extracellular fluid, plasma and red blood cells; it is concentrated in higher amounts in the salivary glands and the gastric mucosa. Much of the iodine is an essential component of two thyroid hormones: triiodothyronine and thyroxine.

The iodine content of most foods depends on the iodine content of the soil in which it was raised. Seafood is rich in iodine, because marine animals are able to concentrate the iodine from seawater. Cod (3 oz) contains 99 mcg of iodine. Milk (3 fluid oz, whole) contains 56 mcg of iodine. Processed foods may contain slightly higher levels of iodine due to the addition of iodized salt or food additives.

The recommended dietary allowance (RDA) is

partly based on the iodine accumulation in the thyroid glands of individuals with normal thyroid function. The RDA for adults is 150 mcg/day. The RDA for pregnant females is 220 mcg/day and 290 mcg/day for breastfeeding. To avoid over-absorption of iodine by the thyroid, adults should not consume more than the tolerable upper intake level (UL) of 1.1 mg per day.

Bibliography

Oregon State University. The Linus Pauling Institute. Micronutrient Information Center. Http://lpi.oregonstate. edu/infocenter

ION An atom(s) that carries a positive or negative charge.

See under ELEMENT; IONIC COMPOUNDS; MINERALS.

IONIC COMPOUNDS See under ELECTRON.

IONIZATION The dissociation of substances into their constituent ions.

IPSILATERAL On the same side.

IRON A metallic element that as an ion in the body is involved in the transport of oxygen and electrons. **Ferrous, reduced iron** is designated as Fe^{2+}. **Ferric, oxidized iron** is designated as Fe^{3+}. About 70% of the iron in the body is needed for hemoglobin and about 5% for myoglobin, cytochromes and enzymes. The remaining 25% is stored mainly in the liver, bone marrow and spleen. One form in which iron is stored in these sites is **ferritin**, a complex chemical compound containing iron and protein. It is found mainly in the liver, spleen and bone marrow.

Iron losses occur through menstruation, sweat, feces and urine. Iron is also lost through the hemoglobinuria and myoglobinuria that follow destruction of red blood cells and muscle cells during exercise. The body's stores of iron in the liver and bone marrow are gradually depleted over a period of years if there is insufficient iron in the diet. When bone marrow stores are depleted, hemoglobin formation depends on iron absorbed from the diet. If the absorption of dietary iron is insufficient, less hemoglobin is formed, thus red blood cell formation is decreased. Eventually, hemoglobin concentration can fall so far as to result in deficiency anemia. **Iron deficiency** has three stages: depletion of iron stores (decreased ferritin), depletion of functional iron (decreased transferrin receptors and decreased erythrocyte protoporphyrin) and iron deficiency anemia (decreased hemoglobin, decreased hematocrit and decreased red cell size). **Transferrin** is a protein that transports iron in the blood. Over 95% of iron in blood serum is bound by transferrin. Transferrin saturation is the extent to which transferrin has vacant iron-binding sites. Low transferrin saturation means that there is a high proportion of vacant iron-binding sites. **Protoporphyrin** is an intermediate in heme biosynthesis, combining with ferrous iron to form **protoheme IX**, the heme prosthetic group of hemoglobin. **Iron deficiency without anemia** entails normal hemoglobin, but low body iron stores. Iron deficiency anemia is an anemia in which iron (and thus hemoglobin) is deficient (less than 13 g/100 mL blood for males or 12g/100 mL for females).

Many athletes, particularly female, are iron depleted, but true iron deficiencies are rare. There is also evidence that some highly trained athletes, especially female long-distance runners, are iron deficient. However, it is not known whether iron deficiency in athletes is due to insufficient iron intake from the diet, an effect of exercise on iron metabolism or a combination of both. Iron depletion does not affect exercise performance, but iron deficiency affects performance through the combined effects of anemia on maximal oxygen uptake and muscle metabolism.

Iron supplementation is not recommended unless serum concentrations of hemoglobin, ferritin, iron and transferrin are measured and the results indicate a state of iron deficiency. The iron status of an individual can only be reliably determined on the combined evidence of several biochemical indices.

Iron supplementation is beneficial to individuals who are deficient in iron, but excessive iron intake can be toxic. It has been suggested that iron balance in male runners requires a dietary intake of 17.5 mg/day of iron, and that menstruating and amenorrheic women require 23 and 17 mg/day of iron, respectively. These figures assume that 10% of ingested iron is absorbed.

Only about 10% of dietary iron is normally absorbed, but it varies according to factors such as an individual's present iron status. The amount of iron in food (or supplements) that is absorbed by the body is influenced by the iron nutritional status of the individual and whether or not the iron is in the form of heme. Because it is absorbed by a different mechanism that nonheme iron, heme iron is more readily absorbed and its absorption is less affected by other dietary factors. Individuals who are anemic or iron deficient absorb a larger percentage of the iron they consume (especially nonheme iron) than individuals who are not anemic and have sufficient iron stores. Heme iron comes mainly from hemoglobin and myoglobin in meat, poultry and fish. Heme iron accounts for only 10 to 15% of the iron found in the diet, but it may provide up to one third of total absorbed dietary iron. The absorption of heme iron is less influenced by other dietary factors than that of nonheme iron. Plants, dairy products, meat and iron salts added to foods and supplements are all sources of nonheme iron. Vitamin C strongly enhances the absorption of nonheme iron by reducing dietary ferric iron (Fe^{3+}) to ferrous iron (Fe^{2+}) and forming an absorbable iron-ascorbic acid complex. Other organic acids such as lactic acid have some enhancing effects on nonheme iron absorption. Phytic acid, present in legumes, grains and rice, is an inhibitor of nonheme iron absorption. Small amounts of phytic acid (5 to 10 mg) can decrease nonheme iron absorption by 50%. The absorption of iron from legumes, such as soybeans, has been shown to be as low as 2%. Polyphenols, found in some fruits, vegetables, coffee, tea, wines and spices, can significantly inhibit the absorption of nonheme iron. This effect is decreased by the presence of vitamin C. Soy protein, such as that found in tofu, has an inhibitory effect on iron absorption that is independent of its phytic acid content.

In the USA, most grain products are fortified with iron. Beef (3 oz, cooked) contains 2.31 mg of iron. Black strap molasses (one tablespoon) contain 3.5 mg of iron.

The recommended daily allowance (RDA) for iron is based on the prevention of iron deficiency and maintenance of adequate iron stores in individuals eating a mixed diet. The RDA for adults (19 to 50 years) is 8 mg (males and postmenopausal females) and 18 mg/day (premenopausal females). The RDA for pregnant women is 27 mg/day; this usually taking a dietary supplement. The RDA for women who breastfeed and are not menstruating is 9 mg a day; and for adolescents who breastfeed, it is 10 mg per day. Breastfed infants between the ages of 7 months and 21 months should be given foods or formula containing additional iron, while those receiving formula also should be given iron-fortified formula or foods. The tolerable upper intake level (UL) for iron is set at 45 mg a day for adults, above which gastrointestinal distress may occur, especially when consuming iron supplements on an empty stomach.

See ANEMIA; IRON; SICKLE CELL TRAIT.

Bibliography

Burke, L.M. and Read, R.S.D. (1993). Dietary supplements in sport. *Sports Medicine* 15(1), 43-65.

Chatard, J-C, Mujika, I., Guy, C. and Lacour, J-R. (1999). Anaemia and iron deficiency in athletes. *Sports Medicine* 27(4), 229-240.

Clarkson, P.M. (1991). Minerals: Exercise performance and supplementation in athletes. *Journal of Sports Sciences* 9, 91-116.

Clement, D.B. and Sawchuk, L.L. (1984). Iron status and sports performance. *Sports Medicine* 1, 65-74.

Food and Nutrition Board, Institute of Medicine (1990). *Nutrition during pregnancy; weight gain, nutrient supplements.* Washington, DC: National Academy Press.

Haymes, E.M. (1987). Nutritional concerns: Need for iron. *Medicine and Science in Sports and Exercise* 19(5), S197-S199.

Newhouse, I.J. and Clement, D.B. (1988). Iron status in athletes. An update. *Sports Medicine* 5, 337-352.

Nielsen, P. and Nachtigall, D. (1998). Iron supplementation in athletes. Current recommendations. *Sports Medicine* 26(2), 207-216.

Oregon State University. The Linus Pauling Institute. Micronutrient Information Center. Http://lpi.oregonstate.edu/infocenter

Selby, G.B. (1991). When does an athlete need iron? *The Physician and Sportsmedicine* 19(4), 96-102.

ISCHEMIA   A condition in which there is decreased blood supply to tissues due to some obstruction of arterial blood flow.

Adenosine plays a central role in the pathophysiology of tissue ischemia. It signals an imbalance between oxygen demand and supply, and it initiates responses to redress such a discrepancy. Besides its property of vasodilation, adenosine possesses anti-platelet and anti-neutrophil activities and provides cytoprotection. During ischemia of the lower limbs, adenosine plays a physiological role by inducing vasodilation and by preventing microcirculatory failure. Exercise training prolongs claudication distance possibly by inducing pulse increases of adenosine and consequently skeletal muscle preconditioning.

See CARDIOVASCULAR DISEASE; PERIPHERAL ARTERIAL DISEASE.

Bibliography

Pasini, F.L., Capecchi, P.L. and Perri, T.D. (2000). Adenosine and chronic ischemia of the lower limbs. *Vascular Medicine* 5(4), 243-250.

ISCHIAL TUBEROSITY   The rough bony projection at the junction of the lower end of the body of the ischium and its ramus. It is the weight-bearing point in the sitting position. It is also the attachment for the sacrotuberous ligaments and is the site of origin of the hamstring muscles.

See under AVULSION FRACTURE.

ISOKINETIC MOVEMENT   A movement performed at a constant angular velocity. Isokinetic exercise involves an accommodating resistance and a fixed speed. In the area of testing and training, isokinetics reached its peak in the 1980s. In the 1990s, researchers and practitioners began emphasizing closed kinetic chain exercises.

Each of the isokinetic systems that are commercially available has its own features, but basically they are all the same in that they have a rotating lever arm which moves in a single plane. The lever arm (that attaches to the subject) moves at a pre-set angular velocity. If the joint center is aligned with the center of rotation of the lever arm, the body segment rotates with the same (constant) angular velocity of the lever arm. Isokinetic machines assume (incorrectly) that the muscles they are testing movement at a constant angular velocity. Most biological joints do not possess a fixed axis of rotation and hence the machine will make errors. The extent of the error will depend on the joint tested and the position of the subject. The angular velocity of many 'normal' activities is far beyond the maximum angular velocity of isokinetic devices, e.g. glenohumeral rotation during throwing is about 6,000 degrees per second whereas most isokinetic machines are limited to about 300 degrees per second. The angular velocity of the knee and ankle just before take off in jumping is about 720 degrees per second.

Before the movement reaches isokinetic values, there will often be a spike at the beginning of the contraction. This is due to **isometric pre-activation**, which is the static tension generated in the muscles before motion (often called '**pre-loading**'). This spike, which has been referred to as the '**impact artefact**' (or '**torque/moment overshoot**'), does not represent muscle performance at the pre-set velocity. A sample rate of 100 measurements per second is adequate for normal isokinetic testing.

Peak torque is the most commonly reported parameter with isokinetic testing. This represents the single highest point on the torque curve. **Rate of torque development** is the time it takes to reach peak torque, predetermined range of motion, or predetermined torque value. **Torque acceleration energy** is a measure of the 'explosiveness' of a muscle action. This can be operationally defined as the total work performed in the first 1/8 second. **Force decay rate** is the downslope of the torque curve. It is reflective of the subject's ability to produce force through the range of motion until the end.

The most effective strength gains from isokinetic exercise have come from a slower training speed (60 degrees per second or less). Training at fast speeds of motion has been found to increase the ability to exert a force rapidly, but not more so than traditional isotonic techniques.

Bibliography

Brown, L.E. (2000, ed). *Isokinetics in human performance*. Champaign, IL: Human Kinetics.

ISOLEUCINE   A six-carbon, essential amino acid. Isoleucine is both glycogenic (glucogenic) and ketogenic, because 4 of its carbons enter the Krebs cycle at succinyl CoA (leading to synthesis of glucose) during degradation and 2 carbons enter at acetyl CoA (leading to synthesis of fatty acids or ketone bodies).

ISOMER   See under CHEMICAL STRUCTURE.

ISOMERASES   See under ENYZMES.

ISOMETRIC MUSCLE ACTION   See under MUSCLE ACTION.

ISOMETRIC TRAINING   A training technique that uses isometric muscle actions. It is of limited value to athletes, because it is specific to the joint angle at which the training is done. It does not improve (and may be detrimental to) the ability to exert force rapidly. It is sometimes used as training to overcome 'sticking points' in the range of movement of a weightlifting exercise. A maximal isometric contraction (sustained long enough to recruit as many muscle fibers as possible) is necessary for an optimal strength improvement.

ISOTHERMAL   Refers to a reaction or process that occurs at a constant temperature.

ISOTONIC   See under MUSCLE ACTION; OSMOLALITY.

ISOTOPES   Forms of a chemical element with atoms that contain the same number of protons and the same number of electrons, but differ in the number of neutrons in nucleus of the atom. Unstable isotopes undergo transitions to a more stable state and, in doing, so, emit radioactivity.

ISOTOPIC DILUTION TECHNIQUE   A method by which the path of a compound can be traced through an organism to its final form and destination. A radioactive isotope is incorporated into a compound that is then introduced into the body. From samples of various tissues taken at intervals, chemical analysis can reveal what compounds are present and in what quantities.

ISOZYME   See under ENZYME.

J

JEJUNUM   The portion of the small intestine between the duodenum and ileum.

JERSEY FINGER An avulsion of the tendon of the *flexor digitorum profundus* muscle from its attachment to the distal interphalangeal joint. It is caused by a sudden, vigorous extension of the distal interphalangeal joint while held in flexion, typically when a player has made an attempt to grab the jersey or equipment of an opposing player in sports such as rugby. Jersey finger presents as an inability to flex the distal interphalangeal joint and it is nearly always the ring finger.

JET LAG A condition that affects many individuals who rapidly traverse three or more time zones. It involves phase shifts in circadian rhythms, hence it may also be referred to as **circadian dysrhythmia**. The exact cause is unknown, but it involves transient dissociation between the environmental time (local time in the new time zone) and internal time (body time due to the internal body clock).

Because the earth is spinning on its axis, for anybody standing on the earth's surface the sun rises in the east and sets in the west and is at its highest point in the sky at noon by local time. These events must occur in the UK after they have taken place in countries to the east, and before they have take place in countries to the west. To overcome this problem, the world has been divided into 24 time zones centered around the Prime Meridian, which is in Greenwich in London (UK) and separated by lines of longitude 15 degrees apart. These time zones determine the relationship between Greenwich Mean Time (GMT) and local time. Traveling to the east means you 'lose time' (in the sense that part of the day appears to have been lost), and to the west that gain it (in the sense that you can relive some hours). Problems arise when you cross several time zones in a short space of time. Adjustment to a westward flight requires individuals to go to bed and wake up later, and their body clock to delay. By contrast, adjustment to an eastward fight requires going to bed and rising earlier, to advance the body clock. The body clock can delay more easily than advance, probably because it tends to run slowly unless it is adjusted each day. As a result, eastward flights, which require the clock to advance, are associated with a longer resynchronization time than the ones to the west (assuming the same number of time zones are crossed). When the time shift approaches 12 hours, adjustment is almost invariably by delay of the body clock.

Napping can work antagonistically by anchoring rhythms in the time zone of departure. A prolonged nap at the time when the individual would be asleep, in the country departed, slows the rate of adjustment to the new local time. Exercise can be used to counteract drowsiness.

Symptoms associated with jet-lag include: fatigue during the new day time, and yet inability to sleep at night; decreased mental performance, particularly if vigilance is required; decreased physical performance, particularly with regard to events that require stamina or precise movement; a loss of appetite, coupled with indigestion and even nausea; and increased irritability, headaches, mental confusion and disorientation. The severity of these adverse effects, and therefore the time required for resynchronization, depends on: the ability to pre-set the biological rhythms prior to flying; the number of time zones crossed; the direction of flight; nutritional status and timing of meals; personality traits; motivation; age; social interaction; and the use of drugs. In general, at least seven days should be allowed for resynchronization to take place.

Two countermeasures to jet lag are: i) to promote sleep and alertness at the appropriate times; and ii) to promote adjustment of the body clock to the new time zone. In both of these, melatonin may have an important role. **Melatonin** is a hormone produced by the pineal gland. The production of melatonin is affected by light. Melatonin and its precursor serotonin have important roles in the sleep-wake cycle, with nocturnal secretions being significantly increased. There is normally a robust circadian rhythm of melatonin secretion, starting at about 21:00 and ending at about 08:00. There is evidence that melatonin can alter the phase of the internal (body) clock, thus endogenous melatonin has been regarded as an internal Zeitgeber. Melatonin secretion is affected by exercise, but it is not clear whether exercise stimulates or depresses secretion of melatonin. The efficacy of melatonin in alleviating the fatigue associated with jet lag is not in dispute. What is less clear, however, is the extent to which the beneficial effects of melatonin extend to promoting performance and mood in the new daytime, and an appropriate adjustment of the body clock. Melatonin ingestion in the morning produces a delay, and in the afternoon and early evening an advance, of the body clock. Melatonin ingestion produces general effects on the body clock similar to those of light, but the timing of its effects is opposite to that of light. Since bright light suppresses melatonin secretion, the effects of light and melatonin reinforce each other. Bright light in the early morning, just after the temperature minimum, advances the body clock directly, but it also has indirect effects through suppression of melatonin secretion, thus preventing the phase-delaying effect that melatonin would exert at this time. Melatonin has no license in Europe or Australia at present. It is available from health-food retailers in the USA, but is not sanctioned for professional prescription.

Whether concentrations of melatonin increase, decrease or remain unaffected by sessions of exercise may be explained by age, fitness status, lighting differences and the time of day that exercise takes place. *See also under* BIOLOGICAL RHYTHMS; HOME ADVANTAGE.

Bibliography

Atkinson, G. et al. (2003). The relevance of melatonin to sports medicine and science. *Sports Medicine* 33(11), 809-831.

Davis, J.O. (1988). Strategies for managing athletes' jet lag. *The Sport Psychologist* 2(2), 154-160.

Loat, C.E. and Rhodes, E.C. (1989). Jet lag and human performance. *Sports Medicine* 8(4), 226-38.

O'Connor, P.J. and Morgan, W.P. (1990). Athletic performance following rapid transversal of multiple time zones: A review. *Sports Medicine* 10(1), 20-30.

Reilly, T., Atkinson, G. and Waterhouse, J. (1997). Travel fatigue and jet lag. *Journal of Sports Sciences* 15, 365-369.

Waterhouse, J., Reilly, T. and Atkinson, G. (1997). Jet lag. *The Lancet* 350, 1611-16.

Waterhouse, J., Reilly, T. and Atkinson, G. (1997). Travel and body clock disturbances. *Sports, Exercise, and Injury* 3, 9-14.

Waterhouse, J., Reilly, T. and Atkinson, G. (1998). Melatonin and jet lag. *British Journal of Sports Medicine* 32, 98-100.

JOGGER'S NIPPLE *See under* CHAFING.

JOINT The union or articulation of two or more bones of the body. There are three types of joint: synarthroses, amphiarthroses and diathroses.

Synarthroses (synarthrodial joints) are fibrous articulations that allow little or no movement to occur. They may be cartilageneous (synchondrosis), ligamentous (syndesmosis) or fibrous (suture). **Amphiarthroses (amphiarthrodial joints)** are bones that are united by either hyaline cartilage, such as that found at the epiphyseal plates, or by fibrocartilage, such as at the pubic symphysis and the intervertebral articulations. The sacro-iliac joint is an amphiarthrodial joint. The sacrum of the vertebral column is connected to the ilium of the pelvis by fibrocartilage.

Diarthroses (synovial joints) are freely movable joints. A synovial joint consists of a cavity enclosed by a capsule of fibrous articular cartilage. The articular cartilage is lined with a **synovial membrane**, which is areolar connective tissue containing elastic fibers and some adipose tissue. Synovial membrane secretes a viscous lubricant called **synovial fluid**, which lubricates the cartilage at joints. The articular cartilage allows smooth gliding of the bone surfaces. A **joint capsule** is a sleeve of connective tissue that envelopes the ends of two bones in a synovial joint. A **simple joint** has only two articulating surfaces. The hip joint is a simple joint. A **compound joint** has three or more articulating surfaces. The wrist is a compound joint. A **complex joint** is a joint with more than two articulating surfaces and with a disc or fibrocartilage. The knee is a complex joint. **Surface joint motion** is the motion between the articulating surfaces of a joint.

A **gliding (plane) joint** consists of the articulation of two plane surfaces, such that only gliding movement is permitted. It is non-axial since it consists of two flat surfaces that slide over each other to allow movement. Examples are the sternoclavicular, acromioclavicular, intercarpal and intertarsal joints.

A **hinge joint (ginglymus)** involves the convex surface of one bone fitting a concave surface of another bone, such that movement is limited to flexion and extension. The elbow, knee, ankle and interphalangeal joints are hinge joints. A hinge joint is uniaxial since it allows movement in one plane (flexion/extension). Examples are the interphalangeal (fingers and thumb), humero-ulnar, tibiofemoral, talofibular and interphalangeal (toes) joints.

A **pivot (trochoid; screw) joint** involves a pivot-like process rotating in the fossa (hole) of another bone. Pivot joints are uniaxial (pronation/supination). The superior and inferior radioulnar joints and the atlantoaxial joint are pivot joints.

A **condyloid (ovoid; ellipsoidal) joint** consists of an oval-shaped condyle fitting into an elliptical cavity. Condyloid joints are biaxial (flexion/extension; abduction/adduction). Examples are the radiocarpal, metacarpophalangeal, metatarsophalangeal and occipitoatlantal joints.

A **saddle joint (reciprocal reception)** involves one articular surface, which is concave in one direction and convex in the other, articulating with another articular surface, which is reciprocally convex-concave so that the bones fit together. A saddle joint is biaxial (flexion/extension; abduction/adduction) with a small amount of rotation also allowed. The trapezium of the carpus and metacarpal of the thumb form a saddle joint.

A **ball-and-socket (spheroid; enarthrodial) joint** consists of the rounded head of one bone fitting into the concave cavity of another. A ball and socket joint is tri-axial (flexion/extension; abduction/adduction; rotation). Examples are the glenohumeral (shoulder) and femoroacetabular (hip) joints. The talonavicular joint is a shallow ball-and-socket joint.

See ARM; ARTHRITIS; CONNECTIVE TISSUE; FLEXIBILITY; HILTON'S LAW; LEG; SPINE.

Bibliography
Levangie, P.K. and Norkin, C.C. (2001). *Joint structure and function: A comprehensive analysis.* 3rd ed. Philadelphia, PA: F.A. Davis Company.

JOINT COMPLIANCE The amount of joint angular deflection per unit of torque increment.

JOINT LAXITY *See under* HYPERFLEXIBILITY.

JOINT MOBILITY The opposite of joint stability.
JOINT, NEUTRAL POSITION The position of a joint where the bones that make up the joint are placed in the optimal position for maximal movement.

JOINT REACTION FORCE The net force acting across a joint. It follows from Newton's 3rd law that there must be an equal and opposite force acting at each joint. It can be calculated given appropriate biomechanical and anthropometric data. Joint reaction force does not reflect a bone-on-bone force across a joint, i.e. the force exerted by the distal bony surface of one segment on the proximal bony surface of the contiguous segment. The actual bone-on-bone force is the sum of the actively contracting muscle forces pulling the joint together and the joint reaction force.

When a system for a free body diagram is defined so that it ends at a joint, the concept of joint reaction force represents the reaction of the adjacent body segment to the forces exerted by the identified system. The normal component is typically directed into the joint surface and represents a compressive force. The two tangential components compose the shear force that acts along the joint surface. The main contributor to joint reaction force is the force due to muscle action.

Bibliography
Enoka, R.M. (2002). *Neuromechanics of human movement.* 3rd ed. Champaign, IL: Human Kinetics.

JOINT STIFFNESS The amount of torque increment per unit of joint deflection.

JONES FRACTURE *See under* METATARSAL FRACTURES.

JUGULAR VEINS   Blood vessels in the neck drain that blood from the head, brain, face and neck.

JUMPER'S KNEE   *See* PATELLAR TENDONOSIS.

JUMPING   A movement that involves a person propelling himself off the ground. It involves a one- or two-foot takeoff with a landing on both feet. Jumping takes three forms: jumping for distance; jumping for height; and jumping from a height. Motor milestones are as follows: jumping down from a low object with both feet can be achieved (2 years); jumping off the floor with both feet (28 months); jumping for distance about 3 feet (5 years); and jumping for height about 1 foot (5 years).

JUVENILE DELINQUENCY   Delinquency is a legal term used to refer to youths whose behavior results in arrest and court action. It is a manifestation of emotional problems. Delinquent adolescents are characterized by various disadvantages, including an increased prevalence of depression and low self-esteem. 40% of all juvenile offenders have learning disabilities and most of them have never received any help for their disabilities. Theories of juvenile delinquency include Labeling, Strain and Differential Association theories.

Labeling theory is based on the premise that delinquents are normal individuals and that if they persist in delinquent behavior, it is due to the negative effects of interaction with authorities. Once an individual has been labeled as a delinquent by authorities, labeling by society as a deviant soon follows. If the individual continues to violate the norms of society, and is repeatedly labeled as a deviant, internalizations of the deviant role will begin to occur. Once acceptance of the role occurs, the individual will become active in fulfilling the role's expectations. Sanctioning is often left to the discretion of social control agents. Labeling theory would predict that an athlete or any other respected youth who is apprehended for participating in some type of delinquent behavior would be more likely to receive favorable treatment by the legal authorities than his peers.

Strain theory is based on the premise that individuals, regardless of social class, prize the middle-class success ethic (the 'American Dream'). Lower class youths, however, are improperly socialized to compete for the goals. This inability to compete, most apparent in the educational system where the mannerisms of lower-class youth make it difficult for them to obtain status or acceptance from teachers and peers, produces tension or strain. Three avenues that a lower class youth could take in attempting to solve this means-goal conflict are: i) acceptance of the challenge of the middle-class system and refusal to accept lower-class status; ii) acceptance of lower-class status and failure to attempt to succeed in the middle-class world; and iii) continued aspirations for middle-class goals, but rejection of all symbols of middle-class life and entry into delinquent subculture. When opportunities for upward mobility have been blocked, sport may function as an alternative means of achieving upward mobility for lower-class adolescents. Problems may occur when the lower-class adolescent places too little emphasis on education and too much emphasis on athletics. The poorly educated athlete will find it extremely difficult to secure employment at an equivalent status level to that enjoyed as a well-educated athlete.

Differential Association theory is based on the premise that deviant behavior is learned within intimate groups through the communication of both the techniques for committing criminal acts and the motivations and rationalizations to justify such actions. If an individual associates with a group that values delinquent behavior more than with groups that sanction deviant behavior, and if the person internalizes the norms of these delinquent groups, then he is likely to become involved in delinquent activities. An athlete's intimate group, at least during the sport season, is likely to be comprised of other players and coaches. A few of the values that are likely to be stressed by this group include hard work, deferred gratification and teamwork. In line with the ideology of athleticism, coaches tend to emphasize character, teamwork and other qualities that might be useful for the athlete long after termination of the athletic career. This theory supports sport participation as a deterrent to delinquency on the basis that sport socialization generally involves internalization of the dominant values and norms of society.

See also CHARACTER BUILDING; CONDUCT DISORDER.

Bibliography

Purdy, D.A. and Richard, S.F. (1983). Sport and juvenile delinquency: An examination and assessment of four major theories. *Journal of Sport Behavior* 6(4), 179-193.

JUVENILE MANIA A disorder characterized by episodes where an affected individual enters into an expansive mood that includes symptoms of extreme agitation and/or an unrealistic exuberance (grandiose ideas and boastfulness). Other symptoms include restlessness, rapidly changing thoughts or ideas, risk taking, sleeplessness and goal-oriented obsessiveness. There is often a family history of bipolar disorder associated with juvenile mania. Some authorities believe that juvenile mania is a variant of attention-deficit hyperactivity disorder rather than a separate and distinct disorder.

See also CONDUCT DISORDER.

K

KALLIKREIN Plasma serine proteases that act on kininogens to produce the proinflammatory kinins, e.g bradykinin.

KARYOTYPE The chromosome complement of a cell or organism.

KERATIN A water insoluble fibrous protein that is the primary constituent of hair, nails and the outer layer of skin.

KERATOCONJUNCTIVITIS Inflammation of the cornea and conjunctiva.

KERATOCONUS A thinning of the cornea, which is the clear outer covering of the front surface of the eye. A thinner cornea is unable to maintain its normal shape and protrudes in the shape of a cone. This distortion causes distorted vision.

KETOACIDOSIS *See* KETOSIS.

KETO ACIDS Compounds that are both a ketone and an acid. Examples are pyruvic acid, acetyl CoA and Kreb's cycle intermediates.

KETOGENIC *See under* KETONE BODIES.

KETONE Any of a class of organic compounds having a carbonyl group linked to a carbon atom in each of two hydrocarbon radicals. Examples are pyruvate and fructose. **Ketonuria** is a high level of ketones in the urine.

KETONEMIA A high level of ketones in the blood.

KETONE BODIES Molecules formed when insufficient carbohydrate is available to completely metabolise fat. The two main ketone bodies are **acetoacetate** and **3-beta-hydroxybutyrate**. **Acetone** is the third, and least abundant, ketone body. Acetone and acetoacetate are ketones, but beta-hydroxybutyrate is not.

Ketogenesis is the process by which excess acetyl CoA from fatty acid oxidation is converted into ketone bodies. Ketogenesis occurs primarily in the liver mitochondria, because of the high levels of beta-hydroxy-beta-methylglutaryl-CoA (HMG-CoA) synthase in that tissue. It is highly active when fatty acid oxidation in the liver produces such an abundance of acetyl CoA that it overwhelms the available supply of oxaloacetate.

When acetyl CoA levels are high, 2 moles of acetyl CoA undergo a reversal of the thiolase reaction to give acetoacetyl CoA. This occurs particularly when levels of oxaloacetate are low, so that flux through citrate synthase is impaired. Acetoacetyl CoA can react, in turn, with a third mole of acetyl CoA to give HMG-CoA, catalyzed by HMG-CoA synthase. When formed in cytosol, HMG-CoA is an early intermediate in cholesterol biosynthesis. In mitochondria, however, HMG-CoA is acted on by HMG-CoA lyase to yield acetoacetate plus acetyl-CoA. Acetoacetate undergoes either NADH-dependent reduction to give D-beta-hydroxybutyrate or, in very small amounts, spontaneous decarboxylation to acetone, which can be smelt on the breath. Acetone is not available as a fuel to any significant extent and is thus a waste product.

After the liver makes ketone bodies, they travel to other tissues via the bloodstream. Tissue cells can convert the ketone bodies back to acetyl CoA for ATP production via the citric acid cycle and the electron transport chain. Ketone bodies are transported from liver to other tissues, where acetoacetate and beta-hydroxybutyrate can be reconverted to acetyl-CoA for energy generation.

The ketone bodies are water-soluble and are transported across the inner mitochondrial membrane as well as across the blood-brain barrier and cell membranes. The body produces small quantities of ketone bodies at all times. Levels of ketone bodies increase during fasting and prolonged exercise. The heart and kidneys prefer acetoacetate to glucose as a fuel source. Other than glucose, ketone bodies are the only effective fuel for the central nervous system. Brain cells can adapt to derive 50 to 75% of their fuel from ketone bodies (principally beta-hydroxybutyrate) after a few weeks of a low supply of glucose.

The term 'ketogenic' means capable of being converted into ketone bodies. In metabolism, fatty acids and some amino acids are ketogenic. Ketogenic amino acids are those amino acids whose carbon atoms are converted to acetyl CoA and/or acetoacetyl CoA when they are degraded for energy. Acetyl CoA and acetoacetyl CoA are precursors of ketone bodies. Leucine is the only completely ketogenic amino acid. Two of its carbons are converted to acetyl CoA, while the other four are converted to acetoacetyl CoA. Lysine, phenylalanine and tyrosine are both glucogenic (glycogenic) and ketogenic. This is because fumarate, an intermediate of the Krebs cycle, and acetoacetate, which leads to acetoacetyl CoA, are the products of their degradation. Isoleucine and threonine are sometimes classified as both glucogenic and ketogenic, but more often as glucogenic.

Bibliography

Laffel, L. (1999). Ketone bodies: A review of physiology, pathophysiology and application of monitoring to diabetes. *Diabetes Metabolism Research and Reviews* 15(6), 412-426.

Mathews, C.K., Van Holde, K.E. and Ahern, K. (2000). *Biochemistry*. 3rd ed. San Francisco, CA: Benjamin/Cummings.

KETONURIA A high level of ketones in the urine.

KETOSIS Ketoacidosis. A medical emergency in which the liver produces more ketones than the peripheral tissues can oxidize and blood levels of ketones reach toxic levels. Metabolic acidosis occurs as a result of lowered pH. Ketosis occurs during starvation, fasting, low carbohydrate diet or uncontrolled Type I diabetes mellitus. Given time, the body can adapt to a very high fat diet and avoid ketosis.

KICKING Imparting force to an object with the foot. Motor milestones are as follows: kicking with the leg straight and little body movement (2 to 3 years); flexing the lower leg on the backswing (3 to 4 years); greater backward and forward swing with definite arm opposition (4 to 5 years); and mature kicking pattern (5 to 6 years).

KIDNEYS Two bean-shaped body organs found behind the 13th rib, posteriorly and somewhat inferiorly on each side of the abdomen. The primary function of the kidneys is to maintain equilibrium by controlling the content and volume of the blood. Filtering about 160 liters of blood per day, the kidneys remove waste products from the blood in the form of urine and conserve water. **Nephrons** in the kidney are able to balance filtration, reabsorption and secretion of various constituents of body fluid. Water makes up about 95% of the total volume of urine, with the remaining 5% consisting of dissolved solutes or waste products such as urea. Urine passes from the kidneys by means of muscle contractions and gravity.

About 3% of American schoolchildren have some history of a kidney or urinary tract disorder. Genital-urinary malformations are second only to congenital blindness and congenital deafness as the most common birth defects in the USA. **Nephritis** is inflammation of the kidney. It is generally caused by an infection. **Bright's disease (acute glomerulonephritis)** causes degenerative changes in the glomeruli, which are small filters in the kidney. It is characterized by proteinuria and hematuria, and sometimes by edema, hypertension and nitrogen retention. About 95% of patients recover from the acute phase of the disease, but if glomerulonephritis becomes chronic then renal damage ensues and, ultimately, kidney failure. Persons with kidney and urinary tract disease need moderate exercise, but not vigorous exercise.

The kidney is susceptible to injury from blunt trauma because of its normal distention by blood. Contusions or even ruptures may occur, but most sports-related renal trauma is mild. Hematuria is the most common presenting sign of renal injury. Exercise-induced hematuria can originate in the kidney, bladder, urethra or prostate.

Chronology

•2004 • After suffering from nephritic syndrome for 10 years, Jonah Lomu, the New Zealand rugby union star, spent a year receiving dialysis, which is method of removing waste products and excess water from the blood when the kidneys are unable to do so. Lomu then received a new kidney from a donor. It was positioned behind the ribcage rather than in the lower abdomen so as to give Lomu a chance of returning to rugby. Lomu was prescribed prednisone as an anti-rejection drug. Prednisone is a corticosteroid that is banned by the World Anti-Doping Agency (WADA). However, Lomu could apply for Therapeutic Use Exemption if he returned to rugby.

Bibliography

Holmes, F.C., Hunt, J.J. and Sevier, T.L. (2003). Renal injury in sport. *Current Sports Medicine Reports* 2(2), 103-109.

KIENBÖCK'S DISEASE Keinböck's syndrome. Avascular necrosis of the lunate. The circulation of the lunate is disrupted; the bone softens and becomes devascularized.

KINANTHROPOMETRY The quantitative interface between structure and function in kinesiology. Mastery of accurate measurement requires rigorous training and strict adherence to specified techniques. A '**criterion anthropometrist**' is one who purportedly does not make systematic errors from a prescribed technique. Most individuals seem to achieve reasonable competence after triple measurement and spot-checking for systematic error with criterion measures on 100 or more subjects. Anthropometric description always refers to the anatomical position. *See also* ANATOMICAL LANDMARKS; ANTHROPOMETRY; PLANES.

Chronology

•1928 • Anthropometric measurements were carried out on athletes at the Olympic Games in Amsterdam.
•1978 • The International Working Group on Kinanthropometry was founded in Brasilia. It was decided to join the International Council of Sport Science and Physical Education (ICSSPE) as an official committee.
•1986 • The International Society for the Advancement of Kinanthropometry (ISAK), which developed from the International Working Group in Kinanthropometry, was founded with the aim of fostering a united approach to kinanthropometry. The techniques adopted by Bloomfield et al. (1994), for example, were consistent with those prescribed by the ISAK Working Group on Standards and Instrumentation and supported by the Laboratory Assistance Scheme of the Australian Sports Commission (adopted for use in Australia in 1993).

Bibliography

Bloomfield, J., Ackland, T.R., and Elliott, B.C. (1994). *Applied anatomy and biomechanics in sport*. Melbourne: Blackwell Scientific.
Eston, R. and Reilly, T. (1996, eds). *Kinanthropometry and exercise physiology laboratory manual*. London: E & FN Spon.
Ross, W.D. et al. (1978). Kinanthropometry landmarks and terminology. In: Shephard, R.J. and Lavellee, H. (eds). *Fitness assessment*. pp44-50. Springfield, IL: Charles C. Thomas.
Ross, W.D. and Marfell-Jones, M.J. (1991). Kinanthropometry. In MacDougall, J.D., Wenger, H.A., and Green, H.J. (Eds). *Physiological testing of the high performance athlete*. pp223-308. Champaign, IL: Human Kinetics.

KINASE An enzyme involved in the phosphorylation of an electron acceptor by ATP.

KINEMATICS The study of the motion of bodies without reference to the forces associated with that motion. **Kinetics** is the study of the motion of bodies with reference to the forces associated with that motion.

KINESIOLOGY A term that literally means the study of movement, but has been used in different ways. Hoffman and Harris (2000) describe kinesiology as the science that studies physical activity (voluntary movement intentionally performed in order to achieve a goal in sport, exercise or any other sphere of life experience). Spheres of physical activity experiences include competition, health, leisure, education, work, self-expression (including dance) and self-sufficiency. Hoffman and Harris (2000) argue that the discipline of kinesiology has evolved primarily from the profession of physical education over the last 50 years.

Brown (2001) states that kinesiology is a term frequently used to describe the entire field of what once was almost universally called physical education and that 'exercise science' has largely supplanted 'sports medicine' as the all-inclusive umbrella term for the discipline that engages in the scientific study of movement. **Exercise science** describes the application of science to the phenomenon of exercise (all human movement, including random or infrequent movement, work, habitual activity, training done for fitness or health, dance, sport and leisure activities).

The American Academy of Kinesiology and Physical Education (AAKPE) defined kinesiology as the study of movement. The term 'kinesiology' also has a narrower meaning, i.e. a discipline concerned with anatomy, physiology and mechanics. In this sense, there are both similarities and differences between kinesiology and biomechanics in that the former includes mechanical aspects, and the latter includes anatomical aspects.

See also ANTHROPOMETRY; SPORTS SCIENCE.

Chronology

•1786 • In Germany, Johann Christoph GuthsMuths succeeded Carl Andre as leader of the Schnepfenthal Educational Institute (that was founded in 1784 by Christian G. Salzmann). GuthsMuths' program included gymnastic skills such as exercises on the climbing mast, horizontal bar, vaulting apparatus, balance beam and rope ladders, and stunts in tumbling. GuthsMuths' manuals were the first published by a practical physical educator. His book *Gymnastics for Youth* (1793) was translated into English in 1800. GutsMuths believed that the theory and practice of gymnastics should be based on knowledge of physiology and medicine.

•1804 • In Sweden, Pehr Henrik Ling was appointed to the University of Lund where he went on to study anatomy and physiology, applying his knowledge to gymnastics. Ling believed that body movements should not be determined by apparatus, as in the German system, but that the apparatus should be designed so as to secure the desired results, whether they were military, educational or rehabilitational. He insisted that medicine and physical education must be allies and that teachers of physical education must have theoretical knowledge as well as practical ability.

•1862 • Captain H. Rothstein, director of the Prussian government's Royal Central Gymnastic Institute, banished the horizontal and parallel bars from the German-based program, because of his beliefs in the 'scientific' Swedish system of gymnastics. Consequently, a commission of medical men was appointed to study the merits of the Swedish and German systems. When the commission recommended that the horizontal and parallel bars should be retained, Captain Rothstein resigned. Prussia then made German gymnastics obligatory in elementary schools.

•1869 • Dudley A. Sargent became the director of Bowdoin College gymnasium, two years before entering the college as a freshman. Upon graduation from Bowdoin in 1875, he assumed the role of instructor of gymnastics at the same time as he was a freshman medical student at Yale. He received his M.D. in 1878.

•1882 • The Central Association of Bodily Education in the Nation and School was organized in Germany. Its aim was the promotion of bodily exercise through gymnastics, skating, swimming, bathing, rowing, games and festivals. This organization was one of the first to appoint a medical section to observe the physical effects of exercise on the individual.

•1885 • The Association for the Advancement of Physical Education was founded by 43 men and 6 women, 10 of whom had a medical degree. It later changed its name to the American Association for the Advancement of Physical Education.

•1890 • Baron Nils Posse founded the Posse Normal School that trained teachers in the Swedish system of gymnastics. In the same year, the Swedish system was formally adopted for all the public schools in Boston. Posse published *The Special Kinesiology of Educational Gymnastics* and was possibly the first person to use the term 'kinesiology.'

•1891 • Wilbur P. Bowen, a math teacher at Michigan State Normal School, who had attended Sargent's Summer School of Physical Education at Harvard for a couple of summers, set up the Department of Physical Education for Men at the University of Nebraska. Bowen began as a wrestling coach at University of California, Berkeley and later became a professor of physical education at Michigan State Normal College.

•1891 • Dudley A. Sargent and George Fitz collaborated to establish a Department of Anatomy, Physiology, and Physical Training at the Lawrence Scientific School of Harvard University. A four-year Bachelor of Science in Anatomy, Physiology and Physical Training was offered, being aimed at those who expected to manage gymnasiums and for those who sought a general education in preparation for studying medicine. In 1897-1898, the practical work was decreased and by 1899 the program was completely pre-medical. The first degree was awarded in 1893, but only eight other students received their degrees before the degree was discontinued.

•1892 • At the Seventh Convention of the American Academy of Physical Education (AAPE), George W. Fitz, president of the Department of Physical Education at the National Educational Association, stated, "We hear much about the theory of physical training and the theory of different systems. What right have we to theories? Physiology has not reached the point where they can say deductively that this should be so and that otherwise. ... As physiologists, we should study the conditions under which the exercises are done, and the results of these exercises upon the system." According to Gerber (1971), Fitz's point was that, while various systems, especially the Swedish, claimed to be scientific, little work had been done to establish the validity of their claims.

•1897 • The Society of College Gymnasium Directors was formed. Dudley A. Sargent was a founding member. It was renamed the National College Physical Education Association for Men (NCPEAM) in 1963.

•1900 • At an international congress of physical education in Paris, three propositions were voted by the delegates (reported to the American Physical Education Review by Thomas D. Wood): i) there should be one fundamental, international basis for physical education, with national application adapted to local conditions; ii) scientific principles are necessary for the application to practical education; and iii) gymnastics must conform to the laws of physiology, psychology, physics and chemistry.

•1903 • The American Association for the Advancement of Physical Education (AAAPE) was renamed the American Physical Education Association (APEA).

•1904 • The American Academy of Physical Education (AAPE) was founded by Luther Gulick, to "bring together those who were doing original scientific work in the field of physical training, and to aid promotion of such work." It was discontinued during World War I.

•1905 • The editor of the *American Physical Education Review*, published by the American Physical Education Association (APEA), pointed to the lack of evidence upon which most claims for the various systems of physical education had been based and emphasized the development of a "consistent and authoritative physiology and hygiene of physical training."

•1912 • Wilbur P. Bowen's *The Action of Muscles in Bodily Movement and Posture* was published. The second edition was named *Applied Anatomy and Kinesiology: The Mechanisms of Muscular Movement*. After revision by several different authors, the latest version is *Kinesiology and Applied Anatomy* by Philip J. Rasch et al. (1989).

•1923 • In Germany, Carl Diem, director of the Berlin College of Physical Education, invited physicians interested in the medical aspects of exercise to organize a medical association for the promotion of physical education. Two years later the Medical Association for the Expansion of Physical Education was founded.

•1924 • The National Association for Physical Education of College Women was founded.

•1925 • David K. Brace outlined a scientific approach for the profession of physical education in the USA. He emphasized tests of intelligence, motor ability, knowledge and techniques, rules, hygiene, performance, achievement and attitudes.

•1926 • The American Academy of Physical Education (AAPE) was founded, for a second time, to encourage and promote the study of educational application of the art and science of human movement. The five original members were Clark W. Hetherington, champion of developmental play and educational athletics; R. Tait McKenzie, physician, scholar and sculptor, who created many pieces of sport art; William Burdick, city recreation specialist and administrator; Thomas A. Storey, physician, health educator and first state supervisor of physical education (New York, 1916); and Jay B. Nash, philosopher of recreation and advocate of the development of the "whole person" through creative leisure.

•1927 • Peter Karpovich, credited with introducing physiology to physical education in the USA, started to establish his research facility at Springfield College, Massachusetts.

•1927 • A pamphlet entitled "The Objectives of American Physical Education Association, 1885-1927" set forth the curricular framework that leaders of the American Physical Education Association (APEA) saw as a necessary guide for the increasing number of undergraduate and graduate level programs in physical education. It stated that the fundamental problems of physical education could best be investigated with a proper understanding of "biology, chemistry, anatomy, physics, physiology, psychology and administrative problems."

•1928 • Pierre de Coubertin established the Bureau Internationale de Pédagogie Sportive in Lausanne to serve as a world center for scientific information on sports and physical education.

•1930 • The American Physical Education Association (APEA) published *Research Quarterly* to promote research within the field of physical education.

•1930 • The Scientific Research Institute for the Study of Physical Education was established within the Moscow Institute of Physical Culture with the aim of cooperative research between the various subdisciplines.

•1941 • Charles H. McCloy, in an editorial of the *Journal of Health and Physical Education*, argued that physical education and health education needed to relinquish their excessively close ties with

education and begin to make independent contributions by conducting their own basic research in the biological and social sciences.

•1945 • McGill University in Canada began offering a four-year course leading to a B.Sc. Degree in Physical Education.

•1946 • In England, the University of Birmingham first included physical education among subjects on offer for the degree of Bachelor of Arts. A study of the history and principles of physical education became the core. The degree was initially offered without honors, but eventually became a full-honors degree.

•1952 • The American Association for Health, Physical Education and Recreation (AAHPER) changed one of its constitutional aims from "acquiring and disseminating accurate information" to "assist in research and experimentation and to disseminate accurate information."

•1954 • *Research Quarterly*, a journal of the American Association for Health, Physical Education and Recreation (AAHPER), started a "Notes and Comments" section to accommodate simple status surveys that previously would have been acceptable as regular articles. This was a response to the belief that "applied" studies were being emphasized to the detriment of "basic" research.

•1962 • The legislature in California passed the Fisher Bill, which created a single-subject teaching credential limiting the teacher to a specific subject field such as physical education. As a result of the Fisher Bill, it took an additional year of college study, a fifth year, before a California teaching credential could be granted. In addition to the additional year of college, the Fisher Bill identified areas of study that are academic and nonacademic. Physical education was classified as nonacademic, but could be classified as academic if certain conditions were met.

•1963 • In The *Education of American Teachers*, James Bryant Conant, former President of Harvard University suggested that graduate programs in physical education should be eliminated if they did not move from studying 'methods' courses to a more rigorous curriculum based on the sciences. This led to reforms that resulted in the many subdisciplines of exercise science. Conant opposed the Fisher Bill.

•1963 • A kinesiology section was formed in the American Alliance for Health, Physical Education and Recreation (AAHPER). It was officially recognized two years later and operated under the new title of Kinesiology Council (Kinesiology Committee, 1972; Kinesiology Academy of the National Association for Sport and Physical Education, 1974).

•1963 • In the USA, the National College Physical Education Association for Men and the National Association of Physical Education for College Women started the journal *Quest* with a commitment to publish "scholarly papers of philosophical and scientific interest."

•1964 • Franklin M. Henry delivered an address before the annual meeting of the National College Physical Education Association for Men titled "Physical Education – An Academic Discipline." This was part of the response by the physical education profession to the Fisher Bill and the arguments of James Conant. In the same year, Henry's paper was also published in *Quest*.

•1965 • The American Academy of Physical Education (AAPE) and the American Association of Health, Physical Education and Recreation (AAHPER) held a conference to "prepare a plan for analyzing the dimensions of physical education as an area of scholarly study and research."

•1978 • The National Association for Physical Education of College Women (NAPECW) and the National College Physical Education Association for Men (NCPEAM) combined to form the National Association for Physical Education in Higher Education.

•1979 • The American Alliance of Health, Physical Education and Recreation (AAHPER) changed its name to the American Alliance of Health, Physical Education, Recreation and Dance (AAHPERD). AAHPERD is now composed of the following six national associations: American Association for Active Lifestyles and Fitness (AAALF), American Association for Health Education (AAHE), American Association for Leisure and Recreation (AALR), National Association for Girls and Women in Sport (NAGWS), National Association for Sport and Physical Education (NASPE) and National Dance Association (NDA). There is also a Research Consortium. There are approximately 26,000 members of AAHPERD.

•1989 • The American Academy of Physical Education (AAPE) resolved that the term 'kinesiology' shall refer to the theoretical and scientific bases of the study of physical activity. The term 'physical education' should be limited to focus on teaching in traditional educational contexts. The AAPE stated, "In American higher education, the term is used to describe a multifaceted field of study in which movement or physical activity is the intellectual focus. Physical activity includes exercise for improvement of health and physical fitness, activities of daily living, work, sport, dance, and play, and involves special population groups such as, children and the elderly; persons with disability, injury or disease; and athletes. Kinesiology is a common name for college and university departments that include many specialized areas of study in which the causes and consequences of physical activity are examined from different perspectives. The specialized areas of study apply knowledge, methods of inquiry, and principles from traditional areas of study in the arts, humanities and sciences. These areas include exercise and sport biomechanics, history, philosophy, physiology, biochemistry and molecular/cellular physiology, psychology, and sociology; motor behavior; measurement; physical fitness; and sports medicine. An interdisciplinary approach involving several of these areas is often used in addressing problems of importance to society. ..."

•1993 • The American Academy of Physical Education (AAPE) changed its name to the American Academy of Kinesiology and Physical Education (AAKPE).

•1993 • The Kinesiology Academy of the American Alliance for Health, Physical Education, Recreation and Dance (AAHPERD) was renamed the Biomechanics Academy of AAPHERD.

Bibliography

Abernethy, B. (2004). *The biophysical foundations of human movement*. 2nd ed. Champaign, IL: Human Kinetics.
American Academy of Kinesiology and Physical Education. Http://www.aakpe.org
Brown, S.P. (2000). *Introduction to exercise science*. Philadelphia, PA: Lippincott Williams & Wilkins.
Hamilton, N. and Luttgens, K. (2002). *Kinesiology. Scientific basis of human motion*. 10th ed. Madison, WI: Brown & Benchmark.
Hoffman, S.J. and Harris, J.C. (2000). *Introduction to kinesiology: Studying physical activity*. Champaign, IL: Human Kinetics.
Housh, T.J. and Housh, D.J. (2000, eds). *Introduction to exercise science*. Boston, MA: Allyn and Bacon.
Kamen, G. (2001). *Foundations of exercise science*. Philadelphia, PA: Lippincott Williams & Wilkins.
Lumpkin, A. (2005). *Introduction to physical education, exercise science, and sport studies*. 6th ed. Boston, MA: McGraw-Hill.
Park, R.J. (1980). The Research Quarterly and its antecedents. *Research Quarterly for Exercise and Sport* 51, 1-22.
Park, R.J. (1987). Physiologists, physicians, and physical educators: Nineteenth century biology and exercise, hygienic and educative. Journal of Sport History 14(1).
Rasch, P.J. and Burke, R.K. (1978). *Kinesiology and applied anatomy*. 6th ed. Philadelphia, PA: Lea and Febiger.
Wade, M.G. and Baker, J.A.W. (1994). *Introduction to kinesiology: The science and practice of physical activity*. Boston, MA: McGraw-Hill.
Wuest, D.A. and Buecher, C.A. (2003). *Foundations of physical education, exercise science, and sport*. 14th ed. Boston, MA: McGraw-Hill.

KINESTHETIC FEEDBACK *See under* PROPRIOCEPTIVE FEEDBACK.

KINETIC CHAIN EXERCISE A kinetic chain involves two or more segments of the body linked together. The **lower-extremity kinetic chain** involves the hip, knee and ankle joints. The **upper-extremity kinetic chain** involves the shoulder, elbow and wrist joints. A distinction can be made between open and closed kinetic chain exercise.

Open kinetic chain exercise is an exercise or movement pattern where the distal aspect of the extremity is not fixed to an object and terminates in free space. An example is the seated knee extension machine found in 'multi-gyms,' where the lower legs and feet are free to move through space, but the feet are fixed to a lever. During knee extension, the tibia glides anteriorly on the femur. During knee flexion, the tibia glides posteriorly on the femur. From 20 degrees of knee flexion to full extension, the tibia rotates externally. From full knee extension to 20 degrees of flexion, the tibia rotates internally.

Closed kinetic chain exercise is an exercise or movement pattern where the distal aspect of the extremity is fixed to an object that is either stationary or moving. An example is the squat, for which the soles of the feet are in contact with the ground. During knee extension, the femur glides posteriorly on the tibia. During knee flexion, the femur glides anteriorly on the tibia. From 20 degrees of knee flexion to full extension, the femur rotates internally on the stable tibia. From full knee extension to 20 degrees of flexion, the femur rotates externally on the stable tibia.

It has been argued that the open- versus closed-kinetic chain dichotomy is inaccurate and confusing. This is because true closed kinetic chain exercise only exists during isometric exercise, since by definition neither the proximal nor the distal segment can move in a closed system. A better dichotomy is kinetic chain exercise versus joint isolation exercise. **Joint isolation exercise** does not take advantage of the secondary stabilizing effect of muscular co-contraction. The squat is a kinetic chain exercise; the multi-gym knee extension is a joint isolation exercise. Both exercises involve contraction of the *quadriceps femoris* muscle group, but the squat involves significantly more contraction of the hamstrings. This hamstring co-contraction helps to neutralize the tendency of the *quadriceps femoris* to cause anterior tibial translation (as happens in isolated *quadriceps femoris* contraction that occurs with the knee extension exercise and which comes about because a shear force is applied perpendicular to the long axis of the tibia (rather than a compressive force being applied axially, as in the squat).

A **joint shear force** is that component of the resultant force transmitted across a joint which tends to transversely displace one joint segment relative to the other. Force acting at the knee joint in a direction parallel to the tibial plateau is a shearing force at the knee. The greatest amount of stress is placed on the ligaments and tendons that prevent the femur from sliding off the tibial plateau. In the last 30 degrees of knee extension, the patellar tendon pulls the tibia forward relative to the femur. This places a lot of stress on the anterior cruciate ligament (ACL), which absorbs nearly 85% of the anterior shear force. This tibiofemoral shear force is maximal in the last few degrees of extension. By moving the contact pad closer to the knee in the knee extension exercise, the shear force can be directed posteriorly, taking the strain off the ACL. The ACL does not prevent anterior tibial translation; along with the posterior cruciate ligament, it acts as a passive guide to the combined rolling and gliding of the femoral condyles on the tibial plateau.

Kinetic chain exercise involves 'pseudo-isometric contraction,' which occurs in the squat because the upward movement involves simultaneous hip and knee extension. As the hip extends, the *quadriceps femoris* lengthen, while the hamstrings shorten, but as the knee extends the *quadriceps femoris* shorten, while the hamstrings lengthen. Joint protection and movement control is enhanced by antagonist co-contraction. Greater antagonist co-contraction is found in trained athletes.

When the barbell is positioned as low as possible on the upper back during a 'back squat,' in order not to fall, the lifter must incline the trunk relatively far forward (i.e. increase trunk flexion), to keep the center of mass of the body plus the bar over the feet. Trunk flexion in the squat increases the torque about the hip joint and decreases the torque about the knee joint by moving the weight and/or center of gravity forward, thereby increasing the involvement of the large hip extensor muscles (especially *gluteus maximus*). There are not only inter-individual differences in torques on a particular exercise, but also intra-individual differences in overcoming resistances of different percentages of the one-repetition maximum. Factors affecting the ability of untrained people to squat with the feet flat on the ground, which is necessary effective co-contraction of the *quadriceps femoris* and hamstring muscles (thus decreasing the risk of knee injury) include: femur length, torso length, height, torso strength, hip flexibility and ankle flexibility. Correct footwear is important for safe squatting. Heavy, wooden-soled, stable, weightlifting shoes with Velcro® straps in addition to laces are designed to prevent excessive pronation of the feet that would force the knees inward, putting stress on structures such as the medial collateral ligaments and menisci. The load that can be used during a full squat tends to be limited by the amount of force that can be generated between the knee angles

of about 95 and 115 degrees (the 'sticking region').
Knee wraps are used as a mechanical ergogenic aid
by many weight trainers and may enable up to 10%
greater weight to be lifted. In the sport of powerlifting, there are rules to limit the ergogenic effect of
knee wraps (e.g. the wrapping must stop 10 cm
above the patella). The wraps may provide direct
assistance in knee extension. Detrimental effects of
wraps, however, include skin damage and chondromalacia. *See also* RESISTANCE TRAINING.

Bibliography

Beynnon, B.D. et al. (1997). The strain behavior of the anterior
cruciate during squatting and active flexion-extension: A comparison of open and closed kinetic chain exercise. *American
Journal of Sports Medicine* 25(6), 823-829.

Chandler, T.J. and Stone, M.H. (1992). The squat exercise in athletic conditioning: A review of the literature. *Chiropractic Sports
Medicine* 6(3), 105-111.

Ellenbecker, T.S. and Davies, G.J. (2001). *Closed kinetic chain exercise. A comprehensive guide to multiple-joint exercises.* Champaign,
IL: Human Kinetics.

Escamilla, R.F. (2001). Knee biomechanics of the dynamic squat
exercise. *Medicine and Science in Sports and Exercise* 33(1), 127-
141.

Kellis, E. (1998). Quantification of quadriceps and hamstring
antagonist activity. *Sports Medicine* 25(1), 37-62.

Palmitier, R.A. et al (1991). Kinetic chain exercise in knee rehabilitation. *Sports Medicine* 11, 402-413.

Wilk, K.E. et al. (1996). Comparison of tibiofemoral joint forces
and electromyographic activity during open and closed kinetic chain exercises. *American Journal of Sports Medicine* 24(4),
518-527.

KINETIC ENERGY *See under* ENERGY.

KINETICS *See under* KINEMATICS.

KININS Polypeptides, formed in the blood from
inactive precursors called kininogens. Kinins cause
increased capillary permeability and venous constriction, along with arterial vasodilation in specific
organs. They serve as chemotactic agents for phagocytes.

KLINEFELTER SYNDROME The most common
chromosomal disorder associated with male hypogonadism and infertility. It is a form of primary testicular failure, with elevated gonadotropin levels arising
from lack of feedback inhibition by the pituitary

gland. It is characterized by hypogonadism (small
testes, azoospermia/oligospermia), gynecomastia at
late puberty, psychosocial problems, hyalinization
and fibrosis of the seminiferous tubules and elevated
urinary gonadotropins.

It is defined classically by a 47,XXY karyotype
with variants demonstrating additional X and Y chromosomes. In general, the extent of phenotypic
abnormalities, including mental retardation, is related directly to the number of supernumerary X chromosomes. Gonadal development is particularly susceptible to each additional X chromosome, resulting
in seminiferous tubule dysgenesis and infertility as
well as hypoplastic and malformed genitalia in
polysomy X males. Moreover, mental capacity
diminishes with additional X chromosomes. Mental
retardation and hypogonadism are more severe in
49,XXXXY than 48,XXXY.

With the 48,XXYY variant, patients typically
have mild mental retardation, tall stature, eunuchoid
body habitus, spare body hair, gynecomastia, long
thin legs, hypergonadotropic hypogonadism and
small testes. Patients with the 48,XXXY variant typically have mild-to-moderate mental retardation,
speech delay, slow motor development, poor coordination, immature behavior, normal or tall stature,
abnormal face (epicanthal folds, hypertolorism, protruding lips), hypogonadism, gynecomastia (33 to
50%), hypoplastic penis, infertility, clinodactyly, and
radioulnar synostosis; and benefit from testosterone
therapy. Patients with 49,XXXYY typically have
moderate-to-severe mental retardation, passive but
occasionally aggressive behavior and temper
tantrums, tall stature, dysmorphic facial features,
gynecomastia and hypogonadism. The 49,XXXXY
variant is characterized by the classic triad of mild-
to-moderate mental retardation, radioulnar synostosis and hypergonadotropic hypogonadism.

In the USA, approximately 1 in 500 to 1,000
males is born with an extra sex chromosome. Over
3,000 affected males are born each year. Most males
born with Klinefelter syndrome go through life
without being diagnosed. Infertility and gynecomastia are the two most common complaints leading to
diagnosis. By late puberty, 30 to 50% of boys with
Klinefelter syndrome manifest gynecomastia, which

is secondary to elevated estradiol levels and increased estradiol/testosterone ratio. The risk of developing breast carcinoma is at least 20 times higher than normal.

Bibliography
Chen, H. (2003). Klinefelter syndrome. Http://www.emedicine.com

KLIPPEL-FEIL SYNDROME Klippel-Feil anomaly. It is a congenital abnormality of the cervical spine characterized by deformity and fusion of adjacent vertebral segments, and may be associated with local cervical instability. Type I is a massive fusion of the cervical spine. Type II is present when the fusion of one or two vertebrae occurs. Type III occurs when thoracic and lumbar spine anomalies are associated with Type I or Type II. It is caused by failure in the normal segmentation or division of the cervical vertebrae during the early weeks of fetal development.

Decreased range of motion in the cervical spine is the most frequent clinical finding with Klippel-Feil syndrome, with rotational loss being more pronounced than the loss of flexion and extension. Other common signs are short neck and low hairline at the back of the head. Associated abnormalities may include scoliosis, spina bifida, anomalies of the kidneys and ribs, cleft palate, respiratory problems, heart malformations and hearing loss. The incidence rate is about 1 in 40,000 live births of which about 60% are girls.

Treatment for Klippel-Feil syndrome is symptomatic and may include surgery to relieve cervical or craniocervical instability and constriction of the spinal cord, and to correct scoliosis. The prognosis for most persons with Klippel-Feil syndrome is good, if the disorder is treated early and appropriately. Activities that can injure the neck should be avoided.

Bibliography
The National Institute of Neurological Disorders and Stroke. Http://www.ninds.nih.gov

KLIPPEL-TRENAUNAY SYNDROME A rare congenital malformation that may include: port-wine stain (cutaneous capillary malformations), soft tissue and bony hypertrophy, and venous malformations and lymphatic abnormalities. Complications include bleeding, cellulitis, venous thrombosis, or pulmonary embolism. Associated abnormalities in other systems, such as gigantism of toes, hand and feet anomalies, lymphedema, or involvement of the abdominal and pelvic organs may also occur. Klippel-Trénaunay syndrome is usually limited to one limb, but may occur in multiple limbs and/or the head or trunk area. Internal organs may be involved. The etiology is unknown and there is no known cure. Pain occurs in about 35% of patients and can discourage sports participation.

Klippel-Trénaunay syndrome can be distinguished from Parkes-Weber syndrome in terms of the hypertrophy and varicosity associated with port-wine staining. Parkes-Weber syndrome is similar, but arteriovenous malformation occurs in association with a cutaneous capillary malformation and skeletal or soft tissue hypertrophy. *See also* STURGE-WEBER SYNDROME.

Chronology
•2001 • In the USA, the Supreme Court ruled that federal disability rights law entitled professional golfer Casey Martin to ride a golf cart between shots while competing in PGA Tour events. Martin experienced pain in his right leg caused by a condition resembling Klippel-Trénaunay syndrome. In 1998, *The Physician and Sportsmedicine* reported that Martin's condition met only one of the three criteria for Klippel-Trénaunay syndrome, venous malformations; but not the other two criteria (port-wine stain, and bony and soft-tissue hypertrophy). Martin played No 3 for Stanford in the National Collegiate Athletics Association (NCAA) championship winning team of 1994 that also included Tiger Woods. After turning professional in 1995, the condition of his right leg grew steadily worse. He could no longer walk a round of golf without great pain. In the first stages of the PGA Qualifying School, competitors are permitted to use carts. However, in the final qualifying stage, and during the Tour itself, the PGA imposes a "walking" rule, requiring competitors to walk from hole to hole. When he reached the final qualifying stage, Martin requested a waiver of the Tour's walking rule. The PGA Tour refused, and in 1997 Martin filed his disability discrimination lawsuit to a federal court in Oregon. The PGA argued that its golf tournaments are not subject to the Americans with Disabilities Act (ADA) even though golf courses are "public accommodations," because the area of the golf course that is restricted to competition is not open to the general public. In reaching its decision, the Court addressed two distinct legal issues, ruling that: The Tour is a "public accommodation" subject to ADA requirements and under those requirements Martin's use of a cart is a "reasonable modification."

Allowing Martin to use a golf cart "is not a modification that would fundamentally alter the nature of the PGA Tour," said Supreme Court Justice John Paul Stevens.

In Feb 2003, Martin was quoted in *Golf Digest* magazine as saying, "My leg was going downhill pretty quick five or six years ago, but now it's kind of leveled off." In 2002, he had surgery in his right leg to improve the circulation. He has only had one full season on the PGA Tour – in 2000 – when his best finish was a tie for 17th in the Tucson Open. In 2004, by mid-July, Martin had earned $15,858 from two PGA Tour events and missed the cut in three Nationwide Tour events.

Bibliography

Schnirring, L. (1998). Casey Martin's case: The medical story. *The Physician and Sportsmedicine* 26(4).

The Klippel-Trénaunay Syndrome Support Group. Http://www.k-t.org

KNEE FLEXION DEFORMITY A condition that is characterized by the legs being permanently bent or contracted in a sitting position. It is common in children with neuromuscular disabilities, such as cerebral palsy, who are confined to a wheelchair. The condition is initially treated with splints and typically requires surgical lengthening of the hamstring tendons, in which their insertions are repositioned. Wheelchair-bound persons should be encouraged to leave their wheelchairs in order to move their knees through the full range of motion.

KNEE JOINT Tibiofemoral joint and patellofemoral joint. The **tibio-femoral joint** is a hinge joint where the condyloid process of the femur articulates with the upper end of the tibia. The movements of flexion, extension, medial rotation and lateral rotation are permitted. Flexion involves decreasing the angle between the femur and the tibia. Muscles that produce **flexion** are: *biceps femoris, plantaris, sartorius, gracilis, popliteus, gastrocnemius, semimembranosus* and *semitendinosus*. Extension involves increasing the angle between the femur and the tibia. Muscles that produce **extension** are: *quadriceps femoris* (*rectus femoris, vastus intermedius, vastus lateralis* and *vastus medialis*). Medial rotation involves inward rotation of the tibia on the femur. Muscles that produce **medial rotation** are: *semitendinosus, semimembranosus, popliteus, sartorius* (after flexion) and *gracilis* (when leg is flexed). Lateral rotation involves outward rotation of the tibia on the femur. A muscle that produces **lateral rotation** is *biceps femoris* (when hip is extended). *See* PATELLOFEMORAL JOINT.

KNEE JOINT, BRACE The four categories of knee braces are knee sleeves, prophylactic knee braces, functional knee braces, and postoperative or rehabilitative knee braces.

Knee sleeves are expandable, slip-on devices usually made of neoprene with a nylon cover. They increase warmth, provide even compression, limit patella movement, and may enhance proprioception. Plain knee sleeves may be used to treat postoperative knee effusions and patellofemoral syndrome. Used in this capacity, the purpose of a knee sleeve is to decrease knee pain. When a knee pad is added, it provides protective cushioning to the patella and anterior knee. When a strap is placed inferior to the patella, it may be used to treat Osgood-Schlatter disease and patellar tendonitis. An **infrapatellar band** is used to decrease the traction forces at the tibial tuberosity. Knee sleeves do not provide ligamentous support and, therefore, are insufficient for the treatment of an unstable knee. Knee sleeves can cause swelling by retaining heat around the knee or by obstructing venous and lymphatic return below the sleeve.

Prophylactic knee braces attempt to prevent or decrease the severity of knee injuries. Prophylactic knee braces are intended to protect the medial collateral ligament from valgus stress applied to the lateral aspects of the extended weight-bearing leg during contact sports such as American football. Prophylactic knee braces are braces with unilateral or bilateral bars, hinges, and adhesive straps. The deformable metal of these braces can absorb some of the impact and decrease the force applied to the medial collateral ligament by 10% to 30%. The American Academy of Orthopedic Surgeons believes that the routine use of prophylactic knee braces currently available has not been proven effective in decreasing the number or severity of knee injuries. In some circumstances, such braces may even have potential to be a contributing factor to injury.

The primary role of **functional knee braces** is to enhance athletic performance by allowing an athlete with an unstable knee to exercise vigorously without pathological subluxation of the knee joint. The pattern of lower-extremity muscle activity during movement is changed, such that less work is done at the knee and more work is done at the hip. There is evidence that some functional knee braces are very effective in controlling abnormal motions under low load conditions, but not under the high loading conditions that occur during many sports.

Rehabilitative knee braces allow protected motion of an injured knee (treated operatively or non-operatively). They are designed to provide a compromise between protection and motion, and are generally more effective in protecting against excessive flexion and extension than in protecting against anterior and posterior motion. The postoperative or rehabilitative brace can be used to protect injured ligaments and control knee flexion / extension angles during the initial healing period. These are most often used during crutch-assisted ambulation immediately after meniscal and/or cruciate ligament injury or surgery. They are used for a short period of time (2 to 8 weeks) after the acute injury or surgery. Advantages of a rehabilitative brace as opposed to a cast or splint include: the ability to adjust the brace for swelling; the ability to remove the brace for serial examinations or icing; and the ability to allow for movement in a controlled range of motion. The American Academy of Orthopedic Surgeons believes that rehabilitative knee braces can be effective in many treatment programs and there is scientific evidence to support this belief.

Bibliography

American Academy of Orthopedic Surgeons (1997). Position Paper. The use of knee braces. Http://www.aaos.org

American Academy of Pediatrics (2001). Technical report: Knee brace use in the young athlete. *Pediatrics* 108(2), 503-507.

Vailas, J.C. and Pink, M. (1993). Biomechanical effects of functional knee bracing. Practical implications. *Sports Medicine* 15(3), 210-218.

KNEE JOINT, BURSAE   The four main bursae that surround the knee are pre-patellar, superficial infra-patellar, deep infra-patellar, and pes anserinus.

Pre-patellar bursitis (housemaid's knee) is the most common injury to bursae. It presents as a superficial swelling on the anterior aspect of the knee.

See also BAKER'S CYST; PES ANSERINUS; POPLITEAL CYST.

KNEE LIGAMENTS   The main four ligaments in the knee are the medial collateral ligament (MCL), lateral collateral ligament (LCL), anterior cruciate ligament (ACL) and posterior cruciate ligament (PCL). MCL and ACL injuries comprise over 95% of knee ligament injuries. Injuries to the PCL account for less than 5% and LCL injuries are rare.

Impact against the lateral side of the knee joint tends to occur in sport when the foot is under load and the knee joint is slightly flexed. The knee joint is forced inwards (i.e. in valgus) and the tibia is rotated externally in relation to the femur, making the medial meniscus and MCL vulnerable to injury. The deep portion of the MCL, which is attached to the meniscus, is short and tight, thus it takes the load before the superficial portion and ruptures first. In a more violent impact, the ACL is also loaded and subsequently tears. In an extremely violent impact, the PCL will also tear. An impact against the medial side of the foot, which forces it laterally in relation to the knee, has the same effect as an impact against the lateral side of the knee. This typically occurs when two soccer players kick the ball at the same time with the inside of their feet.

Impact against the medial side of the knee joint is less common than that against the lateral side, but also tends to occur in sport when the foot is under load and the knee joint is flexed. The knee joint is forced outwards (i.e. in varus) and the tibia is rotated internally in relation to the femur, making the LCL vulnerable to injury. Meniscal injury is less likely than in cases of impact against the lateral side of the knee than the medial side, because the LCL is not attached to the adjacent meniscus. In a more violent impact, the ACL is also loaded and subsequently tears. In an extremely violent impact, the PCL will also tear.

The **anterior cruciate ligament (ACL)** is an extra-articular ligament that runs from the posteriomedial wall of the lateral femoral condyle to the tibial eminence. It is the main ligament resisting anterior tibial translation. It is slack when the knee is flexed and taut when it is fully extended, preventing posterior displacement of the femur on the tibia and hyperextension of the knee joint. When the joint is flexed at a right angle, the tibia cannot be pulled anteriorly because it is held by the ACL. About 80% of ACL ruptures are actually the result of noncontact injury. A noncontact ACL tear always involves a rapid deceleration of the knee joint. A common position that leads to an ACL tear is when the knee is fixed around 20 degrees of flexion, with internal rotation of the thigh, external rotation of the lower leg, pronation of the foot and forward flexion of the torso. Pivoting, cutting or landing awkwardly from a jump in sports such as basketball, soccer and American football are common causes. For effective ACL injury prevention, knee deceleration movements such as landing, cutting and hopping must be included as separate drills. Most noncontact ACL injuries occur with the knee close to full extension. It is therefore possible that the *quadriceps femoris* plays an important role in ACL disruption. Eccentric action of the *quadriceps femoris* can produce forces beyond those required for tensile failure of the ACL. In contrast to the *quadriceps femoris*, the hamstring muscles are ACL agonists or 'stress shielders.' Athletes with hamstrings-to-*quadriceps femoris* strength ratios closer to one suffer fewer noncontact ACL injuries. Overtraining the *quadriceps femoris* relative to the hamstrings is detrimental, because the hamstrings must work with the *quadriceps femoris* during knee joint decelerations to assist the stabilizing role of the ACL. The ACL is also ruptured by hyperextension in combination with internal rotation, but injury from hyperflexion is less common. A higher rate of ACL injuries has been reported in athletes who wear cleats that are placed at the peripheral margin of the sole with a number of smaller pointed cleats positioned interiorly. This cleat arrangement results in a higher torsional resistance than the other cleat designs.

Modern ski binding is much more effective at protecting the ankle and lower leg than the knee. Since 1972, knee injuries in skiing have increased nearly three-fold. ACL sprains are a product of the evolution of the supports system (boots and skis),

but not the release system (bindings). ACL injuries account for about 10% of all skiing injuries. In skiing, most ACL injuries result from internal rotation of the tibia with the knee flexed greater than 90 degrees. **Phantom foot injuries** can occur when the tail of the downhill ski, in combination with the stiff back of the modern ski boot, acts as a lever to apply a unique combination of twisting and bending loads to the knee. Internal rotation of the lower leg relative to the upper leg leads to stretching of the ACL. It is called 'phantom foot' because it involves the tail of the ski, a lever that points in a direction opposite to that of the human foot. Three types of situation can lead to the phantom foot syndrome: getting up while still moving after a fall; attempting a recovery from an off-balance position; and sitting down after losing control. Typically, the uphill arm is back, the skier off-balance to the rear, hips below the knees, uphill ski unweighted, weight on the inside edge of downhill ski tail and the upper body facing the downhill ski. Skiers should: attempt to maintain balance and control; keep the hips above the knees; keep the arms forward; avoid full extension of the legs upon falling; avoid getting up until they have stopped sliding; and avoid landing on the hands. The gait of patients with ACL-deficient knees is characterized by a '**quadriceps-avoidance gait**,' where the amount of hip extensor activity is increased in order to compensate for a lack of knee extensor activity.

Current rehabilitation programs for the ACL use immediate training of range of motion. Weight bearing is encouraged within the first week after an ACL reconstruction. Commonly, the patients are allowed to return to light sporting activities such as running at 2 to 3 months after surgery and to contact sports, including cutting and jumping, after 6 months.

The **medial collateral ligament** (**MCL**) runs from the medial femoral epicondyle to the proximal medial tibia, with a deep band running to the medial meniscus. It is the main ligament resisting valgus stress to the knee. Indirect injuries of the MCL are caused by valgus force, such as when the foot is planted and fixed, and a tackle or block is made against the lateral aspect of the knee that drives the knee medially. During skiing, one ski may become entrapped in the snow, while momentum carries the skier forward. As a consequence, the knee is subjected to a valgus, external rotation.

The **lateral collateral ligament (LCL)** is an extra-articular ligament that runs from the lateral femoral epicondyle to the fibular head. It is the main ligament resisting varus stress to the knee. **LCL** injuries are usually the result of direct varus stress to the knee, generally with the knee extended and the foot planted. The LCL is less vulnerable to injury than the MCL, because the force or blow necessary to damage the ligament must be applied to the medial aspect of the knee in order to force it into a varus position.

The **posterior cruciate ligament (PCL)** is an extra-articular ligament that runs from the anterolateral wall of the medial femoral condyle to the articular surface of the posterior tibial plateau. It is the main ligament resisting posterior tibial translation and it is also the largest and strongest ligament in the knee. It tightens during flexion of the knee joint, preventing anterior displacement of the femur on the tibia or posterior displacement of the tibia on the femur. It also helps prevent hyperflexion of the knee joint. In the weight-bearing flexed knee, the PCL is the main stabilizing factor for the femur. About 50% of PCL injuries are due to 'dashboard injury' from vehicular crashes. An unrestrained vehicle occupant is hurled into the dashboard. With the knee flexed to 90 degrees, the PCL is taut and the posterior capsule is lax. The impact drives the tibia posteriorly and causes rupture of the PCL. In sports, the most common mechanism of PCL injury is a fall on the flexed knee with the foot in plantar flexion; the mechanism is the same as dashboard injury.

The ligaments of Humprey and Wrisberg are meniscofemoral ligaments from the posterior horn of the lateral meniscus to the lateral aspect of the medial femoral condyle. The **ligament of Humphrey** is the anterior meniscofemoral ligament; it arises from the posterior horn of the lateral meniscus, runs anterior to the PCL and inserts at the distal edge of the femoral PCL attachment. The **ligament of Wrisberg** is the posterior meniscofemoral ligament; it extends from the posterior horn of the lateral meniscus to the medial femoral

condyle. The **arcuate ligament** is the posterior third of the lateral capsule of the knee joint. The **arcuate ligament complex** is the arcuate ligament, LCL, *popliteus* muscle and the lateral head of the *gastrocnemius* muscle. It provides significant stability to the posteriolateral corner of the knee. *See also under* GENDER DIFFERENCES.

Bibliography
Boden, B.P., Griffin, L.Y. and Garrett, W.F. (2000). Etiology and prevention of noncontact ACL injury. *The Physician and Sportsmedicine* 28(4), 53-60.
Emerson, R.J. (1993). Basketball knee injuries and the anterior cruciate ligament. *Clinics in Sports Medicine* 12(2), 317-328.
Johnson, S.C. (1995). Anterior cruciate ligament injury in elite Alpine competitors. *Medicine and Science in Sports and Exercise* 27(3), 323-327.
Kvist, J. (2004). Rehabilitation following anterior cruciate ligament injury: Current recommendations for sports participation. *Sports Medicine* 34(4), 269-280.

KNEE MENISCI Two crescent-shaped wedges of fibrocartilage located between the femoral condyles and the tibial plateau. The **lateral meniscus** is more oval-shaped and more mobile than the **medial meniscus**, because it does not have any attachment to the deep posterolateral capsule from which it is separated by the popliteal tendon sheath. The menisci assist joint lubrication and nutrition, improve the congruity of the knee, transmit load, act as shock absorbers (thereby protecting articular cartilage), improve knee joint stability (by deepening the articular surfaces of the tibial plateau) and facilitate control of some rotational movements. The menisci have relatively few radially oriented fibers, and thus are susceptible to shear stresses. The meniscus is torn when it is trapped between the two bone surfaces as torque is applied to the loaded knee (e.g. twisting when rising from a full squat). Mensical injuries often occur in combination with ligament injuries, especially when the medial meniscus is involved. This is partly because the medial meniscus is attached to the medial collateral ligament (MCL) and partly because tackles [in sports such as soccer] are often directed towards the lateral side of the knee, causing external rotation of the tibia. The medial meniscus is about three to five times more likely to be injured than the lateral meniscus. While the medial meniscus is most vulnerable during cases of external rotation of the foot and lower leg in relation to the femur, the lateral meniscus is most vulnerable during internal rotation of the foot and lower leg. Meniscal injuries can also occur as a result of hyperextension and hyperflexion of the knee. Combined injury of the anterior cruciate ligament (ACL), medial collateral ligament (MCL) and medial meniscus is classed as **O'Donoghue's triad** ('unhappy triad').

KNEE, OSTEOCHONDRAL INJURIES
Osteochondral injuries in the knee usually involve the medial facet of the patella or the lateral femoral condyle. Patellofemoral osteochondral injuries are most often the result of a patellar dislocation. Impact, avulsion, shear and rotational force in direct trauma (as opposed to osteochondritis dissecans) are the most common causes of injury to the femoral articular cartilage.

KÖHLER'S DISEASE Asceptic necrosis of the tarsal navicular bone. It can occur in the pre-pubertal child. The cause is unknown.

KREBS CYCLE Tricarboxylic acid cycle. Citric acid cycle. It is a complex cycle of chemical reactions in mitochondrial respiration.

The Krebs cycle involves the transfer of energy carried in the bonds of acetyl CoA to electron-carrier molecules. The molecules receiving the hydrogens and electrons are the coenzymes NAD^+ and FAD, which transfer the hydrogens and electrons to the electron transfer chain for the phosphorylation of ADP to ATP. It is a cycle because a 4-carbon compound (oxaloacetate) joins with a 2-carbon compound (acetyl CoA) to form a 6-carbon compound (citrate), with the ultimate regeneration of the 4-carbon compound. It is called the tricarboxylic acid cycle, because the initial constituents have 3 carboxyl groups. All the reactions take place in the mitochondrial matrix, except the succinate dehydrogenase reaction, which is located in the inner mitochondrial membrane. The Krebs cycle requires the presence of oxygen, but no oxygen is used directly in the reactions.

The Krebs cycle produces most of the energy-rich molecules that ultimately regenerate ATP. One complete turn produces 1 ATP (via GTP), 3 NADH and 1 $FADH_2$. The 1 ATP is produced by substrate-level phosphorylation. 2.5 ATP are generated for each NADH and 1.5 ATP for each $FADH_2$. The total number of ATP produced from one turn of the Krebs cycle is thus, 1 ATP + (3 x 2.5 ATP) + (1 x 1.5 ATP) = 10 ATP. There are two turns of the cycle for each glucose molecule, thus giving 20 ATP.

The series of eight chemical reactions begins and ends with oxaloacetate. In the **citrate synthetase reaction**, 2-carbon acetyl CoA combines with 4-carbon oxaloacetate to yield 6-carbon citrate. This is a condensation reaction. It is moderately exergonic. The CoA is freed and leaves the cycle, becoming available to react with another pyruvate and form a new acetyl CoA or to be used later in the cycle.

In the **aconitase reaction**, the atoms of citrate are rearranged to become isocitrate. It involves a sequential dehydration and hydration reaction. This reaction is endergonic.

In the **isocitrate dehydrogenase reaction**, a pair of hydrogen atoms are removed and accepted by NAD^+, forming NADH. A carbon dioxide molecule is removed, leaving 5-carbon alpha-ketoglutarate. This reaction is an oxidative decarboxylation, and it is exergonic. Isocitrate dehydrogenase is the rate-limiting enzyme.

In the **alpha-ketoglutarate dehydrogenase reaction**, a pair of hydrogen atoms are removed and picked up by NAD^+ and a carbon dioxide molecule is removed. The remaining structure is attached to CoA, forming 4-carbon succinyl CoA. This reaction is an oxidative decarboxylation and it is exergonic.

In the **succinyl CoA synthetase reaction**, coenzyme A is displaced by a phosphate group, which, in turn, is transferred via GTP to ADP to form ATP.

In the **succinate dehydrogenase reaction**, more hydrogen atoms are removed and passed to FAD forming $FADH_2$. Succinate dehydrogenase is tightly bound to the mitochondrial membrane.

In the **fumarase reaction**, water is added and fumarate is converted to malate.

In the **malate dehydrogenase reaction**, a

pair of hydrogen atoms is removed and accepted by NAD^+ forming NADH. This is a highly endergonic reaction. The remaining atoms make up oxaloacetate and the cycle is ready to begin again.

Acetyl CoA from beta-oxidation can enter the Krebs cycle only when fat and carbohydrate metabolism are synchronized. The Krebs cycle requires a steady supply of oxaloacetate. Oxaloacetate can be depleted under conditions such as starvation and very-low carbohydrate diets. This causes acetyl CoA to be converted to ketone bodies. The supply of oxaloacetate can be decreased by the use of some of the Krebs cycle intermediates in biosynthesis. Oxalocetate can be synthesized directly from pyruvate to supply the Krebs cycle. It is said that 'fat burns in a carbohydrate flame,' because carbohydrate (glucose) is the original source of pyruvate.

The terms '**anaplerotic**' and '**cataplerotic**' refer to the addition and loss, respectively, of Krebs cycle intermediates. There are relatively small amounts of each Krebs cycle intermediate, but the Krebs cycle can undergo high rates of turnover, especially during exercise. Therefore, any cataplerotic loss of Krebs cycle material can result in diminished or halted Krebs cycle capacity. To compensate for cataplerotic losses, such as through alpha-ketoglutarate, there must be compensating anaplerotic additions to the Krebs cycle such as by aspartate at oxaloacetate or at fumarate by the action of the purine nucleotide cycle.

Carbon skeletons of amino acids gain access to the Krebs cycle by various pathways, e.g. leucine enters only on acetyl CoA; isoleucine, methionine and valine enter on succinyl CoA.

The activity of rate-limiting enzymes of the Krebs cycle, such as citrate synthetase and succinate dehydrogenase are associated with success in endurance-based sports.

Bibliography

Insel, P., Turner, R.E. and Ross, D. (2004). *Nutrition*. 2nd ed. Sudbury, MA: Jones and Bartlett.

Mathews, C.K., Van Holde, K.E. and Ahern, K. (2000). *Biochemistry*. 3rd ed. San Francisco, CA: Benjamin/Cummings.

KYPHOSIS Thoracic kyphosis. Dorsal kyphosis. A sagittal-plane spinal deformity characterized by excessive flexion. It is usually seen in the thoracic region, where it produces a hunchback posture. It is frequently the result of fatigue or inadequate muscular strength in the extensors of the spine. Thus, poor posture with slouching tends to cause an increase in thoracic kyphosis.

Kyphosis and abducted scapulae are distinctly different conditions, with the former being an increased posterior convexity of the thoracic spine and the latter being a forward deviation of the shoulder girdle. It is not uncommon, however, to find the conditions of thoracic kyphosis, round shoulders, and forward head occurring together. This phenomenon is known as the **kyphosis syndrome**.

See also SCHEURMANN'S DISEASE; THORACIC SPINE.

L

LABYRINTH   Inner ear.

LABYRINTHINE REFLEX   Head-in-space right-ing reflex. A postural reflex that is normal from about 2 months of age and persists throughout life, it is elicited when the body is out-of-upright posture, upside down or leaning. The labyrinthine reflex enables infants to 'right' or elevate the head, thus restoring the head to a position more conducive to breathing and allowing the baby to survive. The head tilts in a direction opposite to the direction the body is tilted, and the entire body follows the head. If an infant is placed in a prone position, breathing may be inhibited to the point of suffocation. Linked to the vestibular motor system, it may be critical to the attainment of upright posture.

In later life, evidence for the labyrinthine reflex can be seen in preparing for takeoff in a standing long jump. As the trunk leans farther forward, the head and neck become more hyperextended. In diving, the labyrinthine reflex must be suppressed con-sciously so that the head may be extended back with the body following it. 'Belly flops' may be attributed to the labyrinthine righting reflex.

Optical (visual) righting reflexes are the same as the head-in-space reactions except that the responses are elicited by visual input instead of vestibular input.

LACERATION   A cut produced by a sharp object. It may leave a smooth or jagged wound through the skin, subcutaneous tissues, muscles and associated nerves and blood vessels.

LACTACID ENERGY SYSTEM   *See under* GLY-COLYSIS.

LACTATE   i) To secrete milk (from the mammary glands). ii) A salt or ester of lactic acid. *See* LACTIC ACID.

LACTATE DEHYDROGENASE DEFICIENCY Glycogenosis type XI. It is a metabolic disease of muscle, with onset during childhood or adolescence. It is inherited as an autosomal recessive trait. Symptoms include exercise intolerance, with muscle damage and urine discoloration possible following strenuous physical activity.

LACTIC ACID   An organic acid that is an end prod-uct of glycolysis. It dissociates into hydrogen ions (H^+) and lactate ions. At normal pH levels, lactic acid is almost completely dissociated immediately to H^+ and lactate. As long as the amount of free H^+ does not exceed the ability of chemical and physio-logical mechanisms to buffer them and maintain pH at a relatively stable level, there are few problems.

The accumulation of H^+ during high-intensity exercise causes metabolic acidosis. About 94% of the H^+ released during exhaustive exercise are as a result of lactic acid. Once in the blood, lactic acid is effec-tively buffered by sodium bicarbonate.

High concentration of H^+ (i.e. low pH) results in: i) pain, when nerve endings located in muscle are stimulated; ii) inactivation of enzymes (especially phosphofructokinase) or changes in membrane transport (either to the carriers in the membrane or to the permeability channels); iii) inhibition of ener-gy substrate availability, because glycogen break-down is slowed by inactivation of glycogen phospho-rylase; iv) decrease in fatty acid utilization as mobi-lization is inhibited; and v) decreased force and velocity of muscle contraction, because actomyosin ATPase is inhibited and H^+ interferes with the actions and uptake of calcium ions.

Lactate is always produced in muscle and other tissues because of the abundance, activity and char-acteristics of cytoplasmic lactate dehydrogenase. The enzyme **lactate dehydrogenase** (LDH) controls the formation of lactate and may regulate the turnover of lactate in the muscle cell. Skeletal mus-cle contains five LDH isoforms.

Lactate production depends on the use of glycogen as a fuel, the formation of pyruvate and the necessity of preserving the redox potential of the cell. Lactate accumulation results when production exceeds clearance. The primary processes in lactate clearance are oxidation, gluconeogenesis and transamination. Research using lactate isotopes has shown that skeletal muscle extracts lactate from the circulation despite a substantial net lactate release and that skeletal muscle has a large capacity for lactate oxidation; these processes being enhanced with exercise. Studies on resting and exercising humans indicate that most lactate (75 to 80%) is disposed of through oxidation, with much of the remainder converted to glucose and glycogen.

Lactate clearance utilizes intracellular and extracellular shuttle systems. Transport across cellular and mitochondrial membranes occurs by facilitated exchange down concentration and pH gradients, utilizing lactate transport proteins known as **monocarboxylate transporters** (**MCTs**). MCT1 is abundant in oxidative skeletal and cardiac muscle fibers. MCT4 is most prevalent in cell membranes of glycolytic skeletal muscle fibers. A distinction can be made between intracellular and extracellular lactate shuttles. The **intracellular lactate shuttle** shows that muscle cells can both produce and consume lactate at the same time. It involves movement of lactate by MCT1 transporters between the cytoplasm where it is produced and the mitochondria. Inside the mitochondria, lactate is oxidized to pyruvate and NAD^+ is reduced to NADH and H^+. The intracellular lactate shuttle permits rapid anaerobic glycolysis. The **extracellular lactate shuttle** moves lactate between tissues. MCT1 and MCT4 move the lactate both out of and into tissues. At the intermuscular level, most lactate moves out of active glycolytic fibers into active oxidative fibers. This can occur either by a direct shuttle between skeletal muscle cells or through the circulation.

Once in the circulation, lactate can also be transported to cardiac cells. During heavy exercise, lactate becomes the preferred fuel for the heart. Circulating lactate can also be transported to the liver for gluconeogenesis.

Endurance training improves muscle capacity for lactate utilization and increases membrane transport of lactate, probably via an increase in MCT1 and perhaps other MCT isoforms as well.

Because of the intracellular lactate shuttle mechanism, lactate produced as a result of glycolysis in the cytosol is balanced by oxidation in the mitochondrion of the same cell. In the steady state, working muscle releases little lactate, so long as mitochondrial respiration is adequate to keep pace with cytosolic lactate production. During steady state exercise conditions, the majority of pyruvate is not converted to lactate, but enters into the mitochondria where it is converted to acetyl CoA by a series of linked enzymes known collectively as **pyruvate dehydrogenase**. This reaction also produces carbon dioxide and NADH. The acetyl CoA can then enter into the Krebs cycle. At the start of exercise, large amounts of lactate are released until the rate of oxygen consumption can rise and balance lactate production and removal. Therefore, working muscle stops releasing lactate and, like the heart, becomes a net lactate consumer.

The concept of **anaerobic threshold** was originally defined as the point where aerobic energy processes alone can no longer meet the skeletal-muscle requirements for ATP. As work is increased above the anaerobic threshold, progressive increases in anaerobic glycolysis must accompany the aerobic metabolism to sustain adequate levels of ATP regeneration. The acceleration of glycolysis leads to an increased lactate production and a consequent metabolic acidosis. The disproportionate increase in ventilation was attributed to excess carbon dioxide resulting from the buffering of the lactic acid. The original concept of anaerobic threshold thus proposed causal links between muscle oxygen insufficiency (anaerobisis), lactate production and changes in pulmonary ventilation. Although inadequate oxygen delivery may facilitate lactic acid production, there is no evidence that lactic acid production above the anaerobic threshold results from inadequate oxygen delivery.

Lactate threshold (LT) is defined as the highest exercise intensity or level of oxygen uptake that is not associated with an elevation in blood lactate concentration. Two lactate thresholds have been distinguished: LT1 and LT2. LT1 generally occurs between 40 and 60% of maximal oxygen uptake. LT2 generally occurs between 80 and 95% of maximal oxygen uptake. LT1 is sometimes equated with a blood lactate concentration of 2 mmol/L. LT2 is sometimes equated with a blood lactate concentration of 4 mmol/L. LT2 is also known as **onset of blood lactic acid** (**OBLA**). Post-exercise values of lactate range from 4 to 19 mmol/L. The higher values result from high volume, moderate load, short-rest period sequences and circuit-type exercise sessions.

Maximal lactate steady state (MLSS) is the highest exercise intensity at which blood lactate remains stable or increases only minimally (less than 1 mmol/L) between 10 and 30 minutes of exercise. It indicates the highest exercise intensity at which a balance exists between the appearance of lactate in the blood and the removal of lactate from the blood during long-term exercise. It is determined by a series of workloads performed on different days. Each succeeding workload gets progressively harder until the blood lactate accumulation increases more or less steadily throughout the test or increases greater than 1 mmol/L after the initial rise and establishment of a plateau in the early minutes.

Ventilatory thresholds are the points at which pulmonary ventilation increases disproportionately with oxygen uptake during graded exercise. Two ventilatory thresholds are commonly identified. The cause of ventilatory thresholds is not understood, but it is likely that a combination of factors are involved (e.g. increasing body temperatures). Lactate thresholds and ventilatory thresholds do not change to the same extent in the same individuals as a result of training, glycogen depletion, caffeine ingestion and varying pedaling rates. The relationship between lactate thresholds and ventilatory thresholds may therefore be primarily coincidental.

The proposed cause-effect relationship between the initial increase in blood lactate and the first disproportionate increase in ventilation was doubted following research with McArdle's disease patients. Blood-borne glucose does not provide a high rate of glucose 6-phosphate production, and therefore glycolytic flux, pyruvate production and lactate production are all low. Since pyruvate is the substrate for the lactate dehydrogenase (LDH) reaction, the exergonic nature of the LDH reaction is decreased. Without muscle glycogenolysis, blood glucose is insufficient to sustain even moderate-intensity steady

state exercise. McArdle's disease patients experience a threshold-like ventilatory response during incremental exercise, but without production of lactic acid. Sometimes the lactate threshold significantly precedes the ventilatory threshold and at other times the ventilatory threshold significantly precedes the lactate threshold. Walsh and Banister (1988) concluded that the two thresholds are not explained by the same mechanism.

Another problem for researchers is that blood lactate concentration does not usually reflect lactate production in active skeletal muscle. This is partly because lactate is produced not only in active muscle, but also in the inactive muscles, the liver and kidneys. The time delay for lactate transfer from the site of production in muscle to the site of blood sampling may be several minutes. Lactate values differ according to the sampling site.

Proposed explanations of lactate thresholds include imbalance between the rate of glycolysis and mitochondrial respiration, decreased redox potential, decreased blood oxygen content and/or lowered blood flow to skeletal muscle. *See also under* ACID-BASE BALANCE; ANAEROBIC ENERGY SYSTEMS; GROWTH; HEART RATE DEFLECTION POINT; OXYGEN DEBT.

Bibliography

Billat, L.V. (1996). The use of blood lactate measurements for prediction of exercise performance and for control of training. Recommendations for long-distance running. *Sports Medicine* 22(3), 157 175.

Billat, V.L. et al. (2003). The concept of maximal lactate steady state: A bridge between biochemistry, physiology and sport science. *Sports Medicine* 33(6), 407-426.

Brooks, G.A. (2000). Intra- and extra-cellular lactate shuttles. *Medicine and Science in Sports and Exercise* 32(4), 790-799.

Gladden, L.B. (2000). Muscle as a consumer of lactate. *Medicine and Science in Sports and Exercise* 32(4), 764-771.

Jacobs, I. (1986). Blood lactate. Implications for training and sports performance. *Sports Medicine* 3, 10-25.

Jones, N.L. and Ehrsam, R.E. (1982). The anaerobic threshold. *Exercise and Sport Sciences Reviews* 10, 49-83.

Jones, A.M. and Carter, H. (2000). The effect of endurance training on parameters of aerobic fitness. *Sports Medicine* 29(6), 373-386.

Katz, A. and Sahlin, K. (1990). Role of oxygen in regulation of glycolysis and lactate production in human skeletal muscle. *Exercise and Sport Sciences Reviews* 18, 1-28.

Loat, C.E.R. and Rhodes, E.C. (1993). Relationship between the lactate and ventilatory thresholds during prolonged exercise. *Sports Medicine* 15(2), 104 115.

McLellan, T.M. (1987). The anaerobic threshold: Concept and controversy. *Australian Journal of Science and Medicine in Sport* 3, 3-8.

Stainsby, W.N. and Brooks, G.A. (1990). Control of lactic acid metabolism in contracting muscles and during exercise. *Exercise and Sport Sciences Reviews* 18, 29-63.

Svedhal, K. and MacIntosh, B.R. (2003). Anaerobic threshold: The concept and methods of measurement. *Canadian Journal of Applied Physiology* 28(2), 299-323.

Van Hall, G. (2000). Lactate as a fuel for mitochondrial respiration. *Acta Physiologica Scandanavia* 168(4), 643-656.

Walsh, M.L. and Banister, E.W. (1988). Possible mechanisms of the anaerobic threshold. *Sports Medicine* 5, 269-302.

Wasserman, K., Van Kessel, A.C. and Burton, B.B. (1967). Interaction of physiological mechanisms during exercise. *Journal of Applied Physiology* 22, 71-85.

Wasserman, K., Whipp, B.J., Koyal, S.N. and Beaver, W.L. (1973). Anaerobic threshold and respiratory gas exchange during exercise. *Journal of Applied Physiology* 35, 236-243.

Weltman, A. (1995). *The blood lactate response to exercise.* Champaign, IL: Human Kinetics.

LACTATE PARADOX   *See under* ALTITUDE.

LACTATE THRESHOLD   *See under* LACTIC ACID.

LACTOSE   A disaccharide composed of glucose and galactose. It is found primarily in dairy products. The enzyme **lactase** is necessary to digest lactose in the small intestine. If lactase is deficient, undigested lactose enters the large intestine. It is fermented by colonic bacteria, which produce short-chain organic acids and gases (including methane). Lactase activity declines with weaning in many ethnic groups. **Lactase maldigestion** is a normal, genetically controlled decrease in lactase activity. It is prevented among 95% African Americans, 100% Native Americans and 12% Caucasian Americans and 75% of the population worldwide.

Bibliography
Insel, P., Turner, R.E. and Ross, D. (2004). *Nutrition.* 2nd ed. Sudbury, MA: Jones and Bartlett.

LAEVOROTATORY   Levorotatory. Rotating the plane of vibration of polarized light to the left (as seen by an observer looking toward the oncoming light). The opposite of laevorotatory is dextrorotatory.

LANDAU REFLEX   Body-in-sagittal plane righting reflex. A postural reflex that develops shortly after the head-in-space reactions are established, and is an extension response of the trunk, hips, knees and ankles that occurs in the prone position when the head is lifted. It is one of the few reactions that are integrated instead of persisting throughout life. It serves a specific developmental function that is not needed after about 3 years of age. The Landau reflex facilitates the change from the flexion posture of infancy to the fully extended prone position with head up and back arched. It overrides the pattern of the symmetric tonic neck reflex (head extended, arms extended, legs flexed) so that the legs can be fully extended at the same time that the head and arms are extended. The ability to maintain a pivot prone position is one of the first milestones in mastering the one-handed reach and grasp from a prone position.

LARYNX   Voice box. It is the organ of voice, containing elastic vocal cords that are the source of the vocal tone in speech. It is comprised of cartilage and is situated in the upper and front part of the neck between the base of the tongue and the trachea (windpipe). **Adam's apple (prominentia laryngea)** is due to the forward protrusion of the thyroid cartilage, the largest and most prominent cartilage of the larynx. It tends to enlarge at adolescence, especially in males. During hyperextension of the neck, it becomes prominent and vulnerable to direct impact forces. High tackles such as in football ('clothesline tackle') or a blow to the neck can also injure the cartilage.

LATENT   Not manifest. It refers to something dormant, but potentially discernible.

LATERAL COLLATERAL LIGAMENT   *See under* KNEE LIGAMENTS.

LATERAL CUTANEOUS NERVE   A pure sensory nerve formed from the L2 and L3 nerve roots. It

enters the lower extremity by passing slightly medial and inferior to the anterior superior iliac spine (ASIS), inferior to the inguinal ligament and superior to the *sartorius* muscle. It supplies sensation to the anterolateral thigh. A hip pointer in American football can injure the lateral femoral cutaneous nerve, usually with neuropraxia only.

LATERAL EPICONDYLITIS   Tendinosis of the common extensor origin at the lateral epicondyle of the elbow. Repetitive microtrauma results in microtears, fibrosis, granulation and mucoid degeneration, with partial failure of the *extensor carpi radialis brevis* tendon. Other tendons that may be affected are those of the *extensor digitorum communis*, *extensor carpi radialis longus* and *supinator* muscles. Because the extensor origin is small, the forces generated by these muscles create high stress. Lateral epicondylitis is related to exercise that increases tensile stress on the wrist extensor and *supinator* muscles, such as the backhand in racquet sports and pitching in baseball. In expert tennis players, risk factors are overuse and muscle imbalances, rather than faulty techniques. Lateral epicondylitis is particularly prevalent in tennis players of the 30 to 50 year age group, for whom risk factors include poor stroke mechanics (e.g. 'leading-elbow backhand syndrome'), insufficient fitness, inappropriate grip size and excessive racquet string tension. A simple method for determining the appropriate grip size is to measure the distance between the midline of the palm of the hand and the tip of the middle finger; this distance should be equal to the grip's circumference. The 'counter force' of a non-elastic band worn just below the elbow is thought to dissipate the forces of muscle contraction over a wider area and thus to help decrease the strain on the lateral epicondyle. The two-handed backhand stroke may help prevent lateral epicondylitis in tennis players.

LATERALITY   *See under* DIRECTIONAL AWARENESS.

LATERALIZATION   *See under* COGNITIVE STYLE.

LAXITY   *See under* HYPERFLEXIBILITY.

LCL   Lateral collateral ligament. *See under* KNEE LIGAMENTS.

LDL   *See under* CHOLESTEROL.

LEADERSHIP   The process of directing and influencing individuals and groups toward goals. It is thus concerned with enhancing the motivation of individuals and groups. Classic styles of leadership are authoritarian, democratic and laissez faire. An **authoritarian (autocratic) leader** makes autonomous decisions and demands group obedience. A **democratic leader** makes decisions after consultation with group members. A **laissez faire** leader exerts minimum control and allows group members to do what they want to.

A distinction can be made between leadership and management. **Management** is primarily concerned with planning, organizing and administration.

Early theories of leadership were based on the notion that a leader has superior personality traits. Later theories emphasized both the personality traits of the leader and situational variables. Fiedler's Contingency theory, for example, proposes that leader effectiveness can be improved by changing either personality or situational factors, with the latter being the easier to change. Leaders are primarily motivated either to develop close and supportive relations with group members (socio-emotive orientation) or to successfully accomplish assigned tasks or goals (task orientation). The situation is defined as the probability of the task being successfully accomplished (controllability). The theory proposes that a task-oriented leader would do best in high control and low control situations, while a socio-emotive oriented leader would do best in situations of moderate control.

The most popular theory of leadership in sport psychology has been Chelladurai's (1978) Multidimensional Model of Leadership in Sport. This involves three aspects of leader behavior: actual leader behavior, leader behavior preferred by the athletes and the leader behavior required in the particular situation. The antecedents of these three aspects consist of the characteristics of the situation, the leader and the athletes. The consequences of these three aspects of leader behavior are performance and satisfaction reported by the athletes. The model predicts that the degree of congruence among the three aspects of leader behavior is positively related to performance and satisfaction. When this model was originally developed, it was conceived that member characteristics influence leadership through the construct of preferred leadership. Members' preferences were presumed to reflect not only their personal needs and desires, but also their judgments about what was appropriate to their situation. Members may, however, lack the intelligence, ability, experience and/or personality disposition to make those kinds of judgments. When members cannot make valid judgments about situational requirements, the leaders must decide for the members. Required leader behavior is thus influenced not only by the contingencies of the situation, but also by member characteristics. There is evidence from research on soccer and basketball that the autocratic style of coaching is preferred both by coaches and players to a greater extent than is commonly believed. The research also suggests that it may be more appropriate to label situations, rather than the leaders themselves, as democratic or autocratic. In contrast to beliefs about autocratic leadership being associated with dictatorship, autocratic style can reflect concern for team members' welfare and provide social support. According to Lyle (2002), the autocratic style within direct intervention is tolerated (and perhaps even welcomed), because of the level of trust generated by a caring, concerned, committed and honest approach in interpersonal behavior more generally.

Contemporary approaches to leadership emphasize concepts like empowerment, vision and shared leadership. **Empowerment** occurs when leaders allow people to develop self-efficacy, self-determination and self-confidence, allowing them to have ownership of themselves and their work. A **vision** is a positive image of the future; it relates to an ideal or desired state. It must be persuasive, attractive and desirable to everyone on the team or organization. Related to vision is a **mission statement**, which refers to the purpose, direction, philosophy and values of an organization. **Shared leadership** means empowering individuals at all levels and giving them the opportunity to take the lead. Shared leadership is becoming more common as the old top-down management structure gives way to flatter, more decentralized forms. The ultimate leader of an organization ('the boss') can be regarded as a coordinator of specialists, who share the leader's vision and bring their own creativity to it. Any attempt to control their input will decrease their quality.

A distinction can be made between transactional and transformational leaders. While the **transactional leader** motivates subordinates to perform as expected, the **transformational leader** typically inspires followers to do more than originally expected. Transformational leaders demonstrate: charisma (providing vision and a sense of mission, instilling pride and gaining respect as well as trust); inspiration (communicating high expectations, using symbols to focus efforts and expressing important purposes in simple ways); intellectual stimulation (promoting intelligence, rationality and careful problem solving); and individualized consideration (giving personal attention, treating people individually, coaching and advising).

See also COACHING BEHAVIORS; INTRINSIC MOTIVATION.

Bibliography

Bennis, W. and Nanus, B. (1985). *Leaders: The strategies for taking charge*. New York: Harper and Row.

Bennis, W.G., Spreitzer, G.M. and Cummings, T.G. (2001). *The future of leadership: Today's top leadership thinkers speak to tomorrow's leaders*. San Francisco, CA: Jossey-Bass.

Chelladurai, P. (1984). Leadership in sports. In: Silva, J.M. and Weinberg, R.S. (eds). *Psychological foundations of sport*. pp329-339. Champaign, IL: Human Kinetics.

Chelladurai, P. (1990). Leadership in sports: A review. *International Journal of Sport Psychology* 21(4), 328-354.

Chelladurai, P. and Doherty, A.J. (1998). Styles of decision making in coaching. In Williams, J.M. (ed). *Applied sport psychology: Personal growth to peak performance*. 3rd ed. pp115-126. Mountain View, CA: Mayfield.

Covey, S.R. (1989). *The 7 habits of highly effective people*. New York: Simon and Schuster.

Daft, R.L. and Marcic, D. (2001). *Understanding management*. 3rd ed. Fort Worth, TX: Harcourt College Publishers.

Lyle, J. (2002). *Sports coaching concepts. A framework for coaches' behavior*. London: Routledge.

Nanus, B. (1992). *Visionary leadership: Creating a compelling sense of direction for your organization*. San Francisco: Jossey-Bass.

LEAN BODY MASS Body mass minus fat mass. Now termed fat-free mass.

See under BODY COMPOSITION.

LEARNED HELPLESSNESS *See under* ATTRIBUTION THEORY.

LEARNING A relatively permanent change in behavior potential in a particular situation due to previous experience and practice of that situation, but excluding changes due to maturation or temporary conditions (such as fatigue, injury or effect of drugs). Learning is not observed directly, but is inferred from changes in performance. **Performance** is thus observable behavior. Performance is temporary, but learning is relatively permanent. A **learning curve** is obtained by plotting a graph of measured changes in learning performance over time. **Skill acquisition** involves changes that occur due to both maturation and learning.

See MOTOR LEARNING; MOTOR SKILLS.

LEARNING DISABILITIES The official term of federal legislation in the USA is severe learning disabilities, but it is nearly always shortened to learning disabilities. These are disorders in one or more of the basic psychological processes involved in understanding or in using language, spoken or written, which may manifest itself in an imperfect ability to listen, think, speak, read, write, spell or perform mathematical calculations. Such disorders include conditions such as **dyslexia** (a severe reading disorder, presumed to be of neurological origin) and **developmental aphasia** (impairment of ability to communicate presumed to be of neurological origin). Learning disability involves an IQ of 70 or higher, and a severe discrepancy between intellectual ability and academic achievement in one or more areas. A score that is 1.5 or more standard deviations below average on a standardized academic achievement test is generally accepted as proof of a severe discrepancy.

About 2 million students in the USA are classified as having learning disability and receive special education services. This represents about 47% of all students in special education and 4 to 5% of the total school-age population. Famous people with learning disabilities include Sir Winston Churchill, Nelson Rockefeller and Albert Einstein.

Conditions that are often associated with learning disabilities are attention deficit hyperactivity disorder (ADHD) and developmental coordination disorder. A higher-than-average percentage of persons with learning disability have perceptual-motor, motor coordination and other movement-related problems.

Signs that may indicate learning disabilities include: inconsistent school performance; difficulty in short-term memory; short attention span; letter and number reversals; poor reading; frequent confusion about directions and time; personal disorganization; impulsive and/or inappropriate behavior; failure on written tests, but high scores on oral exams (or vice versa); speech problems; difficulty in understanding and following instructions; poor coordination in gross motor activities, such as walking, and/or in fine motor activities, such as tying a shoe lace; and difficulty with interpretation of nonverbal behavior.

There are two distinct movement subtypes of learning disabilities. First, language impaired with subtle motor difficulties, mainly in information processing. This subtype tends to prefer visual learning. Second, visual-spatial-motor impaired with obvious perceptual-motor problems and clumsiness. This subtype mainly has problems with mathematics, although language can be impaired also. Auditory input tends to be the preferred learning modality.

It has been hypothesized that poor motor performance and/or poor social skills lead to exclusion from games, creating a vicious cycle of decreasing participation, decreasing competence, a deterioration of self-worth and increasing social maladjustment.

Individuals with learning disabilities can be taught to compensate and overcome their learning problems. There is limited experimental evidence to support the view that structured physical activity programs, with an embedded social skills training component, can be an effective method of enhancing both actual motor ability and self-perception of physical and academic competence.

Chronology

•1964 • The Association for Children with Learning Disabilities was founded. It is now the Learning Disabilities Association of America.

•1972 • Claudine Sherill wrote a chapter on learning disabilities for Hollis Fait's *Special Physical Education*. In order to do this, she worked with parents and professionals from the Association for Children with Learning Disabilities.

Bibliography

American Psychiatric Association. (1994). *Diagnostic and statistical manual of mental disorders*. 4ᵗʰ ed. Washington,

Bluechardt, M.H., Wiener, J. and Shephard, R.J. (1995). Exercise programmes in the treatment of children with learning disabilities. *Sports Medicine* 19(1), 55-72.

Learning Disabilities Association of America. Http://www.ldanatl.org

Learning Disabilities Association of California. Http://www.ldaca.org

Sherill, C. (2004). *Adapted physical activity, recreation, and sport: Crossdisciplinary and lifespan*. 6ᵗʰ ed. Boston, MA: McGraw-Hill.

LECITHIN Phosphatidylcholine. It is a phospholipid that occurs naturally in a variety of foods such as eggs. It can be synthesized by humans from choline and is contained in every cell in the body. It is responsible for maintaining the surface tension of the cell membrane, thus controlling what enters and leaves the cell. It is also responsible for transmitting nerve impulses and messages through or from the cell. In foods, lecithin is a blend of phospholipids with different nitrogenous components. Lecithin facilitates the mixing of hydrophobic components with water. It forms water-soluble packages called **micelles** that suspend fat-soluble compounds in watery media. *See* MEMBRANE LIPIDS.

LEG *See under* SKELETON.

LEGG-PERTHES' DISEASE *See* PERTHES' DISEASE.

LEG LENGTH **True leg length** is measured using an X-ray on a grid scale, with foot pronation corrected, as the distance from the anterior superior iliac spine to the medial malleolus. **Apparent leg length** is measured as the distance from the umbilicus to the medial malleolus.

Leg length discrepancy can be structural (anatomical shortening or lengthening of bone), functional (the result of soft tissue shortening or relaxation causing compensatory changes in the lower limb) or environmental (often caused by the camber of the road when running). Leg length discrepancy may be a risk factor for stress fractures, medial collateral ligament injuries, patellar subluxation, plantar fasciitis and hyperpronation. Neely (1998) argues that a discrepancy of greater than 1 cm in the lengths of the left and right legs should be considered a functionally significant leg length discrepancy, and thus in need of correction. In such a case, a built up shoe or orthotic insertion may be indicated. Biomechanical alterations that may occur as a result of leg length discrepancy include: i) pelvic tilt to the shorter side, followed by compensatory lumbar scoliosis and compression of the intervertebral disc on the concave (inner side) of the curve; ii) increased abduction of the hip in the longer leg; iii) excessive pronation of the foot (on either the longer or shorter side); iv) secondary increased genu valgus; and vi) lateral rotation of the leg.

Bibliography

Neely, F.G. (1998). Biomechanical risk factors for exercise-related lower limb injuries. *Sports Medicine* 26(6), 395-413.

LEISURE Time that is not spent engaged in paid or unpaid employment (work), sleep and essential personal or domestic chores.

Chronology

•1930 • The theme of American Education Week was "The Wise Use of Leisure, the Enrichment of Human Life, and Adult Education."

•1932 • The American Association for Health and Physical Education (AAHPE) appointed two committees to study how physical education could contribute to youth leisure-time activities and at the same time combat the social evils of commercial recreation that had developed during the prosperous years. The two committees concluded that physical educators should place more emphasis on skills with recreational potentials.

•1935 • In Britain, the Central Council of Recreative Physical Training was founded by the Ling Physical Education Association and the National Association of Organizers and Lecturers in

Physical Education. It was a voluntary organization with the aim of encouraging the development of all forms of games, sports, outdoor activities and dancing as part of post-school recreation. In 1944, it was renamed as the Central Council of Physical Recreation.

• 1936 • A report by the British Medical Association's committee for physical education, which had been appointed in 1934, stated that schools had contributed little to the leisure-time activities of Britain's youth. It also stated that provisions for physical exercise and recreation left much to be desired.

• 1937 • During debate of the Physical Training and Recreation Bill in Britain, Labour Party politicians accused the Government of providing physical education for the masses, while the upper classes enjoyed lavish facilities at their public schools. In 1938, the Physical Training and Recreation Act became law, providing grants for development of physical education and recreation.

• 1945 • The National Association of Organizers of Physical Education stated that the Swedish system of gymnastics adopted by the British had the following aims: a) secure and maintain high standards of bodily health, physique and vigor; b) develop qualities of character, high social ideals and team spirit, e.g. hardihood, courage, perseverance, fair play and friendliness; c) foster an appreciation of the joy of physical fitness; d) cultivate quick and accurate coordination of thought and action; e) develop easy, graceful bodily movement and poise; f) develop general motor skill and specialized recreational and occupational skills; g) help to correct bodily distortions due either to heredity or environment; h) provide opportunities for self expression and self testing; and i) encourage the pursuit of wholesome leisure-time activities.

• 1947 • A grant was made by the Athletic Institute to help sponsor a National Facilities Conference at Jackson's Mill, West Virginia. The Athletic Institute was founded in 1946 as a non-profit organization of sporting good companies for the advancement of athletics, physical education and recreation. 54 outstanding educators, park and recreation leaders met with architects, engineers, and city planners to prepare a guide for planning facilities for health, physical education and recreation programs.

• 1974 • The American Association for Health, Physical Education and Recreation (AAHPER) was reorganized into seven associations, one of which was the American Association for Leisure and Recreation. It is now one of eight associations of the American Association for Health, Physical Education, Recreation, and Dance (AAHPERD).

Bibliography

Cordes, K.A. and Ibrahim, H.M. (2003). *Applications in recreation and leisure. For today and the future*. 3rd ed. Boston, MA: McGraw-Hill.

LENGTH

LENGTH The Standard International unit is the metre (m). One metre is the length of the path traveled by light in a vacuum during $1/299,792,458$ of a second. 1 m = 1.094 yard = 3.281 feet = 39.370 inches. 1 yard = 0.914 metre; 1 foot = 0.305 metre;

1 inch = 0.0254 metre. 1 mile = 1609 meters = 1.609 kilometers. *See under* STATURE.

LENGTH-TENSION RELATIONSHIP The relationship between the length of the sarcomere and the tension developed by the muscle fiber. When the muscle fiber is stretched beyond its normal resting length, smaller portions of the thick and thin myofilaments overlap within the sarcomere. This decreases the potential number of cross-bridge interactions, and thus the force-producing capacity of the muscle. When the muscle fiber is excessively shortened, the opposing thin filaments overlap and interfere with cross-bridge formation near the center of the sarcomere. Again, the force-producing capacity of the muscle is decreased.

Under most *in vivo* conditions, the length-tension relationship is of little consequence in muscle force production, because sarcomere length is maintained within the optimal range by the muscle attachments to the skeletal system. However, the angle of muscle attachment and the joint angle can significantly influence the fraction of total muscle force available for movement of the limb throughout its range of motion. For limb movement, the force-producing capacity of muscle is maximized when the long axis of the muscle is parallel to the direction of movement.

Bibliography

American College of Sports Medicine (2001). *ACSM's resource manual for Guidelines for exercise testing and prescription*. 4th. Philadelphia, PA: Lippincott Williams and Wilkins.

LEPTIN A protein hormone that is produced and secreted mainly by adipocytes. Smaller amounts of leptin are also secreted by cells in the epithelium of the stomach and by cells in the placenta. Leptin stimulates lipid metabolism and increases energy expenditure.

Disturbances in secretion of leptin, due to a defective obesity gene, impair the ability of the hypothalamus to sense satiety. It interacts with leptin receptors in the hypothalamus where animal studies show that it suppresses appetite and increases energy expenditure. When obese experimental animals that do not reproduce leptin are given the hormone, their weight normalizes.

A few rare cases of genetic leptin deficiency or abnormal leptin receptors have been identified in humans with profound overeating and weight gain. Leptin deficiency appears to be inherited as an autosomal recessive trait. In general, however, human obesity is associated with increased leptin levels. In fact, obesity seems to be associated with leptin insensitivity.

The diurnal rhythm of leptin depends on the availability of energy and, more specifically, of carbohydrate. Leptin is regulated by the tiny flux of glucose through the hexosamine biosynthesis pathway.

Leptin levels positively correlate with body mass index in humans and are disproportionately lowered in the presence of fasting. The diurnal rhythm of leptin concentration is suppressed in response to low energy intake. Low leptin levels have been reported in amenorrheic women and the typical diurnal pattern of leptin concentration in these women is absent. Nutritional restriction may be an important causal factor in the hypoestrogenism observed in these athletes.

It is possible that exercise-associated decreases in leptin may be due to alterations in nutrient availability or nutrient flux at the level of the adipocytes.

Bibliography

Hilton, L.K. and Loucks, A.B. (2000). Low energy availability, not exercise stress, suppresses the diurnal rhythm of leptin in healthy young women. *American Journal of Physiology: Endocrinology and Metabolism* 278, E43-E49.

Hulver, M.W. and Houmard, J.A. (2003). Plasma leptin and exercise: Recent findings. *Sports Medicine* 33(7), 473-482.

Schutz, Y., Flatt, J.P. and Jéquier, E. (1989). Failure of dietary fat intake to promote fat oxidation: A factor favoring the development of obesity. *American Journal of Clinical Nutrition* 50, 307-314.

Wang, H., Storlien, L.H. and Huang, X.F. (2002). Effects of dietary fat types on body fatness, leptin, and ARC leptin receptor, NPY, and AgRP mRNA expression. *American Journal of Physiology: Endocrinology and Metabolism* 282, E1352-E1359.

LES AUTRES   From the French term for 'the others.' It is used in sport to refer to people with a range of disabilities, such as dwarfism, which do not fit into traditional classification systems of the established disability groups. There are two major ways in which athletes with *les autres* conditions are classified for sport: i) the number of affected limbs and the severity of the condition; and ii) assessment of the athlete's range of motion. *Les autres* athletes currently compete in events of the US Cerebral Palsy Athletic Association.

LESBIANISM   *See under* GENDER.

LEUCINE   *See under* AMINO ACIDS.

LEUCOCYTES   *See* LEUKOCYTES.

LEUKOCYTES   Leucocytes. White blood cells. Neutrophils, eosinophils and basophils are **granulocytes**, because they have cytoplasmic granules (protein-containing vesicles). 60 to 80% of leukocytes are granulocytes. Monocytes (c. 5%) and lymphocytes (c. 30%) are **agranulocytes**, but this is a misnomer because they do actually have cytoplasmic granules.

Neutrophils and eosinophils (1.5%) are phagocytes. **Phagocytes** are cells that envelop and digest bacteria, cells, cell debris and other small particles. About half of the neutrophils in the vascular compartment do not circulate freely, but are instead loosely attached (electrostatically) to the inner walls of large-diameter veins, especially veins in the pulmonary circuit. The fluid shear stresses that accompany the increased cardiac output of exercise strip these cells free; epinephrine also triggers this 'release.' Following moderate exercise, the concentration of neutrophils becomes more than doubled. **Eosinophils** release toxins where there is an allergic reaction or parasite infection. There are two rare types of asthma that trigger a high eosinophil count in the blood. One of these types of asthma, **bronchopulmonary aspergillosis**, is a serious allergic reaction to a common fungus that can grow in the lungs. The other type, **Churg-Strauss syndrome**, involves numbness or weakness as a result of nerve damage in one or more parts of the body.

Basophils (less than 1%) are phagocytes. Basophils release mediators, such as histamine, heparin, platelet-activating factor and serotonin, in order to produce inflammation at the site of an infection or allergic reaction. The main purpose of inflammation is to attract leukocytes and the soluble mediators they produce.

Monocytes are phagocytes. A **macrophage (histiocyte)** is a large phagocyte derived from a monocyte. Of the numerous types of phagocytes, macrophages play the largest role in removing debris and foreign material.

Lymphocytes are a set of granular leukocytes. There are three major types of lymphocyte: B- cells, T-cells and null cells. **B-cells** are derived from bone marrow, and convert to plasma cells and memory cells. **Plasma cells** produce antibodies. **Memory cells** provide long-lasting immunity. **T cells** are produced in bone marrow and are so named because they are processed in the thymus gland before entering the lymph nodes. Unlike the B-cells and phagocytes, however, which prey on the antibodies of exposed pathogens, the T-cells target the exposed antigens of infectious organisms that penetrate cells to reproduce and interfere with cell function. There are four types of T-cells: cytotoxic, helper, suppressor and memory. **Cytotoxic (killer) T-cells** rupture and destroy foreign and virus-infected cells. **Helper T cells** secrete interleukin–1 and gamma-interferon. **Suppressor T cells** decrease the function of other T cells. **Memory T-cells** come from T-cells and they are stored for specific antibodies. **Null cells** lack cell membrane components that are characteristic of B-cells and T-cells, and are mostly large, granular lymphocytes known as natural killer cells. **Natural killer cells** recognize and kill certain human cells, virally-infected cells and some micro-organisms. Viruses, unlike bacteria, must enter cells to reproduce, and by killing virus-infected cells, natural killer cells limit the production of new viruses in the body. The activities of natural killer cells can be enhanced by the cytokine interleukin-2, and by antibodies, which are produced by T-cells and plasma, respectively, during specific immune responses. *See under* IMMUNITY.

LEUKOTRIENES Biochemical mediators released from mast cells, eosinophils and basophils that contract airway smooth muscle, increase vascular permeability, increase mucus secretions, and attract and activate inflammatory cells in the airways.
See also under EICOSANOIDS.

LEVER A simple machine that magnifies speed or force of a movement. A rigid bar which rotates about a fixed point (**axis**; **pivot**; **fulcrum**) with a force (effort) to move it and a resistance (load) to be overcome by it. In the body, a bone or system of bones acts as a lever. The axis passes through a joint. One or more muscles are inserted on the bone, and force is caused by contraction of those muscles. The **point of resistance** is the center of gravity of the body segment being moved plus the center of gravity of any external resistance. The relative arrangement of the axis, the point of force and the point of resistance determine the type of lever.

The **force arm** is the perpendicular distance from the axis to the line of force. The **resistance arm** is the perpendicular distance from the axis to the point of resistance. The **mechanical ratio** (amount of leverage) is the ratio of the force arm to the resistance arm. When the force arm is larger than the resistance arm, the lever is called a **force lever**, because it favors the application of force while sacrificing speed. When the resistance arm is larger than the force arm, the lever is called a **speed lever**, because it favors speed while sacrificing force.

Three types of lever system can be distinguished: first, second and third class. Most of the levers in the human body are either first or third class, with the third-class levers being most prevalent.

A **first-class lever** has the axis between the point of force and the point of resistance. The first-class levers in the human body have their axis close to the point of force, the force arm is shorter than the resistance arm, and they are therefore speed levers. There are few first-class levers in the musculoskeletal system, because the body levers are not generally arranged with the axis of rotation between the muscle attachment and the resistance. Agonists and antagonists can create a first-class lever. An example is extension of the head: the load is the weight of the head and the tension of the antagonists, the *splenius* muscle provides the effort to extend the head, and the fulcrum is the atlanto-occipital joint.

A **pulley** is a simple machine that alters the

direction of a force application. It is typically a wheel-type device with a rope running over it. In the human body, pulleys are a type of first-class lever seen in the action of certain bony prominences in the body and are represented by tendons that wrap over parts of bones and change the line of pull of a muscle (e.g. the lower tendon of the *peroneous longus* muscle wraps around a protruding part of the lower end of the fibula). A pulley functions to change the direction of force. During knee extension, the angle of pull of the *quadriceps femoris* muscle group is changed by the riding action of the patella on the condylar groove of the femur. The angle of pull of the *gracilis* is increased by means of the bulging medial condyles, both above and below the knee joint, over which the tendon passes before it attaches to the tibia. The *peroneus longus* muscle passes behind the lateral malleolus, before it turns under the foot to attach to the first cuneiform and the base of the first metatarsal bone. It is therefore able to plantar flex the foot at the ankle. If it passed in front of the lateral malleolus, its angle of pull would be shifted in front of the ankle joint and it would then dorsal flex the foot at the ankle.

A **second-class lever** has the point of resistance between the axis and the point of force. Second-class levers are always force levers. The use of a wheelbarrow entails a second-class lever system, but there are few examples of second-class lever in the human body. The push up is an example of the total body acting as a second-class lever: the foot is the axis; the weight of the body at the center of gravity is the point of resistance; and the reaction force of the ground pushing against the hands is the point of force.

A **third-class lever** has the point of force between the axis and the point of resistance. Third-class levers are always speed levers. The swing of a lacrosse stick is an example of a third-class lever system: the axis is at the grip end of the stick with the left hand, the point of force is applied by the right hand lower down the stick and the point of resistance is the weight of the stick and ball. *See* TORQUE.

LIFE SKILLS *See under* SPORTS PSYCHOLOGY.

LIFT *See under* DRAG; MAGNUS EFFECT.

LIFTING *See under* INTRA-ABDOMINAL PRESSURE; POSTURE.

LIGAMENTS Strong bands of connective tissue that are relatively inelastic and serve to connect bones. They are pliant and allow freedom of movement, but at the same time limit movement that would damage the joint. Ligaments display viscoelastic behavior.
See also SPRAIN.

LIGAND (i) An atom, a group of atoms or a molecule that binds to a metal ion. (ii) An atom, a group of atoms or a molecule that binds to a macromolecule (a molecule of high molecular weight).

LIGASES *See under* ENZYME.

LIGHTNING A discharge of atmospheric electricity, accompanied by a vivid flash of light, commonly from one cloud to another, but sometimes from a cloud to the earth. A cloud-to-ground lightning flash is the product of the buildup and discharge of static electric energy between the charged regions of the cloud and the earth. The negatively charged lower region of the cloud induces a positive charge on the ground below. **Thunder** is created when lightning quickly heats the air around it.

The **stepped leader** comes down from the thunder cloud. It is an invisible pathway made by the negatively charged particles, as they are attracted to the ground. The **upward streamer** shoots up from the ground to meet the stepped leader. It is a positively charged stream, which is the electricity visible to our eyes. Once the upward streamer and stepped leader meet, the upward streamer forms **a return stroke**. This fills in everywhere in the air that was negatively charged by the stepped ladder, as it explodes up to the cloud, and is what is seen as lightning. The **dart leader** is another negatively charged stroke, visible to the eye, which heads toward the ground once more. This time, it travels only down the main channel of the stepped leader (middle of the previous stroke). The **second return stroke** once more goes up the channel made by the dart leader and occurs less than a second after the first return stroke.

Lightning kills approximately 100 people and injures hundreds more each year. Worldwide, approximately 2000 thunderstorms and 50 to 100 lightning flashes occur every second. Usually, lightning is associated with cumulonimbus (thunder) clouds, but may occur in nimbostratus clouds, snowstorms, or in the erupting gas of an active volcano. Approximately 5% of deaths from lightning are golf-related.

Lightning tends to strike tall objects because, although the earth's normal electrical field runs in equipotential planes parallel to its surface, these planes are elevated over trees, hills and tall buildings. Lightning causes injury through five basic mechanisms: direct strike, flash discharge, contact, ground current (step voltage) and blunt trauma. **Direct strikes** occur when the victims are outside and often carrying metal objects, such as an umbrella. Metal worn in the hair, such as a hairpin, increases the chance of a direct strike, compared with a metal object worn lower on the body. Although not always fatal, direct strikes are associated with high morbidity because they frequently involve the head. **Flash discharge** from another struck object may occur when someone seeks shelter beneath a tree that is subsequently struck by lightning. Because the resistance to direct current flow in the air between the tree and victim is less than that of direct current flow in the tree, and lightning seeks the path of least resistance, it will jump from the tree to the victim. This type of injury ('**splash injury**') also occurs from person to person when several people are standing close together. **Contact injury** occurs when a person is touching an object that is either directly hit or splashed by lightning. **Ground current injury** causes mass casualties in fields or other open areas. Severity of ground current injuries decreases with distance from the point of the lightning strike. Ground is a good insulator, while a person is a good conductor. Therefore, a person standing with his feet spread may create a potential difference large enough to create a circuit between the legs and ground. This type of injury, with its increased electrical conduc-

tion, may account for the high mortality (30%) of lightning victims with leg burns. **Blunt trauma** occurs as a result of lightning current causing violent muscular contractions that throw its victims many meters from the strike point.

The only acute cause of death from lightning injury is cardiac arrest. The direct current of lightning depolarizes the entire myocardium at once, causing a single systolic contraction followed by a variable period of asystole (primary cardiac arrest). The anoxic brain damage that can occur if the person is not rapidly resuscitated can be devastating. If a lightning-strike victim presents in asystole or respiratory arrest, it is critical to initiate cardiopulmonary resuscitation (CPR) as soon as safely possible. A lightning-strike victim may be unconscious, with fixed and dilated pupils and cold extremities and cardiopulmonary arrest. Once stopped, the heart will most likely spontaneously restart, but breathing centers in the brain may be damaged. Respiratory arrest lasts longer than cardiac arrest, leading to secondary asystole from hypoxia. Therefore, those who are 'apparently dead' should be treated first, by promptly initiating CPR. Damage to the central nervous system accounts for the second most debilitating group of lightning injuries. Injuries to the central nervous system from lightning include amnesia and confusion, immediate loss of consciousness, weakness, intracranial injuries (e.g. epidural and subdural hematomas) and brief aphasia after regaining consciousness. Lighting can also injure the eyes. Intraocular lesions such as cataracts may result.

Safe shelter includes a building with four solid walls, electrical and telephone wiring, and plumbing, all of which aid in grounding a structure. Showering, bathing, standing near household appliances (such as dishwashers) and talking on landline telephones are not safe. Injury from acoustic damage can occur via explosive static from the earpiece caused by a nearby lightning strike. Cordless or cellular telephones are safer to use when emergency help is needed. A fully enclosed vehicle, with a metal roof and windows completely closed, is also considered a good shelter. Care should be taken not to touch any part of the metal framework of the vehicle while inside it during lightning. Rain shelters may actually increase the risk of lightning strike via a side flash and cause injury to the occupants. In the absence of good shelter, the lowest elevation area and/or a dense area of trees or bushes should be sought. On golf courses, the following should be avoided: solitary trees; small rain and sun shelters; large, open areas; wet areas; elevated areas; all metal objects, including golf clubs, golf cars, fences, electrical and maintenance machinery; and power lines. If sudden, close-in lightning does not permit evacuation to a safer place, a 'baseball catcher's position,' with feet together and hands on knees, should be adopted. This position is intended to minimize the probably of a direct strike by both lowering the person's height and minimizing the area in contact with the surface of the ground.

A flash-to-bang count of at least 30 seconds is strongly recommended as a determinant of when to suspend or postpone athletic or recreational activities. The flash-to-bang method is based on the fact that light travels faster than sound, which travels at a speed of approximately 1.61 km (1 mile) every 5 seconds. A flash-to-bang count of 30 seconds equates to a distance of 6 miles. A typical thunderstorm moves at a rate of approximately 40.23 km (25 miles) per hour. 30 minutes allow the thunderstorm to be about 10 to 12 miles from the area, minimizing the probability of a nearby, and therefore dangerous, lightning strike. Lightning can strike far from where it is raining, even when the clouds begin to clear and show evidence of blue sky.

The lightning-safety policy should identify the safe structure or location specific to each venue. This information will enable individuals to know where to go in advance of any thunderstorm situation and appreciate how long it takes to get to the specific safe location from each field or event site. There should be criteria to describe the suspension and resumption of athletic or recreational activities. The United States Golf Association (USGA) emphasizes that players in a competition have the right to stop play if they think that lightning threatens them, even though the committee may not have authorized it specifically by signal.

According to the basic principles of tort law in the USA, an individual has a duty to warn others of dangers that may not be obvious to a guest or subordinate of that person. An institution has the duty to warn spectators, invited guests and participants if conditions are such that lightning activity may be an imminent danger in the immediate area.

Chronology
•1753 • Benjamin Franklin invented the lightening rod.
•1975 • Lee Trevino and Jerry Heard were struck by lightning at the Western Open on the Professional Golfer's Association (PGA) Tour.
•1998 • At a soccer match in the Republic of Congo, 11 members of a team were killed by lightning.

Bibliography
Cherington, M. (2001). Lightning injuries in sport: situations to avoid. *Sports Medicine* 31(4), 301-308.
Edlich, R. (2003). Burns, lightning injuries. Http://www.emedicine.
National Lightning Safety Institute. Http://www.lightningsafety.com
United States Golf Association. Http://www.usga.org
Walsh, K.M. et al. (2000). National Athletic Trainers' Association (NATA) position statement: Lightning safety for athletics and recreation. *Journal of Athletic Training* 35(4), 471-477.

LIMB DEFICIENCIES Congenital limb deficiencies or acquired deficiencies (i.e. amputations). Acquired amputations occur more often in adults than in children. Ischemia from vascular disease, usually due to complications from diabetes, is the most common cause of amputations. Causes of acquired amputation in children include trauma, cancer, infection and vascular conditions such as gangrene. Under trauma, the leading causes of amputations are farm and power tool accidents, vehicular accidents and gunshot explosions. Most of these occur in the age group from 12 to 21 years. Approximately 150,000 amputations are performed annually in the USA.

Congenital limb deficiencies occur about twice as frequently as acquired amputations. Lower limb amputations are more common than upper limb amputations. **Dysmelia** refers to absence of arms or legs. **Phocomelia** refers to absence of middle segment of limb, but with intact proximal and distal portions (the hands or feet are attached directly to shoulder or hips, respectively). The cause of congenital limb deficiencies is seldom known. The drug **thalidomide** was used as a sedative and sleeping pill in the 1960s. Women who took thalidomide in early pregnancy, even a single dose, gave birth to children with severe birth defects, such as phocomelia. Thalidomide was subsequently banned worldwide.

International sport classifications distinguish between limb deficiencies (congenital amputations) and acquired amputations. Limb deficiencies are considered *les autres* conditions. Persons with lower limb deficiencies can compete in wheelchair sports, ambulatory sports with prostheses like Flex-Foot, or activities that can be done without prostheses like swimming and high jumping. A **prosthesis** is a substitute for a missing body part. Persons with upper-limb deficiencies compete in sports such as soccer. Age of prosthetic fitting is an important factor in subsequent development of motor skills. Upper-extremity prostheses are usually fitted when the child develops good sitting balance, usually between 8 and 10 months of age. Lower-extremity prostheses are fitted when the child begins to pull up to a stand, usually between 10 and 15 months. As the child grows, the prostheses must be periodically replaced (every 15 to 18 months for an upper-extremity prosthesis and about every 12 months for a lower-extremity prosthesis). Gaits used by people with prostheses are called hop-skip running and leg-over-leg running. **Hop-skip running** entails the following sequence: stepping forward on the good leg, hopping on the good leg while swinging through the prosthetic leg, switching weight to the prosthetic side and immediately transferring weight to the good leg. **Leg-over-leg running** is similar to the able-bodied reciprocal running pattern, but there is a slight asymmetry in stride length and time spent on each foot. Flex-Foot and other lightweight prosthetic devices permit leg-over-leg running.

Bibliography

Sherill, C. (2004). *Adapted physical activity, recreation and sport. Cross disciplinary and lifespan.* 6th ed. Boston, MA: McGraw-Hill.

LIMBIC SYSTEM   *See under* BRAIN.

LINEAR MOTION   Translation. Motion in a straight line. It is motion in which all parts of the body travel along parallel paths.

LINEBACKER'S SPUR   *See under* HUMERUS.

LINKED SYSTEM   *See under* RIGID BODY.

LIPID PEROXIDATION   *See under* FREE RADICALS.

LIPIDS   A group of organic compounds that are insoluble in polar solvents, such as water but that dissolve readily in non-polar solvents such as chloroform. **Simple lipids** are neutral fats (e.g. triglycerides) and waxes (e.g. bees wax). **Compound lipids** are phospholipids (phosphatidates, e.g. lecithins), glycolipids (e.g. cerebrosides) and lipoproteins (e.g. chylomicrons). **Derived lipids** are fatty acids (e.g. palmitic acid), steroids (e.g. cholesterol) and hydrocarbons (e.g. terpenes).

The main lipids found in blood are cholesterol, phospholipid and triglyceride. These lipids circulate in the plasma bound to proteins. As lipoprotein complexes, the otherwise insoluble lipids are made soluble, thus enabling their transport into and out of the plasma.

LIPOGENESIS   *See* FATTY ACID SYNTHESIS.

LIPOIC ACID   Alpha-lipoic acid. An endogenous thiol that is present in very small quantities in animal tissues and is a necessary cofactor in energy producing reactions in the mitochondria, lipoic acid helps to convert pyruvate to acetyl CoA. It is generally bound to an enzyme complex that renders alpha-lipoic acid unavailable as an antioxidant. Alpha-lipoic acid is reduced to dihydrolipoic acid, which is a potent antioxidant against all major reactive oxygen species. Dihydrolipoic acid is also an important agent in recycling vitamin C during periods of oxidative stress and can be an effective glutathione substitute.

Alpha-lipoic acid can be consumed in the diet and has no known toxic side effects. Most alpha-lipoic acid in food is derived from lipoamide-containing enzymes and is bound to the amino acid lysine (lipoyllysine). Animal tissues that are rich in lipoyllysine include kidney, heart and liver, while plant sources that are rich in lipoyllysine include spinach, broccoli and tomatoes. It has been hypothesized that most dietary alpha-lipoic acid is absorbed as lipoyllysine, and free alpha-lipoic acid has not been detected in the circulation of humans who are not taking alpha-lipoic acid supplements.

Bibliography
Spriet, L.L. and Gibala, M.J. (2004). Nutritional strategies to influence adaptations to training. *Journal of Sports Sciences* 22, 127-141.

LIPOLYSIS   The catabolism (breakdown) of lipids into fatty acids and glycerol. During submaximal exercise, the main source of lipid for metabolism is not blood or adipose tissue, but intramuscular stores of lipid. Within skeletal muscle, triglycerides are stored in lipid droplets. A special intracellular lipase enzyme, hormone-sensitive lipase, is activated by cAMP and sequentially releases free fatty acid molecules from the glycerol backbone of triglycerides. Another lipase enzyme, lipoprotein lipase, is attached to the endothelial lining of blood vessels and catabolizes lipids from blood lipoprotein molecules. The free fatty acid molecules can then be catabolized by muscle, while the remaining glycerol molecule is circulated to the liver. Long-chain (greater than 15 carbons) free fatty acids must be modified by the addition of co-enzyme A (CoA) for transport into the mitochondria where they are then catabolized in a metabolic pathway called beta-oxidation. The metabolism of carbohydrate and lipid is identical after acetyl CoA formation.

The stimulation of adipose tissue lipolysis during exercise occurs primarily via activation of beta-receptors in adipocytes as a result of increased plasma concentration of epinephrine. During aerobic exercise, the fat from adipose tissue is broken down in order to mobilize fatty acids. The free fatty acids are transported from the adipose tissue to muscle tissue. After entering the muscle tissue, the energy levels of the fatty acids is raised before entry into the mitochondria where beta-oxidation takes place. *See* FATTY ACIDS.

LIPOMAS   Noncancerous, fatty tumors.

LIPOPROTEIN   A conjugated protein containing a lipid or a group of lipids. Lipoproteins carry lipids in the watery fluids of the body. Increased lipid content decreases the density of lipoproteins. *See under* CHOLESTEROL.

LIPOPROTEIN LIPASE   *See* ABDOMINAL OBESITY; CHOLESTEROL; LIPOLYSIS.

LIPOSUCTION   Lipoplasty. Suction-assisted lipectomy. It is the process of removing unwanted fat from specific areas of the body, including the abdomen, hips, buttocks, thighs, knees, upper arms, chin, cheeks and neck. Liposuction involves inserting a sharp, hand-held instrument (cannula) through an entrance wound in the patient's skin. Powered by a vacuum pump or aspirator, the suctioned fat passes through the cannula into a hose that then deposits the fat into bags, bottles, or other containers. **Tumescent liposuction** involves injecting large volumes of a solution directly into areas of excessive fatty deposits. The diluted solution usually contains a local anesthetic and epinephrine to shrink capillaries and prevent blood loss.

It is the extra-abdominal fat that is commonly removed in liposuction. The more dense, superficial fat is less commonly removed because it is tightly packed with nerves and blood vessels. It is dangerous to attempt liposuction on intra-abdominal fat due to the high risk of puncturing abdominal organs. Liposuction may decrease cellulite, but it is unlikely to eliminate it.

Bibliography
American Society of Dermatologic Surgery. Http://www.asds-net.org

LITTLE LEAGUER'S ELBOW   *See under* ELBOW JOINT, THROWING INJURIES.

LITTLE LEAGUER'S SHOULDER   A stress fracture of the proximal humeral physis. It is an overuse injury seen in young athletes who perform overhead throwing activities.

During the acceleration phase of throwing or pitching, the shoulder is subject to rapid internal rotation as the forearm and hand are whipped forward. During this phase, in adults, the internal rotators of the shoulder may be injured or there may be spontaneous (and usually spiral) fractures of the shaft of the humerus. In children and adolescents, this phase may cause widening and absorption of the proximal humeral epiphysis and a stress fracture from sudden internal rotation may result.

LIVER   A body organ located in the upper right quadrant of the abdomen that is responsible primarily for blood glucose regulation, the regulation of blood lipoprotein concentration and the catabolism of many molecules produced in other tissues.

Glycogenolysis in the liver involves the activation of the enzyme phosphorylase and is therefore similar to skeletal muscle. In the liver, however, the hormone glucagon also induces an increase in intracellular cAMP, similar to epinephrine, which contributes to the stimulation of glycogenolysis during low blood glucose conditions. Subtle differences exist between skeletal muscle and liver metabolism in the Krebs cycle. Carbohydrate catabolism in the liver can support the Krebs cycle intermediates by resupplying malate, and hence oxaloacetate. A continual supply of oxaloacetate is crucial for incorporating acetyl CoA molecules into the Krebs cycle, especially during conditions of low glucose and high lipid catabolism. The reactions of lipid metabolism that produce acetyl CoA are similar in liver and skeletal muscle; the main difference in metabolic regulation occurs after acetyl CoA formation. There are enzymes in the liver that can convert acetyl CoA to ketone bodies.

 A direct blow to the upper right quadrant can lead to contusion. Pain may be referred to the inferior angle of the right scapula. Systemic diseases such as hepatitis can enlarge the liver, making it more susceptible to injury. An enlarged liver (hepatomegaly) is a contraindication for sports participation.

See also BILE; CORI CYCLE; GLUCOSE-ALANINE CYCLE.

LOAD   i) The weight that is supported by a structure. ii) The burden placed on a machine. iii) Application of an external force to a body. A load is defined in terms of its magnitude, location, direction, duration, frequency, variability and rate. Normal functional loading is termed '**use**,' whereas repeated overload is '**overuse**.' *See* OVERUSE INJURIES.

LOCOMOTION   The act of moving from place to place. Vision is important for locomotion in a straight line. Reflexes have important regulatory functions during human locomotion. The function of a given reflex pathway changes dynamically throughout the locomotor cycle. While all reflexes act in concert to a certain extent, generally cutaneous reflexes at to alter swing limb trajectory to avoid stumbling and falling. It appears that cutaneous reflexes stabilize human gait against external perturbations produced by an uneven surface in stance or obstacles encountered during swing. Stretch reflexes act to stabilize limb trajectory and assist force production during stance. Load receptor reflexes are shown to have an effect on both stance phase body weight support and step cycle timing.

After neurotrauma or in disease, reflexes no longer function as during normal locomotion, but still have the potential to be clinically exploited in gait modification regimens.

See GALLOPING; RUNNING; WALKING.

Bibliography

Danion, F., Boyadjian, A. and Marin, L. (2000). Control of locomotion in expert gymnasts in the absence of vision. *Journal of Sports Sciences* 18, 809-814.

Zehr, E.P., Stein, R.B. and Komiyama, T. (1998). Function of sural nerve reflexes during human walking. *Journal of Physiology* 507(1), 305-314.

Zehr, E.P. and Stein, R.B. (1999). What functions do reflexes serve during human locomotion? *Progress in Neurobiology* 58(2), 185-205.

LOMBARD'S PARADOX   When rising from a chair, the extensor torque produced at the hip by the hamstrings is in excess of the flexor torque produced at the hip by the *rectus femoris*. Similarly, at the knee, the extensor torque of the *quadriceps femoris* dominates the flexor torque of the hamstrings. The *quadriceps femoris* and hamstring muscles, both bi-articular muscles, contract simultaneously during the sit-to-stand motion. The paradox concerns the activity of a bi-articular muscle when the required torque at one joint is in the opposite direction to that caused by the muscle. The paradox can be explained with respect to the relative moment arms of the hamstrings and *rectus femoris* at either the hip or the knee, and their effects on the magnitude of the moments produced by either muscle group at each of the two joints. Muscles cannot develop different amounts of force in their different parts. Therefore the only way for hip extension and knee extension to occur simultaneously in the act of standing (or eccentrically in the act of sitting) is for the net moment to be an extensor moment at both the hip and knee joints. The antagonists produce a net knee extension moment, even if they develop identical forces, because their moment arms around the knee are unequal; the moment arm of the *rectus femoris* at the knee exceeds that of the hamstrings.

Bibliography

Lombard, W.P. and Abott, F.M. (1907). The mechanical effects produced by contraction of individual muscles of the thigh of the frog. *American Journal of Physiology* 20, 1-60.
Rasch, P.J. (1978). *Kinesiology and applied anatomy*. 7th edition. Philadelphia: Lea and Febiger.

LOOSE BODIES   Pieces of tissue that are loose in a joint. Loose bodies may be congenital or acquired. Acquired loose bodies at the elbow are often the result of injuries such as osteochondritis dissecans or valgus extension overload syndrome. In the knee, loose bodies cause mechanical symptoms of locking and recurrent effusions.

LORDOSIS   Swayback. An abnormal accentuation of the normal curve that is normally present, to a minor degree, in the lumbar region of the spine. It produces excessive concave curvature. A compensatory kyphosis develops to balance the increased concavity. True lordosis is usually associated with anterior tilt of the pelvis. Tight hip flexors and weak abdominal muscles contribute to the anterior tilt, while the gluteal muscles and hamstrings are too weak to counteract the anterior tilt. An increased lumbar curve is associated with hyperextension of the knees. It is thought that this often precipitates the development of lordosis.

The opposite of lordosis, clinically, is **flat back**.

It is a decrease or absence of the normal anteroposterior curve. The pelvic inclination is less than normal, with the pelvis held in posterior tilt. The lower back muscles are weak. The hip flexors, especially the *psoas major*, are weak and lengthened. The hamstrings are abnormally tight. Flat back is normal in all children until the age of 3 or 4 years, when they begin to exhibit lordosis. *See also under* ABDOMINAL OBESITY.

LOU GEHRIG DISEASE   *See* AMYOTROPHIC LATERAL SCLEROSIS.

LOW BACK PAIN   Lumbago. Low back pain is second only to the common cold in the most common complaints seen in primary care. At least 80% of the population suffers at least one episode in their lifetime and in as many as 50% of cases the problem will recur within the following 3 years. Without treatment, 60% of low back pain sufferers go back to work within a week and nearly 90% return within 6 weeks. 5 to 10% of patients suffer chronic low back pain. There is strong evidence that aerobic exercise can play a role in decreasing the incidence of low back injury. One of the objectives of Healthy People 2010 in the USA is to decrease activity limitation due to chronic back conditions.

There are many causes of low back pain, including: herniated nucleus pulposus; low back strain or sprain; spondylolysis; spinous or transverse process fracture; spinal stenosis; ankylosing spondylitis; Scheuermann's disease; abdominal aortic aneurysm; and sacroiliac joint dysfunction. Of the 80% who experience low back pain at some time in their lives, however, about 97% of the pain stems from mechanical injury to muscles, ligaments or connective tissue.

Lower-extremity muscle tightness, especially tight hip flexors or tight hamstring muscles, is common with low back pain. **Tightness of the hip flexor muscles** (e.g. *iliopsoas* and *rectus femoris*) results in excessive anterior tilt and increased lumbar lordosis. These factors lengthen the hip extensors (e.g. *gluteus maximus* and hamstrings), placing them at a mechanical disadvantage and causing early recruitment of the lumbar extensor muscles (*erector spinae*). Treatment consists of stretching the hip flexors and strengthening the hip extensors. **Tightness of the hamstring muscles** causes excessive posterior pelvic tilt and decrease lumbar lordosis. These factors place the back extensors at a mechanical disadvantage and also make the spine less resilient to axial (compressive) loads. Treatment is aimed at stretching the back extensors.

Repetitive movements, common in sport, can fatigue the supporting structures of the lumbar spine and overload the viscoelastic tissues that protect the intervertebral disks and ligaments. Combined movements (especially flexion and rotation) carry the highest injury potential. Excessive flexion is detrimental for most people, as is sedentary posture. Flexion causes the nucleus pulposus to shift posteriorly and press against the annulus fibrosus at its thinnest, least-buttressed place. In some people, this leads to disk herniation, but in other people it just leads to pain. When the lumbar spine is in neutral lordosis, the extensor musculature is responsible for creating the extensor moment and at the same time provides a posterior shear force that supports the anterior shearing action of gravity on the upper body and the hand-held load. The joint shear forces are approximately 200 N. With spinal flexion, the strained interspinous ligament complex imposes an anterior shear force on the superior vertebra. The joint shear forces are likely to exceed 1,000 N. Thus, using muscle to support the moment in a neutral posture rather than being fully flexed with ligaments supporting the moment greatly decreases the shear loading. The margin of safety is much larger in the compression mode than in the shear mode because the spine can safely tolerate well over 10,000 N in compression, but 1,000 N of shear causes injury with cyclic loading.

Athletes who participate in sports involving repeated and forceful hyperextension of the spine (such as gymnastics) may suffer from spondylolysis or facet joint inflammation and impingement.

In a study comparing the spinal motion of six male professional golfers with low back pain and six without low back pain, it was found that golfers with low back pain tended to flex their spines more when addressing the ball and used significantly greater left side bending (lateral flexion) on the backswing.

Muscle fatigue can cause reflex muscle spasm and pain. Pain results from mechanical or chemical irritation of nociceptive nerve fibers. In the lower back, these pain receptors are located in the outer third of the intervertebral disk, the facet joint capsule, the anterior and posterior longitudinal ligaments, and the musculoligamentous supporting structures of the lumbar spine.

The clinical practice guidelines of the Agency for Health Care Policy and Research of the federal government in the USA, published in 1994, de-emphasize the role of bed rest, narcotic painkillers and surgery. Bed rest appears to have no advantage in most cases and can compromise recovery. Exercise is the central element of modern conservative treatment. During the first two weeks after symptoms begin, low-stress activity such as walking, biking or swimming is recommended even if the activities make the symptoms a little worse. Non-prescription pain relievers, such as aspirin and ibuprofen, work as well as prescription painkillers and muscle relaxants, and cause fewer side effects. There is a lack of evidence to support the effectiveness of traction, acupuncture, massage, ultrasound and transcutaneous electrical neural stimulation (TENS). Surgery helps only 1 in 100 people with acute low back problems. There are four absolute indications for back surgery: cauda equina syndrome, intractable pain (with appropriate corroborative radiographic findings), progressive neurologic deficit and new-onset incontinence (fecal or urinary). Spinal manipulation by a chiropractor or other therapist can be helpful when symptoms begin. Manipulation is contraindicated in disk herniations and, when used, should always be used with other appropriate rehabilitative components.

See also LUMBAR-PELVIC RHYTHM; POSTURE.

Bibliography

Drezner, J.A. and Herring, S.A. (2001). Managing low-back pain. Steps to optimize function and hasten return to activity. *The Physician and Sportsmedicine* 29(8), 33-43.

Healthy People 2010. Http://www.healthypeople.gov

Kuritzky, L. and White, J. (1997). Low back pain: Consider extension education. *The Physician and Sportsmedicine* 25(1), 23-30.

Lindsay, D. and Horton, J. (2002). Comparison of spine motion in elite golfers with and without low back pain. *Journal of Sports Sciences* 20(8), 599-605.

McGill, S.M. (2001). Low back stability: From formal description to issues for performance and rehabilitation. *Exercise and Sport Sciences Reviews* 29(1), 26-31.

McGill, S. (2002). *Low back disorders: Evidence-based prevention and rehabilitation*. Champaign, IL: Human Kinetics.

Norris, C.M. (2000). *Back stability*. Champaign, IL: Human Kinetics.

Shipple, B.J. (1997). Treating low-back pain. Exercise knowns and unknowns. *The Physician and Sportsmedicine* 25(8), 51-66.

LOWER LEG   The tibia and fibula serve as a rigid link between the knee and ankle. The lower leg has four compartments (anterior, lateral, superficial posterior and deep posterior) that are defined by nonelastic osseofascial boundaries. Each compartment contains specific muscles, nerves and vessels. The **anterior compartment** consists of the following muscles: *tibialis anterior*, *extensor hallucis longus*, *extensor digitorum longus* and *peroneus tertius*. All are dorsal flexors; the first two are inverters, the last two are everters. The **lateral compartment** consists of the following muscles: *peroneus longus* and *peroneus brevis*. Both are plantar flexors and everters. The **superficial posterior compartment** consists of the following muscles: *gastrocnemius*, *plantaris* and *soleus*. All three are plantar flexors, the first two are also knee flexors. The **deep posterior compartment** consists of the following muscles: *flexor hallucis longus*, *flexor digitorum longus*, *tibialis posterior* and *popliteus*. The first three are plantar flexors and inverters. The *popliteus* has no action at the ankle or foot; it flexes and medially rotates the leg. *See also* ANKLE JOINT; FOOT.

LOWER LEG, COMPARTMENT SYNDROME
Increased intracompartmental pressure in the lower leg that interferes with microvascular flow and causes tissue ischemia and pain. It may be acute or chronic. 85% of **acute compartment syndrome** cases are caused by severe trauma-associated fractures or dislocations of the leg. Most of the remainder is caused by a significant and prolonged increase in exercise intensity, while a small number are caused by vascular injury or prolonged externally applied pressure. An acute compartment syndrome is a surgical emergency that requires immediate fasciotomy in order to avoid permanent ischemic contracture.

Chronic compartment syndrome mainly affects endurance athletes who walk or run, and involves elevation of intra-muscular pressure and pain during exercise with return to baseline after exercise. It can be the result of muscle hypertrophy, through increased training, exceeding the compartment's inherent volume. During exercise, small blood vessels dilate in order to increase the blood flow and thus increase the bulk of the muscle. The resulting increase in intra-muscular pressure causes ischemia and thus a relative lack of oxygen. Fluid that results from the metabolic changes, such as the formation of lactic acid, leads to edema within the muscle. This further increases intra-muscular pressure and ischemia. This vicious circle continues until exercise is ceased. Anatomical factors such as fascial thickening may be a risk factor for chronic compartment syndrome.

LOWER LEG PAIN   'Shin splints' is an umbrella term that refers to any lower leg pain. **Posteriomedial pain** is caused by tibial stress reaction that can develop into a stress fracture, medial tibial stress syndrome or deep posterior compartment compression syndrome. **Tibial pain** is caused by tibial stress reaction (that can develop into a stress fracture) or injury to the pes anserine tendon or bursa. **Tibial stress reaction** is a stress reaction in which the tibia adapts to stress placed on it. **Anterior tibial compartment pain** is caused by muscle strains, tendon injury and lateral compartment compression syndrome. **Fibular pain** is caused by fibular stress reaction (that can develop into a stress fracture) and biceps tendon injury at the head of the fibula. **Posterior pain** is caused by muscle strains, tendon injury, thrombophlebitis and posterior compartment compression syndrome of either the superficial or deep posterior compartment.

Miscellaneous causes of lower leg pain include: popliteal artery entrapment syndrome, varicose veins, interosseus membrane calcification, fascial herniae, and pain referred from the lower back.

Nerves involved in compressive syndromes of the leg include: i) the superficial peroneal nerve as it exits the fascia of the lateral compartment; ii) the deep peroneal nerve as it enters the anterior compartment through the intermuscular septum; iii) the peroneal nerve as it enters the fibula tunnel at the origin of the *peroneus longus* muscle; and iv) the sural nerve in the calf.

Bibliography

Touliopolous, S. and Hershman, E.B. (1999). Lower leg pain. Diagnosis and treatment of compartment syndromes and other pain syndromes of the leg. *Sports Medicine* 27(3), 193-204.

LUMBAGO *See under* LOW BACK PAIN.

LUMBAR Of the lower back.

LUMBAR-PELVIC RHYTHM The relationship between lumbar and pelvic movement. During forward flexion in standing, when the legs are straight, movement of the pelvis on the hip is limited to about 90 degrees of hip flexion. Further forward flexion, enabling the person to touch the ground, must occur at the lumbar spine. Movement into a fully flexed position from standing posture is initiated by the abdominal and *iliopsoas* muscles. It is continued by the force of gravity acting on the trunk and controlled by eccentric movement of the *erector spinae* muscles. *Erector spinae* activity increases up to 50 to 60 degrees of flexion as the trunk flexes at the lumbar vertebrae. The lumbar vertebrae discontinue their contribution to trunk flexion while movement continues as a result of the contribution of anterior pelvic tilt, and this is controlled by eccentric contraction of the hamstring and *gluteus maximus* muscles. As the trunk moves deeper into flexion, the activity in the *erector spinae* diminishes to total inactivity in the fully-flexed position. This is called the **'flexion relaxation response.'** In this position, trunk flexion is controlled by the posterior ligaments and the passive resistance of the elongated *erector spinae* muscles. It does not occur in all individuals and occurs later in the range of movement when weights are carried. Controlled animal studies show that static lumbar flexion develops creep in the associated viscoelastic tissues and elicits spasms and modification of muscle function. Solomonow et al. (2003) showed experimentally in humans that static lumbar flexion is an activity that constitutes an occupational risk factor for the development of low back disorder.

In a study of males and females, the *erector spinae* were active through a significantly larger angle during flexion and initiated activity significantly earlier during extension after static flexion. Females demonstrated more pronounced changes than males. Muscle spasms were recorded in more than half of the subjects during the static flexion period. Creep developed during a short static lumbar flexion elicited significant changes in the muscular activity pattern of the 'flexion-relaxation response.' The muscles seem to compensate for the loss of tension in the lumbar viscoelastic tissues, while spasms suggest that some micro-damage was incurred to the viscoelastic tissues. McGorry et al. (2001) found that the flexion-relaxation response is ubiquitous in the *erector spinae* of the lumbar region and is present in the hamstrings and lower thoracic *erector spinae*, although not consistently in all subjects.

Dissociation of lumbar movement from pelvic movement is essential for healthy functioning of the body. For lumbar-pelvic rhythm to function correctly, the movement of the pelvis on the hip should be at least equal to the movement of the lumbar spine on the pelvis. People with a history of low back pain are often unable to move the pelvis on the hip. *See also* SWISS BALL.

Bibliography

McGill, S. (2002). *Low back disorders: Evidence-based prevention and rehabilitation*. Champaign, IL: Human Kinetics.

McGorry, R.W. et al. (2001). Timing of activation of the erector spinae and hamstrings during a trunk flexion and extension task. *Spine* 26(4), 418-425.

Norris, C.M. (2000). *Back stability*. Champaign, IL: Human Kinetics.

Solomonow, M. et al. (2003). Flexion-relaxation response to static lumbar flexion in males and females. *Clinical Biomechanics* 18(4), 273-279.

LUMBAR SPINE INJURIES *See* LOW BACK PAIN; SCIATICA; SPONDYLOLYSIS; SPONDYLOLISTHESIS.

LUMEN The space in the interior of a tubular structure such an artery or intestine.

LUMINOUS FLUX The flow of light, which produces a visual sensation, measured in lumens.

LUNG   The lungs are the main organs of external respiration in the human body, situated one on each side of the chest (thoracic) cage, which is a closed compartment separated from the abdomen by the diaphragm and surrounded at the neck by muscles and connective tissue. The **pleural space** consists of two thin membranes located between the lungs and the chest wall. On entering the lungs, the **bronchi** divide into a large number of smaller branches called **bronchial tubes** and **bronchioles**. Each bronchiole ends in an elongated saccule called the **atrium**. On the surface of each atrium there are alveoli. An **alveolus** is a minute air-filled sac found in the lung and surrounded by blood vessels. The exchange of oxygen and carbon dioxide takes place through the surfaces of the millions of alveoli. Gas moves across the blood-gas interface in the lung by diffusion. Small **pores of Kohn** within each alveolus allow for even dispersion of surfactant over the respiratory membrane to decrease surface tension for easier alveolar ventilation. The pores also provide for gas exchange between adjacent alveoli, thus sustaining indirect ventilation of alveoli that are damaged or blocked from chronic obstructive lung diseases such as emphysema. In pulmonary disease, gas transfer capacity at the alveolar-capillary membrane may be impaired by: i) the build up of a pollutant layer that 'thickens' the alveolar membrane and/or ii) a decrease in alveolar surface area.

LUNG COMPLIANCE   Distensibility of the lungs; the ease with which they can be expanded. The more the lung expands for a given increase in transpulmonary pressure, the greater is its compliance.

LUNG DISEASE   *See* CHRONIC OBSTRUCTIVE PULMONARY DISEASE.

LUPUS   A chronic inflammatory disease that can affect various parts of the body, especially the skin, joints, blood and kidneys. For most people, lupus is a mild disease affecting only a few organs. In others, it may cause serious and even life-threatening problems. There are three types of lupus: discoid, systemic and drug-induced. **Discoid (cutaneous) lupus** is always limited to the skin. It is identified by

a rash that may appear on the face, neck and scalp. In approximately 10% of patients, discoid lupus can evolve into the systemic form of the disease, which can affect almost any organ or system of the body. **Systemic lupus** is usually more severe than discoid lupus, and can affect almost any organ or organ system of the body. **Drug-induced lupus** occurs after the use of certain prescribed drugs, such as hydralazine (used to treat hypertension) and procainamide (used to treat irregular heart rhythms). Genes on chromosome 6 called immune response genes have been associated with lupus. Hormonal factors may explain why lupus occurs more frequently in females than in males.

The increase of disease symptoms before menstrual periods and/or during pregnancy support the belief that hormones, particularly estrogen, may somewhat regulate the way the disease progresses.

Bibliography
National Institute of Arthritis and Musculoskeletal and Skin Disorders. Http://www.niams.nih.gov
The Lupus Foundation of America. Http://www.lupus.org

LUTEINIZING HORMONE   *See under* GONADOTROPIC HORMONES.

LYASES   *See under* ENZYMES.

LYME DISEASE   An infection caused by *Borrelia burgdorferi*, a type of bacterium called a spirochete that is carried by deer ticks. Ticks are not insects, but arachnids, a class of arthropods, which also includes mites, spiders and scorpions. Ticks are parasites that feed by latching onto an animal host, embedding their mouthparts into the host's skin and sucking its blood. There are over 850 tick species, about 100 of which are capable of transmitting diseases. Ticks are responsible for at least 9 different known diseases in the USA. Lyme disease is the most common arthropod-borne illness in the USA. More than 150,000 cases have been reported to the Centers for Disease Control and Prevention since 1982. *Borrelia burgdorferi* infects other species of ticks, but is known to be transmitted to humans and other animals only by the deer tick (black-legged tick) and the related Western black-legged tick. The prevalence of Lyme disease in the northeast and upper mid-west in the USA is due to the presence of large numbers of the deer tick's preferred hosts – white-footed mice and deer – and their proximity to humans. Lyme disease is spreading slowly along and inland from the upper east coast, as well as in the upper Midwest and the northern California and Oregon coast. Up to 50% of adult ticks in certain areas of the northeast infected with *Borrelia burgdoferi*.

An infected tick normally cannot begin transmitting the spirochete until it has been attached to its host about 36 to 48 hours. Three stages of Lyme disease are recognized. Stage 1 infections occur 3 to 30 days after the initial exposure. Approximately 75% of patients experience erythema migrans, which is a rash, usually at the site of the tick bite. This stage is often associated with constitutional symptoms such as fever, myalgias, arthralgias and headache. Stage 2 occurs weeks to months after the initial infection, and there may be neurologic or cardiac involvement as well as malaise, myalgias and arthralgias. The most common cardiac manifestation is AV nodal block. Stage 3 occurs months to years later and can involve the synovium, nervous system and skin. If caught early, Lyme disease is treatable with antibiotics. Late-stage Lyme disease does not respond as well. Arthritis occurs in the majority of previously untreated patients. It usually involves several large joints, especially the knee.

Preventive measures include wearing long pants and other protective clothing, wearing tick repellant, checking for ticks, and knowing tick removal methods. Ticks hide in shady, moist, leaf litter, but also cling to tall grass, shrubs and low tree branches. Ticks can attach themselves almost anywhere on the body, but prefer creases like the armpit, groin, or back of the knee. The chances of Lyme disease transmission are low if the tick can be removed quickly. To remove a tick, it should be grasped with fine-point tweezers at the place of attachment, as close to the skin as possible. The tick should not be pricked, crushed or burned. The Lyme Disease Foundation indicates that there are two competing opinions as to whether or not to remove the mouthparts of the tick, if they break off in the skin. One opinion is that they should be removed, because they can cause a secondary infection; the other opinion is that the mouthparts should be left to come out on their own as the skin sloughs off.

Bibliography

Lyme Disease Foundation. Http://www.lyme.org

Wang, D.H. and Goodman, J.L. (1997). Joint pain and swelling: Could it be Lyme arthritis? *The Physician and Sportsmedicine* 25(2).

LYMPH A fluid derived from interstitial fluid that travels through the lymphatic system. It consists of water, electrolytes, proteins and other substances. It is transported in lymphatic channels from the tissues to the blood. The fluid portion of lymph is called **plasma**.

LYMPHADENOPATHY Any disease process affecting one or more lymph nodes.

LYMPHANGIOMA A well-circumscribed nodule or mass of lymphatic vessels or channels, that varies in size.

LYMPHATIC SYSTEM A system of small vessels, ducts, valves and organized tissue. It is a circulatory system that bypasses the liver, before delivery to the blood stream. Unlike the vascular system, the lymphatic system has no pumping organ. There is smooth muscle in vessel walls and one-way valves. It joins the bloodstream via two ducts in the neck. Its vessels pick up and transport most end products of fat digestion.

LYMPH NODES Small glands clustered in the neck, armpits, abdomen, and groin that supply infection-fighting cells to the bloodstream and filter out bacteria and other antigens.

LYMPHOCYTES *See under* LEUKOCYTES.

LYMPHOID TISSUE Lymphatic tissue. It is a network of cells through which lymph flows and is the site of lymphocyte production. **Central lymphoid tissues** are bone marrow and the thymus. **Peripheral lymphoid tissues** are the spleen, lymph nodes, tonsils, adenoids, appendix and regions in the lining of the gastrointestinal tract. See under IMMUNITY.

LYMPHOKINES　Soluble proteins produced by lymphocytes acting as messengers in the cell-mediated immune response. Lymphokines may be interleukins or gamma-interferon.
　See CYTOKINES.

LYSINE　An essential, mainly ketogenic six-carbon amino acid. It is an important constituent of collagen and elastin.

LYSIS　*See under* CYTOTOXIC REACTIONS.

LYSOSOMES　Small spherical organelles containing digestive enzymes that degrade intracellular debris and extracellular debris that has been taken into the cell.

LYSOZYME　One of a class of enzymes that dissolves the cell wall of bacteria.

M

MACHINE   A device for doing work whereby a mass (load) may be moved by a much smaller force (effort) than the weight of the load. The ratio of the distance moved by the effort to the distance moved by the load is the **velocity ratio** of the machine. The ratio of the load to the effort is the **force ratio** (**mechanical advantage**) of the machine. The ratio of the work done on the load to that done by the effort is the **efficiency** of the machine. It is equal to the ratio of mechanical advantage to velocity ratio. A **frictionless (perfect) machine** would have an efficiency of unity (one). *See* LEVER; PULLEY; WHEEL AND AXLE.

MACROCYTES   *See under* ANEMIA.

MACROMINERAL   *See under* MINERAL.

MACROMOLECULES   Large molecules made from many smaller units by anabolism. Examples include proteins, nucleic acids and polysaccharides. These macromolecules have amino acids, nucleotides and monosaccharides, respectively, as building blocks.

MACROPHAGE   *See under* LEUKOCYTES.

MACULA   A structure in the center of the retina that is responsible for the fine, detailed central vision used in reading and color vision. **Macular edema** is a common complication of diabetic retinopathy.

MACULAR DISEASE   There are many forms of macular disease, with many different names. **Age-related maculophathy (macular degeneration)** is a degenerative disorder of the central retina typically with an age of onset after the fifth decade. It is the most common cause of blindness in the western world for people over the age of 55 years. A distinction can be made between dry and wet macular degeneration. In the **dry form**, the layer of macular cells that sense light become thinner and some cells break down. It is usually discovered by difficulty with reading, but rarely causes the total loss of reading vision. In the **wet (neovascular) form**, new blood vessels grow under the macular and leaking fluid causes nearby cells to die. There may be blank spots in the field of vision or straight lines may appear to be wavy.

Only the later stages of age-related maculopathy (either form) result in moderate or severe loss of vision. The only proven treatment for the wet form is focal laser photocoagulation. Less than 20% of lesions are eligible for laser treatment at clinical presentation and even in these the benefit is modest.

Stargardt disease is the most common form of inherited juvenile macular degeneration. It is characterized by a decrease of central vision with a preservation of peripheral vision. It is usually diagnosed in persons under the age of 20 years, when decreased central vision is first noticed. It is nearly always inherited as an autosomal recessive trait. Mutations in the ABCR gene, which cause Stargardt disease, produce a dysfunctional protein that cannot perform this energy transport. As a result, the photoreceptor cells in the retina degenerate and vision loss occurs.

Bibliography
Macular Disease Society (UK). Http://www.maculardisease.org

MAGNESIUM   A metallic element which, as a 'macromineral' in the human body, is important for activating enzymes, especially in glycolysis, Krebs cycle, fatty acid oxidation and amino acid metabolism. It is a co-factor for the enzymes that hydrolyze ATP and ADP, and transfer their phosphate groups to acceptor molecules. ATP is always present as a magnesium-ATP complex. Magnesium is involved in protein synthesis, being necessary for the activation of amino acids by aminoacyl-tRNA synthetase and the attachment of mRNA to the ribosome. Magnesium is found in high concentrations in bone and intracellular fluid. 50% of total magnesium is found in bone and 25% is found in muscle. It also plays a role in nerve conduction. Under certain conditions, exercise appears to lead to magnesium depletion and may worsen a state of deficiency when magnesium intake is inadequate.

Hypermagnesemia (excessive magnesium in the blood) occurs following short-term, high-intensity exercise as the consequence of a decrease in plasma volume and a shift of cellular magnesium resulting from acidosis. Prolonged submaximal exercise, however, is accompanied by hypomagnesemia. A mechanism for the observed decrease in plasma magnesium concentration after long-term physical exercise could be a shift of magnesium into the red blood cells. Magnesium status is adequate for most athletes and there is no evidence that magnesium supplements can enhance performance. Low dietary intakes, as found in many female athletes, coupled with increased urinary losses with exercise, may eventually lead to a magnesium deficiency.

Because magnesium is part of chlorophyll, the green pigment in plants, green leafy vegetables are rich in magnesium. Unrefined grains and nuts also have high magnesium content. Spinach (half a cup, chopped, cooked) contains 78.3 mg of magnesium. Banana (one medium) contains 34.2 mg of magnesium.

The recommended dietary allowance (RDA) for adults (31 years and older) is 420 mg (males) and 320 mg/day (females).

Bibliography

McDonald, R. and Keen, C.L. (1988). Iron, zinc and magnesium nutrition and athletic performance. *Sports Medicine* 5, 171-184

Newhouse, I.J. and Finstad, E.W. (2000). The effects of magnesium supplementation on exercise performance. *Clinical Journal of Sports Medicine* 10(3), 195-200.

Oregon State University. The Linus Pauling Institute. Micronutrient Information Center. Http://lpi.oregonstate.edu/infocenter

MAGNETIC RESONANCE IMAGING

A scanning technique that creates a visual image, using electromagnetic fields to determine the spatial localization of protons, to see inside the body. It is especially useful for visualizing soft tissue.

In a study of mental imagery in six golfers using magnetic resonance imaging, decreased brain activation was found to occur with increased golf skill level for the supplementary motor area and cerebellum with little activation of the basal ganglia. The golfers were asked to mentally rehearse their golf swings from a first person perspective, i.e. they used 'internal imagery.'

Bibliography

Ross, J.S. et al. (2003). The mind's eye: Functional MR imaging evaluation of golf motor imagery. *American Journal of Neuroradiology* 24(6), 1033-1034.

MAGNUS EFFECT

The curve in the path of a spinning object, such as a ball, caused by a pressure differential on either side of the ball. One side of the ball spins against the airflow, causing the boundary layer to slow down that side. On the other side of the ball, because it is moving in the same direction as the airflow, the boundary layer speeds up. By Bernoulli's principle, this results in a pressure differential on either side of the ball. The ball is deflected laterally towards the direction of the spin or the side on which there is a lower pressure area.

In a basketball shot, backspin decreases the air pressure above the ball and increases it below the ball. This creates an aerodynamic lift force (the **Magnus force**) that is perpendicular to the axis of rotation of the spinning basketball. This slows the forward speed of the ball even before it hits the rim and it will descend more vertically than a no-spin shot (bank shot).

In baseball, the curveball deflects toward the direction of the rotation on a smooth trajectory. A curveball with less speed will curve more, because it takes longer to get to the plate and consequently has more time to deflect. An effective curveball has to break both horizontally and vertically. To throw a curve ball, the ball is gripped by the seams with the thumb on one side and with the middle and index fingers on the other. The ball is thrown like a fastball except as the ball is released, a downward snapping of the wrist in conjunction with the fingers imparts a twelve-to-six o'clock rotation on the ball. If the pitcher throws properly, the back of his hand will be facing the batter at the end of the motion. The ball will break down and away from a right-handed batter if thrown by a right-handed pitcher.

Chronology

•1853 • Heinrich Gustav Magnus first explained how sideways force would be generated on a spinning sphere. A surface layer of air, called the boundary layer, is picked up. This creates a difference in pressure and air speed on different sides of the ball. When a spinning ball is moving forward, one side is turning in the direction of the flight, the other away from it. On the side turning away from the direction of flight, more air 'sticks' in the boundary layer and it must move past the ball relatively faster than the air on the other side. Following Bernoulli's (1738) theorem, the result is less pressure on the side where the air is moving fastest.

•1997 • In a World Cup match against France, Roberto Carlos of Brazil took a free kick 35 yards from the French goal. He hit the ball with the outside of his left foot, sending it to the right of the human wall, apparently well away from the goal mouth. Having reached a peak velocity of 85 mph, the ball then suddenly swerved left into the goal. Between 60 mph and 80 mph critical changes in turbulence can occur. Thus, the ball may have slowed to enable the turbulence around it to alter suddenly causing the Magnus effect.

Bibliography

Zumerchik, J. (1997, ed). *Encyclopedia of sports science*. New York: Macmillan Library Reference.

MAISONNEUVE FRACTURE *See under* ANKLE LIGAMENTS; TIBIA-FIBULAR FRACTURE.

MALAISE A feeling of discomfort or uneasiness that is often the first indication of an infection or other disease.

MALALIGNMENTS *See under* MISALIGN-MENTS.

MALATE-ASPARTATE SHUTTLE *See under* MITOCHONDRIAL MEMBRANE SHUTTLES.

MALIGNANT i) Resistant to medical treatment. It refers to a condition with high mortality. ii) *See under* NEOPLASM.

MALLET FINGER Closed rupture of the distal extensor tendon of the finger at or near its insertion on the terminal phalanx. An injury that is caused by a sudden flexion force on the distal interphalangeal joint while the finger is actively extended, e.g. when a player is poised to catch a ball. As a result, the tendon of the *extensor digitorum* muscle may be avulsed from the distal phalanx, with or without a piece of bone. The counterpart of mallet finger is jersey finger.

MALLET TOE Flexion posture of the distal interphalangeal joint. It is a deformity that occurs when the joint at the end of the toe cannot straighten. It is often caused by bone and muscle imbalances. It may occur as an isolated disorder, or along with hammer toe. Mallet toe is common in diabetics with peripheral neuropathy. Shoes with a high and broad toe box are recommended for people suffering from forefoot deformities such as mallet toes.

MALTODEXTRINS Dextrins. Glucose polymers produced from the hydrolysis of corn starch. Maltodextrin molecules are larger than maltose (a disaccharide), but smaller than the starch molecules from which they are derived. Maltodextrins are often added to carbohydrate-electrolyte drinks. *See* FLUID REPLACEMENT.

MALTOSE *See under* CARBOHYDRATE.

MANAGEMENT *See under* LEADERSHIP.

MANGANESE A metallic element that, as a 'trace element,' is part of the mineral apatite in bone, where about 25% of the body's manganese is found. Manganese is also found in tissues that have a high concentration of mitochondria. It is a component of several enzymes and a co-factor for several enzymes, including the antioxidant enzyme, manganese-superoxide dismutase. This antioxidant enzyme is located in the mitochondria and is responsible for eliminating superoxide radicals produced by oxidative phosphorylation.

Rich sources of manganese include whole grains, nuts, leafy vegetables and teas. Foods high in phytic acid, such as beans, seeds, nuts, whole grains and soy products; or foods high in oxalic acid, such as spinach, may slightly inhibit manganese absorption. Although teas are rich sources of manganese, the tannins present in tea may moderately decrease the absorption of manganese. Whole wheat bread (one slice) contains 0.65 mg of manganese. Spinach (half a cup, cooked) contains 0.84 mg of manganese. The adequate intake for adults is 2.3 mg (males) and 1.8 mg/day (females). The tolerable upper intake level (UL) is set at 11 mg for adults, based on a research showing that no adverse health effects occurred when this amount was consumed on a chronic basis. Neurological side effects have been observed in persons consuming 15 mg per day.

Bibliography
Oregon State University. The Linus Pauling Institute. Micronutrient Information Center. Http://lpi.oregonstate.edu/infocenter

MANIC DEPRESSION *See* BIPOLAR DISORDER.

MANIPULATION   Use of the hands. **Intrinsic movements** involve coordinated movements of the individual digits used to manage an object already in the hand. **Extrinsic movements** involve displacing both the hand and the in-hand object through movements of the upper limb. A **simple synergy** occurs when all hand movements in which the action of all the digits, including the thumb, are similar. A **reciprocal synergy** occurs when a combination of movements involving the thumb and other involved digits reciprocally and simultaneously interact to produce relatively dissimilar movements.

MARCH FRACTURE   A stress fracture of the 2nd or 3rd metatarsal. It is known as a 'march fracture,' because it is common in foot soldiers. It is the most common stress fracture.

MARFAN SYNDROME   A connective tissue disorder that affects many organ systems, including the skeleton, lungs, eyes, heart and blood vessels. It is an autosomal dominant disorder stemming from defects in the FBN1 gene that encodes fibrillin-1. **Fibrillin** is a large glycoprotein that is a calcium-binding component of certain connective tissue microfibrils. In 25% of people, Marfan syndrome develops due to a spontaneous mutation.

Prevalence of Marfan syndrome is at least 1 per 5,000 in the general population. It is estimated that 200,000 people in the USA have Marfan syndrome or a related connective tissue disorder.

Skeletal manifestations of Marfan syndrome include scoliosis, pectus deformity, loose jointedness and disproportionate growth that usually results in tall stature. About 50% of people with Marfan syndrome have dislocation of the ocular lens. People with Marfan syndrome are often near sighted (myopic).

The major risks to an athlete with Marfan syndrome are cardiovascular problems arising from the two primary defects: aortic root dilation and mitral valve prolapse. The aorta is generally wider and more fragile in patients with Marfan syndrome. This widening is progressive and can cause leakage of the aortic valve or tears (dissection) in the aorta wall. When the aorta becomes greatly widened, surgical repair is necessary. The risk of sudden death increases as aortic root diameter increases. Treatment with beta-blockers limits the progression of aortic dilation. Various surgical techniques are possible.

Bibliography
Marfan Association UK. Http://www.marfan.org.uk
National Marfan Foundation. Http://www.marfan.org
Pyeritz, R.E. (2001). Disorders of vascular fragility. Implications for active patients. *The Physician and Sportsmedicine*. 29(6), 53-59.

MARIJUANA   A preparation of leafy material from the cannabis plant, containing the drug delta-9 tetrahydrocannabinol (THC). Marijuana is the most frequently used illegal drug in the USA. It can be smoked or mixed with a food or drink and consumed orally. **Hash** (**hashish**) is a more concentrated form of the plant that is up to ten times more powerful than marijuana. After intake, THC undergoes metabolism to an inactive metabolite (8-11-DiOH-THC) and also to a highly active metabolite (11-OH-delta-9-THC). The half-life of THC is approximately 4 hours. The long life of the active metabolite is explained by the incorporation of the compound in lipid storage depots and similar storage sites in muscle tissue. 30 to 60% of THC, in all forms, is excreted in feces; the remaining amount is excreted in urine.

For one cigarette smoked, maximal blood concentrations are normally obtained after 3 to 8 minutes, the onset of action on the central nervous system is observed in approximately 20 minutes and peak effect in 2 to 4 hours. Duration of action for psychological effects is 4 to 6 hours.

THC binding sites are distributed widely throughout the brain. The density of these sites is highest in the basal ganglia and cerebellum. They are moderately dense in the hippocampus and cortex. A number of brain neurochemical changes seem to occur after THC penetrates the blood-brain barrier, including an increase in the synthesis of catecholamines, increased GABA and increased sensitivity of brain cells to dopamine. Marijuana affects the brain's reward system by enhancing the processes that produce reward that is the 'high' sought by the user. It appears that stimulation of THC receptor sites in the brain activates the same parts of the brain that are stimulated by opiates, such as heroin and morphine. The drug **naloxone** blocks the actions of opiates, and has also been found to block the effects of marijuana. Marijuana produces both excitation and depression of the central nervous system. The cholinergic changes in the hippocampal region of the brain may be linked to memory and perceptual dysfunction. It is thought that the euphoria, and distortion of time and space, is related to the release of serotonin.

Marijuana use has contributed to more motor vehicle crashes than any drug except alcohol. After smoking one marijuana cigarette, driving skills are impaired for the next four to six hours. It affects the driver's judgment, concentration, slows down the eyes' ability to adjust to changes in light and distorts perception of time and space.

Other adverse effects of marijuana use include: headaches and dizziness; disturbances with short-term memory and learning; trouble with thinking and problem solving; loss of coordination; hilarity without cause; paradoxical hyperalertness; and paranoia and anxiety or panic attacks. It is also associated with increased appetite (the 'munchies'). People who eat marijuana may experience nausea and vomiting. Heavy marijuana users suffer greater cognitive impairment. At very high doses, marijuana can produce severe psychotic symptoms such as hallucinations and delusions. Sperm count is lower among chronic marijuana users than non-users. Young

women are at an increased risk of infertility due to chronic marijuana use.

There are long-term risks to health, including chronic bronchitis. Marijuana contains more than 400 chemicals, many of which are considered carcinogenic when smoked. The amount of tar inhaled by marijuana smokers and the level of carbon monoxide absorbed are three to five times greater than among tobacco smokers. This may be due to marijuana users inhaling more deeply and holding the smoke in the lungs. Teenagers who already smoke cigarettes and drink alcohol are more likely to use marijuana.

Heavy marijuana use can inhibit ovulation and disrupt the menstrual cycle in women. It can decrease sperm counts in men. Long-term marijuana use decreases sexual function.

Common marijuana withdrawal symptoms include restlessness, loss of appetite, insomnia, weight loss and shaky hands.

According to data from the 1998 National Household Survey on Drug Abuse, more than 72 million Americans (33%) aged 12 years and older have tried marijuana at least once in their lifetime. In the USA, marijuana is classified as a Schedule I drug by the Federal Drug Agency (FDA), i.e. it has a high potential for abuse, has no currently accepted medical use in the USA and it has no safe level of use under medical supervision. In 1996, medical use of marijuana was approved by statewide ballot initiatives in California and Arizona, thus setting up a dichotomy between state and federal law. THC, available in pill form as Marinol®, is a Schedule II drug (i.e. legal only with a prescription and is considered to have less potential for abuse than Schedule I or II drugs) that can be effective in relieving nausea and/or restoring appetite to some chemotherapy and AIDS patients. Adverse effects of Marinol® include somnolence (drowsiness), dizziness, euphoria and paranoid reactions. Anxiety and heart palpitations may also occur. When used in higher doses, amnesia, ataxia and hallucinations have been reported.

Doping with marijuana is tested by means of urinalysis of 11-nor-delta-9-tetrahydrocannabinol-9-carboxylic acid (carboxy-THC), the main metabolite of delta-9-tetrahydrocannobinol (THC). Because

THC is absorbed by and stored in fatty tissue in the body, it can be detected by a urine test for up to one month after marijuana is smoked (and even longer in chronic abusers). Exposure to secondhand marijuana smoke can lead to a positive result on a drug test, because THC is released into the air when marijuana is smoked.

In 1989, the International Olympic Committee (IOC) included marijuana in its list of prohibited drugs under the title of classes of prohibited substances in certain circumstances. Cannabinoids now form a category of substances prohibited by the World Anti-Doping Agency (WADA) in all sports. Concentrations of greater than 15 ng/mL in confirmatory analytical procedures are considered doping by WADA.

Chronology
•2,700 BC • Marijuana was used in the Chinese Empire in the treatment of malaria and rheumatism.
•1998 • The Canadian snowboarder Ross Rebagliati was stripped of his gold medal after he was drug tested and found to have 17.8 nanograms of marijuana per liter of urine. The International Ski Federation has a limit of 15 nanograms before declaring a positive. Rebagliati claimed that he was a victim of passive smoking at a party prior to the Olympics and his gold medal was subsequently reinstated. Marijuana can remain in the urine for up to four weeks, but David Cowan, director of the IOC-accredited laboratory at King's College (London) said that research into the effects of passive smoking showed that to reach the level of 15 nanograms, researchers had been forced to wear goggles to protect their eyes from the effects of the smoke. Rebagliati could not be stripped of his medal, because the International Ski Federation and the International Olympic Committee (IOC) did not have an agreement regarding testing for marijuana at the Games.

Bibliography
Campos, D.R., Yonamine, M. and de Moraes Moreau, R.L. (2003). Marijuana as doping in sports. *Sports Medicine* 33(6), 395-399.
Daly, R.C. (2002). Cannabis compound abuse. Http://www.emedicine.com
Hayden, J.W. (1991). Passive inhalation of marijuana smoke: Critical review. *Journal of Substance Abuse* 3, 85-90.
Wagner, J.C. (1991). Enhancement of athletic performance with drugs. An overview. *Sports Medicine* 12(4), 250-65.
World Anti-Doping Agency. Http://www.wada-ama.org

MASS   The amount of matter contained in an object. It is a measure of a body's resistance to being accelerated. The Standard International unit is the kilogram (kg). The US Customary unit is pound mass (lbm). 1 kg = 2.24 lbm; lbm = 0.453 kg.

MASS ACTION EFFECT   *See under* LACTIC ACID.

MASS ACTION LAW   *See under* CHEMICAL REACTIONS.

MASSAGE   Sports massage incorporates a wide range of manipulative techniques including rubbing, kneading and tapping of body parts. It is used before exercise as a substitute for, or supplement to, conventional warm up and stretching. After a game or training session, it is used with the aim of accelerating elimination of waste products from muscles. As a method of treatment for injuries, it is used to promote the treatment of strained muscles, to decrease edema, for pain relief and for breaking down adhesions in an old injury. There is evidence that vigorous massage has modest effects on local blood flow. The mechanism for this effect is most likely related to pressure changes produced by massage, rather than the release of any active vasodilatory substance.

There is little or no scientific evidence to support the claim that oxygen transport, metabolic processes or endorphin release are substantially influenced by massage. There is little scientific evidence that massage has any significant impact on the short- or long-term recovery of muscle function following exercise. There is some evidence that post-exercise massage may alleviate symptoms of delayed-onset muscle soreness. Contraindications to massage include pathology of a circulatory, dermatological or cardiac nature.

Chronology
•1984 • The US Olympic Committee made massage available to American athletes in the Olympic Games.

Bibliography
Benjamin, P.J. and Lamp, S.P. (1996). *Understanding sports massage*. Champaign, IL: Human Kinetics.
Cafarelli, E. and Flint, F. (1992). The role of massage in preparation for and recovery from exercise. *Sports Medicine* 14(1), 1-9.
Ernst, E. (1998). Does post-exercise massage treatment reduce delayed onset muscle soreness? A systematic review. *British*

Journal of Sports Medicine 32(3), 212-214.

King, R.K. (1993). *Pre-performance massage*. Champaign, IL: Human Kinetics.

Samples, P. (1987). Does 'sports massage' have a role in sports medicine? *The Physician and Sportsmedicine* 15, 177-183.

Tiidus, P.M. (1997). Manual massage and recovery of muscle function following exercise: A literature review. *Journal of Orthopaedic and Sports Physical Therapy* 35(2), 107-112.

Tiidus, P.M. (1999). Massage and ultrasound as therapeutic modalities in exercise-induced muscle damage. *Canadian Journal of Applied Physiology* 24(3), 267-278.

MASS FLOW The mass of a fluid in motion, which crosses a given area in a given time.

MASS REFLEX A withdrawal response, triggered by a minor noxious stimulus, accompanied by a massive response of the autonomic nervous system that may include evacuation of the bladder and bowel.

MASS SPECTROMETERS *See under* OXYGEN UPTAKE, MEASUREMENT OF.

MAST CELLS Cells found in connective tissue that help signal the early events of inflammation by releasing histamine.

MASTOCYTOSIS A condition characterized by excessive accumulation of mast cells in various body organs and tissues. The cause is unknown.

MATERIALS Four basic groups of materials are metals (e.g. aluminum, steel, titanium), ceramics (e.g. glass, concrete), polymers (e.g. rubber, plastic, synthetic fibers) and composites (e.g. wood, graphite, fiber glass). **Composites** are mixtures of two materials, usually fibers or powders of one material in a matrix of another. **Fiberglass** is comprised of glass fibers in a matrix of polyester resin. **Graphite** composites are made from carbon fibers in epoxy resin. One advantage of a multi-material composite, as opposed to a single material, is that it allows equipment to be customized to meet particular stress requirements. Usually, this entails strengthening the equipment to withstand both tensile stress and compressive stress, in addition to torsion and shearing.

Recurve bows, originally made by Turks and now used in target archery, are relatively small but have a high ratio of draw length to bow length, i.e. the limbs can be drawn back much farther, relative to the overall length of the bow. The Turkish bow was composed of animal sinew, which was effective against tensile forces, and horn that resisted compressive forces.

Until the 1990s, skis were manufactured as either a soft, flexing ski for soft and deep snow or a stiff, rigid ski for the packed snow on which most competitions take place. Using new composite materials, however, skis can be manufactured with both rigidity and flexibility to perform well under most conditions.

Selecting materials for sports equipment involves trade-offs among elasticity, strength and weight.

A vaulting pole requires elasticity (to maximize the amount of energy returned to the vaulting athlete as the bent pole gradually straightens), strength (to minimize breakage) and lightness (to maximize approach velocity). A vault causes both compression on the side nearer the athlete and tension on the side farther away from the athlete. When a bamboo vault broke in two, the splitting started from the tension force on the far side of the pole. Aluminum poles were developed in the 1940s. Like composite poles, aluminum poles have a high Young's modulus (stiffness) and thus low energy loss (i.e. they transfer energy efficiently). A fiberglass pole, consisting of up to 12 layers of glass fiber wrapped around a thin metal cylinder, is slightly thicker around the middle, where it bends most, and tapered towards the ends. Fiberglass poles, introduced in the 1960s, allow a higher handhold, significantly increasing the height an athlete can reach. Such poles are effective at transforming a large fraction (c. 90%) of the athlete's initial kinetic energy into gravitational potential energy, through the intermediary of elastic potential energy. The yield strength of the fiberglass composite is comparable to the aluminum pole that it replaced, but the fiberglass composite is much lighter. The latest poles contain a mixture of fiberglass and carbon fiber.

See also ELASTIC MODULUS; STRUCTURE.

Chronology

•1957 • Bob Gutowski used an aluminium pole to set a world record of 4.78 meters in the pole vault. Gutowski's record was broken in the same year by Don Bragg, who used a steel pole to clear 4.80 meters.

•1961 • The first world record was set using fiberglass was set. Used as early as 1948, the fiberglass pole came to prominence after it was used in the 1956 Olympic Games.

•1962 • Marine corporal John Uelses used a newly-designed fiberglass pole to reach the hitherto "unreachable" height of 16 feet.

•1972 • At the US Olympic trials, Bob Seagren set a world record in the pole vault of 18 feet 5.25 inches using a fiberglass pole. A month before the Olympic Games, the fiberglass pole was banned by the International Amateur Athletics Federation (IAAF) due to its limited availability. Seagren was Olympic champion at the 1968 Olympics (17 feet, 8 and _ inches), but finished second in the 1972 Olympic Games.

Bibliography

Easterling, K.E. (1992). *Advanced materials in sports equipment: How advanced materials help optimise sporting performance and make sport safer*. London: Chapman and Hall.

Zumerchik, J. (1997, ed). *Encyclopedia of sports science*. New York: Macmillan Library Reference.

MATTER   Anything that occupies space and has mass.

MATURATION   *See under* GROWTH.

MAXILLA   Upper-jaw bone. *See under* TEMPOROMANDIBULAR JOINT.

MCARDLE'S DISEASE   Myophosphorylase deficiency. Myophosphorylase deficiency. Glycogenosis type 5. A rare carbohydrate processing disorder, involving lack, or defective function, of the skeletal muscle enzyme phosphorylase. Onset of McArdle's disease occurs between childhood and adolescence with symptoms including muscle cramps that usually occur after exercise. Intensive exercise can cause muscle destruction and possible kidney damage. It is inherited as an autosomal recessive trait. A person with McArdle's disease may tolerate light-to-moderate exercise, such as walking on level ground, but strenuous exercise will usually bring on symptoms quickly.

MCL   Medial collateral ligament. *See under* KNEE LIGAMENTS.

MECHANICAL ADVANTAGE   *See under* MACHINE.

MECHANICS   *See under* BIOMECHANICS.

MECHANORECEPTORS   Specialized nerve endings that respond to mechanical stimuli such as touch, pressure, compression, stretch and vibration. The function of mechanoreceptors is to transduce some form of mechanical deformation into a frequency-modulated neural signal that is transmitted via afferent and efferent pathways.

Touch, pressure and vibration are classified as separate sensations, but the same types of receptors detect them. The **touch** sensation results from stimulation of tactile receptors in the skin; **pressure** sensation results from deformation of deeper tissues; and **vibration** sensation results from rapidly repetitive sensory signals. All the different tactile receptors are involved in detection of vibration, though different receptors detect different frequencies.

Ruffini endings, located in joint capsules, respond to change in joint position and velocity of movement of the joint. They have a low threshold for activation and are slow adapting. **Ruffini corpuscles**, located in the individual joint ligaments, are slower adapting and have a higher threshold for activation. **Pacinian corpuscles**, located in joints capsules and connective tissue, respond to pressure created by muscle and detect joint acceleration. They also respond to pain and are quick adapting with a very low threshold for activation.

A **cutaneous receptor** is a sensory receptor that is sensitive to such stimuli as skin displacement, pressure on the skin and temperature. These receptors include Pacinian corpuscles, Merkel disks, Meissner corpuscles and Ruffini endings. A **Meissner corpuscle** is a cutaneous mechanoreceptor that is sensitive to local, maintained pressure. A **Merkel disk** is a cutaneous mechanoreceptor that is sensitive to local vertical pressure.

Distributed everywhere in the skin and in all tissues, **free nerve endings** respond to many somatic sensory modalities but adapt slowly. **Thermoreceptors** are mainly free nerve endings. There are warm spots and cold spots in the skin. The cold receptors are located near the surface of the skin; the warm receptors are deeper and therefore their latency is longer. The number of cold receptors is three to ten times higher than the number of warm receptors. **Nociceptive free nerve endings** are situated in muscle, ligament and cutaneous tissue. They are sensitive to touch, pressure and pain.

See also GOLGI TENDON ORGANS; MUSCLE SPINDLES; PROPRIOCEPTIVE FEEDBACK.

MEDIA   *See under* COMMERCIALISM.

MEDIAL   Toward or relating to the mid-line of the body.

MEDIAL COLLERAL LIGAMENT   *See under* KNEE LIGAMENTS.

MEDIAL EPICONDYLITIS   'Golfer's elbow.' It is tendinosis of the common flexor-pronator origin adjacent to the medial epicondyle. The pathology is generally at the interface of the *pronator teres* and *flexor carpi radialis* muscles, but may also affect the *flexor carpi ulnaris* muscle. In golf, the common flexor origin of the right elbow (in a right-handed player) is placed under valgus stress at, or near, the top of the backswing and proceeds through the downswing to just before impact with the ball. In tennis, it results from excessive loading during the forehand and service strokes. In elite tennis players, it is usually caused by the 'American twist' serve, in which the wrist is flexed at the same time as the forearm is pronated. The twist serve, which imparts a combination of topspin and some sideways rotation, is used frequently for second serves and may spin at greater than 4,000 rpm (often twice as great as the first serve). On the forehand stroke, attempting to hit the ball with exaggerated topspin is a risk factor, because it involves excessive pronation. It occurs frequently in throwing (e.g. javelin), which includes a high-velocity valgus extension mechanism. Ulnar nerve symptoms are present in 60% of medial epicondylitis cases. Medial epicondylitis is about one fifth as frequent as lateral epicondylitis.

MEDIAL TIBIAL STRESS SYNDROME   It is the most common cause of exertional leg pain in athletes, especially in those participating in repetitive activities (especially jumping and running). Pain usually starts after exercise and is relieved by rest. Korkola and Amendola (2001) use the term medial tibial stress syndrome to refer to periostitis of the posteromedial tibia or as a synonym for periostitis. Detmer (1986) classified medial tibial stress syndrome into three distinct entities: periostitis, deep posterior compartment syndrome and tibial stress fracture. Although these conditions are related and may coexist, they should be considered three distinct diagnoses.

One theory of medial tibial stress syndrome implicates periosteal traction. This theory is limited in a number of ways, however; e.g. by the fact that the injury site coincides with only small areas of the origins of implicated muscles (*soleus* and *flexor digitorum longus*) and fascia (deep crural). An alternative theory is that chronic repetitive loads induce tibial bending and precipitate stress injury at the site, about which maximum bending occurs.

Risk factors include: changes in surface; shoes; technique; prolonged, intensive training on hard surfaces; rear foot varus; genu valgus; excessive forefoot pronation; and high instep.

Bibliography
Beck, B.R. (1998). Tibial stress injuries. An aetiological review for the purposes of guiding management. *Sports Medicine* 26(4), 265-279.

Detmer, D.E. (1986). Chronic shin splints: Classification and management of medial tibial stress syndrome. *Sports Medicine* 3(6), 436-446.

Korkola, M. and Amendola, A. (2001). Exercise-induced leg pain. *The Physician and Sportsmedicine* 29(6), 35-50.

MEDIAN NERVE   A nerve that receives contributions from both medial (C8, T1 roots) and lateral cords (C5-C7 roots). The nerve travels distally across the medial aspect of the arm and enters the forearm between the two heads of the *pronator teres* muscle. It then travels underneath the *flexor digitorum superficialis* muscle and gives off a purely motor branch, the anterior interosseus nerve, as it passes. The main trunk of the median nerve then travels distally down the forearm and through the carpal tunnel. The median nerve, along with eight flexor tendons, runs through the carpal tunnel on the volar surface of the wrist. It is the sensory nerve to the radial three and one-half fingers of the hand, and it also provides motor innervation of the thenar muscles. The extensible borders formed by the carpal bones and the flexor retinaculum preclude an increase in the size of the carpal tunnel.

See also ANTERIOR INTEROSSEUS SYNDROME; PRONATOR TERES SYNDROME.

MEDIASTINUM The median partition of the thoracic cavity.

MEDITATION A set of procedures designed to produce relaxation and an altered state of consciousness, which is associated with religious or spiritual beliefs, such as Zen Buddhism. A variety of techniques are used, e.g. control of breathing, focusing of attention on some object, unusual body postures, imagery and repetition of sound patterns (audibly uttered or imagined). Transcendental Meditation is based on ancient Hinduism, and was popularized by the Maharishi Mahesh. Benson's (1975) 'Relaxation Response' has been described as Transcendental Meditation without the mystical overtones.

See AUTOGENIC TRAINING; BIOFEEDBACK; HYPNOSIS; MIND-BODY EXERCISE; PROGRESSIVE RELAXATION; PSYCHOLOGICAL SKILLS TRAINING.

Bibliography
Benson, H. (1975). *The relaxation response*. New York: Morrow.

MEDIUM CHAIN TRIGLYCERIDES Fats that have fatty-acid chains of 6 to 12 carbon atoms long and contain 8.2 calories per gram as opposed to the 16 to 22 carbon atoms and 9.5 calories per gram of long-chain triglycerides. The fatty acids of medium-chain triglycerides are more soluble in water than long-chain triglycerides allowing the body to absorb them easier. Normal long-chain triglycerides enter the blood 3 to 4 hours after ingestion and are bound to chylomicrons. Medium-chain triglycerides are transported directly from the small intestine to the liver by the main portal vein. They are then converted to ketones that the muscles can use for energy. They diffuse into muscle rapidly, because they do not require the transport mechanisms that limit the rate

of uptake of long-chain fatty acids. Medium-chain triglycerides are oxidized at a rate comparable to exogenous glucose. Clinically, medium-chain triglycerides are used to treat malabsorption disorders. Medium-chain triglycerides increase thermogenesis via brown fat. Dietary supplements containing medium-chain triglycerides are sold on the basis that they can increase energy expenditure and decrease body fat. Evidence from research on rats has found that feeding medium-chain triglycerides increases energy expenditure and leads to smaller deposition in storage fat. There is some evidence that feeding medium-chain triglycerides increases thermogenesis in humans. It has been proposed that medium-chain triglycerides may enhance 'ultra-endurance' by either sparing the intra-muscular lipid and carbohydrate stores, or by augmenting the rate of utilization of extra-muscular lipid when the intra-muscular pool becomes depleted. There is no convincing evidence, however, to support an ergogenic effect of medium-chain triglycerides ingestion prior to exercise. Furthermore, most individuals cannot consume more than 30 g of ingested medium-chain triglycerides without experiencing severe gastrointestinal discomfort and diarrhea. Medium-chain triglycerides are not recommended for individuals who have diabetes or liver disease. Increased mobilization of free fatty acids would not seem to be of any value for untrained people, because their mobilization of free fatty acids normally exceeds the ability of the muscles to oxidize free fatty acids.

Bibliography
Berning, J.R. (1996). The role of medium-chain triglycerides in exercise. *International Journal of Sport Nutrition* 6(2), 121-133.
Hawley, J.A. and Hopkins, W.G. (1995). Aerobic glycolytic and aerobic lipolytic power systems. A new paradigm with implications for endurance and ultra-endurance events. *Sports Medicine* 19(4), 240-250.
Jeukendrup, A.E., Saris, W.H. and Wagenmakers, A.J. (1998). Fat metabolism during exercise: A review. Part III: Effects of nutritional interventions. *International Journal of Sports Medicine* 19(6), 371-379.

MEDULLA *See under* ADRENAL GLANDS; BRAIN.

MEGADOSE   10 or more times the recommended amount of a nutrient or drug.

MEGAKARYOCYTE   A huge cell in the bone marrow that produces blood platelets.

MEGALOBLASTS   *See under* ANEMIA.

MELATONIN   *See under* JET LAG.

MEMBRANE LIPIDS   Polar lipids. These are major components of cell membranes. The most abundant membrane lipids are the phospholipids, including choline. *See* LECITHIN.

MEMORY CELLS   *See under* LYMPHOCYTES.

MENARCHE   *See under* MENSTRUAL CYCLE.

MENINGES   The three membranes that cover the spinal cord: arachnoidea, dura mater and pia mater.

MENISCI   *See under* KNEE MENISCI.

MENOPAUSE   *See under* ESTROGENS; MENSTRUAL CYCLE.

MENSTRUAL CYCLE   It is the monthly cycle of changes in the hypothalamus, pituitary gland, ovaries, uterus and other parts of females. It involves the gonadotropic hormones, estrogens and progesterone. **Menarche**, the beginning of menstrual function, usually begins between the ages of 12 to 15 years. Each menstrual cycle usually lasts 28 to 30 days, ceasing only during pregnancy or lactation. At 45 to 50 years of age, the menstrual cycle ceases altogether. **Menopause** occurs when a whole year has passed without menstruation. After menopause, 1% of bone is lost each year until the end of life. This is due to osteoporosis.

The three major phases of the menstrual cycle are the proliferation, secretory and menstrual phases. The **proliferation phase** prepares the uterus for fertilization and lasts about 10 days. A hypothalamic-releasing factor (follicle stimulating hormone-releasing factor) causes the release of follicle-stimulating hormone from the pituitary gland, initiating the growth of one Graafian follicle in the ovaries and its consequent increased production of estrogens. High estrogen levels eventually inhibit the release of follicle stimulating hormone-releasing factor and luteinizing hormone-releasing factor from the hypothalamus, decreasing follicle-stimulating hormone and luteinizing hormone output. About two days prior to ovulation, there is a marked increase in output of luteinizing hormone from the pituitary gland. This induces the rupture of the Graafian follicle from which an ovum is discharged about 15 days before the next menstrual period. The proliferation phase ends when the ovum is released from the Graafian follicle.

The **secretory phase** involves a thickening of the endometrium as the uterus prepares for pregnancy. It lasts 10 to 14 days. After the escape of the ovum from the ruptured follicle, blood fills up the follicle and the corpus luteum (a mass of cells found in the ruptured Graafian follicle) secretes progesterone. This stimulates the growth and secretion of the endometrial glands of the uterus during the fourteen days before menstruation.

The **menstrual (flow) phase** lasts 4 to 5 days (days 28 to 4 in a normal menstrual cycle). **Menstruation** involves the shedding of the endometrium. If there is no pregnancy, the menstrual cycle repeats immediately as follicle stimulating hormone-releasing factor is released again. If pregnancy occurs, maintenance of the corpus luteum is sustained for a short period by luteinizing hormone and then by human chorionic gonadotropin, which is secreted by the implanted blastocyst and later by the placenta. A **blastocyst** is a hollow ball of cells that later becomes the embryo and then the fetus.

The **ovarian cycle** consists of two phases: the follicular and luteal phases. The **follicular phase** corresponds to the menstrual and proliferation phases of the menstrual cycle. It ends on day 14 of a 28-day menstrual cycle when ovulation occurs. The **luteal phase** corresponds to the secretory phase of the menstrual cycle.

The prevalence of menstrual cycle alterations in athletes is considerably higher than in non-athletes. Irregular menses have been reported to range from 1 to 66% among athletes, compared with 2 to 5% of the general population. In women who have been ovulating regularly, the most prevalent change with training is a decrease in normal pre-menstrual symptoms (such as breast enlargement or tenderness) followed by a shortening of the luteal phase. **Luteal suppression** may be an intermediate condition between menstrual regularity and secondary amenorrhea in athletes. Alternatively, it may be the endpoint of a successful adaptation to exercise training.

Personal best performances have been achieved during all phases of the menstrual cycle. Best performances tend to occur in the immediate postmenstrual days, while worst performances occur during the pre-menstrual interval (days 25 to 28 of a normal cycle) and the first few days of menstrual flow. Some women suffer **premenstrual syndrome** (PMS) and experience depression, edema, sore and swollen breasts, low back pain and unexplained fatigue. **Menorrhagia (**excessive flow) may be a contraindication for exercise. Time to exhaustion at sub-maximal exercise intensities shows no change over the menstrual cycle. There is some research evidence of a higher cardiovascular strain occurring during moderate exercise in the mid-luteal phase. During prolonged exercise in hot conditions, a decrease in exercise time to exhaustion is shown during the mid-luteal phase, when body temperature is elevated. Increased progesterone and estradiol levels during the luteal phase lead to a net fluid retention, because of a complex interaction of renin, angiotensin and aldosterone. This does not seem to have a significant overall effect on performance.

Even when hormone concentrations are measured, the possible effects of the menstrual cycle on exercise performance may be obscured by a combination of differences in timing of testing, the high inter- and intra-individual variability in estrogen and progesterone concentration, the pulsatile nature of their secretion and their interaction.

See also AMENORRHEA; ESTROGENS; ORAL CONTRACEPTIVES.

Chronology
•1877 • In her book, *The Question of Rest for Women During*

Menstruation, Mary Putnam Jacobi argued that women did not need to refrain from physical activity during menstruation. The *Journal of Nervous and Mental Diseases* gave Jacobi's monograph a glowing review, noting the thoroughness and use of extensive statistical evidence and familiarity with important scientific and medical works. The reviewer could find little to disagree with, except Jacobi's contention that women's "motor apparatus" was not inferior to that of the men's, and that women were inherently intellectually inferior.

•1894 • Celia Mosher, an assistant in hygiene at Stanford University, conducted research that supported her battle for dress reform in women (e.g. abandonment of stiff corsets). Mosher showed that women were able to enjoy orgasms and that corsets and restrictive Victorian clothing affected menstruation and distorted the body's internal organs.

•1922 • An article entitled "The Influence of Games on the Sex Health of Girls" by Mary Stansfield discussed the relation of strenuous activity to menstrual functioning and childbirth.

Bibliography
Arena, B. et al. (1995). Reproductive hormones and menstrual changes with exercise in female athletes. *Sports Medicine* 19(4), 278-287.

Baxter-Jones, A.D. (1994). Menarche in intensively trained gymnasts, swimmers and tennis players. *Annals of Human Biology* 21(5), 407-415.

Easton, R.G. (1984). *The regular menstrual cycle and physical activity*. Champaign, IL: Human Kinetics Publishers.

Janse de Jonge, X.A. (2003). Effects of the menstrual cycle on exercise performance. *Sports Medicine* 33(11), 833-851.

Lebrun, C.M. (1993). Effect of the different phases of the menstrual cycle and oral contraceptives on athletic performance. *Sports Medicine* 16(5), 295-304.

Loucks, A.B. (1990). Effects of exercise training on the menstrual cycle: Existence and mechanisms. *Medicine and Science in Sports and Exercise* 22(3), 275-280.

Marti, B. (1991). Health effects of recreational running in women. Some epidemiological and preventive aspects. *Sports Medicine* 11(1), 20-51.

Prior, J.C., Vigna, Y.M. and McKay, D.W. (1992). Reproduction for the athletic woman. New understandings of physiology and management. *Sports Medicine* 14(3), 190-9.

Shangold, M.M. (1988). Gynecological concerns in exercise and training. In: Shangold, M. and Mirkin, G. (eds). *Women and exercise: Physiology and sports medicine*. pp186-194. Philadelphia: FA Davis.

Sinning, W.E. and Little, K.D. (1987). Body composition and menstrual function in athletes. *Sports Medicine* 4, 34-45.

MENTAL DISORDERS   In the USA, the American Psychiatric Association (APA) is the professional organization that assumes responsibility for publishing the reference book on mental disorders, the *Diagnostic and Statistical Manual of Mental*

Disorders, which is used by all of the disciplines related to medicine, by courts of law and by insurance companies. Major categories in the latest version of this reference book, (DSM-IV) are: (i) disorders usually first diagnosed in infancy, childhood or adolescence, including mental retardation, attention deficit disorders and development problems; (ii) delirium, dementia, amnesia and other cognitive disorders resulting from brain damage, degenerative diseases such as syphilis or Alzheimer's, toxic substances, or drugs; (iii) substance-related disorders associated with excessive use of, or withdrawal from, alcohol and other drugs; (iv) schizophrenia and other psychotic disorders, characterized by delusions, hallucinations, and severe disturbances in thinking and emotion; (v) mood disorders; (vi) anxiety disorders; (vii) eating disorders; (viii) somatoform disorders, which involve physical symptoms (e.g. fatigue) for which no organic cause can be found; (ix) dissociative disorders, including dissociative amnesia, in which important events cannot be remembered after a traumatic event, and dissociative identity disorder, characterized by the presence of two or more distinct identities or personalities; (x) sexual and gender identity disorders, including problems of sexual (gender) identity, such as transsexualism (wanting to be the other gender) or problems of sexual performance (such as premature ejaculation or lack of orgasm); (xi) impulse control disorders, involving an inability to resist an impulse to perform some acts that is harmful to the individual or to others, such as pathological gambling, stealing (kleptomania), setting fires (pyromania) or having violent rages; and (xii) personality disorders. Additional conditions that may be a focus of clinical attention include "problems in living," such as bereavement, academic difficulties, spiritual problems and acculturation problems.

DSM-IV lists 10 conditions that are usually first diagnosed in infancy, childhood, or adolescence: i) mental retardation; ii) learning disorders; iii) developmental coordination disorder; iv) communication disorders; v) pervasive developmental disorders; vi) attention deficit and disruptive behavior disorders; vii) feeding and eating disorders (pica and rumination); viii) tic disorders; ix) elimination disorders (encopresis and enuresis); and x) other disorders (e.g. separation anxiety disorder, stereotypic movement disorders).

With each new edition of the *Diagnostic and Statistical Manual of Mental Disorders*, the number of mental disorders has grown. The first edition contained about 100 diagnoses; whereas DSM-IV contains nearly 400 diagnoses of mental disorders. There are a number of problems with the manual, including the danger of over-diagnosis. Since attention-deficit hyperactivity disorder was added to the manual, it has become the fastest-growing disorder in the USA, where it is diagnosed at least ten times as often as it is in Europe. Critics argue that child and youth behavior is being pathologized. Diagnostic labels have a powerful effect, and can create self-fulfilling prophecies. Each edition of the manual adds more everyday problems, e.g. "religious or spiritual problem," thus serious mental disorders may be confused with normal problems. An example of this concerns **dissociative identity**, commonly known as **multiple personality disorder**, which is marked by the apparent appearance within one person of two or more distinct personalities, each with its own name and traits. It could simply be an extreme form of the ability to present different aspects of one's personality or self to others. Diagnosis of multiple personality disorder was first included in the manual in 1980. In the USA, 6,000 cases were reported by 1986 and more than 40,000 cases by 1995. It has been argued that clinicians who believe in the prevalence of multiple personality disorder may actually be creating the disorder in their clients through the use of suggestive techniques such as hypnosis.

See also MENTAL HEALTH; PSYCHIATRY.

Bibliography

American Psychiatric Association (1994). *Diagnostic and Statistical Manual of Mental Disorders*. 4th ed. Washington, DC: American Psychiatric Association.

Wade, C. and Tavris, C. (2003). *Psychology*. 7th ed. Upper Saddle River, NJ: Prentice Hall.

MENTAL HEALTH Exercise has been found to be associated with improvements in aspects of mental health such as mood and self-esteem, although a causal link has not been established. There is evidence that 20 to 40 minutes of vigorous exercise results in improvements in state anxiety and mood that can last for several hours, but light exercise has little effect. These transitory changes occur in both individuals with normal or elevated levels of anxiety, but appear to be limited to aerobic forms of exercise.

The **Hyperthermic theory** may explain the 'feeling-better' effect of exercise. It concerns the elevation in body temperature associated with exercise and the resultant effects on the brain brought about by the hypothalamus. It is proposed that the hypothalamus detects the elevation in core temperature and then inhibits the thalamus. This results in decreased activation of the cerebral cortex, which leads to pleasant feelings of relaxation. Excessive exercise in activities such as running and swimming, however, can result in a negative emotional state. Bahrke and Morgan's (1978) **Distraction theory** proposes that being distracted from stressful stimuli, or taking 'time out' from one's daily routine, is responsible for the anxiety decrease seen with exercise. Another theory is that exercise activates the release of catecholamines, which in turn are associated with euphoric and positive mood states.

Although people with depression tend to be less physically active than those who are non-depressed, increased aerobic exercise or strength training has been shown to decrease depressive symptoms significantly. Habitual physical activity has not been shown to prevent the onset of depression. Anxiety symptoms and panic disorder also improve with regular exercise, and beneficial effects appear to equal meditation or relaxation.

Exercise can be used to treat mild-to-moderate depression. Aerobic exercise seems to be effective in improving general mood and symptoms of depression and anxiety in both healthy individuals and psychiatric patients. In general, acute anxiety responds better to exercise than does chronic anxiety. There are almost no contraindications for psychiatric patients to participate in exercise programs, provided they are free from cardiovascular diseases and acute infectious diseases. However, little is known about the effects of exercise in psychiatric disease other than those in depression and anxiety disorders. See also QUALITY OF LIFE.

Bibliography

Bahrke, M.S. and Morgan, W.P. (1978). Anxiety reduction following exercise and meditation. *Cognitive Therapy and Research* 2, 323-33.

Biddle, S., Fox, K. and Boutcher, S. (2000, eds). *Physical activity and psychological well being*. London: Routledge.

Boutcher, S. (1993). Emotion and aerobic exercise. In: Singer, R. Murphy, M. and Tennant, L.K. (eds). *Handbook of research on sport psychology*. pp799-814. New York: MacMillan.

International Society of Sport Psychology (1992). Physical activity and psychological benefits: A position statement. *International Journal of Sport Psychology* 23(1), 86-91.

Kety, S.S. (1966). Catecholamines in neuropsychiatric states. *Pharmacological Review* 18, 787-798.

Martinsen, E.W. (1990). Benefits of exercise for the treatment of depression. *Sports Medicine* 9(6), 380-389.

Meyer, T. and Broocks, A. (2000). Therapeutic impact of exercise on psychiatric diseases: Guidelines for exercise testing and prescription. *Sports Medicine* 30(4), 269-279.

O'Neal, H.A., Dunn, A.L. and Martinsen, E.W. (2000). Depression and exercise. *International Journal of Sport Psychology* 31(2), 110-135.

Paluska, S.A. and Schwenk, T.L. (2000). Physical activity and mental health: Current concepts. *Sports Medicine* 29(3), 167-180.

Schwenck, T.L. (1997). Psychoactive drugs and athletic performance. *The Physician and Sportsmedicine* 25(1), 32-46.

Weyerer, S. and Kupfer, B. (1994). Physical exercise and psychological health. *Sports Medicine* 17(2), 108-116.

MENTAL PRACTICE Covert (rather than overt) practice of a skill in that no actual movement occurs. It involves the use of imagery and verbal thoughts. In addition to its use in sports skill learning and performance preparation, mental practice can be used as part of stress management (e.g. when an athlete is injured) and for problem solving in competitive situations. There is evidence to suggest that mental practice is better than no practice, and that mental practice in combination with physical practice is even better. During physical practice, the athlete should attend to the feel of the movement, so that kinesthetic imagery can be well developed.

A number of theories have been proposed to explain mental practice. Cognitive theories include the Symbolic Learning theory; psychophysiological theories include the Psychoneuromuscular theory.

According to the **Symbolic Learning theory**, mental practice gives the performer the opportunity to rehearse a sequence of movements as symbolic components of the task. It is proposed that mental practice will be most effective in activities with a high degree of cognitive components, such as floor gymnastics. Mental practice gives the performer the opportunity to rehearse the temporal and spatial elements of a skill. Attempts can be made to predict the consequences of each action and rule out inappropriate responses. The symbolic elements of an unfamiliar task can be learned from task instructions, observational learning (modeling) and initial physical practice. The theory predicts that mental practice effects can occur at all stages of learning, but the relevant processes may differ according to the stage of learning. During the early stages of learning, mental practice may give the performer an approximate schema of the symbolic elements of the task. Feedback during practice may enable the schema to be more fully developed. In the late stage of learning, mental practice will be more concerned with overall strategy and performance rehearsal.

The **Psychoneuromuscular theory** is based on the premise that neuromuscular efference patterns during imagined (covert) movement should be identical to those patterns during the same overt movement, but decreased in magnitude. It is proposed that only a small, localized efference from imagery is required for visual and kinesthetic feedback to be available to the motor cortex in order to further enrich the motor memory. Suinn (1980) reported that the electrical activity of skiers' muscles recorded by electromyography during mental practice mirrored the ski terrain. Peak muscle activity during mental practice of skiing was associated with turns and rough sections, just as it would in real skiing. Rather than being localized, the minute innervations associated with mental practice may be spread more generally throughout the whole body or a whole limb. The functional significance of the minute innervations may be for setting the arousal level and other factors necessary for optimal performance. The minute innervations may help 'prime' the muscles in preparation for performance. It may also allow attention to be narrowed or focused to block out task-irrelevant cognitive activity.

Bibliography

Feltz, D.L. and Landers, D. (1983). The effects of mental imagery and mental rehearsal to performance of a motor or motor task: A meta-analysis. *Journal of Sport Psychology* 5, 25-57.

Grouios, G. (1992). Mental practice: A review. *Journal of Sport Behavior* 15(1), 42-59

Murphy, S.M. (1994). Imagery interventions in sport. *Medicine and Science in Sports and Exercise* 26(4), 486-494.

Suinn, R.M. (1980). Psychology and sport performance: Principles and applications. In: Suinn, R.M. (ed.) *Psychology in sports: methods and applications*. pp26-36. Minneapolis, MI: Burgess.

MENTAL RETARDATION Substantial limitations in certain personal capabilities; it is manifested as significantly sub-average intellectual functioning; it exists concurrently with related disabilities in two or more of the following adaptive skill areas: communications, self care, home living, social skills, community use, self direction, health and safety, functional academics, work and leisure; and it begins before the age of 18 years (American Association on Mental Retardation, AAMR, 1992). The AAMR policy is not to classify mental retardation in terms of IQ, but rather to distinguish between mild and severe mental retardation based on level of function within adaptive skills. Prevalence of mental retardation is generally estimated as 3% of the total population. The USA has about 7.5 million citizens with mental retardation and there are about 156 million individuals in the world with mental retardation.

Most mental retardation is caused by multiple factors, some biological and some environmental. The three major causes of mental retardation are Down syndrome, fetal alcohol syndrome and fragile X syndrome, but no clear etiology can be determined for approximately 30 to 40% of cases. About 20% of individuals with mild mental retardation have seizures. In contrast, over 50% of individuals with severe mental retardation have seizures. Infants who are **small for gestational age** [by two standard deviations] experience growth retardation from inadequate nutrition *in utero* and are at high risk of having mental retardation.

A much larger percentage of people with severe mental retardation than people in the general population have serious emotional disturbances. These individuals might be taking psychotropic drugs (e.g. antipsychotics) to treat stereotypic behaviors (e.g. hand flapping), self-injurious behavior, aggressive behavior, social withdrawal and many other problems.

Depending on the severity of the disability, infants and toddlers with mental retardation exhibit various developmental delays. Boys with mental retardation are shorter with wider hips. Most persons with severe mental retardation do not learn to walk before the age of 3 years. Cognitive delays may influence reaction time, movement time, acquisition of fundamental movement patterns, physical fitness, and complex motor skill development. Persons with mental retardation tend to be overweight or obese, and this condition affects both motor performance and predisposition to physical activity. Even when persons are actively involved in sport programs, fitness is lower than that of peers without mental retardation. In severe mental retardation, the aim should be increased exercise tolerance instead of cardiorespiratory endurance. Common side effects of mental retardation that affect physical activity involvement are lethargy, hypersensitivity to sunlight, and balance problems.

Many individuals with mental retardation are nonambulatory and/or have speech difficulties, because they have cerebral palsy. The 'institutional' walk of the nonathletic child with mental retardation is characterized by a shuffling gait with legs wide apart and externally rotated for balance. Body alignment is in a total body slump. Club hands and feet are also common. Those with mild mental retardation can learn to use wheelchairs and experience success in various wheelchair sports. The Special Olympics has wheelchair events, because many people with mental retardation also have cerebral palsy or other orthopedic impairments. The more severe the mental retardation, the lower the communication level. Some individuals with severe mental retardation who cannot communicate verbally learn to use manual signs or other communication devices.

Many persons with mental retardation exhibit problems of over-exclusive or over-inclusive attention. Over-exclusive attention, normal until about age 6 years, is focusing on one aspect of a task with restricted visual scanning and incidental learning. Over-inclusive attention, normal from about age 6 to 12 years, is responsiveness to everything, rather than attending only to relevant cues.

Persons with mental retardation have long-term memory equal to that of peers, but they have many problems with short-term memory. Whereas persons without mental retardation use spontaneous rehearsal strategies, persons with mental retardation are unlikely to do so. Research shows that they can use rehearsal strategies, when carefully taught, but even then, they lag behind peers in spontaneity of application and generalization.

Teachers and coaches should use modeling, verbal rehearsal, self-talk and imagery. Tactile cues are often useful, e.g. tapping a person on the shoulder to cue timing of a movement. Persons with mental retardation do not use feedback as fully as normal peers and need more trials than normal peers and instruction in smaller chunks (i.e. overlearning and extended practice).

See also SAVANTISM.

Chronology

•1846 • Edward Seguin, a leader in the residential school movement for individuals with mental retardation, published *Idiocy and Its Diagnosis and Treatment by the Physiological Method*.

•1848 • The first residential institution for persons with mental retardation in the USA was organized in Massachusetts.

•1961 • President John F. Kennedy appointed the first President's Panel on Mental Retardation. His older sister Rosemary had mental retardation.

•1963 • In the year that President John F. Kennedy was assassinated, his sister Eunice Kennedy Shriver started a summer day camp for children and adults with mental retardation at her home in Maryland.

•1965 • Eunice Kennedy Shriver was keynote speaker at the American Alliance of Health, Physical Education and Recreation (AAHPER) conference in Dallas. Her challenge to professionals was the beginning of awareness of the needs of people with mental retardation. The AAHPER Project on Recreation and Fitness for the Mentally Retarded was formed with a grant from the Jospeh P. Kennedy, Jr. Foundation. This project was the forerunner of the Unit on Programs for the Handicapped, which lasted from 1968 to 1981.

•1968 • Together with the Chicago Park District, the Kennedy Foundation planned and underwrote the 1st International Special Olympics Summer Games, held in Chicago's Soldier Field, with 1,000 athletes with mental retardation. Later that year, Special

Olympics, Inc. was established as a not-for-profit charitable organization. Special Olympics is founded on the belief that people with mental retardation can, with proper instruction and encouragement, learn, enjoy, and benefit from participation in individual and team sports, adapted as necessary to meet the needs of those with special mental and physical limitations.

•1987 • The Developmental Disabilities and Bill of Rights Act Amendments (P.L. 100-146) were passed by Congress. The original law was the Mental Retardation Facilities and Community Mental Health Centers Construction Act of 1963 (P.L. 88-164). The Act was amended in 1990 (P.L. 101-496) and in 1994 by the Developmental Disabilities Assistance and Bill of Rights act of 1994.

•2002 • In the USA, the Surgeon General released a report, *Closing the Gap: A National Blueprint to Improve the Health of Persons with Mental Retardation*. The report outlines the findings of the first-ever Surgeon General's Conference on Health Disparities and Mental Retardation held at Georgetown University in Washington, DC in 2001. The impetus for the conference came from a Senate Hearing on the subject at the 2001 Special Olympics World Winter Games.

Bibliography

American Association on Mental Retardation. Http://www.aamr.org

Shapiro, D. and Dummer, G.M. (1999). Perceived and actual basketball competence of adolescent males with mild mental retardation. *Adapted Physical Activity Quarterly* 15(2), 179-190.

Sherill, C. (2004). *Adapted physical activity, recreation, and sport: Crossdisciplinary and lifespan*. 6th ed. Boston, MA: McGraw-Hill.

Winnick, J.P. (2000, ed). *Adapted physical education and sport*. 3rd ed. Champaign, IL: Human Kinetics.

MENTAL TOUGHNESS

MENTAL TOUGHNESS In sports psychology, it is a somewhat nebulous concept that relates to an athlete's motivation and ability to cope with the demands of the sport. Jones et al. (2002) identified twelve mental toughness attributes: (i) having an unshakable self-belief in your ability to achieve your competition goals; (ii) having an unshakable self-belief that you possess unique qualities and abilities that make you better than your opponents; (iii) having an insatiable desire and internalized motives to succeed; (iv) bouncing back from performance setbacks as a result of increased determination to succeed; (v) thriving on the pressure of competition; (vi) accepting that competition anxiety is inevitable and knowing that you can cope with it; (vii) not being adversely affected by others' good and bad performances; remaining fully-focused in the face of personal life distractions; switching a sport focus on and off as required; remaining fully-focused on the task at hand in the face of competition-specific distractions; pushing back the boundaries of physical and emotional pain, while still maintaining technique and effort under distress (in training and competition); and regaining psychological control following unexpected, uncontrollable events (competition-specific).

A golf boom, a change in the perception of traditional roles and Se Ri Pak's breakthrough rookie season has driven the Korean female golfing movement. Mental toughness is one of several traits posited by Shin and Nam (2004) to explain the success of Korean golfers on the LPGA tour.

Bibliography

Jones, G., Hanton, S. and Connaughton, D. (2002). What is this thing called mental toughness? An investigation of elite sport performers. *Journal of Applied Sport Psychology* 14, 205-218.

Shin, E.H. and Nam, E.A. (2004). Culture, gender roles, and sport. The case of Korean players on the LPGA Tour. *Journal of Sport & Social Issues* 28(3), 223-244.

MESENCHYMAL CELLS *See under* CONNECTIVE TISSUE.

MESENTERY A double layer of peritoneum that encloses the organs and connects them to the abdominal wall. It contains the arteries and veins that supply the intestines. The small bowel mesentery anchors the small intestine to the back of the abdominal wall. There are also mesenteries to support the sigmoid colon, appendix, transverse colon, and parts of the ascending and descending colon.

MESOMORPHY *See under* SOMATOTYPE.

MESOSTERNALE An anatomical landmark that is the point located on the corpus sterni (body of the sternum), at the intersection of the mid-sagittal plane and the horizontal (transverse) plane at the mid-level of the fourth chondrosternal articulation, i.e. the mid-point of the sternum at the level of the center of the articulation of the fourth rib with the sternum.

MET Metabolic equivalent. *See under* ENERGY EXPENDITURE.

METABOLIC ACIDOSIS *See under* ACID-BASE BALANCE.

METABOLIC EQUIVALENT A multiple of the resting metabolic rate. It is an expression of energy cost relative to an individual's resting energy expenditure. One MET is equal to resting oxygen uptake, which is approximately 3.5 mL/kg/min. For any particular physical activity, the MET rating is the energy cost of an activity divided by resting energy expenditure. METs can be used to indicate exercise intensity, but are not used as commonly as target heart rate and ratings of perceived exertion.

Sleeping or lying awake quietly in bed is 0.9 MET; sitting quietly watching television is 1.0 MET; standing quietly is 1.2 METs; making the bed is 2 METs; ironing is 2.3 METs; sweeping the floor is 4 METs; and scrubbing the floor is 5.5 METs. Sexual activity is 1.5 METs (active, vigorous effort); 1.3 METs (general, moderate effort); and 1.0 (passive, light effort, kissing, hugging).

Walking and carrying light objects less than 25 lb is 3 METs at 2.5 mph; 4 METs at 3 mph; and 4.5 METs at 3.5 mph. Walking on the level ground at less than 2 mph is 2.5 METs; at 2 mph is 3 METs; at 3 mph is 3.5 METs; at 4 mph is 4 METs (very brisk); and at 4.5 mph (very, very brisk) is 4.5 METs.

Running at 5 mph (12-minute mile) is 8 METs; at 6 mph (10-minute mile) is 10 METs; at 8 mph (7.5 minute mile) is 13.5 METs; and at 10 mph (6-minute mile) is 16 METs.

Cross-country skiing at 2.5 mph (slow or light effort) is 7 METs; 4.0 to 4.9 mph (moderate speed and effort) is 8 METs; 5.0 to 7.9 mph (brisk speed, vigorous effort) is 9 METs; and greater than 8 mph (racing) is 14 METs.

Swimming laps with slow, moderate or light effort, is 8 METs; and by using freestyle, fast, with vigorous effort is 10 METs.

Bicycling at less than 10 mph is 4 METs; 10 to 11.9 mph (slow, light effort) is 6 METs; 12 to 13.9 mph (moderate effort) is 8 METs; 14 to 15.9 mph (fast, vigorous) is 10 METs; and 15 to 19 mph (rac-

ing) is 12 METs.

See also ENERGY EXPENDITURE.

Bibliography

Ainsworth, B.E. et al. (1993). Compendium of physical activities: Classification energy costs of human activities. *Medicine and Science in Sports and Exercise* 25, 71-80.

Ainsworth, B.E. et al. (2000). Compendium of Physical Activities: An Update of Activity Codes and MET Intensities. *Medicine and Science in Sports and Exercise* 2000 (32 Supp. 9), S498-S516.

METABOLIC PATHWAY A set of chemical reactions that take place in a definite order to convert a particular starting molecule into one or more specific products.

METABOLIC RATE *See under* ENERGY EXPENDITURE.

METABOLIC SYNDROME Syndrome X. Insulin resistance syndrome. A cluster of metabolic disorders manifesting four categories of abnormality: atherogenic dyslipidemia (elevated triglycerides, increased LDL cholesterol and decreased HDL cholesterol), increased blood pressure, elevated plasma glucose and a prothrombotic state. Metabolic syndrome may indicate a predisposition to diabetes, hypertension and heart disease. As defined by the National Cholesterol Education Program, men with metabolic syndrome are 2.9 to 4.2 times more likely to die of coronary heart disease than healthy men. Mortality from cardiovascular disease is 2.6 to 3 times higher in men with metabolic syndrome than healthy men. Metabolic syndrome was first described in 1988. In 2002, the Center for Disease Control and Prevention estimated that as many as 47 million Americans may exhibit metabolic syndrome.

According to the National Cholesterol Education Program guidelines, patients with metabolic syndrome have at least three of the following criteria: abdominal obesity (waist girth of more than 40 inches in men or 35 inches in women); high triglyceride level (150 mg/dL or higher); low HDL cholesterol (less than 40 mg/dL in men or 50 mg/dL in women); high blood pressure (130/85 mm Hg or higher); and impaired fasting glucose value (110 mg/dL or higher).

Insulin resistance may lie at the heart of the metabolic syndrome. 10 to 25% of the adult population may be insulin resistant to some degree. Elevated serum triglycerides are commonly associated with insulin resistance and represent a valuable clinical marker of the metabolic syndrome. Abdominal obesity is a clinical marker for insulin resistance.

It seems that metabolic syndrome has a central neuroendocrine origin in the form of enhanced engagement of the hypothalamic-pituitary-adrenal axis. Here the peripheral endocrine perturbations act as triggers for both abdominal obesity and the metabolic abnormalities.

Various therapeutic approaches for the patient with metabolic syndrome should be implemented to decrease the risk of cardiovascular disease events. These interventions include decreasing obesity, increasing physical activity and the use of drugs to manage dyslipidemia. Pharmacologic therapy consists of statins, fibrates, ACE inhibitors and thiazolidinediones, all of which can decrease the risk and incidence of coronary artery disease. **Thiazo-lidinediones** are classes of drugs that decrease the concentration of glucose in the blood. Immediate treatment of metabolic syndrome is essential because these patients quickly develop diabetes.

See also CARDIAC SYNDROME X; HYPER-LIPIDEMIA.

Bibliography

Bjorntorp, P., Holm, G., Rosmond, R. and Folkow, B. (2000). Hypertension and the metabolic syndrome: Closely related central origin? *Blood Pressure* 9(2-3), 71-82.

Carroll, S. and Dudfield, M. (2004). What is the relationship between exercise and metabolic abnormalities? A review of the metabolic syndrome. *Sports Medicine* 34(6), 371-418.

Grundy, S.M. (1999). Hypertriglyceridemia, insulin resistance, and the metabolic syndrome. *American Journal of Cardiology* 83(9B), 25F-29F.

Lakka, H.M. et al. (2002). The metabolic syndrome and total and cardiovascular disease mortality in middle-aged men. *Journal of the American Medical Association* 288, 2709-2716.

Scott, C.L. (2003). Diagnosis, prevention and intervention for the metabolic syndrome. *American Journal of Cardiology* 92(1A), 35i-42i.

METABOLISM   The chemical processes that take place in a living system. **Catabolism** is the breaking down of organic compounds from complex to simple with the release of energy. **Anabolism** is the building up of organic compounds from simple to complex using energy released by catabolism. *See* ENERGY EXPENDITURE.

METABOLITE   Any substance that is involved in metabolism.

METACARPALE RADIALE   An anatomical landmark that is the most lateral point of the distal head of the 2nd metacarpal of the outstretched hand (i.e. on the radial side of the hand).

METACARPALE ULNARE   An anatomical landmark that is the most medial point on the distal head of the 5th metacarpal of the outstretched hand (i.e. on the ulnar side of the hand).

METACARPALS   These are the long bones of the hand that articulate with the carpal bones proximally and the proximal phalanges distally at the metacarpophalangeal (MP) joint. The collateral ligaments of the MP joint insert onto the proximal phalanges. They are taut in flexion and relaxed in extension.

METACARPALS, FRACTURES   Fractures of the metacarpal bones are especially common among handball players, and may be caused by vigorous extension of the fingers (e.g. during shooting when a player's hand hits the covering arm of an opposing player) or as a result of a direct blow. Metacarpal head fractures occur most commonly in the 2nd finger. Metacarpal neck fractures are traditionally termed '**boxer's fractures,**' but rarely occur in professional boxers. Instead, they occur during informal fights at the 5th metacarpal.

Bennett's fracture is a fracture-dislocation of the first metacarpal base; it is really a dislocation in which the small medial fragment of the proximal metacarpal is left in the joint, where it is held by the attachment of the volar ligament. It results from an axial force applied when the metacarpal bone is in flexion. One cause of Bennett's fracture is a poorly delivered punch in boxing. A **reverse Bennett's fracture** ('baby Bennett') is a fracture of the base of the 5th metacarpal.

METACARPO-PHALANGEAL JOINT It is a shallow condyloid joint that depends on its collateral ligament-volar plate complex for stability. The **volar plate** is a dense fibrous band that protects the metacarpo-phalangeal joint and is also an attachment site for the flexor tendon sheath, which keeps the flexor tendons tight to the bone, preventing bowstringing. The clinical ramification of tendon bowstringing is that the grip is weakened, flexion is incomplete and stiff joints can ensue. The deep transverse metacarpal ligament further reinforces the volar plate. The metacarpo-phalangeal joint is protected laterally by the collateral ligaments and the intervolar plate ligaments. The lateral bands (the lumbrical and interosseus muscles) also act as partial checkreins to lateral instability. Dorsally, the capsule, the extensor tendons and the sagittal bands secure the joint.

The movements of flexion, extension, abduction and adduction are permitted. Most of the muscles moving the thumb have *pollicis* in their name. Most of the muscles moving the fingers have *digiti* in their name. The recessed position of the metacarpo-phalangeal joint within the web space, coupled with the protection afforded by adjacent fingers, provides additional stability. The metacarpo-phalangeal joint of the thumb, however, remains unprotected and is frequently injured. Injury to the collateral ligaments of the finger metacarpo-phalangeal joints is not common, but injury to the thumb's ulnar collateral ligament occurs frequently. **Skier's thumb (gamekeeper's thumb)** is a rupture (sprain) of the ulnar collateral ligament of the 1st metacarpo-phalangeal joint. It is caused by forced abduction with the metacarpo-phalangeal joint in near extension, such as when Alpine skiers fall onto their outstretched hand with the thumb in an abducted position. To prevent this injury, skiers should use poles without straps or avoid using straps that are already attached to poles. In cross-country skiing, the strap is grasped between the palm of the hand and the pole grip; thus 'skier's thumb' may occur during a forceful pole plant. It may occur in other sports, such as in ice hockey, when a player's stick gets trapped, forcing the thumb backwards. **Ulnar collateral ligament sprain** can also result from hyperextension of the 1st metacarpo-phalangeal joint, such as when a collision occurs between two athletes. The **Stener lesion**, associated with skier's thumb, is the interposition of the adductor aponeurosis between the ends of the torn collateral ligament. Tears of the radial collateral ligaments of the thumb and finger metacarpo-phalangeal joints are less frequent than tears of the ulnar collateral ligaments, but they do occur in the athlete. The radial collateral ligaments, most commonly those of the 3 ulnar fingers, are torn during forced abduction when the metacarpo-phalangeal joint is flexed.

Dorsal dislocations of the metacarpo-phalangeal joint are caused by forced hyperextension of a digit in a fall on an outstretched hand. As the joint is forced into hyperextension, the large volar metacarpal head tears through the proximal aspect of the volar plate. If the distal portion of the torn volar plate becomes interposed between the proximal phalanx and the head of the metacarpal, the dislocation is complex (complete); if it is not interposed, the dislocation is simple. Dorsal metacarpo-phalangeal joint dislocations typically occur in football and basketball. Volar dislocations of the metacarpo-phalangeal joint are rare. **Volar plate fractures** are the result of hyperextension, with a small fragment of bone being avulsed from the volar aspect of the base of the proximal phalanx. A **Wilson fracture** refers to a volar plate injury to the middle phalanx of a finger.

See also BOXER'S KNUCKLE; HAND; JERSEY FINGER, MALLET FINGER; TRAPEZIO-METACARPAL JOINT; ULNAR DIGITAL NERVE.

METAPHYSIS *See under* EPIPHYSEAL GROWTH PLATE.

METAPLASIA The transformation of one differentiated cell type into another. A condition in which there is a change of one adult cell type to another similar adult cell type.

METASTASIS Transfer of the causal agent (cell or micro-organism) of a disease from a primary focus to a distant focus via the blood or lymphatic vessels.

METATARSALE FIBULARE An anatomical landmark that is the most lateral point on the head of the 5th metatarsal when the subject is standing.

METATARSALE TIBIALE An anatomical landmark that is the most medial point on the head of the 1st metatarsal of the foot when the subject is standing.

METATARSAL FRACTURES A fracture of one or more of the metatarsal bones, especially the 5th metatarsal. It is the most common of all the fractures that can affect the foot. A typical cause of fracture is the foot being trodden on during a ball sport. The most common fracture of the 5th metatarsal base is an avulsion fracture. It often occurs in conjunction with an inversion sprain, and is due to contraction of the *peroneus brevis* muscle.

A **Jones fracture** is a transverse fracture of the diaphysis of the base of the 5th metatarsal. It may begin as a stress fracture, becoming a complete fracture with an inversion injury; or may be an acute injury resulting from abnormal loading of the lateral part of the foot as the heel is elevated and the metatarso-phalangeal joints are extended. Jones fractures are common in athletes, especially those between the ages of 15 and 21 years.

Metatarsal stress fractures appear related to either hypermobility or hypomobility of the foot. *Pes cavus* is also a risk factor, because the foot may not be able to pronate sufficiently to absorb the forces generated by the ground on the foot and lower leg, thus increasing stress across the metatarsal arch with the 2nd and 3rd metatarsals being affected.

METATARSALGIA Pain over the metatarsal heads without any other obvious diagnosis. The 2nd metatarsal head is most frequently involved. With hyperpronation, the forces move medially, and the 2nd metatarsal may assume an excessively large percentage of the force. It can be caused by anything that puts extra stress on the front of the foot, such as being overweight, high-heeled shoes, pes cavus, claw toes, hammer toes, bunions, interdigital neuroma or tarsal tunnel syndrome.

METATARSO-PHALANGEAL JOINTS Condyloid joints formed between the metatarsals and phalanges. The proximal articulating surface is the head of the metatarsal. The distal articulating surface is the base of the phalange. The movements permitted are abduction/adduction and flexion/extension. See also FOOT; GOUT; TURF TOE.

Bibliography
Loretta, B. and Chou, M.D. (2000). Disorders of the first metatarsophalangeal joint. Diagnosis of great-toe pain. *The Physician and Sportsmedicine* 28(7), 32-45.

METATARSUS ADDUCTUS *See* FOREFOOT VARUS.

METHIONINE An essential, glucogenic (glycogenic), five-carbon amino acid. It is the precursor of taurine, which combines with acetyl CoA to form one of the bile salts, taurocholate.

MICROCEPHALUS *See under* BRAIN.

MICROGRAVITY An environment that will impart to an object a net acceleration that is small compared with that produced by Earth at its surface. In the context of space travel, microgravity refers to what astronauts feel in space flight during orbit around the earth, when the rocket's altitude exceeds about 100 miles at a velocity of about 17,500 mph. The main physical stressors from space travel are decreased hydrostatic pressure gradients within the cardiovascular system and decreased weight loading on muscles. Physiological changes include decreased red blood cell mass and plasma volume. Decrease in total body water, and greater proportional decrease of extracellular volume, indicates increased cellular volume that may contribute to in-flight cephalic edema (swollen head). Astronauts suffer negative energy balance on most space missions, because of increased energy demands of space flight and decreased food intake.

During short space flights (1 to 14 days), 40 to 70% of astronauts and cosmonauts exhibit in flight neurovestibular effects including postural illusions, sensations of tumbling or rotation, nystagmus, dizziness and vertigo. During long space flight (more than

14 days), vestibular disturbances are the same as for shorter missions.

During the first few days in microgravity, fluid shifts from the lower body to the upper body. In the absence of gravity, no linear, downward head-to-foot acceleration forces act on the body. Total fluid volume also decreases, which in turn decreases the work effect of the heart. Continued microgravity exposure decreases overall heart size, mainly from decreased left ventricular volume (especially left ventricular end-diastolic volume).

Without gravity, normal biologic functions become more susceptible to short- and long-term maladaptations, such as **space motion sickness**, which is similar to motion sickness on Earth, with symptoms including headache, dizziness, disorientation, loss of appetite, malaise, nausea, vomiting, gastrointestinal disturbances and fatigue. 70% of astronauts and cosmonauts on their first flight are affected by space motion sickness. Motion sickness symptoms appear early in flight and subside or disappear in 2 to 7 days. Space motion sickness was first reported on the Apollo and Skylab missions where astronauts had greater freedom of movement. Astronauts did not experience spatial disorientation during the flight of Mercury and Gemini missions, because mobility and peripheral vision were restricted. Of pharmacological intervention for space motion sickness, 'Scope-dex' has been found to minimize the symptoms. It contains a combination of scopalmine and amphetamine. On reentry after short-duration missions, space motion sickness can manifest as **general reentry syndrome**, which involves vertigo, nausea, instability and fatigue induced by reimposition of increased head-to-foot acceleration forces on the body during reentry and landing.

During space missions that last twelve months, there is altered muscular coordination patterns, delayed-onset muscle soreness, and generalized muscular fatigue and weakness. Each month, there is a 1% loss in weightbearing bone mass. A residual deficit in bone mineral density of the calcaneus has been observed in astronauts 5 years after repeated exposures to microgravity. There are decreases in lean body mass, muscle volume and muscle strength.

In particular, there is atrophy of skeletal muscles that support posture and locomotion. In-flight workouts are required to counteract the adverse changes associated with microgravity, and have included the use of treadmills, bicycle ergometers, rowing machines and resistance training machines. The Space Cycle™ is a self-powered human centrifuge that produces artificial gravity as a person rotates about the shaft while pedaling. It is thus a countermeasure to the adverse physiological effects of prolonged human exposure to spaceflight micro gravity. Pedaling the Space Cycle™ propels a centrifuge in a curvilinear motion about a fixed central shaft that is rigidly fixed within the spacecraft. In order to provide sufficient recovery from space motion sickness, astronauts are advised not to engage in exercise during the first 48 to 72 hours.

In the post-flight period, astronauts experienced post-flight dehydration and weightlessness, with a decrease in orthostatic tolerance and exercise tolerance.

Bibliography
Kreitenberg, A. et al. (1998). The Space Cycle™ self powered human centrifuge: A proposed countermeasure for prolonged human space flight. *Aviation and Space Environmental Medicine* 69, 66-72

MICROTRAUMA Destruction of a small number of cells caused by the additive effects of repetitive forces.

MICTURITION Voiding. Urination. The process used to eliminate urine from the bladder. The internal and external urethral sphincters regulate storage and emptying of the bladder. The smooth muscle fibers of the bladder are known collectively as the **detrusor muscle**. The neck of the bladder, the area that surrounds the urethral opening, contains an **internal urethral sphincter**. The smooth muscle fibers of this sphincter involuntarily control the discharge of urine from the bladder. The **external urethral sphincter** lies below the internal sphincter and is made up of smooth muscle mixed with skeletal muscle of the pelvic floor (pelvic diaphragm). It enables voluntary control of intra-abdominal pressure to prevent urine leakage.

The **urethra** is a small tube that leads from the floor or neck of the urinary bladder to the outside of the body. In women, the urethra is about 1.5 inches long and is found in the front wall of the vagina. The **urethral orifice (meatus)** is the outside opening of the urethra and is located between the clitoris and the vaginal opening. In men, the urethra is about 8 inches long. When it leaves the bladder, it passes downward through the prostate gland, the pelvic muscles and finally through the length of the penis until it ends at the urethral orifice or opening at the tip of the glans of the penis.

The bladder has somatic, parasympathetic and sympathetic innervation. The **pudental nerve** is the somatic component of bladder innervation and innervates the external urethral sphincter, which normally contracts during transient increases in intra-abdominal pressure, such as occurs with coughing. The parasympathic nerve fibers are stimulated when the individual has the urge for micturition. When stimulated, the detrusor muscle contracts resulting in elevated intravesicular pressure. The internal urethral sphincter relaxes when it is innervated by the sympathetic nervous system.

As urine accumulates in the bladder, distension of the bladder walls activates stretch receptors there. Impulses are transmitted via visceral afferent fibers to the sacral region of the spinal cord, setting up spinal reflexes that initiate increased sympathetic outflow to the bladder. This produces temporary inhibition of the detrusor muscle and internal urethral sphincter; pudental motor fibers are activated, stimulating contraction of the external urethral sphincter. When about 200 to 300 ml of urine has accumulated, afferent impulses are transmitted to the brain and the individual feels the urge to void. Contractions of the bladder become more frequent and urgent. If the individual chooses to empty the bladder, voiding reflexes are initiated. Visceral afferent impulses activate the micturition center of the dorsolateral pons, which signals the parasympathetic neurons to stimulate contraction of the detrusor muscle and relaxation of the internal and external sphincters. This allows urine to be expelled from the bladder. If the person chooses not to void, the micturition reflex can be overridden; reflex bladder

contractions subside within a minute or so and urine continues to accumulate. Because the external urethral sphincter (and the *levator ani*) is under voluntary control, the person can choose to keep it closed and postpone bladder emptying temporarily. After a further 200 to 300 ml has accumulated in the bladder, the micturition reflex occurs again. If the person again chooses not to void, then it is damped once more. Eventually the urge to void becomes irresistible and micturition occurs, voluntarily or involuntarily. Contraction of the diaphragm and abdominal muscles can increase the volume of urine voided by increasing intra-abdominal pressure, which increases the pressure on the bladder for micturition.

Urinary continence is maintained as long as intra-urethral pressure remains higher than the pressure within the cavity of the bladder (**intravesical pressure**). When intra-abdominal pressure is increased, urinary continence is normally maintained, because urethral pressure rises more than pressure within the bladder cavity as a response to the increased intra-abdominal pressure. Continence when a person is asleep results from the unconscious inhibition of the detrusor muscle.

During infancy, micturition is under involuntary control. Voiding occurs whenever the bladder is sufficiently full to activate the stretch receptors. The internal urethral sphincter prevents dribbling of urine between each voiding. Between the ages of 2 and 3 years, the pontine micturition center develops in the lower part of the brain, so as to facilitate the development of conscious bladder control and toilet training.

See also AGING; URINARY INCONTINENCE.

Bibliography
Germann, W.J. and Stanfield, C.L. (2001). *Principles of human physiology*. San Francisco, CA: Benjamin Cummings.
Marieb, E.N. (2002). *Anatomy and physiology*. San Francisco, CA: Benjamin Cummings.

MID-CARPAL JOINTS *See under* INTERCARPAL JOINTS.

MID-TARSAL JOINTS Transverse tarsal joint. Chopart's joint. The mid-tarsal joint comprises two joints: the talonavicular joint and the calcaneocuboid joint. The proximal articulating surfaces are (talonavicular) distal talus and (calcaneocuboid) distal calcaneus. The distal articulating surfaces are (talonavicular) proximal navicular and (calcaneocuboid) proximal cuboid. The midtarsal joint has an oblique and longitudinal axis. These axes do not necessarily correspond to talonavicular or calcaneocuboid articulations. Movements permitted are gliding and inversion/eversion. When the calcaneus is everted, the axes of the talonavicular and calcaneocuboid joints are parallel, thus motion can occur at the midtarsal joint. When the calcaneus is inverted, the axes are not parallel and motion at the midtarsal joint is limited.

The **talocalcaneonavicular joint** is the talonavicular joint and the subtalar joint.

MIDLINE   An imaginary, straight, vertical line drawn from the mid-forehead through the nose and the umbilicus to the floor.

MIGRAINE   *See under* HEADACHE.

MIND-BODY EXERCISE   Physical activity combined with mindfulness or a meditative mindset, with an emphasis on proprioceptive awareness, posture, breathing, self monitoring of perceived effort, and a focus on the present moment. Methods of exercise such as tai chi and yoga have spread rapidly throughout the fields of health, fitness and rehabilitation. Tai chi and yoga are based on Eastern mysticism, which assumes that a vital life force or energy (chi) unifies mind, body and nature. **Hatha yoga** is a form of exercise based on the belief that the body and breath are intimately connected with the mind. By controlling the breath and holding the body in steady poses or 'asanas,' yoga improves flexibility and promotes relaxation and mind-body harmony.

Tai chi chuan involves low velocity, low impact exercise and is especially popular in the USA with older adults. The choreographed movements ('forms') resemble a slow graceful dance and were designed to mimic animal movements such as that of the snake. It is based on the Taoist belief that good health results from balanced chi.

Many of the claimed benefits for these activities are not supported by clinical evidence, and, as alternative therapies they carry legal and professional ramifications. Ives and Sosnoff (2000) concluded that there is insufficient scientific evidence to support replacing conventional medical treatments with somatic methods. However, they also stated that, in certain instance, mind-body exercise can offer some benefits not easily obtained with traditional exercise. For example, tai chi has been shown to be more effective than traditional exercise in preventing falls in the elderly.

Bibliography

Cheng, J. (1999). Tai Chi Chuan. A slow dance for health. *The Physician and Sportsmedicine* 27(6), 109-110.

Ives, J.C. and Sosnoff, J. (2000). Beyond the mind-body exercise hype. *The Physician and Sportsmedicine* 28(3), 67-81.

Wolf, S.L., Coogler, C. and Xu, T. (1997). Exploring the basis for Tai Chi Chuan as a therapeutic exercise approach. *Archives of Physical Medicine and Rehabilitation* 78(8), 886-892.

MIND-BODY RELATIONSHIP   *See under* PHYSICAL EDUCATION.

MINERALOCORTICOIDS   *See under* CORTICOSTEROIDS.

MINERALS   In nutrition, elements that are inorganic nutrients required by the human body in very small amounts. There are 'macrominerals' and 'microminerals.'

Macrominerals are required at levels of at least 100 mg per day. Macrominerals that are generally accepted as being 'essential' (required daily in the diet) are calcium, chlorine, magnesium, phosphorus, potassium, sodium and sulfur.

Microminerals ('**trace elements**') are required at levels of less than 100 mg per day. Trace elements generally accepted as being 'essential' are chromium, cobalt, copper, fluorine, iodine, iron, manganese, molybdenum, selenium and zinc. Other trace elements include arsenic, boron, cadmium, lead, lithium, nickel, silicon, tin and vanadium.

Minerals dissolved in the aqueous fluids of the body as ions are often called **electrolytes**. Salts, acids and bases are electrolytes. Positive ions (cations) in body fluids include sodium, potassium, calcium and magnesium ions; negative ions (anions) include chloride, bicarbonate, phosphate and sulfate ions.

Electrolytes are important in the control of fluid exchange between cells and their external fluid environment, particularly in establishing the necessary electrical gradients across cell membranes. The electrical difference between the inside and the outside of the cell is required for the transmission of nerve impulses, the functioning of glands and the contraction of muscle. Electrolytes are also important in maintaining acid-base balance.

Poor diet seems to be the main reason for any mineral deficiencies found in athletes, although in certain cases exercise could contribute to the deficiency. In cases of deficiency, mineral supplementation may be important to ensure good health. There is little evidence of any beneficial effects of mineral supplementation on athletic performance.

Bibliography

Clarkson, P.M. (1991). Minerals: Exercise performance and supplementation in athletes. *Journal of Sports Sciences* 9, 91-116.

Haymes, E.M. (1991). Vitamin and mineral supplementation in athletes. *International Journal of Sport Nutrition* 1(2), 146-69.

McDonald, R. and Keen, C.L. (1988). Iron, zinc and magnesium nutrition and athletic performance. *Sports Medicine* 5, 171-184

MISALIGNMENTS Malalignments. Deviations from the ideal alignment of bones. A distinction can be made between normal and ideal alignment. Normal alignment is a measure of what occurs on average in the population and is not necessarily the same as the ideal alignment.

Compensation refers to a change of structure, position or function of a body part in an attempt to adjust or neutralize the abnormal force of a deviation of structure, position or function of another part.

See FEMORAL TORSION; FEMORAL VALGUS; FEMORAL VARUS; FLAT FEET; FOREFOOT ABDUCTION; FOREFOOT VALGUS; FOREFOOT VARUS; REARFOOT VALGUS; REARFOOT VARUS; TIBIAL TORSION; TIBIAL VALGUS; TIBIAL VARUS.

MITOCHRONDRIA Small structures in the cytoplasm of cells containing enzymes that are involved in respiration. There are about 2000 mitochondria in a human cell. Mitochondria have their own DNA, and are thus self-replicating. Mitochondrial DNA (mtDNA) mutations often cause deficient function in the electron transfer chain. When a need for more ATP arises, mitochondria split in half and then grow to their former size. The inner membrane is folded into tubules called **cristae**; this increases the area for the electron transport chain.

MITOCHONDRIAL MEMBRANE SHUTTLES

Special carrier molecules that transfer high-energy electrons from NADH in the cytosol across the outer mitochondrial membrane. The carrier molecules may deliver the high-energy electrons at the beginning of the electron transport chain or farther along. If the NADH produced from glycolysis is to be used as an electron and proton donor in the electron transport chain, there must be a means to transfer this molecule and its electrons and protons into the mitochondria. In addition, there must be a means to transfer the ADP from the cytosol into the mitochondria, as well as the ATP produced in the mitochondria to the cytosol, because ADP and ATP are large, charged molecules (therefore, neither molecule can diffuse through the inner mitochondrial membrane). A specific transport protein called **ADP-ATP translocase** facilitates the movement of ADP and ATP between the cytosol and mitochondria. The function of the translocase requires the binding of a cytosolic ADP and a mitochondrial ATP, resulting in the coupled entry of ADP into the mitochondria and exit of ATP. To support the electrochemical changes that occur with the transport of charged molecules from the mitochondria, specialized transport systems exist that essentially return or remove charge to or from the mitochondria, thus requiring less ATP expenditure to maintain the mitochondrial membrane potentials. The two main methods of electron and proton transfer from the cytosol to the mitochondria are the glycerol phosphate shuttle and the malate-aspartate shuttle.

The **malate-aspartate shuttle** works as follows. In the cytosol, there is coupled oxidation of

NADH to NAD$^+$ and reduction of oxaloacetate to malate. Malate enters the mitochondria via a transporter. Once in the mitochondria, malate is oxidized to oxaloacetate, regenerating NADH. NADH passes its electrons directly to the electron transport chain. The **glycerol phosphate shuttle** is also a pathway for the regeneration of NAD$^+$ from NADH, so that glycolysis may continue. NADH is generated in the cytoplasm during glycolysis when glyceraldehyde 3-phosphate is oxidized. NADH must be oxidized to NAD$^+$ by the electron transport chain so that more glyceraldehyde 3-phosphate can be processed. The mitochondrial membrane is impermeable to both NADH and NAD$^+$, therefore electrons are transferred to dihydroxyacetone phosphate to form glycerol 3-phosphate, which is able to cross the membrane. Once in the mitochondria, the dihydroxyacetone phosphate is reformed by an FAD-linked enzyme and diffuses back into the cytosol, to complete the glycerol phosphate shuttle. The FAD that accepts the electrons in the mitochondria yields only about 1.5 ATP from the electron transport chain whereas the NADH would have yielded about 2.5 ATP.

Until recently it was assumed that the malate-aspartate shuttle did not exist in skeletal muscle, but does exist in liver, kidney and myocardium. However, it seems that both shuttles exist in skeletal muscle and that the malate-aspartate shuttle is more operable in endurance-trained muscle.

Bibliography
Houston, M.E (2001). *Biochemistry primer for exercise science.* 2nd ed. Champaign, IL: Human Kinetics.

Robergs, R.A. and Roberts, S.O. (2000). *Fundamental principles of exercise physiology.* Boston, MA: McGraw-Hill.

MITOCHONDRIAL MYOPATHY A metabolic disease of muscle with onset during early infancy or adulthood. Symptoms include generalized muscle weakness, flaccid neck muscles and inability to walk. There may be seizures, deafness, loss of balance and vision, and mental retardation. Progression and severity varies widely. Inheritance is by the maternal mitochondrial gene (mtDNA).

Bibliography
Muscular Dystrophy Association. Http://www.mdausa.org

MITRAL VALVE The atrioventricular valve on the left side of the heart. It consists of two flaps or leaflets which normally open and shut in a coordinated way to allow blood to flow only in one direction from the left atrium to the left ventricle.

MITRAL VALVE PROLAPSE Barlow's syndrome. Click-murmur syndrome. Floppy-valve syndrome. A congenital heart disease in which there are abnormalities of valvular connective tissue, resulting in redundancy and/or thickening of valve leaflets. This leads to various degrees of dispensability, poor leaflet opposition and subsequent prolapse. One or both leaflets of the mitral valve protrude into the left atrium during the systolic phase of ventricular contraction.

A pronounced mid-systolic click, with or without late systolic murmur, usually indicates the presence of this disorder. Occurrence of systolic murmur in individuals with mitral valve prolapse is about 32%. Cases of mitral valve prolapse with a murmur and not just an isolated click have a general mortality rate that is increased by 15-20%.

Mitral valve prolapse may be associated with valve infection, arrhythmias and atypical chest pain. It may be present in people with other connective tissue diseases, such as Marfan syndrome and Ehlers-Danlos syndrome.

Mitral valve prolapse occurs in 4 to 7% of the population and is approximately three times more common in females. Most cases of mitral valve prolapse are inherited as an autosomal dominant trait. Diagnoses of mitral valve prolapse increased in the 1990s, because of its association with endocarditis, atherosclerosis and muscular dystrophy. 60% of persons with mitral valve prolapse have no symptoms, but 40% experience profound fatigue during mild physical activity.

In general, mitral valve prolapse is a benign disorder, but it may account for the majority of isolated cases of mitral regurgitation, 90% of cases of ruptured chordae tendinae, 40% of strokes in young patients, and 10 to 15% of cases of endocarditis.

Mitral regurgitation (mitral insufficiency) occurs when a large amount of blood leaks backward through the defective valve instead of continuing in the normal direction. Mitral regurgitation can result in thickening or enlargement of the heart wall, caused by the extra pumping required to compensate for the backflow of blood. Mitral valve prolapse is the most common cause of mitral valve regurgitation. Those with leaflet thickening and redundancy seem to be at highest risk for developing regurgitation.

Between 3% and 5% of cardiac-related deaths during exercise are attributed to mitral valve prolapse. Several factors have been identified in those who progress to sudden death, including severe mitral regurgitation, severe valve abnormalities without regurgitation, and increased heart weight.

Athletes with mitral valve prolapse, and without any of the following criteria, can engage in all competitive sports: history of syncope, documented to be arrhythmogenic in origin; family history of sudden death associated with mitral valve prolapse; repetitive forms of sustained and nonsustained supraventricular arrhythmias, particularly if exaggerated by exercise; moderate-to-marked mitral regurgitation; or a prior embolic event. Athletes with mitral valve prolapse, and one or more of the aforementioned criteria, can participate in only low-intensity competitive sports.

Medications are generally not necessary for mitral valve prolapse, but beta-blockers may be helpful if palpitations are severe. Aerobic exercise should be encouraged for all patients with mitral valve prolapse.

Bibliography

Joy, E. (1996). Mitral valve prolapse in active patients: Recognition, treatment, and exercise recommendations. *The Physician and Sportsmedicine* 24(7), 78-86.

Plewa, M.C. (2002). Mitral valve prolapse. Http://www.emedicine.com

MIXED VENOUS BLOOD   *See under* VEIN.

MIXING CHAMBER   *See under* OXYGEN UPTAKE, MEASUREMENT OF.

MOBILITY   *See* JOINT MOBILITY.

MODEL   An idealized or simplified representation of one or more objects, phenomenon, process or system. The type of model chosen depends largely on what problem is being tackled or what questions are being asked. When a model comprises equations describing a system, the model may be used to perform simulated experiments to address questions about the system. Engineers construct miniaturized versions of machines and structures prior to construction of the full-size version. Biomechanical models are typically physical or mathematical. Physical models include anthropometric models (crash-test dummies).

See also FINITE ELEMENT MODELING; RHEOLOGICAL MODELS.

MODELING   i) Use of a model. ii) See under BONE. iii) A technique for demonstrating a learning task. See under MOTOR LEARNING.

MOIETY   i) One of two approximately equal parts. ii) One of two parts.

MOLE   The molecular weight of a substance expressed in grams. It is the basic unit of amount of substance adopted under the Standard International system of units. A mole of any substance contains the same number of elementary particles as there are atoms in 12 grams of the 12C isotope of carbon. There are two stable (i.e. nonradioactive) isotopes of carbon, known as carbon 12 and carbon 13. The difference between these two isotopes is the presence of an additional neutron in the nucleus of the 13C atom, so that this isotope is a little heavier than the 12C isotope. In general the ratio of 13C to 12 C is approximately 1 to 99.

One mole can also be expressed as Avogadro's number, which is 6.02×10^{23} of any elementary particles (atoms, molecules or ions).

Molarity (M) expresses the concentration of, or number of moles of, substance in a liter of solution. A mole of any atoms has a mass in grams equal to the **atomic weight** of an element, which is the weighted average of the atomic masses of the different isotopes of an element. **Molecular weight** is the sum of the atomic weights of the atoms in the molecules that form a compound. For example, the atomic weight of carbon is 12. Thus, one mole of carbon weighs 12 g. The molecular weight of carbon dioxide is 44; thus one mole of carbon dioxide weighs 44 g. The molecular weight of glucose ($C_6H_{12}O_6$) is 180 g [(6x12) + (12x1) + (6x16)]. Thus a one molar solution of glucose will contain 180 g of glucose per liter of glucose solution, expressed as 1 M or 1 mole/liter. A millimole (mM) contains one millimole per liter. The molecular weight of lactic acid is 90. If the blood lactic acid concentration is 10 mM, there is 900 mg of lactic acid per liter of blood. *See also* OSMOLALITY.

MOLECULE *See under* ELEMENT.

MOLYBDENUM An element that, as a 'trace element' in the human body, is found in the liver, kidneys, bones and skin. It functions as a component of several redox enzymes including xanthine oxidase that catalyzes the breakdown of purines. Rich sources of molybdenum in food include legumes, such as beans. The recommended dietary allowance (RDA) for adults is 45 mcg/day. The tolerable upper intake level (UL) was set at 2 mg based on studies showing impaired reproduction and growth in animals at high levels of chronic intake.

Bibliography
Oregon State University. The Linus Pauling Institute. Micronutrient Information Center. Http://lpi.oregonstate.edu/infocenter

MOMENT In vector terms, moment is the vector (cross) product of force and distance. The Standard International units are Newton meters (N.m). The US Customary units are pound force feet (lbf.ft). *See under* TORQUE.

MOMENT ARM Lever arm. It is the perpendicular distance from the point of application of a force to the axis of rotation.

MOMENT OF INERTIA Rotational inertia. It is the rotational equivalent of mass in its mechanical effect. It is a measure of the resistance offered by a body to angular acceleration. It is the sum of the products formed by multiplying the mass of each element of a figure by the square of its distance from a specified axis of rotation. **Polar moment of inertia** is the moment of inertia with respect to a point. **Axial moment of inertia** is the moment of inertia with respect to an axis. The Standard International unit is the kilogram metre squared ($kg.m^2$). The US Customary unit is the slug inch squared ($sl.in^2$).

Unlike mass, for which there is only one value, a new value exists for moment of inertia for each new axis that is chosen. The heavier the body, the greater is its moment of inertia. The more a body's mass is distributed away from the center of gravity, the greater its moment of inertia.

The **parallel axis theorem** states that the moment of inertia about any axis equals the moment with respect to the parallel centroidal axis plus the mass times the square of the distance between the axes.

Radius of gyration is an abstract concept sometimes used for the estimation of moment of inertia of body segments. It is the square root of the ratio of the moment of inertia of a body about a given axis to its mass. It is a measure of the distribution of a body's mass about an axis of rotation. It is the distance from the axis of rotation to a point where the body's mass could be concentrated, without altering its rotational characteristics.

In archery, stabilizers increase the moment of inertia of the bow. These stabilizers are metal rods that are usually screwed into the back of the bow handle. This is analogous to a tight-rope walker holding a long stick horizontally for stability; the stabilizers increase the force necessary for the bow to twist in the archer's hand.

The moment of inertia of a snowboard is lower than that of two skis. It is both lighter and closer to the rider's axis of rotation. Snowboards are thus easier to turn. In snowboarding, the feet are placed to the rear and to the heel side of the board's center of gravity. Unlike the skier, whose feet are close together, the snowboarders feet are wide enough apart to give him more control over his turns.

Chronology

•1974 • A patent for enlarging the width of the head of a tennis racket was granted in 1974. It was known that by increasing the width, the 'polar moment of inertia' would also increase thus reducing the effect of off-center hits. In 1976, Howard Head's Prince Classic became the first successfully marketed wide-headed racket.

Bibliography

Zumerchik, J. (1997, ed). *Encyclopedia of sports science.* New York: Macmillan Library Reference.

MOMENT OF MOMENTUM   *See* ANGULAR MOMENTUM.

MOMENTS, PRINCIPLE OF   *See under* EQUILIBRIUM.

MOMENTUM   Quantity of motion calculated as mass multiplied by velocity. The principle of **conservation of linear momentum** states that the linear momentum of a system remains constant in the absence of external forces (i.e. from outside the system) or if such forces cancel each other out. The Standard International units are kilogram meters per second (kg.m/s). The US Customary units are foot pounds per second (ft.lb/s).

MONOCYTE   *See under* LEUKOCYTES.

MONONUCLEOSIS   *See under* CHRONIC FATIGUE SYNDROME; SPLEEN.

MONOSACCHARIDES   *See under* CARBO-HYDRATES.

MONTEGGIA FRACTURE   *See under* ELBOW FRACTURES.

MOOD DISORDERS   Affect disorders. Mood disorders may be **bipolar** (mood shifts from mania to depression, and vice versa) or **unipolar** (usually episodes of extreme depression). **Manic episodes** are defined as the presence (for at least one week) of: hyperactivity and restlessness; decreased need for sleep; unusual talkativeness; distractibility manifested as abrupt, rapid changes in activity or topics of speech; inflated self esteem; and excessive involvement in such high-risk activities as reckless driving, buying sprees, sexual indiscretions and quick business investments. **Depressive episodes** include loss of interest or pleasure in almost all usual activities; too much sleep or insomnia; poor appetite and significant weight loss; low self esteem; chronic fatigue; diminished ability to think, concentrate and make decisions; and recurrent thoughts of death and suicide.

Children with depression tend to withdraw and must be coaxed into activity. Some individuals with mania channel their energy into intense periods of productivity. About 1 person in 100 has severe manic-depressive illness, and an equal number has milder variants. The average age of onset is 18 years, and both sexes are affected equally. Major depressive illness is twice as likely to affect women.

Lithium is the drug of choice in manic-depressive illness, and a wide variety of antidepressants are used for depression. Common side effects of lithium are skin rashes, generalized itching, hair loss, headache, dizziness, weakness, blurred vision, fine hand tremor, unsteadiness, nausea and diarrhea.

A mood disorder can be very serious and carries a high risk of suicide.

See also JUVENILE MANIA.

Bibliography

American Psychiatric Association (1994). *Diagnostic and Statistical Manual of Mental Disorders.* 4th ed. Washington, DC: American Psychiatric Association.

MOOD STATE   An emotional condition that persists for a period of time, but is transitory compared to personality traits.

Many studies on athletes using a self-report inventory called the **Profile of Mood States** have found the '**iceberg profile**,' which consists of scores falling well below population norms for tension, depression, anger and fatigue, but above the norm on vigor and esteem-related affect.

An iceberg profile does not necessarily imply that positive mental health leads to success; success in sport may lead to more positive mood profiles and enhanced mental health. Rowley et al. (1995) concluded that successful athletes possess a mood profile only slightly more positive than less successful athletes, calling into question the utility of the Profile of Mood States for predicting athletic success. Use of the Profile of Mood States to track mood changes in athletes during a competitive season has found that variations in the iceberg profile generally reflect overtraining.

Bibliography

Cockerill, I.M., Nevill, A.M. and Lyons, N. (1991). Modeling mood states in athletic performance. *Journal of Sports Sciences* 9, 205-212.

LeUnes, A. and Burger, J. (2000). Profile of mood states research in sport and exercise psychology: Past, present and future. *Journal of Applied Sport Psychology* 12, 5-15.

LeUnes, A. (2000). Updated bibliography on the profile of mood states in sport and exercise psychology research. *Journal of Applied Sport Psychology* 12, 110-113.

Morgan, W.P. et al. (1987). Psychological monitoring of overtraining and staleness. *British Journal of Sports Medicine* 21, 107-114.

Rowley, A.J. et al. (1995). Does the Iceberg Profile discriminate between successful and less successful athletes? A meta analysis. *Journal of Sport & Exercise Psychology* 17(2), 185-199.

MORALITY *See under* CHARACTER BUILDING.

MORBIDITY It refers to a state of illness or disease. A **disease** is an interruption, cessation or disorder of body function, system or organ. **Comorbidity** is a term used in epidemiology to indicate the coexistence of two or more disease processes.

MORO REFLEX A primitive reflex that is present at birth and persists until about 4 months of age. It acts as an infant's 'flight or fight' reaction. It can be elicited in a number of ways, such as placing the palm of the hand under the infant's head and then suddenly, but gently, lowering the head a few inches. This leads to extension of the arms, fingers and legs. It contributes to the development of extensor and abductor strength of the upper extremities, and serves as a propping and parachute reactions. The Moro reflex should be inhibited by about 4 months of post-natal life and replaced by the startle reflex. Failure to integrate the Moro reflex causes inappropriate emotional reactions in childhood, such as throwing a tantrum. Retention of the Moro reflex

into adulthood is associated with the 'flight or fight reaction' and psychological problems such as mood swings and anxiety.

Two-sided absence of the Moro reflex at birth suggests damage to the central nervous system. One-sided absence of the Moro reflex suggests the possibility of a fractured clavicle or injury to the brachial plexus, which can occur because of birth trauma. Conditions associated with brachial plexus injury include Erb's palsy. Paralysis on one side of the body may also produce an asymmetrical Moro reflex.

MORQUIO SYNDROME MPS-IV. Morquio-Brailsford syndrome. It is an inherited disease belonging to the group of mucopolysaccharide storage diseases. It is inherited as an autosomal recessive trait. **Type A MPS-IV** is characterized by the absence of the enzyme galactosamine-6-sulfatase and the excretion of keratan sulfate in the urine. **Type B MPS-IV** results from deficiency results from deficiency of the enzyme beta galactosidase. Symptoms of MPS-IV include large head (macrocephaly), knock knees, short stature, hypermobile joints, abnormal development of many bones including the spine, abnormally short trunk and neck, severe kyphosis and compression of the spinal cord that can lead to weakness or paralysis. It occurs in 1 out of 40,000 to 200,000 births. There is no specific treatment for Morquio syndrome.

Bibliography

National Mucopolysaccharide Syndrome Society, Inc. Http://www.mpssociety.org

MORTALITY A population's death rate.

MORTON'S NEUROMA Morton's toe. Plantar interdigital neuroma. A perineural fibrosis of the plantar nerve that is due to repetitive irritation of the nerve. It commonly affects one interspace, most commonly between the 3rd and 4th toes. It involves compression of the bifurcation of the neurovascular bundle between the metatarsal heads. It is usually due to a shearing force caused by a hypermobile foot with excessive pronation during heel-off in the stance phase, just as the toes are in maximal dorsal flexion prior to take-off. Another cause is tight-fitting shoes with a narrow toe box. The treatment usually involves exercises and inserting an arch support in the shoes.

MOSAICISM This refers to a **chimera**, which is tissue containing 2 or more genetically distinct cell types or an individual composed of such tissues. This is usually found as a variation in the number of chromosomes in the body's cells. One cause is development of a new mutation during the early embryonic growth of a fetus, which affects some, but not all cells. Another cause is **gonadal mosaicism** in which a mutation occurs in a developing fetus' egg or sperm cells. With trisomy, the chromosomal anomaly occurs in every body cells; but with mosaicism the chromosomal anomaly occurs in only some cells.

MOTILITY Capability of motion. Contractility. It refers to the ability to move spontaneously.

MOTION ANALYSIS In the biomechanics of sport, technology for motion capture and analysis has developed rapidly since the early 1990s. Cine film analysis has become largely redundant with the development of video with high sampling rates and short exposure times. For studying impacts in sport (e.g. golf clubface on ball), video cameras, such as the Spin Physics SP2000 Motion Analysis System have been used to record at sampling rates of up to 2,000 full pictures per second or 12,000 partial pictures per second. Mechanical or electronic shuttering enables exposure times in the order of 0.0001 second, resulting in little noise during a 'freeze frame.'

Optoelectronic systems that enable three-dimensional (3D) analysis of human movement with automatic digitizing and data processing have vastly cut down the time needed to gain results. Companies, such as Vicon Motion Systems and Motion Analysis Corporation, use high-resolution digital strobe technology cameras that interface directly with a microcomputer to enable light to be reflected from 'passive markers' (i.e. no electrodes or wires) on the subject into each camera. The markers are spherical or hemispherical, and are covered in retroreflective paper. Strobe lights can be either visible light, near infra-red light (to not interfere with certain equipment signals) or fully infra-red light (so as not to interfere with lighting conditions or visibility). Through pattern recognition, the shape of the detected light source is compared with the expected shape. Some optoelectronic systems (e.g. Selspot) use 'active markers,' which consist of electronic transmitters such as infra-red, light-emitting diodes.

The Vicon 612 system has powerful, automated software that allows 12 cameras and 50 markers to be used for data capture, with data being processed quickly. It has a feature called "Pipeline" that enables all the steps of one or more routine experiments to be stored, so that the process is automated, from capture through to analysis in a single step. It takes raw camera data, converts it to 3D coordinates, performs editing features (such as gap filling and filtering) and then, if required, runs a biomechanical model for joint-based output of kinematic and kinetic parameters. Vicon systems can reach accuracy levels of less than +/-0.1 mm. Accuracy of automatic digitization depends on many factors, e.g. the number of cameras, placement of cameras and marker placement. A larger number of cameras allow a greater space to be captured for motion analysis or for increased accuracy to be gained from a given space. With high-resolution cameras, small markers can be used even in large collection volumes and since smaller markers produce cleaner data, due to decreased possibility of one marker obscuring another, the result is better data. Accuracy of the reconstructed 3D position of a marker also depends on many factors, e.g. accuracy of calibration and quality of the direct linear transformation of a marker's 2D coordinates on the video to its 3D location in space.

A further development was the Vicon iQ, an integrated software system that keeps all information intact throughout all processes of "Pipeline" and uses it intelligently to automatically resolve any problems or ambiguities as they arise.

The Vicon MX 40 was the first 4 million-pixel motion capture camera. The MX40 camera processes the sensor's images at up to 166 frames per second, and higher at decreased resolution. The more pixel resolution that the marker reflection creates in the sensors image the more accurately the relative two-dimensional position of the particular marker in the two-dimensional field can be calculated. The pixel resolution and rate of recording are inversely related, so that the higher the resolution used, the lower the capture rate. The Eagle Digital Camera (Motion Analysis Corporation) has a resolution of 1.3 million pixels up to 500 frames per second.

The latest motion capture systems have real-time capabilities that allow users to see capture results with little or no perceptible time delay, as the subject is performing a specific task. The signals from digital cameras go directly to the tracking computer via an Ethernet connection. This streamlined system of motion capture from camera to computer means less hardware and less potential for equipment problems. The Talon Viewer (Motion Analysis Corporation), for example, provides real-time, streamed viewing of a skinned character during a motion capture session. It works with Skeleton Builder to create a binding form the motion capture data to the character's skeleton (which is exported from an animation package using Animation plug-ins).

The **direct linear transformation (DLT) method** (Abdel-Aziz and Karara, 1971) determines the relationship between the image space and each of the digitized views and does not depend on knowing the location or orientation of the cameras, the distance of the cameras to the subject, or any information about the camera or projection lenses such as focal length.

Chronology

•1881 • Eadweard J. Muybridge and Etienne J. Marey met in Paris to begin collaborating in the study of motion.
•1882 • Marey designed and built what was to become the world's first portable motion picture camera. He designed a camera in the shape of a rife, which he used to take pictures of birds in flight.
•1884 • Muybridge produced more than 100,000 plates of humans and animals in a great variety of motions in a study conducted at University of Pennsylvania.
•1887 • Muybridge published *Animal Locomotion: An Electrophotographic Investigation of Consecutive Phases of Animal Movement*, an 11-volume work with more than 20,000 photographs.

•1901 • A year after the Olympic Games in Paris, Etienne J. Marey reported to the Academy of Sciences on the work of a Committee on Physiology and Hygiene. He claimed that his chronophotographs had revealed the technical secrets of champions. According to Höberman (1992), Marey's investigations represented the most advanced sports physiology of this period.
•1931 • Harold E. Edgerton developed the stroboscope for use in ultra-high speed and still photography.
•1938 • Harold E. Edgerton perfected multi-flash photography of athletes in action. By 1940, sports photography was revolutionized by Edgerton's technique, which allowed the camera to capture high-speed motion and preserve an unprecedented degree of detail. Electronic flash photographs of sports events were regularly published in major newspapers after 1940.
•2004 • Using 50 cameras with the Eagle Digital System to cover a 50 foot x 50 foot volume, Motion Analysis Studios captured up to six athletes simultaneously, at 120 frames per second, for a Nike television commercial which premiered on Monday Night Football.

Bibliography

Abdel-Aziz, Y.I. and Karara, H.M. (1971). Direct linear transformation from comparator coordinates into object space coordinates in close-range photogrammetry. *Proceedings of the Symposium on Close-Range Photogrammetry*. pp1-18. Falls Church, VA: American Society of Photogrammetry.

Bartlett, R. (1997). *Introduction to sports biomechanics*. London: E & FN Spon.

Kreighbaum, E. and Barthels, K.M. (1996). *Biomechanics: A qualitative approach*. 4th ed. Needham Heights, MA: Allyn and Bacon.

Motion Analysis Corporation. Http://www.motionanalysis.com

Nigg, B.M. and Herzog, W. (1999, eds). *Biomechanics of the musculoskeletal system*. Chichester, UK: John Wiley.

The Complete History of the Discovery of Cinematography. Http://www.precinemahistory.net

VICON Motion Systems. Http://www.vicon.com

MOTION SICKNESS A condition that involves a mismatch of sensory inputs, including those from vestibular apparatus, visual system and proprioceptors, and comparison of those inputs with the individual's expectations derived from previous experience. Motion sickness occurs most commonly with acceleration in a direction perpendicular to the longitudinal axis of the body, which is why head movements away from the direction are so provocative. Vertical oscillatory motion at a frequency of 0.2 Hertz (corresponding to a roll rate on a ship of 5 seconds) is most likely to cause motion sickness.

Nausea and vomiting are the most common symptoms of motion sickness. In response to visual and vestibular input, increased levels of dopamine stimulate the medulla oblongata's chemoreceptor trigger zone, which in turn stimulates the vomiting center within the reticular formation. The vomiting center is also directly stimulated by motion and by high levels of acetylcholine.

Actual movement is not necessary to produce symptoms of motion sickness. Symptoms can result from purely visual stimuli, such as from a flight simulator, with the degree of motion sickness seeming related to how well the visual stimulus simulates motion.

Children under the age of 2 years are rarely affected by motion sickness, but susceptibility increases with age, peaking between 4 and 10 years, and then gradually declining. Females tend to be more susceptible than males, regardless of age, with pregnancy, menses and use of oral contraceptives increasing susceptibility. A high level of aerobic fitness is associated with increased susceptibility, possibly because of increased parasympathetic tone. Recent ingestion of food has also been associated with increased susceptibility.

Drugs to prevent or lessen motion sickness can be subdivided into anti-dopaminergics, anti-cholinergics and anti-histamines. Anti-dopaminergic drugs include promethazine hydrochloride (e.g. Anergan) that has anti-histamine, anti-cholinergic and sedative effects. Anti-cholinergic drugs include the anti-muscarinic scopolamine hydrobromide (Transderm-Scop), or hyoscine, which is delivered via a cutaneous patch. Scopolamine prevents motion-induced nausea by inhibiting vestibular input to the central nervous system, resulting in an inhibition of the vomiting reflex. It may also have a direct action on the vomiting center. Scopolamine is contraindicated in patients at risk of narrow-angle glaucoma and should be discontinued immediately if pain occurs. Antihistamines include meclizine hydrochloride, a histamine-receptor blocker. The benefit derived from antihistamines is probably due to their intrinsic anti-cholinergic properties, rather than their antihistamine properties. Meclizine is contraindicated in patients with respiratory problems (e.g. chronic bronchitis), glaucoma or enlarged prostate.

In a study of 22 elite field athletes, half of whom practiced both discus and hammer, it was found that 59% reported dizziness while throwing the discus, but none while throwing the hammer. Because several individuals practiced both sport, these results exclude the hypothesis of individual susceptibility to dizziness. During hammer throwing, visual bearings can be used more easily than during discus throwing. Moreover, there is a loss of plantar afferents and generation of head movements liable to induce motion sickness.

See also under MICROGRAVITY.

Bibliography
Germann, W.J. and Stanfield, C.L. (2001). *Principles of human physiology*. San Francisco, CA: Benjamin Cummings.

Perrin, P. et al. (2000). Dizziness in discus throwers is related to motion sickness generated while spinning. *Acta Otolaryngology* 120(3), 390-395.

MOTIVATION   The direction, intensity and persistence of behavior. **Survival behavior** is regulated by physiological systems that operate according to the principle of homeostasis. The hypothalamus plays an important role in survival behavior such as feeding and drinking. The intensity of motivation has classically been explained with concepts like tensions, physiological needs and their resulting drive states, and psychological needs. The construct of arousal has also been used in this context. Direction of motivation has been explained with concepts like intentions and goals. There have been many theories to explain behavior that is not necessary for pure survival.

See also ACHIEVEMENT MOTIVATION; ATTRIBUTION THEORY; EXERCISE ADHERENCE; GOAL; GOAL ORIENTATION; INTRINSIC MOTIVATION; PERFECTIONISM; SELF EFFICACY; SPORT COMMITMENT.

MOTOR BEHAVIOR   A field of study that emphasizes the behavioral analysis of skilled movement. *See* MOTOR LEARNING; MOTOR SKILLS.

MOTOR CONTROL   An area of study that is concerned with the neural and biomechanical aspects of movement.

Bibliography

Latash, M.L. (2002, ed). *Progress in motor control. Volume 2. Structure-function relations in voluntary movements*. Champaign, IL: Human Kinetics.

Rose, D.J. (1997). *A multilevel approach to the study of motor control and learning*. San Francisco, CA: Benjamin Cummings.

Rosenbaum, D.A. (1991). *Human motor control*. London: Academic Press.

MOTOR CORTEX *See under* BRAIN.

MOTOR DEVELOPMENT An area of study that is concerned with the changes that occur in human movement throughout the lifespan.

Developmental directions may be cephalocaudal or proximodistal. These directions should not be viewed as being operational at all levels of development or in all individuals. In the context of both growth and maturation, **cephalocaudal** means 'from the head to the tail;' the head experiences greater growth earlier than the rest of the body. **Gross motor development** begins with head control and proceeds downward (i.e. in a cephalocaudal direction). Voluntary control of the head or neck may gradually become apparent by the end of the first month. This is then followed by lifting of the chest (2 months); sitting without support, but with an acute forward lean (5 months); self-supported sitting position in either a prone or supine position (7 months); and onset of standing progression and pull from a sitting to a standing position (9 months).

Crawling precedes creeping in the progression of movement acquired for prone locomotion. Creeping normally begins from 7 to 9 months of age, but most children do not creep efficiently until the first year of age. **Crawling** is a form of locomotion in which the body is kind of dragged along the supporting surface, but **creeping** is an elevated, highly efficient form of locomotion. Many children who have learned to walk often revert to creeping when they have the desire to move more quickly. Some normal babies never creep or crawl at all; they sit around until they learn to stand up. Early crawling makes no difference to later motor development. Infants who are put to sleep on their stomach may crawl somewhat earlier than those put to sleep on their backs. There is a substantial increase in the risk of **sudden infant death syndrome (crib death)** that comes with sleeping face down. If assisted with considerable support, a child can walk as early as 8 months. It is rare, however, that independent walking occurs at 8 months. Around 10 months the child can walk with much less support. By 11 months, the child can walk when led by another person and by 12 months, the child can walk unassisted.

Proximodistal means 'from proximal to distal.' It applies especially to human prenatal growth. The human evolves from the **neural groove**, a tiny elongated mass of cells that eventually forms the spinal cord. Proximal muscle groups become functional before the more distal, e.g. a child learns to catch with shoulders, upper arms and forearms before catching with fingers. Movements performed at midline (in front of body) are easier than those that entail crossing midline (to left or right of body). This is referred to as **proximodistal coordination**. With aging, cephalocaudal and proximodistal processes reverse themselves.

Bilateral movement patterns (both limbs moving simultaneously) are the first to occur in the human infant, followed by **unilateral movement patterns** (e.g. right arm and left leg moving simultaneously) and then cross-lateral patterns (e.g. right and left arm moving simultaneously). This is referred to as **bilateral-to-crosslateral motor coordination**.

Differentiation is the gradual progression from gross, immature movement to precise, well-controlled, intentional movement of children and adults. As muscle systems become differentiated, they also become integrated, i.e. more capable of functioning together. **Integration** involves bringing various opposing muscle and sensory systems into coordinated interactions with one another. Integration involves the neural process of laying over, inhibiting or suppressing reflexes and stereotypies. When reflexes and stereotypies do not disappear in infancy, they are classified as pathological. Integration is never total or complete; abnormal reflex activity is recognizable in clumsy movement at all ages. Under fatigue and stress conditions, integration sometimes breaks down. Like differentiation, integration tends to be reversible with aging.

Abnormal motor development refers to severe conditions in which some of the motor skills are dominated by reflexes due to failure of some reflexes to be integrated. **Delayed motor development** refers to slowness in achieving motor milestones.

See under AGING; DEVELOPMENTAL COORDINATION DISORDER; MOTOR LEARNING; MOTOR SKILL; OVERFLOW; REFLEXES; SELF CONCEPT; SPINE.

Bibliography

Cech, D.J. and Martin, S. (2002, eds). *Functional movement development. Across the lifespan.* 2nd ed. Philadelphia, PA: W.B. Saunders Co.

Gallahue, D.L. and Ozmun, J.C. (2002). *Understanding motor development. Infants, children, adolescents, adults.* 5th ed. New York, NY: McGraw-Hill.

Gormly, A.V. (1997). *Lifespan human development.* 6th ed. South Melbourne, Australia: Wadsworth.

Haywood, K.M. and Getchell, N. (2004). *Life span motor development.* 4th ed. Champaign, IL: Human Kinetics.

Motor Development Task Force (1995). *Looking at physical education from a developmental perspective. A guide to teaching.* Reston, VA: National Association for Sport and PE.

Payne, V.G. and Isaacs, L.D. (2005). *Human motor development. A lifespan approach.* 6th ed. Boston, MA: McGraw-Hill.

Sherill, C. (2004). *Adapted physical activity, recreation and sport. Cross disciplinary and lifespan.* 6th ed. Boston, MA: McGraw-Hill.

MOTOR LEARNING

A field of study concerned with the learning of motor skills.

Fitts and Posner's (1967) model of learning has been applied to motor learning. Three stages can be identified in the learning of a skill. First, there is the cognitive (early) stage, when task relevant instruction is important and the learner is concerned with how different components of the skill are interrelated. Verbal commands play an important role at this stage. Second, there is the associative (intermediate) stage, when the learner makes fewer errors and there is a strengthening of the interrelationships between components of the skill. Third, there is the autonomous (final) stage, which is characterized by automatization. There is less reliance on verbal commands at this stage.

Modeling may be enhanced if a learner watches a 'learning model' rather than an 'expert model.' This may be explained in terms of the learner being able to focus on the processes of skill learning, especially those associated with 'trial-and-error,' i.e. how the learner attempts to perform the task, how feedback is used and how adjustments are made on the next trial. Cognitive theories of modeling are based on the premise that the learner translates the observed movement information into a cognitive code that the person stores in memory and uses when the observer performs the skill. Noncognitive theories assume that the visual system is capable of automatically processing the observed movement that constrains the motor control system to act accordingly, so that the learner does not need to use cognitive processes.

Guidance involves passive learning procedures, ranging from physically pushing and pulling the learner through a movement sequence, to preventing incorrect movements by physical limitations on apparatus. There is evidence that guidance can be beneficial when interspersed with active practice trials. Guidance is often used in sports such as gymnastics to minimize risk of injury and decrease fear when learning a new skilled movement.

The **part method of learning** involves breaking down information into smaller units to be learned separately and then recombined to perform the whole skill. **Fractionization** involves practicing individual limbs first for a skill, such as the breaststroke in swimming, which involves the asymmetric coordination of the arms or legs. Practice should begin with the hand or arm that must perform the more difficult or complex movement. **Segmentation** involves separating the skill into parts and then practicing the parts in a progressive and cumulative manner (practice one part, then practice that part with the next part, etc). **Simplification** is a variation of a whole practice strategy that involves decreasing the difficulty of the whole skill or different parts of the skill.

Verbal labels and visual imagery can add meaningfulness to movement by: decreasing the complexity of verbal instructions; helping to change an abstract, complex array of movement to a more concrete, meaningful set of movement; and directing the individual's attentional focus to the outcome of the performance. For limb-positioning movements, people typically associate end location of a movement with a body part and use that as a cue to aid their recall performance. People will also spontaneously associate the end location of limb positions with well-known objects, such as a clock face, to aid recall. *See* EXPERTISE; FEEDBACK; MOTOR DEVELOPMENT; MOTOR SKILL; PRACTICE; REFLEXES.

Bibliography

Annett, J. (1985). Motor learning: A review. In: Heuer, H., Kleinbeck, U. and Schmidt, K.U. (eds). *Motor behaviour: Programming, control and acquisition*. Berlin: Springer.

Blandin, Y. and Proteau, L. (2000). On the cognitive basis of observational learning: Development of mechanisms for the detection and correction of errors. *Quarterly Journal of Experimental Psychology* 53A, 846-867.

Fitts, P.M. and Posner, M.I. (1967). *Human performance*. Belmont, California: Brookes-Cole.

Glencross, D.J., Whiting, H.T.A. and Abernethy, B. (1994). Motor control, motor learning and the acquisition of skill: Historical trends and future directions. *International Journal of Sport Psychology* 25, 32-52.

Hodges, N.J. and Franks, I.M. (2002). Modeling coaching practice: The role of instruction and demonstration. *Journal of Sports Sciences* 20(10), 793-811.

Kluka, D.A. (1999). *Motor behavior: From learning to performance*. Englewood, Colorado: Morton Publishing Co.

Magill, R.A. (2004). *Motor learning and control*. 7th ed. Boston, MA: McGraw-Hill.

McCullagh, P. and Caird, J.K. (1990). Correct and learning models and the use of model knowledge of results in the acquisition and retention of a motor skill. *Journal of Human Movement Studies* 18, 107-116.

McCullagh, P. (1993). Modeling: Learning, developmental, and social psychological considerations. In Singer, R., Murphey, M. and Tennant, L.K. (eds). *Handbook of research on sport psychology*. pp106-126. New York: MacMillan.

McCullagh, P. and Meyer, K.N. (1997). Learning versus correct models: Influence of model type on the learning of a free-weight squat lift. *Research Quarterly of Exercise and Sport* 68, 56-61.

Piek, J.P. (1998, ed). *Motor behavior and human skill*. Champaign, IL: Human Kinetics.

Rose, D.J. (1997). *Multilevel approach to the study of motor control and learning*. San Francisco, CA: Benjamin Cummings.

Schmidt, R.A. and Lee, T.D. (1999). *Motor control and learning. A behavioral emphasis*. 3rd ed. Champaign, IL: Human Kinetics.

Schmidt, R.A. and Wrisberg, C.A. (2004). *Motor learning and performance*. 3rd ed. Champaign, IL: Human Kinetics.

Thomas, J.R. (1997). Sport and exercise psychology. In: Massengale, J.D. and Swanson, R.A. (eds.). *The history of exercise and sport science*. pp203-292. Champaign, IL: Human Kinetics.

Wightman, D.C. and Lintern, G. (1985). Part-task training strategies for tracking and manual control. *Human Factors* 27, 267-283.

Williams, A.M. and Hodges, N.J. (2004, eds). *Skill acquisition in sport. Research, theory and practice*. London: Routledge.

MOTOR LEARNING, THEORIES OF Models of closed-loop control and open-loop control have been used to explain motor learning. **Open-loop control** refers to a mode of system control that does not depend on feedback. Traffic lights provide an everyday example of open-loop control. A theoretical construct concerned with open-loop control of movement is a **motor program**, which is a plan for a movement sequence that is stored in the central nervous system. The plan, rather than ongoing feedback, controls the movement. The founder of the motor program hypothesis was K.S. Lashley, who observed during World War I soldiers with gunshot wounds to the spinal cord, which produced de-afferentation (i.e. cut off sensory feedback from limbs). These wounded soldiers never made a mistake in the direction of voluntary movement when blindfolded, and their accuracy in the extent of the movement compared favorably with fit soldiers. **Closed-loop control** is a mode of system control in which feedback from action is compared against a reference of correctness to give an error signal that acts as a stimulus for future action. The home thermostat is an everyday example of a system under closed-loop control, i.e. negative feedback control. When the temperature in the house reaches the level set on the thermostat, the heating turns off. When the temperature drops below the set level, the heating turns on again.

Adams (1971,1976) proposed a **Closed-Loop theory of motor learning**. The feedback from a response is compared with a reference mechanism to a desired value of feedback. Discrepancies between the feedback and the reference value become the source of error correction. Two different forms of memory are proposed: the perceptual trace and the memory trace. The **perceptual trace** is the memory of the feedback associated with a specific movement in the past, against which incoming feedback is compared. It grows in strength each time the response is produced accurately. Feedback, in the form of knowledge of results, is necessary when the correct perceptual trace has been established. The **memory trace** is concerned with the selection and initiation of a response from the store of alternative responses. Like the perceptual trace, it grows as a function of accurate response production.

Schmidt (1975) criticized Adams' theory and proposed a **Schema theory of motor learning**. A **schema** is a memory construct that is constructive in nature, rather than merely reproductive. It is unlikely that the great range of movements that are performed by a tennis player, for example, could be produced from a finite store of fixed motor responses, as suggested by Adams' Closed-Loop theory. Schema theory proposes that there is a motor response mechanism that consists of a set of operational rules (algorithms) that has been acquired from learning. The set of operational rules is called the schema. It is proposed that there is a separate schema for each particular class of movement under consideration. Skill is determined by the efficiency of the schema. The schema is constructed on the basis of certain types of information, such as limb positions, which are stored after each movement. The 'strength' of the schema is a function of the number of learning trials in which there is feedback (in the form of knowledge of results) and the variability of practice. **Practice variability** refers to the variety of movement and context characteristics a person experiences while practicing a skill. To produce a motor response, there is a '**general motor program**' that allows the production of a number of similar movements of a given class. All movements with the same phasing and relative forces are produced by the same general motor program. These movement characteristics are thought to constitute invariant elements. It is also assumed that programs can be executed with different response specifications (parameters). The most important of these parameters are temporal duration, speed, absolute force and movement size. The time to change a tennis ground stroke to a lob (presumably requiring a different program and parameters) in response to a visual stimulus has been estimated as about 600 milliseconds, whereas the time required to change

the direction or length of the ground stroke (presumably only requiring new parameters) has been estimated to be about 400 milliseconds (Roth, 1988).

It seems that the extent to which each mode of control is used in a particular skill depends on a number of factors, such as skill level. Highly skilled performance often seems to be predominantly under open loop control.

In contrast to the theories of Adams and Schmidt, Bernstein (1967) adopted a non-cognitive approach to motor learning. The learning of movements is viewed in terms of exploiting non-muscular forces, such as gravity. In other words, the control of movement cannot be viewed simply in terms of a control center in the brain issuing commands that are sent to the muscles, which then contract and move the bones. Information from movement detectors in joints and connective tissues is used during movement and is involved in feedback loops. These loops are not controlled by the control center in the brain, but are controlled by nervous tissue located outside the brain and spinal cord. Bernstein used the notion of '**degrees of freedom**' to refer to the number of variables that need to be controlled when body movement is produced. Bones can move in one or more directions, and their movement is limited by joint structure and connective tissues. The more directions of movement permitted by a joint, then the more degrees of freedom it has. Also, the more muscles that can move the bones of a particular joint, the more degrees of freedom it has. If the degrees of freedom can be decreased, then control of a motor skill becomes simpler. During the early stages of learning, a person can decrease the degrees of freedom in at least two ways. The first way is by keeping one or more joints rigidly fixed, in a robotic-like manner. The second way is by moving two or more joints together in a closely time-phased manner. As learning proceeds, there is a gradual release of the rigid control of degrees of freedom. There are two successive stages in this release. In the first stage, the control becomes less rigid and there is the emergence of various non-muscular forces. These include forces due to gravity, changes in the ease with which the limbs can be rotated and changes in the reactive forces that one joint exerts against another. Depending on contextual factors such as plane of movement and the particular muscles innervated, the movement of one segment in a limb (such as the arm) will tend to cause movement of another segment in that limb (such as the hand). In the second stage, the non-muscular forces are fully incorporated into the sequence of movement. This makes the movement more economical.

Bernstein's (1967) approach can be classed under ecological psychology, which focuses on the interaction between mind, body and environment. Following the work of Gibson (1966, 1979) visual perception is defined as the detection of invariants in the optical array. A person does not need to detect, process and interpret environmental information like a computer. Lee et al (1982) showed how invariants in the optical array are involved in the coordination and control of the take-off in long jumping.

Chronology
•1932 • In *Remembering: A Study in Experimental and Social Psychology*, Frederic C. Bartlett of Cambridge University stated "Suppose I am making a stroke in a quick game, such as tennis or cricket... I do not, as a matter of fact, produce something absolutely new, and I never merely repeat something old. The stroke is literally manufactured out of the living visual and postural 'schemata' of the movement and their interrelations." Bartlett's concept of the schema had an impact later on theories of knowledge representation in cognitive psychology and also on theories of motor learning.
•1964 • A text entitled *Movement Behavior and Motor Learning* published by B.J. Cratty of UCLA was the first textbook devoted solely to motor behaviour and learning.

Bibliography
Adams, J.A. (1976). Issues for a Closed Loop theory of motor learning. In: Stelmach, G.E. (ed). *Motor control: Issues and trends*. pp87-105. New York: Academic Press.
Bernstein, N. (1967). *The coordination and regulation of movement*. Oxford: Pergamon Press.
Gibson, J. (1966). *The senses considered as perceptual systems*. Boston: Houghton Mifflin.
Gibson, J. (1979). *The ecological approach to visual perception*. Boson: Houghton Mifflin.
Latash, M.L. (1998, ed). *Progress in motor control. Bernstein's traditions in movement studies*. Champaign, IL: Human Kinetics.
Lee, D.N., Lishman, J.R. and Thompson, J.A. (1982). Regulation of gait in long jumping. *Journal of Experimental Psychology: Human Perception and Performance* 8, 448-459.

Magill, R.A. (2004). *Motor learning and control. Concepts and applications*. 7th ed. Boston: MA: McGraw-Hill.
Schmidt, R.A. (1975). *A Schema theory of discrete motor skill learning*. Psychological Review 82, 225-260.
Vereijken, B., Van Emmerik, R.E.A., Whiting, H.T.A. and Newell, K.M. (1992). *Free(z)ing degrees of freedom in skill acquisition*. Journal of Motor Behavior 24, 133-142.

MOTOR LEARNING, TRANSFER OF **Positive transfer** occurs when previous experience facilitates performance of a skill in a new context or the learning of a new skill. **Negative transfer** occurs when previous experience hinders or interferes with performance of a skill in a new context or the learning of a new skill. **Zero transfer** occurs when previous experience has no influence on performance of a skill in a new context or learning of a new skill.

Asymmetric transfer occurs when a person learns a skill using one limb before learning it with the contralateral limb. **Symmetric transfer** occurs when the amount of transfer is similar when either limb is used first. **Bilateral transfer** is the transfer of a skill learned on one side of the body to the other side. The acquisition of a particular skill involving the left hand is enhanced if that skill has already been learned with the right hand. It is generally accepted that bilateral transfer is asymmetric, but there is controversy as to whether this asymmetry favors transfer from the preferred to nonpreferred limb, or vice versa. The traditional view is that there is a greater amount of transfer when a person practices initially with the preferred limb, i.e. a greater amount of transfer occurs from the preferred to the nonpreferred limb.

Bibliography
Magill, R.A. (2004). *Motor learning and control. Concepts and applications*. 7th ed. Boston: MA: McGraw-Hill.

MOTOR NEURONS Effector neurons. Nerve cells, located in the anterior horn of the gray matter of the spinal cord, which conduct impulses from the central nervous system to muscles or glands. *See* MOTOR UNITS; NERVOUS SYSTEM.

MOTOR PROGRAM In terms of motor control, a motor program can be defined as a set of muscle commands that are structured before the motor acts begin and that can be sent to the muscles with the correct timing so that the entire sequence can be carried out in the absence of peripheral feedback. From a cognitive perspective, a motor program is a memory representation that stores information needed to perform an action.

See under MOTOR LEARNING, THEORIES OF.

Bibliography

Brooks, V. (1986). *The neural basis of motor control*. Oxford: Oxford University Press.

MOTOR SKILL A skill involving significant movement of one or more joints of the body. By **skill** is meant the capability to perform a particular task. The 'building blocks' of skills are abilities. The defining characteristics of skill are effectiveness and flexibility. **Effectiveness** refers to the accuracy of response and economy of effort. **Flexibility** refers to being able to deal with many different circumstances.

A **gross motor skill** is one involving large muscle groups. A **fine motor skill** is one involving only small muscle groups. A **closed skill**, such as trampolining, is one in which the environment of the activity does not change significantly. An **open skill**, such as rugby, is a skill in which the environment of the activity is constantly changing. Anticipation and timing accuracy are important in open skills. A **discrete skill**, such as throwing a ball, has clearly defined beginning and end points. A **continuous skill**, such as running, has arbitrary beginning and end points. **Sport skills** involve social, perceptual, cognitive and motor skills. Physical fitness is important for sport skills; training involves both physical fitness and skill. Some skills, such as walking, are acquired as a result of normal maturational processes through much training and practice. Other skills, such as the tennis serve, are learned.

Phylogenetic skills are resistant to external environmental influences; examples include rudimentary manipulative tasks of reaching, grasping and releasing objects. **Ontogenetic skills** depend primarily on learning and environmental opportunities, require practice and are influenced by culture.

Rudimentary movements are voluntary movements typically mastered during infancy (0 to 2 years) and are primarily reflex in nature. The developmental sequence, temporally, is in the following order: stability, locomotion and manipulation.

Fundamental movement skills can be classed as stability, locomotion and manipulation. Stability can be categorized as either axial (bending, stretching, twisting, turning and swinging) or postural (inverted supports, body rolling, starting, stopping, dodging and balancing). Fundamental movement skills for locomotion can be categorized as having one element (e.g. walking, running, leaping, jumping and hopping) or as having two or more elements (e.g. galloping, sliding, skipping and climbing). Manipulation can be categorized as propulsive (throwing, kicking, punting, striking, volleying, bouncing and rolling) or absorptive (catching and trapping). By the age of 6 years, most children have the potential to perform at the mature stage of most fundamental movement patterns and to begin the transition to the specialized movement phase.

Specialized movement skills are mature fundamental movement patterns that have been refined and combined to form sport skills and other specific and complex movement skills.

Early childhood (3 to 5 years) is characterized by limited fundamental movement skills. It has been found that only 20% of 4 year-old children are proficient at throwing and 30% at catching. This lack of catching skill may be due to lack of visual maturity rather than lack of coordination. It is not until the age of 6 or 7 that the eye has developed a mature spheroid shape. Childhood (6 to 9 years) is characterized by continued development in fundamental skills. Postural and balance skills will have reached adult patterns by about the age of 7 years. Running improves to mature levels by about the age of 8 years. Children rely on verbal commands accompanied by visual demonstrations. Attention span is still relatively short and there is a tendency for children to attend to objects or events regardless of their relevance. During late childhood (10 to 12 years), both fundamental and transitional skills improve. Attention becomes more selective.

The **Bruininks-Oserestsky Test of Motor Proficiency** is a norm-referenced test battery of eight subtests comprised of 46 items relating to gross and fine motor skills. It is aimed at children of ages 4½ to 14½ years. The tests and their purposes are as follows: bead stringing (eye-hand coordination and dexterity), target throwing (eye-hand coordination as related to throwing), marble transfer (finger dexterity and speed of hand movement), back and hamstring stretch (flexibility), standing long jump (strength and power of lower legs and thighs), face down to standing (speed and agility), stationary balance with eyes open and closed (static balance), basketball throw (explosive arm and shoulder strength), ball striking (striking coordination), target kicking (eye-foot coordination) and agility run (ability to change directions quickly).

See ATTENTION-DEFICIT HYPERACTIVITY.

Chronology
•1959 • The Research Council of the American Association for Health, Physical Education and Recreation (AAHPER) recognized the need to standardize skills tests on a national level and initiated the Sports Skills Test Project.

Bibliography
Gallahue, D.L. and Ozmun, J.C. (1997). *Understanding motor development*. Madison, WI: Brown & Benchmark.

Haywood, K.M. (1993). *Lifespan motor development*. 2nd ed. Champaign, IL: Human Kinetics.

Nelson, M.A. (1991). Developmental skills and children's sports. *The Physician and Sportsmedicine* 19(2), 67-79.

MOTOR UNIT A single motor neuron and the muscle fibers it innervates. A muscle fiber either contracts to its present maximum ability (dependent on factors such as its stores of energy) or not at all ('**All-or-none law**'). All muscle fibers within the same motor unit will consist of the same fiber type. Typically, slow-twitch motor units innervate between 10 and 180 muscle fibers. Fast-twitch motor units innervate between 300 and 800 muscle fibers. According to the **Size Principle of Motor Unit Recruitment**, for graded movements representing submaximal muscle actions, motor units with smaller motor neurons (slow-twitch motor units) will be recruited before those with larger motor neurons (fast-twitch motor units). In ballistic movement involving rapid alternating movements, however, there appears to be synchronous or concurrent activation of the motor unit pool, whereby fast-twitch motor units are recruited along with slow-twitch motor units. This synchronous firing has also been shown to occur as a result of weight training. There is evidence that in athletic performance requiring a wide range of muscular output, fast-twitch motor units may be recruited before slow-twitch motor units in vigorous muscle action.

Increased motor unit synchronization enables greater force to be generated and increased efficiency in application of force. Increased recruitment of high-threshold motor units enables increased rate of force development and increased ability to train high-threshold motor units. Activation of high-threshold motor units for a long period of time enables increased time over which maximal force can be maintained. Synchronized motor unit firing rates lead to smooth acceleration. It also leads to greater power and increases the time during which high muscle tension can be maintained.

High-intensity strength training is associated with a more rapid recruitment of motor units and an increased firing rate of motor neurons. Furthermore, a more synchronized discharge of the motor neurons enables activation bursts to discharge a greater number of muscle fibers in a shorter period of time. These adaptations lead to significant improvement in rate of force development and therefore power production.

Motor unit remodeling is a normal, continual process involving motor end-plate repair and reconstruction. Remodeling progresses by select denervation of muscle fibers, followed by terminal sprouting of axons from adjacent motor units. Motor units remodeling gradually deteriorates in old age.

Bibliography
Schmitbleicher, D. (1992). Training for power events. In: Komi, P.V. (ed). *Strength and power in sport*. pp381-395. Oxford: Blackwell Scientific Publishers.

Siff, M.C. (2000). Biomechanical foundations of strength and power training. In Zatsiorsky, V. (ed). *Biomechanics in sport. Performance enhancement and injury prevention. Vol. IX of the Encyclopedia of Sports Medicine*. pp103-139. Oxford: Blackwell Science.

MOUNTAIN SICKNESS *See under* ALTITUDE.

MOUTHGUARD A resilient plastic device that is placed inside the mouth to protect against injuries to the teeth, lacerations to the mouth, and fractures and dislocations of the jaw. An athlete is 60 times more likely to sustain dental injuries when not wearing a mouthguard. The American Dental Association recommends wearing custom-fitted mouthguards for the following sports: acrobatics, basketball, boxing, field hockey, football, gymnastics, handball, ice hockey, lacrosse, martial arts, racquetball, roller hockey, rugby, shot putting, skateboarding, skiing, skydiving, soccer, squash, surfing, volleyball, water polo, weightlifting and wrestling.

See also HEAD INJURIES; TEETH.

Bibliography
Sports Dentistry Online. Http://www.sportsdentistry.com

MOVEMENT Changes in joint angles and/or changes in the position of the body as a whole. A **movement pattern** is an organized series of related movements. **Active movement** involves voluntary muscle contractions to move a joint. A **maximum-force movement** occurs when the agonists contract with maximum force. There are two types of maximum-force movement: continuous-force and ballistic. **Continuous-force movement** occurs when near-maximum force is applied throughout the range of movement. **Ballistic movement** occurs when brief contractions of the agonist initiate movement and then the movement continues under the momentum of the limb(s) without continued muscular contraction. Ballistic movement is a combination of active and passive movement. **Passive movement** takes place without continuing [active] muscle contraction and may be manipulative, inertial or gravitational. **Manipulation** occurs when the motive force is another person or an outside force other than gravity. **Inertial movement** is a continuation of pre-established movement, with no concurrent motive muscular contraction. Inertial movement is considered to include frictional influences (e.g. air resistance) and other deceleratory elements.

Examples are the glide phase of the breaststroke, sliding into a base, and the horizontal component of the free flight of a jump. **Gravitational movement** is a special case of manipulative movement. Examples include free fall, the vertical component of the free flight of a jump, and relaxed pendulum movements in gymnastics. **Whiplike movement** is the acceleration of the end point of a moving kinematic chain induced by the deceleration of the proximal segments.

When analyzing motion, an understanding of planes and axes enables the observer to select the best position from which to observe and record a motion.

See ELECTROMYOGRAPHY; FORCE; FORCE PLATFORM; MUSCLE ACTION; SUMMATION OF VELOCITY PRINCIPLE; TORQUE.

Bibliography
Zatsiorsky, V.M. (2002). *Kinetics of human motion*. Champaign, IL: Human Kinetics.

MRI *See* MAGNETIC RESONANCE IMAGERY.

MUCOID Any of several glycoproteins similar to mucin.

MUCOPOLYSACCHARIDES These are the polysaccharide components of glycosaminoglycans (proteoglycans).

MUCOPOLYSACCHARIDOSIS A group of inherited lyosomal storage disorders caused by the body's inability to produce certain enzymes. Each disorder is caused by deficiency of one of ten specific lysosomal enzymes, resulting in an inability to metabolize mucopolysaccharides or glycosaminoglycans into simpler molecules. The accumulation of these large, undegraded mucopolysaccharides or glycosaminoglycans in the cells of the body causes a number of physical symptoms and abnormalities. Three of these disorders are Hunter's syndrome, Hurler's syndrome and Morquio's syndrome.

Bibliography
National MPS (Mucopolysaccharidoses/Mucolipidoses) Society, Inc. Http://www.mpssociety.ca

MUCOPROTEIN Any of a group of organic compounds, occurring mainly in mucous secretions, that consist of a complex of proteins and glycosaminoglycans.

MUCOSA Mucous membrane. It is the moist tissue that lines certain organs and body cavities, such as the nose, mouth and lungs. In the digestive tract, there is also a layer of smooth muscle supporting the mucosa. Mucosa generally contains glands that secrete **mucus**, a thick, viscous fluid that acts as a lubricant and a means of protection for cells.

MUCOUS MEMBRANE *See* MUCOSA.

MUCUS *See under* MUCOSA.

MULTANGUM MAJOR *See* TRAPEZIUM.

MULTANGUM MINOR *See* TRAPEZOID.

MULTIPLE DISABILITIES In the USA, these are defined by federal legislation as concomitant impairments (such as mental retardation-blindness, mental retardation-orthopedic impairment etc), the combination of which causes such severe educational needs that they cannot be accommodated in special education programs solely for one of the impairments.

MULTIPLE SCLEROSIS An autoimmune disease in which it seems the body mistakes portions of nerve covering (myelin) for a virus and therefore releases substances that cause myelin to disintegrate. 30 to 60% of new clinical attacks occur shortly after a cold, influenza or other viral illness. **Sclerosis** means hardening and it refers to the scar tissue that replaces the disintegrating myelin.

The most common symptoms are extreme fatigue, heat intolerance, hand tremors, loss of coordination, numbness, general weakness, double weakness, double vision, slurred speech, staggering gait, and partial or complete paralysis.

Multiple sclerosis occurs about twice as frequently in women as in men. In the USA, there are about 400,000 persons with multiple sclerosis, with an estimated 2.5 million worldwide. Age of onset is typically between 20 and 40 years. Symptoms usually last 4 to 12 weeks and then gradually disappear, leaving various degrees of disability. Some individuals with multiple sclerosis have only one or two attacks in a lifetime, recover well and never become disabled. About 25% have frequent attacks, but recover sufficiently to lead normal lives. Others become more and more disabled with each attack, and eventually become wheelchair users with highly individual profiles of motor and sensory disturbances, pain, fatigue, and bladder or bowel disorders. In this progressive type of multiple sclerosis, spasticity, tremors and paralysis can occur in the later stages.

The type of physical activity that can be undertaken in multiple sclerosis depends on the extent of demyelination and the presence of pain, spasticity, tremors, muscle weakness, ataxia, impaired sensation, chronic fatigue and heat intolerance. Some individuals with multiple sclerosis are active in wheelchair basketball and tennis.

A unique aspect of multiple sclerosis is heat intolerance. Exposure to heat and humidity intensifies problems caused by demyelination and results in rapid fatigue. Any activity that substantially raises the body's core temperature is contraindicated. Thus swimming in cool water is especially recommended. Morning exercise is recommended, because the body temperature is normally lowest in the morning and higher in the afternoon. An emphasis should be placed on preventing loss of motion, which would result in permanent contractures, and preserving strength and endurance. Moderate physical activity on a regular basis significantly decreases nonactivity-related fatigue. Aquatic activities are suitable, but the water temperature should remain between 80 and 90 degrees Fahrenheit.

Bibliography

Apatoff, B.R. (1998). Multiple sclerosis and exercise. In Jordan, B., Tsairis, P. and Warren, R.F. (eds). *Sports neurology*. 2nd ed. Pp309-314. Philadelphia, PA: Lippincott-Raven.

National Multiple Sclerosis Society. Http://www.nmss.org

Sherill, C. (2004). *Adapted physical activity, recreation and sport. Cross disciplinary and lifespan*. 6th ed. Boston, MA: McGraw-Hill.

Winnick, J.P. (2000, ed). *Adapted physical education and sport*. 3rd ed. Champaign, IL: Human Kinetics.

MURMUR An auscultatory sound, benign or pathological. **Auscultation** involves listening for sounds produced with the body, using the unaided ear or via an instrument such as a stethoscope. **Heart murmurs** are sounds brought about by the increased turbulence in the blood flow through the heart, arteries or veins. The increased turbulence is usually caused by mechanical insufficiency of a valve or restriction of a valvular orifice as a result of disease. **Systolic murmurs** are murmurs that occur during systole and are further described as early systolic, mid-systolic, late systolic, or holosystolic. **Diastolic murmurs** occur during diastole. **Continuous murmurs** occur through both the systolic and diastolic cycles.

Normal (innocent) heart murmurs are heard in about 50% of normal infants and do not reflect abnormalities of the heart. **Abnormal (pathologic) heart murmurs** are heard in patients with certain heart diseases (e.g. stenosis, regurgitation and ventricular septal defect). There is no known method to prevent heart murmurs.

MUSCLE In kinesiology, the term 'muscle' usually refers to **skeletal muscle**. There are two other types of muscle in the human body: smooth muscle and cardiac muscle. The three major functions of [skeletal] muscle are: motion, postural support and heat production during cold stress. Muscle is comprised of approximately 75% water, 20% protein, and the remainder of other substances such as enzymes, lipids and carbohydrates. It is made up of bundles of muscle fibers (**fasciculi**). A **muscle fiber** is a long, narrow, multi-nucleated cell bound by a membrane called the **sarcolemma**. The muscle fibers, the fasciculi and the whole muscle are each surrounded by connective tissue.

Each muscle fiber is made up of **myofibrils**, consisting of thick and thin filaments. The thin filaments overlap the thick filaments and are joined to a transverse structure: the **Z line**. Actin and myosin make up 85% of the myofibrillar complex. **Thin filaments** are comprised mainly of actin, but also tropomyosin, troponin and nebulin. **Nebulin** is found adjacent to actin and is believed to control actin linkage within a thin filament. **Thick fila-**

ments are comprised mainly of myosin, but also C protein, M protein and myomesin. **C protein** is involved in holding the tails of the myosin in the correct spatial arrangement. The sarcomere region containing the myosin filaments is the **A band**. The A band spans the length of the thick filament. The Z lines bind the **sarcomeres**, which are the functional units of the myofilaments. **Alpha-actinin** attaches actin filaments together at the Z disk. **Desmin** links Z lines of adjacent myofibrils together. The relatively dense zone in the center of the A band is the **M band**, which helps keep the thick filaments connected in the sarcomere. **Myomesin** is an M band protein that functions to keep the thick and thin filaments in their correct spatial arrangement. The center of the A band contains the **H zone**, which does not contain actin filaments. **I bands** are the spaces between the A bands of adjacent sarcomere and contain actin filaments. Strands of titin extend along each thick filament from the M line to each Z line, thereby anchoring the thick filaments in their proper position relative to the thin filaments. **I bridges** span the gaps between titin and thin filaments.

T tubules are organelles that carry the action potential that enables muscle contraction from the sarcolemma to the interior of the cell. T-tubules are continuous with the sarcolemma and protrude into the sarcoplasma of the cell. The T-tubules form **triads** with the sacs of the **sarcoplasmic reticulum**, which is a tubular system that encircles each myofibril. In a relaxed muscle fiber, the sarcoplasmic reticulum stores calcium ions.

Muscle contraction can partly be explained by the **Sliding Filament theory**, which proposes a sliding of the thin filaments toward the centers of the thick filaments. The I bands shorten and the distance between Z lines decreases. The force for the sliding of the thin filaments is provided by rotation of the heads of myosin molecules at the ends of the thick filaments. Splitting of ATP by an enzyme in the heads of the myosin (myosin ATPase) provides the energy for their rotation, enabling attachment of the cross bridges between the thick and thin filaments. The release of calcium from the sarcoplasmic reticulum triggers the contraction. The release of calcium is triggered when a nerve impulse reaches the sarcoplasmic reticulum. The calcium ions inhibit the cross-bridge blocking action of the troponin-tropomyosin system.

ATP serves two main functions during skeletal muscle contraction. It disconnects actin from myosin and is hydrolyzed by the S-1 portion of the myosin molecule. In contracting skeletal muscle, ATP binds to the actin-myosin complex, causing actin and myosin to dissociate. When it does, ATP is hydrolyzed by myosin into ADP and a phosphate, which then allows actin and myosin to reassociate. Actin acts as a catalyst for ATP hydrolysis by S-1. The rate-limiting step of the entire sequence is the release of the reaction products from myosin, so that actin increases the ATP hydrolysis rate by speeding the release of hydrolysis products from myosin.

The Sliding Filament theory can be understood by using an analogy to the way in which a rowing crew propels the boat through water. The boat can be thought of as the thick filament and the water as the thin filament; the oars form the cross bridges and the crew provide the ATP. As the oars dip into the water (attachment) their shape changes and the boat is drawn along. The oars are then lifted from the water (detachment) and the stroke is repeated. The attachment and detachment of the cross bridges continues as long as there are sufficient calcium ions to inhibit the troponin-tropomyosin system (this will be the case as long as the muscle is being stimulated), and as long as ATP is available. In the absence of ATP, the cross bridges remain coupled and the muscle remains in contraction (rigor). A **cross-bridge cycle** is the sequence of events from the time a cross bridge first attaches to actin to the time when it binds again and repeats the process.

The greater the number of sarcomeres aligned in series in a given length of muscle, the more actin and myosin will be simultaneously sliding past one another and the greater the rate of muscle contraction. The force generated by individual fibers is determined by: the summation of contractions, the number of sarcomeres in parallel, and the length of the individual sarcomeres. The force generated by the whole muscle is determined by: the force generated by individual fibers and the number of active fibers.

Muscle tissue cannot lengthen actively, but it can be passively stretched. When a muscle is stretched under tension during eccentric muscle action, the actin and myosin filaments slide apart and elastic energy is stored in the cross-bridge linkages. The greater the muscular tension, the more actin and myosin filaments are linked. In isometric contractions, the number of cross bridges remains constant. Titin is primarily responsible for the sarcomere's resting tension. The theoretical limit of the sarcomere's elongation, while still maintaining at least one cross bridge between the thick and thin filaments, exceeds 50% of its resting length.

Overall, the tension developed in a muscle depends upon the number of fibers recruited, the relative size of the muscle, muscle temperature, muscle fatigue, the stretch-shortening cycle, length-tension relationship, force-velocity relationship and tension-time relationship.

Unlike other genes, which are generally switched on and off by the indirect action of signaling molecules such as hormones, muscle genes are regulated largely by mechanical stimulation.

Chronology

•1664 • William Croone's *De Ratione Motus Musculorum* concluded from nerve section experiments that the brain must send a signal to the muscles to cause contraction.

•1791 • Luigi Galvani's *Commentary on the Effects of Electricity on Muscular Action* was probably the first explicit statement on the presence of electrical potentials in nerve and muscle. Galvani noted that an electric current applied to the muscle or nerve would cause a contraction of the muscle of a frog.

•1954 • In *Nature*, two papers independently proposed the 'sliding filament' mechanism of muscle contraction. Andrew F. Huxley and Ralph Niedergerke showed that the width of 'A bands' in muscle fibers remains constant during contraction, suggesting a 'sliding filament' model in which myosin filaments run the length of the 'A band' and actin filaments slide into the A band. Hugh E. Huxley (not a relative of Andrew) and E. Jean Hanson also established the sliding filament mechanism and constancy of the A-band width.

Bibliography

Clarke, M. (2004). The sliding filament at 50. *Nature* 429, 145, 13 May.

Lieber, R.L. (2002). *Skeletal muscle structure, function, and plasticity. The Physiological basis of rehabilitation.* 2nd ed. Philadelphia, PA: Lippincott Williams & Wilkins.

McComas, A.J. (1996). *Skeletal muscle: Form and function.* Champaign, IL: Human Kinetics.

McArdle, W.D., Katch, F.I. and Katch, V.I. (1996). *Exercise physiology: Energy, nutrition and human performance*. Philadelphia, PA: Lippincott, Williams & Wilkins.

Newsholme, E., Leech, A. and Duester, G. (1994). *Keep on running. The science of training and performance*. Chichester, W. Sussex: John Wiley.

MUSCLE ACTION   The development of muscle tension. This term can be applied to any type of tension development, regardless of whether a muscle is lengthening, shortening or maintaining the same length. In mechanical terms, muscle can exert a tensile force, but not a compressive force. This tensile force can, however, be transmitted along a segment and exert a compressive bone-on-bone force.

Eccentric muscle action involves muscle lengthening under tension. This lengthening occurs when the external force acting on the segment to which a muscle is attached causes a net moment that is greater than the moment that is being developed by the muscle and its synergists. When a muscle is forcibly lengthened from an isometric muscle action, the attached cross-bridges are stretched, and this increases the average force exerted by each cross-bridge. Motor unit synchronization is enhanced during eccentric muscle action. Eccentric muscle action is capable of generating greater force than either concentric or isometric muscle action. Concentric muscle actions generate the least force. Although muscle force is greater during a voluntary eccentric muscle action, the electrical activity (as shown by electromyography) is substantially less than during a concentric muscle action. Eccentric muscle actions are more energy efficient than concentric or isometric. Downhill running involves a significant reliance on eccentric muscle actions of the leg muscles. Most downward movements, unless they are rapid, are controlled by an eccentric action of antagonist muscles. Lowering into a squat position involves hip and knee flexion that is controlled by the eccentric action of the hip and knee extensors. The total force output in a lowering action is the result of both muscular torques and gravitational torques. There appear to be heightened levels of feedback from muscle spindles during eccentric muscle actions. This may be necessary to achieve the precise match between the muscle and load torques that enables the individual to perform a controlled lowering of an inertial load with eccentric muscle action. Relative to concentric muscle actions, eccentric muscle actions may provide a more effective stimulus for hypertrophy, which might be mediated by a differential control (transcription vs. translation) of protein synthesis.

Concentric muscle action involves an active shortening (contracting) of muscle under tension, and a decrease in the distance between the two ends of a muscle. This shortening occurs when the net moment developed by a muscle and its synergists is greater than the moment caused by the external forces acting on the segment to which the muscle is attached.

Isotonic muscle action involves the production of a constant force. For *in vivo* muscle actions, the term is also commonly used both when the joint moment is constant over a range of motion and when a constant load is being moved through a distance. Because of the leverage effects at the joint, the force developed by the muscles in both these cases will actually be changing, rendering them non-isotonic.

Isometric muscle action involves no change in muscle length. This condition probably does not exist, because the contractile components of a muscle shorten at the expense of the elastic structures in series even when the joint crossed by the muscle is fixed. Isometric usually refers to the joint rather than the muscle, i.e. the action of a muscle when no change exists in the distance between its points of attachment. A **maximum voluntary contraction** is the maximum output of a muscle or a group of muscles during voluntary, isometric muscle action. (*See also* ISOMETRIC TRAINING.)

Isokinetic muscle action involves a constant rate of shortening or lengthening of the muscle. As joint geometry makes this impossible to determine *in vivo*, it usually refers to either a constant velocity of the load being lifted or resisted, or to a constant angular velocity of the joint. As muscle usually shortens or lengthens at varying rates and tension, isokinetic muscle action is useful only in certain situations (e.g. when testing muscles under standardized conditions – *see* ISOKINETIC MOVEMENT).

A **spurt muscle** is one that possesses a line of pull across a joint such that it favors torque. Spurt muscles have their proximal attachments at a distance from the joints about which they act, while their distal attachment(s) is near the joint. They direct the greater part of their force across the bone rather than along it and provide the force that acts along the tangent to the curve traversed by the bone during movement. A **shunt muscle** has a line of pull across a joint that is oriented predominantly along the long axis of a bone and thus acts mostly as a joint stabilizing force. The muscles do, however, provide the increase in centripetal force required in rapid or resisted movements. Shunt muscles have their proximal insertions near the joints on which they act and their distal insertions at a distance from them, so that the greater part of their contractile force is directed along the bones. When a muscle acts on two joints, it is usually a shunt muscle to one and a spurt to the other. The *biceps brachii* is a shunt muscle for the shoulder joint and a spurt muscle at the elbow. In some cases, the role of the muscle may be changed when the direction of muscle action (lengthening or shortening) is reversed.

For a particular movement, a skeletal muscle may function as an agonist, antagonist or synergist. An **agonist** (**prime mover**) causes rotational movements at joints by producing torque. **An antagonist** muscle produces the opposite movement to that of the agonist muscle. Muscles with opposite actions at joints are antagonists. With respect to a particular plane of movement, the muscles whose lines of application are on opposite sides of a joint axis are antagonists. When the agonist contracts, the antagonist must relax. This is usually accomplished by reciprocal inhibition. **Co-contraction (coactivation)** involves the simultaneous contraction of agonists and antagonists. Only muscles acting on a single joint are assumed to be true antagonists. **Synergist** actions include assisting, guiding, stabilizing (fixating) and neutralizing. **An emergency muscle** may be used to designate an assistant mover that is called into action only when an exceptional amount of total force is needed. A **guiding muscle** works to divert the moving body part from the agonist's exact line of action, e.g. the hip adductors allow for diagonal movement of the leg in kicking a soccer ball. The long head of the *biceps brachii*, for example, is not often called into action in the performance of shoulder joint abduction, but it may assist that action in times of great need. A **neutralizing muscle** helps cancel out, or neutralize, extra motion from the agonist muscles to ensure that the force generated works within the desired plane of motion. Neutralizers are either helping or true synergists. **Helping synergy** occurs when two or more muscles have a common action in one plane, but opposing actions in other planes. In the sit up exercise, the right and left external oblique muscles both cooperate in flexing the spine, since each is a prime mover for this action. Their lateral and rotation tendencies, in opposite direction, are mutually counteracted, or neutralized and the resultant motion is pure vertebral flexion. **True synergy** occurs when one muscle contracts statically to prevent any action in one of the joints traversed by a contracting two-joint or multi-joint muscle. *Extensor digitorum longus* and *tibialis posterior* act in true synergy to extend the distal interphalangeal joints without moving the ankle and subtalar joint. A **fixating (stabilizing)** muscle provides support to enable the rest of the body to remain stable when movement is generated by agonist muscles. Stabilizing function works to fix a particular body part(s), to allow other muscle to act from or upon it, e.g. fixing the neck so that the shoulder girdle can be elevated. In the ideal case, a fixator or stabilizer muscle will be acting isometrically, although in practice, there is a slight motion in the 'stabilized' part to continuously adjust the stabilization to the requirements of the desired motion. A good example of fixating occurs in the floor push-up exercise. The abdominal muscles contract isometrically during push-ups to prevent an undesirable sagging of the body in the hip and trunk region, thus counteracting the action of gravity on the hip and vertebral column.

See also KINETIC CHAIN EXERCISE; MUSCLE ACTION, MULTI-JOINT.

Bibliography

Basmajian, J.V. and DeLuca, C.J. (1985). *Muscles alive: Their function revealed by electromyography*. 5th ed. Baltimore, MD: Williams & Wilkins.

Cavanagh, P.R. (1988). On 'muscle action' vs. 'muscle contraction.' *Journal of Biomechanics* 21, 69.

Enoka, R.M. (2002). *Neuromechanics of human movement*. 3rd ed. Champaign, IL: Human Kinetics.

Lieber, R.L. (2002). *Skeletal muscle structure, function, and plasticity. The Physiological basis of rehabilitation*. 2nd ed. Philadelphia, PA: Lippincott Williams & Wilkins.

Smith, L.K., Weiss, E.L., and Lehmkuhl, L.D. (1996). *Brunnstrom's clinical kinesiology*. 5th ed. Philadelphia: F.A. Davis.

Zajac, F.E. and Gordon, M.E. (1989). Determining muscle's force and action in multi-articular movement. *Exercise and Sport Sciences Reviews* 17, 187-230.

MUSCLE ACTION, MULTI-JOINT Many muscles cross more than one joint. According to the axiom that a muscle tends to perform all of its possible actions when it contracts, a multi-joint muscle will tend to cause movement at each joint it crosses. A muscle acts to accelerate not only the joints it spans, but the unspanned joints as well. The *soleus* exerts only an ankle extensor torque, yet it can accelerate the knee into extension with more vigor than it accelerates the ankle into extension. When humans stand with their feet flat on the floor, the *soleus* acts with twice as much power to accelerate the knee into extension than it does the ankle. The *gastrocnemius* exerts both ankle-extensor and knee-flexor torques. It can act to extend the ankle and flex the knee, flex the ankle and flex the knee, or extend the ankle and extend the knee. A muscle's action can vary among motor tasks, and even during a single motor task, because it depends on the position of the body and on the muscle's interaction with external objects (such as the ground). The effectiveness of a multi-joint muscle in causing movement at any joint crossed depends on: the location and orientation of the muscle's attachment, relative to the joint; the tightness or laxity present in the musculotendinous unit; and the actions of other muscles that cross the joint.

Multi-joint (multi-articular) muscles can continue to exert tension without shortening. When mono-articular (single-joint) muscles contract, however, their shortening is accompanied by a corresponding loss of tension. In quick movements of the limbs, mono-articular muscles rapidly lose their tension. Multi-articular muscles invoke a mechanical coupling of the joints that facilitates a rapid release of stored elastic energy in the muscle-bone lever system. They save energy by allowing positive (concentric) work to be done at one joint and negative (eccentric) work to be done at the adjacent joint. In walking, the cooperative actions of the mono-articular and multi-articular muscles appear to supplement each other in order to produce efficient movement. Tendinous action, belt-like action and pulley action are characteristics attributed to multi-articular muscles, because these muscles cannot cause a full range of motion simultaneously at each joint on which they act.

A bi-articular (two-joint) muscle cannot act as a one-joint muscle without the assistance of other muscles and unless one of the joint actions is stabilized by other muscles (or by some external force). The kinetic effect of the muscle on the second joint is decreased.

A distinction can be made between concurrent and countercurrent movements. A **concurrent movement** occurs when bi-articular muscles act on each other in such a way that they do not lose length, thus maintaining their tension. When the hip and knee flex simultaneously, or extend simultaneously, the muscle contracts yet does not lose as much of its length as two mono-articular muscles would if performing the same action. A **countercurrent movement** occurs when one bi-articular muscle of an antagonistic pair shortens at both ends, while the other bi-articular muscle lengthens. Simultaneous hip flexion and knee extension shortens the *rectus femoris* at both ends, while stretching the hamstrings at both ends.

See also LOMBARD'S PARADOX; MUSCLE INSUFFICIENCY; PSOAS PARADOX.

Bibliography

Hamilton, N. and Luttgens, K. (2002). *Kinesiology. Scientific basis of human motion*. 10th ed. Madison, WI: Brown & Benchmark.

Lieber, R.L. (2002). *Skeletal muscle structure, function, and plasticity. The Physiological basis of rehabilitation*. 2nd ed. Philadelphia, PA: Lippincott Williams & Wilkins.

Rasch, P.J. (1978). *Kinesiology and applied anatomy*. 7th edition. Philadelphia: Lea and Febiger.

MUSCLE ATROPHY Decrease in size of muscle. Some muscles (primarily anti-gravity muscles) atrophy tremendously with disuse while their antagonists do not atrophy much at all. The same muscle fiber within different muscles may atrophy to different extents. Different types of the same muscle fibers within the same muscles may atrophy to different extents. It is possible that each muscle fiber has a 'set point' regarding the level of activity that will maintain its mass.

See also BED REST; IMMOBILIZATION.

Bibliography
Lieber, R.L. (2002). *Skeletal muscle structure, function, and plasticity. The Physiological basis of rehabilitation.* 2nd ed. Philadelphia, PA: Lippincott Williams & Wilkins.

MUSCLE ATTACHMENTS   The **origin** is the attachment of a skeletal muscle that is closer to the midpoint or midline of the body, i.e. it is more proximal. The **insertion** is the attachment that is further away from the midpoint or midline of the body, i.e. it is more distal. The origin should not be viewed as the bony attachment that does not move when the muscle contracts. Muscles pull equally on both ends so that both attachment sites receive equal forces. Both bones do not move when a muscle contracts, because of the difference in the mass of the two bones or segments to which the muscle is attached or in the stabilizing force of adjacent muscles. To demonstrate the invalid nature of defining the origin as the bony attachment that moves, consider the *psoas major* muscle that can cause hip flexion and movement of the thigh (such as in leg raises), but also trunk flexion and movement of the spine (such as in sit ups). The origin (more proximal) of the *psoas major* is the bodies of the last thoracic and all of the lumbar vertebrae; the insertion is the lesser trochanter of the femur. Thus, which bone remains stationary, and which one moves, depends on the purpose of the movement. In a pull up, the upper arm moves toward the forearm; whereas in a barbell curl, the forearm moves toward the upper arm. Most precision movements require that the proximal bone be stabilized, while the distal bone performs the movement.

See also BREATHING MUSCLES; PSOAS PARADOX.

MUSCLE BALANCE   The strength, power or endurance of one muscle or muscle group relative to another muscle or muscle group. A consequence of many sporting activities is that strength is increased in one muscle group without a concomitant increase in its antagonist. The stronger the agonist becomes, the greater is the stress that the antagonist is placed under as a joint stabilizer. It can be argued that the antagonist should then be trained for reasons of performance enhancement and injury prevention. Muscle balance is also an issue in the context of rehabilitation from injury. There is no consensus on specific ratios for muscle balance, but a common heuristic for knee extension/flexion strength is a ratio of 3-to-2. Muscle imbalance generally refers to a lack of flexibility in the most active muscle-tendon groups and an overpowering of the more passive, antagonistic groups.

See also KINETIC CHAIN EXERCISE.

MUSCLE BIOPSY   *See under* MUSCLE FIBER TYPES.

MUSCLE CONTRACTION   *See under* MUSCLE ACTION.

MUSCLE CONTUSION   An injury that results from an external force sufficient to cause muscle damage. There are two types of muscle contusion: intermuscular and intramuscular hematoma. **Intermuscular hematoma** is a hemorrhage occurring along intermuscular septal or fascial sheaths. **Intramuscular hematoma** is a hemorrhage occurring within muscle tissue, and is associated with a scar, myositis ossificans and acute compartment syndrome secondary to hemorrhage.

MUSCLE ENDURANCE   Local muscle endurance. *See under* ENDURANCE.

MUSCLE FIBER ARRANGEMENT   The force that a muscle can exert is proportional to its **physiological cross section**, a measure that accounts for every fiber and whose size depends on the number and thickness of the fibers. Physiological cross-sectional area (and therefore maximum muscle tension) is not simply proportional to muscle mass. The arrangement of the material is of critical importance. Muscle fiber shortening and rotation occur simultaneously during muscle contraction. Fiber angle can change by as much as 45 degrees depending on the particular muscle and specific movement. **Longitudinal muscles** have fibers that lie parallel to the long axis of the muscle. Examples are *sartorius* and *rectus abdominis*. Longitudinal muscles can exert force over a longer distance than muscles such as those of the pennate type with shorter fibers. **Quadrate (quadrilateral) muscles** are usually flat and have parallel fibers. Examples are *pronator quadratus* and the *rhomboids*. **Triangular (fan) shaped muscles** are relatively flat with fibers that radiate from a narrow attachment at one end to a broad attachment at the other end. An example is the *pectoralis major*. **Fusiform (spindle) shaped muscles** are usually rounded shaped and tapered at either end with parallel muscle fibers and fascicles that run the length of the muscle. Examples are *brachialis* and *brachioradialis*.

Penniform muscles, the most common type of skeletal muscles, are feather shaped, shorter and run at an angle relative to the line of pull of the muscle. The fiber force is in a different direction to the muscle force. **Angle of pennation** is the angle at which the muscle fibers attach to the tendon; there may be more than one angle of pennation with a particular muscle. The greater the angle of pennation, the smaller is the effective force that is transmitted to the tendon(s) to move the attached bone(s). Pennate arrangements allow greater packing of muscle fibers, i.e. more muscle fibers per unit of muscle volume, and therefore generation of more force than fusiform muscles of the same size. Penniform muscles thus produce slower movements and are not capable of producing movement through as large a range of movement. **Unipenniform** muscles have a series of short, parallel, featherlike fibers extend diagonally from the side of a long tendon, making it look like a wing feather. Examples are the *extensor digitorum longus* and *tibialis posterior*. **Bipenniform** muscles have a long central tendon with fibers extending diagonally in pairs from either side of the tendon and resemble a symmetrical tail feather. Examples are the *flexor hallucis longus* and *rectus femoris*. **Multipenniform** muscles have several tendons

with the muscle fibers running diagonally between them. An example is the mid-deltoid.

MUSCLE FIBER TYPES   Over 95% of normal muscle fibers can be classified into one of three categories, obtained from histochemical assay: fast glycolytic (FG), fast oxidative glycolytic (FOG) and slow oxidative (SO). Others include fast (F), fast oxidative (FO), slow (S), slow glycolytic (SG) and slow oxidative glycolytic (SOG). Slow fibers are also known as **type I muscle fibers**; fast fibers are **type II muscle fibers**.

Slow oxidative (SO) fibers have a small diameter, high capillary density, low contractile force, high aerobic capacity, low anaerobic capacity and are the most fatigue resistant. **Fast oxidative glycolytic (FOG) fibers (type IIa)** have the largest diameter, high capillary density, fast contraction, high contractile force, medium aerobic capacity, medium anaerobic capacity and medium fatigability. **Fast glycolytic (FG) fibers (type IIb)** have a large diameter, low capillary density, fast contraction, high contractile force, low aerobic capacity, high anaerobic capacity and are the most fatigable. FG muscle fibers produce lactate whether oxygen is present or not. This is due to high activity of the muscle type (M-type) lactate dehydrogenases in the cytosol and as a result of low mitochondrial density. More FG fibers are recruited as exercise intensity increases. This change in recruitment pattern appears to coincide well with the change in blood lactate level.

The muscles of elite endurance athletes can be comprised of as much as 80% of slow fibers. Elite strength athletes can have as much as 80% of fast fibers. It is not known the extent to which such composition is genetically determined.

Slow fibers function predominantly during submaximal exercise, whereas fast fibers are recruited as exercise intensity approaches maximal oxygen uptake and/or glycogen stores are depleted. Sprint training leads to the preferential use of fast fibers. Male (but not female) sprinters have larger fast fibers than untrained controls. Endurance training increases triglyceride stores adjacent to mitochondria; slow fibers have greater triglyceride stores than fast fibers. Creatine phosphate activity and ATP levels are higher in fast than slow fibers. Endurance training decreases creatine phosphate and ATP depletion at submaximal workloads, but also increases concentrations of creatine phosphate and ATP.

Muscle fiber type is determined using **biopsy**, which involves the extraction of small samples of tissue for histological or biochemical analysis. A hollow needle is inserted into a muscle through a small incision in the skin and fascia. By inserting a stylet into the needle, a small sample of muscle is excised within the needle. After removing the needle, the sample is quick frozen before analysis. *See* MOTOR UNIT; MUSCLE GROWTH.

Bibliography

Abernethy, P.J., Thayer, R. and Taylor, A.W. (1990). Acute and chronic responses of skeletal muscle to endurance and sprint exercise. A review. *Sports Medicine* 10(6), 365-389.

Billeter, R. and Hoppeler, H. (1992). Muscular basis of strength. In: Komi, P.V. (ed). *Strength and power in sport.* pp39-63. Oxford: Blackwell Scientific Publications.

MUSCLE FUNCTION *See* MUSCLE ACTION.

MUSCLE GROWTH, EXERCISE-INDUCED

The major mechanism by which muscle increases in size is by an increase in cross-sectional area of muscle fibers (**hypertrophy**). Heavy resistance training results in hypertrophy of skeletal muscle with the size of fast-twitch fibers increasing more readily and at a faster rate than slow-twitch fibers. This increase is a direct result of increased contractile protein, as evidenced by an increase in both the area and number of myofibrils. Interstitial connective tissue also increases in proportion to the increase in fiber area. A distinction can be made between sarcoplasmic and myofibrillar hypertrophy. Myofibrillar hypertrophy is tension induced, whereas sarcoplasmic hypertrophy is fatigue induced. **Sarcoplasmic hypertrophy** is elicited mainly by local muscular fatigue. The sarcoplasmic increase is predominantly composed of interfibrillar fluid (including non-contractile proteins), mitochondria, glycogen, ATP and creatine phosphate stores. Muscle fibers also show large increases in capillarization. Although the cross-sectional area of the muscle increases greatly, there is a decrease in fiber density, causing a loss in force production but an increase in fatigue tolerance. This form of hypertrophy is largely found in bodybuilders. **Myofibrillar hypertrophy** results principally from an increase in the cross-sectional area of the contractile region. It results in a larger muscle fiber with a greater density of contractile fibers. Because of the increase of actin-myosin cross-bridges, a muscle fiber that undergoes myofibrillar hypertrophy exhibits greater tensile strength and contractile force. This form of hypertrophy is mostly found in elite Olympic weightlifters and powerlifters.

There is some evidence (mainly from animal research) that an increase in the number of muscle fibers (**hyperplasia**) is another mechanism for increase in muscle size. It is possible that the development of new fibers may only occur when muscle is stretched to an extent that muscle fibers degenerate. However, it may only occur in young, developing muscle. It is possible that hyperplasia may be an adaptation to resistance training that occurs when some fibers reach a theoretical upper limit in cell size. If hyperplasia does occur, it probably accounts for less than 10% of the increase in muscle size.

One theory to explain hyperplasia is activation of satellite cells. In skeletal muscle, **satellite cells** are muscle stem cells under a muscle fiber's basement membrane that serve as muscle cell precursors. The **basement membrane (basal lamina)** is a fibrous layer of connective tissue that surrounds the sarcolemma. Although activation of satellite cells and subsequent generation of new fibers are generally thought to occur in response to fiber injury or death, new muscle fibers may be formed as an adaptation to mild damage caused by intensive resistance training. Activation of skeletal muscle via specific types, intensities and durations of functional use stimulates otherwise dormant satellite cells to proliferate and differentiate to form new fibers. Fusion of satellite cell nuclei and their incorporation into existing muscle fibers probably enables the muscle fiber to synthesize more proteins to form additional myofibrils. This most likely contributes directly to muscle hypertrophy with chronic overload and may stimulate transformation of existing fibers from one type to another. A variety of extracellular signal molecules, primarily peptide growth factors (e.g. insulin-like growth factor) govern satellite cell activity and possibly exercise-induced muscle fiber proliferation and differentiation.

See also MUSCLE PUMP; PROTEIN SYNTHESIS.

Bibliography
Kelley, G. (1996). Mechanical overload and skeletal muscle fiber hyperplasia: A meta-analysis. *Journal of Applied Physiology* 81(4), 1584-1588.

MacDougall, J.D. (1992). Hypertropy or hyperplasia? In: Komi, P.V. (ed). *Strength and power in sport*. pp230-238. Oxford: Blackwell Scientific Publications.

Sevilla, A.L.C. (2003). Hypertrophy and hyperplasia: Adaptations of muscular tissue to various resistance training protocols. Http://home.hia.no/~stephens/hypplas.htm

Taylor, N.A.S. and Wilkinson, J.G. (1986). Exercise-induced skeletal muscle growth, hypertrophy or hyperplasia? *Sports Medicine* 3, 190-200.

MUSCLE INJURY   Acute injuries to skeletal muscle include strains, avulsions, muscle contusions, delayed-onset muscle soreness and contractures. Complications of muscle injury include scar tissue formation, myositis ossificans, and the fact that muscle ruptures may mimic tumors.

MUSCLE INSUFFICIENCY   The inability of a multi-joint muscle (e.g. bi articular muscle) to effectively move each of its crossed joints simultaneously. A distinction can be made between passive and active insufficiency. **Passive insufficiency** is a phenomenon characterized by the difficulty of bi-articular (two-joint) muscles to be stretched sufficiently to permit a full range of movement in both joints simultaneously. For example, the hamstrings do not permit full extension of the knee if the hip is also extended because the muscles are stretched at the knee end, but are not stretched at the hip end. In other words, a position of hip extension and knee flexion creates passive insufficiency of the *rectus femoris*. **Active insufficiency** refers to the phenomenon whereby bi-articular muscles cannot exert enough tension to shorten sufficiently and cause full range of movement in both joints at the same time. For example, when hip extension and

knee flexion occur simultaneously, the hamstring muscles cannot shorten sufficiently to produce full hyperextension of the hip, while also producing full extension at the knee. In other words, a position of hip flexion and knee extension creates active insufficiency of the *rectus femoris*.

Bibliography
Gajdosik, R.L., Hallett, J.P., and Slaughter, L.L. (1994). Passive insufficiency of two-joint shoulder muscles. *Clinical Biomechanics* 9, 377-378.

Kreigbaum, E. and Barthels, K. (1996). *Biomechanics: A qualitative approach for studying human movement*. 4th ed. London: Allyn and Bacon.

MUSCLE, PATHOLOGY   *See* MYOPATHIES.

MUSCLE PUMP   The flow of water into muscle tissue during exercise due to increased blood concentration and pressure within the muscle. Plasma leaks from blood vessels (mostly capillaries) into interstitial spaces between muscle cells and blood vessels. The higher amount of fluid outside the muscle cells, compared to inside, creates a flow of fluid into muscle cells. The muscle pump is thought to be an important process in the growth of muscle, because of its effect on the muscle's microstructure.

MUSCLE RUPTURE   *See* MUSCLE STRAIN.

MUSCLE SORENESS   Two types of muscle soreness caused by exercise are immediate and delayed muscle soreness. **Immediate muscle soreness** involves soreness that arises during or immediately after exercise, but soon disappears when exercise is stopped. The decrease in blood flow to muscle caused by forceful muscle contractions, is thought to hinder the removal of metabolic by-products such as lactic acid. The build up of these by-products and lack of oxygen may cause pain by stimulating nerve endings. Cramp can be a type of immediate muscle soreness.

Delayed-onset muscle soreness appears 24 to 48 hours after exercise and may persist for several days. It is caused by severe, unaccustomed exercise, particularly involving eccentric muscle actions or a sharp increase in training intensity. The soreness is typically most evident at the muscle/tendon junction initially, then spreading throughout the muscle. Muscle soreness is experienced as a dull aching pain combined with tenderness and stiffness. It can affect athletic performance by causing a decrease in flexibility, shock attenuation and peak torque. Alterations in muscle sequencing and recruitment patterns may also occur, causing unaccustomed stress to be placed on the muscle and tendons. It usually subsides within 5 to 7 days following exercise.

No effective way has been found to decrease soreness once it has occurred, but some success has been reported using static stretching or neuromuscular electrical stimulation. There is some research evidence that if pain is suppressed with anti-inflammatory medication, muscle function is compromised.

A variety of theories have been proposed to explain delayed-onset muscle soreness. According to the **Tissue Damage theory**, muscle fibers and/or surrounding connective tissues are damaged by exercise. The resulting swelling (edema) causes stimulation of nerve endings. Exercise-induced skeletal muscle damage includes the release of intracellular proteins and an increase in skeletal muscle protein turnover. The disruption of the Z lines probably results from damage to the nebulin and titin protein stabilization of the actin and myosin molecules of the Z line proteins. About 12 hours later, macrophages and lymphocytes infiltrate the damaged muscle region. This results in the destruction of the damaged region of muscle. It is thought that chemicals released through the immune response induce the symptoms of swelling. The repair of damaged muscle resulting in hypertrophy may be an important mechanism for protection against further exercise-induced damage. Recovery from even a single bout of exposure to eccentric muscle actions may protect the muscle from the same damage during a second bout of eccentric muscle actions, but the processes involved remain to be elucidated. A repeated bout of similar eccentric exercise results in less damage and is referred to as the 'repeated-bout effect.' It is possible that the repeated-bout effect occurs through the interaction of various neural, connective tissue and cellular factors that are specific to the nature of the eccentric exercise bout and the muscle groups involved.

Tissue damage is the most likely explanation for the increased serum enzyme activities following prolonged weight-bearing activities that cause marked delayed-onset muscle soreness. The serum activities of those enzymes found especially in muscle, such as creatine kinase, increase in proportion to the intensity and duration of the preceding exercise, peaking 24 hours after exercise. Weight-bearing exercises that include eccentric muscular actions, such as downhill running, induce the greatest increases in serum enzyme activities. In non-weight bearing exercise, such as swimming and cycling, that does not include eccentric muscular actions, serum enzyme activities increase very little. Daily training or competition of more than two hours duration in weight-bearing exercise produces chronically elevated serum enzyme activities.

There is growing evidence that free radicals play an important role as mediators of skeletal muscle damage and inflammation. During normal conditions, free radicals are generated at a low rate and are dealt with by scavenger and antioxidant systems. During exercise, the greatly increased rate of free radical production may lead to cell membrane damage. This could initiate the skeletal muscle damage and inflammation caused by severe exercise.

Bibliography

Abraham, W.M. (1977). Factors in delayed muscle soreness. *Medicine and Science in Sports and Exercise* 9, 11-20.

Armstrong, C.B. (1986). Muscle damage and endurance events. *Sports Medicine* 3, 370-381.

Armstrong, R.B., Warren, G.L. and Warren, J.A. (1991). Mechanisms of exercise-induced muscle fibre injury. *Sports Medicine* 12(3), 184-207.

Cheung, K., Hume, P. and Maxwell, L. (2003). Delayed onset muscle soreness: Treatment strategies and performance factors. *Sports Medicine* 33(2), 145-164.

Cleak, M.J. and Eston, R.G. (1992). Delayed onset muscle soreness: Mechanisms and management. *Journal of Sports Sciences* 10, 325-341.

Evans, W.J. and Cannon, J.G. (1991). The metabolic effects of exercise-induced muscle damage. *Exercise and Sport Sciences Reviews* 19, 99-125.

McHugh, M.P. et al. (1999). Exercise-induced muscle damage and potential mechanisms for the repeated bout effect. *Sports Medicine* 27(3), 157-170.

MacIntyre, D.L., Reid, W.D. and McKenzie, D.C. (1995). Delayed muscle soreness. The inflammatory response to muscle injury and its clinical implications. *Sports Medicine* 20(1), 24-40.

Sjordin, B., Westing, Y.H. and Apple, F.S. (1990). Biochemical mechanisms for oxygen free radical formation during exercise. *Sports Medicine* 10(4), 236-254.

MUSCLE SPASM It is a sudden, involuntary muscle twitch.

MUSCLE SPINDLES Sense organs located within skeletal muscle and stimulated by muscle stretch. Muscle spindles signal the absolute amount of stretch and the rate of change of stretch in a particular muscle. They may also be stimulated by pressure and vibration. **Extrafusal fibers** are innervated by alpha motor neurons. About one third of all the motor neuron fibers that enter a muscle have no connection with extrafusal muscle fibers, but instead innervate the intrafusal fibers of the muscle spindle. The **intrafusal fibers** are attached to tendon or to the endomysium of a fasciculus of extrafusal muscle fibers. They are not innervated by alpha motor neurons from a spinal level, but rather are innervated independently by **gamma motor neurons** whose activity is controlled by the descending pathways from the brain. The **gamma efferent system** is under voluntary control (gamma bias) and functions to adjust the muscle spindle length by causing the intrafusal fibers to contract. It receives signals whenever the **alpha motor system** stimulates the extrafusal fibers. Thus a balance is maintained between the length of the extrafusal and intrafusal fibers. Activity from brain centers often causes simultaneous contraction of both extrafusal and intrafusal fibers, thereby ensuring that the spindle is sensitive to stretch at all muscle lengths.

A distinction can be made between bag and chain intrafusal fibers. A **nuclear bag fiber** is an intrafusal fiber in which the nuclei cluster in a group. A **nuclear chain fiber** is an intrafusal fiber in which the nuclei are arranged end to end. The nuclear bag fibers are innervated by type Ia afferent fibers. Stretching the *quadriceps femoris* muscle quickly evokes a discharge in the type Ia fibers (phasic response). The nuclear chain fibers are innervated by the type II afferent fibers and are more numerous than the type Ia afferent fibers. The type II afferent fibers are not very sensitive to the dynamic stage of muscle lengthening, but do respond to tonic (static) lengthening of the muscle fibers. The tonic stretch reflex involves discharge from the type II afferent fibers that increases the tone of extensor (antigravity) muscles. The tonic stretch reflex is important for maintaining erect body posture.
See also under MECHANORECEPTORS; STRETCH REFLEX.

MUSCLE STRAIN Muscle rupture. Muscle tear. An injury in which there is strain of skeletal muscle. A distinction can be made between compression and distraction ruptures. A **compression rupture** occurs as a result of direct impact; the muscle is pressed against the underlying bone, e.g. when a soccer player's knee hits the thigh of another player, and heavy intramuscular bleeding may result. A **distraction rupture** is an indirect injury caused by overstretching or overload, and often occurs in the superficial parts of muscles or at their attachments (especially the *quadriceps femoris*, *gastrocnemius* and *biceps brachii*). Distraction ruptures occur frequently in sports that require rapid acceleration (concentric work), sudden deceleration (eccentric work) and during acceleration-deceleration movements such as jumping. *See also* ADDUCTOR MUSCLE STRAIN.

MUSCLE TEAR *See* MUSCLE STRAIN.

MUSCLE TONE Tonus. It is the state of continued, partial contraction of muscles that helps to maintain posture, blood pressure and other functions. The muscle spindles are important for muscle tone to be maintained. Resting muscle tone has passive and active components. The **active component** involves a constant state of activity by a small portion of the muscle fibers caused by stretch reflexes that innervate the alpha motor neurons. It is thought that there is not a constant contraction of the same fibers, but rather a 'rotation of duty' among many different motor units. The **passive component** is determined by the elasticity of muscle and connective tissues, plus the tissue turgor (the pressure with which body fluids tend to distend their surrounding tissues).

At birth, the muscle tone of the anterior groups is better developed than that of the posterior groups. This is evident in the curled (flexed) postures of infants during their first weeks. Each time that infants are placed on their backs, the muscle tone shifts to strengthen the extensor muscle responses. The flexor and extensor postural tone gradually matures so that body parts can act independently.

See also HYPERTONIA; HYPOTONIA; POSTURE.

Bibliography

Payne, V.G. and Isaacs, L.D. (2005). *Human motor development. A lifespan approach*. 6th ed. Boston, MA: McGraw-Hill.

MUSCLE TWITCH The mechanical response of a muscle to a single, brief, low-level stimulus. The latent period lasts a few milliseconds when excitation-contraction occurs, but no tension is developed. This can be regarded as the time to take up slack in the elastic elements. The contraction period lasts 10 to 100 milliseconds (depending on the muscle fiber composition); it is the time from onset of tension development to peak tension. If the tension developed exceeds the resisting load, the muscle will shorten. In the relaxation period that follows, the tension drops to zero.

MUSCULAR DYSTROPHY A group of inherited conditions in which there is a progressive wasting and weakening of muscle. All the muscular dystrophies are caused by genetic faults. About 250,000 persons in the USA have muscular dystrophy. Of these, 50,000 use a wheelchair. It is about five times more common in males than females.

There are more than twenty types of muscular dystrophy, but those having the highest incidence are Duchenne, facioscapulohumeral and limb girdle types.

Mutations in the DMD gene cause the **Duchenne** and **Becker** types of muscular dystrophy. The DMD gene makes a protein called **dystrophin**, which helps to stabilize and protect muscle fibers and may play a role in chemical signaling within cells. Mutations in the DMD gene alter the structure or function of dystrophin, or prevent any functional dystrophin from being produced. As a result, muscle fibers become damaged with repeated use. The damaged fibers weaken and die over time, leading to the muscle weakness and heart problems characteristic of Duchenne and Becker muscular dystrophies. Duchenne and Becker muscular dystrophies are inherited in an X-linked recessive pattern. Males are affected by X-linked recessive disorders much more frequently than females. With X-linked inheritance, fathers cannot pass X-linked traits to their sons. In about two thirds of cases, an affected male inherits the mutations from a mother who carries one altered copy of the DMD gene. The other one third of cases probably result from new mutations in the gene. Females who carry one copy of a DMD mutation may have some signs and symptoms related to the condition, but these are typically milder than the signs and symptoms seen in affected males.

Most boys affected by Duchenne muscular dystrophy develop the first signs of difficulty in walking at the age of 1 to 3 years. By about 8 to 11 years, boys become unable to walk. Survival beyond the late twenties is rare. The risk of Duchenne muscular dystrophy is about 1 in 3,500 male births. Symptoms include generalized weakness and muscle wasting that affects the limb and trunk muscles first. The disease progresses slowly, but it will affect all voluntary muscles. There may be hypertrophy of calf muscles and, occasionally, of the *deltoid*, *infraspinatus* and *vastus lateralis*. The hypertrophy occurs when quantities of fat and connective tissue replace degenerating muscle fibers, which progressively become smaller, fragment and then disappear.

Becker muscular dystrophy appears in adolescence or adulthood. The symptoms are almost identical to Duchenne muscular dystrophy, but often much less severe. There may be significant cardiac problems. Becker muscular dystrophy progresses at a slower and more variable rate than Duchenne muscular dystrophy with survival well into mid- to late-adulthood.

Facioscapulohumeral muscular dystrophy is caused when the number of copies of a particular sequence of DNA is decreased below a certain level.

The gene for facioscapulohumeral muscular dystrophy is at one end of each copy of chromosome 4. One copy of this particular pair is faulty. The pattern of inheritance is autosomal dominant. The age of symptom onset and severity of facioscapulohumeral muscular dystrophy seems to correlate broadly with the extent of the DNA rearrangement on chromosome 4. It appears in childhood to early adulthood and affects both genders equally. The prognosis is good and life span is normal. It is indicated by progressive weakness of face, shoulder and arm muscles. The scapular muscles are often very weak, making it difficult to lift the arms. About 10 to 20% of people eventually require a wheelchair, but up to a third remain unaware of symptoms at least into old age. A common feature of facioscapulohumeral muscular dystrophy is an asymmetry of muscle weakness.

Limb girdle muscular dystrophy can occur at any time from age 10 years or after. Males and females are affected equally. The earliest symptom is usually difficulty in raising the arms above shoulder level or awkwardness in climbing stairs. Limb girdle muscular dystrophy usually progresses slowly with cardiopulmonary complications often occurring in the later stages of the disease. There are many different types of limb-girdle muscular dystrophy, so named because generally they cause weakness in the shoulder and pelvic girdle. The two main groups of limb girdle muscular dystrophy are Type I (autosomal dominant) and Type 2 (autosomal recessive). About 90% of limb girdle muscular dystrophy is Type 2.

Children with muscular dystrophy should receive instruction in some relatively sedentary recreational activities (e.g. fishing) that will carry over into the wheelchair years. The role of exercise training in the management of patients with myopathic disorders is controversial. Low-to moderate-intensity resistance and aerobic training may be recommended in slowly progressive myopathic disorders. In rapidly progressive myopathies, such as Duchenne muscular dystrophy, the use of high-resistance and eccentric training should be avoided. Exercise regimens should be started in the early stages of the disease, while there is still a substantial amount of trainable muscle fibers.

Bibliography

Ansved, T. (2001). Muscle training in muscular dystrophies. *Acta Physiologica Scandanavia* 171(3), 359-366.
Ansved, T. (2003). Muscular dystrophies: Influence of physical conditioning on the disease evolution. *Current Opinion in Clinical Nutrition and Metabolic Care* 6(4), 435-439.
Genetics Home Reference. Http://ghr.nlm.gov
Muscular Dystrophy Association. Http://www.mdausa.org
Muscular Dystrophy Campaign. Http://www.muscular-dystrophy.org
Sherill, C. (1998). *Adapted physical activity, recreation and sport. Cross disciplinary and lifespan.* 5th ed. Boston, MA: McGraw-Hill.

MUSCULAR ENDURANCE Local muscle endurance. *See under* ENDURANCE.

MUSCULOTENDINOUS JUNCTION The connection between a muscle and its tendon.

MUTATION Chemical modification of a gene such that one or more of the bases in the DNA is deleted or altered or a new base is inserted, thus changing the base sequence. As a consequence, the protein coded by the gene is either produced with an altered amino acid sequence or is not produced at all. For example, sickle cell anemia is a mutation that confers protection from another disease (malaria) as well as causing the primary disease (hemolytic anemia).

A **spontaneous mutation** is a mutation that occurs in the absence of any known mutagenic agent.

MYALGIC ENCEPHALOMYELITIS *See under* CHRONIC FATIGUE SYNDROME.

MYASTHENIA GRAVIS The most common primary disorder of neuromuscular transmission. The usual cause is an acquired immunological abnormality, but some cases result from genetic abnormalities at the neuromuscular junction. It is now understood to be an autoimmune disease. In the USA, the prevalence of myasthenia gravis is estimated at 14 per 100,000 of the population. It appears from childhood to adulthood. Symptoms include weakness and fatigability of the muscles of the eyes, face, neck, throat, limbs and/or trunk. Weakness of the extraocular and lid muscles of the eye occurs in about 50% of cases, resulting in drooping of the eyelid (ptosis) and double vision (strabismus). Abnormalities of the thymus gland are associated with myasthenia gravis. Disease progression varies. Drug therapy or removal of the thymus gland is often effective.

Muscle weakness makes it difficult to carry out activities of daily living. Physical fitness training is important to counteract the early onset of fatigue during activities.

Bibliography
Mysasthenia Gravis Foundation of America. Http://www.mysasthenia.org
Winnick, J.P. (2000, ed). *Adapted physical education and sport*. 3rd ed. Champaign, IL: Human Kinetics.

MYELIN   *See under* NERVOUS SYSTEM.

MYELITIS   i) Inflammation of spinal cord. ii) Inflammation of bone marrow

MYOADENYLATE DEAMINASE DEFICIENCY
A metabolic disorder of muscle affecting ATP synthesis. It is inherited as an autosomal recessive trait. It may cause exercise intolerance, cramps and muscle pain. In many cases, however, no symptoms will be experienced.

MYOCARDIAL CONTRACTILITY   The intrinsic property of the myocardium (heart muscle) that gives it the ability to contract.

MYOCARDIAL CONTUSION   An injury caused by blunt chest trauma that compresses the heart between the sternum and spine. The right ventricle is often injured, because it lies directly posterior to the sternum. Red blood cells and fluid leak into the surrounding tissues, thereby decreasing circulation to the heart muscle. This leads to local cellular damage and necrosis of the heart tissue.

MYOCARDIAL INFARCTION   Heart attack. Acute myocardial infarction is the necrosis of cardiac myocytes resulting from prolonged myocardial ischemia, caused by complete coronary artery occlusion lasting at least 60 minutes. Depending on how much cardiac muscle is damaged, a person can die or be disabled from a myocardial infarction. Myocardial infarction and/or myocardial ischemia, if extensive-

ly distributed in the heart, may lead to left ventricular dysfunction (chronic heart failure). Coronary artery disease causes approximately 1 million myocardial infarctions per year in the USA.

Sometimes a coronary artery temporarily contracts or goes into spasm. This causes the artery to narrow and blood flow to part of the heart muscle decreases or stops. A spasm can occur in normal-appearing blood vessels as well as in vessels that are partly occluded by atherosclerosis. Drugs such as cocaine can cause a life-threatening spasm. A severe spasm can cause a heart attack. Rarely, a heart attack can occur when a blood clot from inside a diseased heart breaks loose and lodges in a healthy or narrowed coronary artery.

Signs of a heart attack are: chest pain or discomfort lasting more than 3 to 5 minutes or that goes away and comes back; the pain is not relieved by rest, changing position or medication, and it may spread to the shoulder, arm, back, neck or jaw; dyspnea; nausea; sweating or changes in skin appearance; dizziness or unconsciousness; and ache, heartburn or indigestion.

Bibliography
American College of Sports Medicine (2001). *ACSM's resource manual for Guidelines for Exercise Testing & Prescription*. 4th ed. Philadelphia, PA: Lippincott Williams & Wilkins.
American Heart Association. Http://www.americanheart.org

MYOCARDIAL ISCHEMIA   A pathological condition in which blood flow to the myocardium is decreased below the amount needed to provide adequate amounts of oxygen to match the needs of the heart for ATP production. It results in oxygen deprivation accompanied by inadequate removal of metabolites. Ischemia may result in hypoxia, accumulation of toxic metabolites and acidosis.

MYOCARDIUM   *See* CARDIAC MUSCLE.

MYOCLONUS   A fleeting burst of muscular excitation or relaxation, resulting in a synchronous quick jerk of a muscle or group of muscles. Myoclonus is a symptom in a wide variety of nervous system disorders such as Alzheimer's disease, Creutzfeldt-Jakob disease, epilepsy, multiple sclerosis and Parkinson's disease. Examples of normal myoclonus are hiccups and the jerks that some people experience while drifting off to sleep.

See also RESTLESS LEG SYNDROME.

Bibliography
The Myoclonus Research Foundation. Http://www.myoclonus. com

MYOFASCIAL PAIN SYNDROME   A muscular pain disorder involving regional pain referred from trigger points localized within the myofascial structures or distant from the pain sites.

MYOFIBRIL   *See under* MUSCLE.

MYOGENIC   Muscle related.

MYOGLOBIN   A heme protein, abundant in skeletal and cardiac muscle, which provides intramuscular storage and acts as an oxygen carrier. Each myoglobin molecule has only one iron atom, while hemoglobin has 4 iron atoms. It has a greater affinity for oxygen than hemoglobin. It binds and releases oxygen at low oxygen pressures much more readily than hemoglobin. However, it is usually only during heavy exercise (when the partial pressure of oxygen falls to about 20 mm Hg or less) that myoglobin releases its oxygen. The greatest quantity of oxygen is released from myoglobin when the partial pressure of oxygen falls below 5 mm Hg. The oxygen binding affinity of myoglobin is not affected by carbon dioxide and tem-perature, thus there is no Bohr effect. **Myoglobinuria** refers to myoglobin in the urine. It is seen to some degree with intensive exercise.

MYOMECTOMY   Surgical removal of a myoma. A **myoma** is a benign neoplasm of muscular tissue.

MYOPATHIES   A group of disorders that can be classified as muscular dystrophies, inflammatory myopathies (dermatomyositis, polymyositis and inclusion body myositis), motor neuron diseases (e.g. amyotrophic lateral sclerosis, spinal muscular atrophies), diseases of the neuromuscular junction (e.g. myasthenia gravis), myopathies due to endocrine abnormalities (e.g. hyperthyroid or hypothyroid myopathy), diseases of the peripheral nerve (e.g. hereditary motor and sensory neuropathy and Friedreich's ataxia), other myopathies (e.g. central core disease) and metabolic diseases of muscle (e.g. phosphorylase deficiency, phosphofructokinase deficiency, mitochondrial myopathy, myoadenylate deaminase deficiency, carnitine deficiency and lactate dehydrogenase deficiency).

MYOPLASTICITY   The capacity of skeletal muscle for adaptive change

MYOSITIS OSSIFICANS   See under HETERO-TOPIC OSSIFICATION.

MYOTATIC REFLEX   *See* STRETCH REFLEX.

N

NAD⁺ Nicotinamide adenine dinucleotide. It is an oxidizing-reducing (redox) co-enzyme. The reduced form is expressed as **NADH**. NAD^+ is a major electron acceptor in the conversion of energy from fuel nutrients into ATP. NAD^+ serves as a coenzyme for the dehydrogenases, which are enzymes that remove two hydrogen atoms from their substrates. One of the protons is released into the surrounding medium and the other proton and the two electrons are transferred to the coenzyme, which becomes NADH. NAD^+ is composed of nicotinamide, D-ribose (a five-carbon sugar), phosphoric acid and adenine (a purine base).

See also ELECTRON TRANSPORT CHAIN.

NADPH A co-enzyme of niacin. It is a modified form of NADH that provides reducing power and free energy for many anabolic reactions. $NADP^+$ is the oxidized form.

See PENTOSE PHOSPHATE PATHWAY.

NANDROLONE *See under* ANDROGEN SUPPLEMENTS.

NARCISSICISM *See under* PSYCHIATRY.

NARCOTIC *See under* DRUG; OPIATE.

NASAL DILATOR *See under* BREATHING.

NASAL INJURIES Due to their prominence and relative thinness, the bones of the nose are the most frequently fractured bones in the face. Nasal injuries are common in sports where protective faceguards are not worn. *See* EPISTAXIS.

NASOPHARYNX *See under* PHARYNX.

NATIONALISM Shared feelings of attachment to symbols that identify the members of a given population as belonging to the same overall community. Coakley (2003) states that many people in the USA use sport events as sites for reaffirming their collective sense of "we-ness" as Americans. **Globalization** refers to the long-term processes of social change that involve relationships between nation-states and the use of power on an international level. Consumerism and the promotion of capitalist expansion have become more important since the end of the Cold War. Athletes and teams are now associated with corporate logos as well as nation-states. Global political processes are also associated with other aspects of sports, such as the migration patterns of elite athletes and the production of sporting goods. Political issues are raised when athletes cross national borders to play their sports, and when transnational corporations produce sports equipment and clothing in labor-intensive poor nations, in order to sell those items in wealthy nations.

Media coverage of international sports influences the formation of national identities, ideas about the 'national character' of people from other countries and international political processes. The media provide 're-presentations' of selected versions of reality that are grounded in the power relations of society as a whole. Sports are 're-presented' to viewing audiences through video technology used to create dramatic and stylized images and messages for the purpose of entertaining viewers and maintaining sponsors. *See* COMMERCIALISM.

Chronology

•1772 • In *Treatise on the Government of Poland*, Jean Jacques Rousseau emphasized the role of exercise and competitive games in the development of character and national unity in Poland: "A gymnasium for physical exercise should be established in every college. ... the function of games is not merely to occupy children, and to give them a strong physique or free and agile movements, but to accustom them early to discipline, equality, fraternity and cooperation."

•1936 • Hitler turned the Olympic Games into a propaganda show to legitimate Nazism. Germany won 89 medals, 23 more than the USA, and more than four times as many as any other country won. It was rumored that as a concession to the Nazis, the USA dropped two Jewish sprinters from the 400-metre relay. The Black US runner Jesse Owens won gold medals in the 100 meters, 200 meters, 4 x 100 meters and the long jump. Hitler personally attended the

first day of the track and field competition. He personally congratulated the German athlete Hans Woellke who became the first German to win a gold medal in the Olympics since 1896. Throughout the rest of the day, Hitler continued to receive all Olympic champions in his VIP box. The following day, Comte Baillet-Latour, the chairman of the International Olympic Committee (IOC) told Hitler that he had violated Olympic protocol by having winners paraded to his box. Hitler apologized and subsequently refrained from congratulating any of the winner, German or otherwise. It was on this day that Owens won his gold medals. In his autobiography, *The Jesse Owens Story*, it is stated that Hitler had stood up and waved to him. US President Franklin D. Roosevelt refused to see Owens at the White House, nor sent him a letter of congratulations. Owens later remarked that it was Roosevelt, not Hitler, who snubbed him. In 1976, Jesse Owens was awarded the Presidential Medal of Freedom, the highest honor the USA can bestow upon a civilian, by President Ford.
•1948 • The Communist Party in the Soviet Union resolved that all organizations to take steps "to ensure a rise in Soviet athletic records so that within the next few years Soviet athletes may beat world records in all major sports." In the 1952 Olympic Games, the Soviet Union's 22 gold medals were second only to the USA's 40 gold medals.
•1976 • The East German medal count in the Olympics was 40, 25 and 25 for gold, silver and bronze, respectively, in contrast to 9, 6 and 7 in the 1968 Olympic Games. Subsequently there were accusations that many East German athletes used banned drugs. Erich Honecker, the East German leader, asserted, "Our state is respected in the world because of the excellent performance of our athletes."
•1992 • In Japan, Akebono (formerly Chad Rowan), an American sumo wrester, was voted into the rank of yokozuna (grand champion) by the Yokozuna Promotion Council. He became the 64th yokozuna in over three hundred years of sumo wrestling, but not without objections from many Japanese people who felt that Japan might lose control of a celebrated part of its own culture if such an honor was not reserved for native Japanese.

Bibliography

Coakley, J.J. (2004). *Sport in society. Issues and controversies.* 8th. Boston, MA: Irwin McGraw-Hill.

Eitzen, D.S. and Sage, G.H. (2003). *Sociology of North American sport.* 7th ed. Boston, MA: McGraw-Hill.

Maguire, J. et al. (2002). *Sport worlds: A sociological perspective.* Champaign, IL: Human Kinetics.

NATURAL KILLER CELLS   *See under* LEUKOCYTES; IMMUNITY.

NATURAL SELECTION   *See under* EVOLUTION; HEREDITY.

NAVICULAR BONE   i) A bone with which the head of the talus articulates on the medial side of the foot. ii) Os naviculare. *See* SCAPHOID.

NEBIVOLOL   *See under* BETA-BLOCKERS.

NEBULIN   *See under* MUSCLE.

NECKING   *See under* PLASTIC DEFORMATION.

NECK INJURIES   Cervical spine injuries. These injuries usually result from the neck being forced into hyperflexion or, less commonly, hyperextension, often combined with rotation. Most severe injuries from hyperflexion and hyperextension (with or without rotation) result in spinal cord damage from a fracture and/or a dislocation. In American football, the most common mechanism of neck injury is flexion-compression. When the neck is slightly flexed, the normal cervical lordosis disappears and the cervical vertebrae are aligned axially. As a result, the cervical spine is devoid of the curvature required for energy-absorbing bending and the cervical structures must receive all of the loading energy. When the cervical structures are unable to absorb the loading energy, failure of the intervertebral disks, vertebral body and processes, or spinal ligaments may occur. This, in turn, leads to further flexion or rotation of the cervical spine. As a result, vertebral dislocation may occur and there will be a risk of impinging the spinal cord or spinal nerves.
See also ATLANTO-OCCIPITAL FUSION; BRACHIAL PLEXOPATHIES; BURNER; KLIPPEL-FEIL ANOMALY; SPEAR-TACKLER'S SPINE; TORTICOLLIS; WHIPLASH.

NECK LIGAMENTS   The primary ligaments of the neck are ligamentum flavum, ligamentum nuchae, alar ligaments, transverse ligament of the atlas, anterior longitudinal ligament and posterior longitudinal ligament. The **ligamentum flavum** secures the lamina of the adjacent vertebrae and prevents excessive motion of one vertebra upon another. It also maintains the tension on the capsule of the facet joint, thus preventing the capsule from becoming entrapped in the joint. The **ligamentum nuchae** runs from the external occipital protuberance to the posterior spinous processes of the seven cervical vertebrae, below which it becomes the supraspinous and interspinous ligaments. The **alar ligaments** join the skull with the axis, and limit lateral flexion and rotation of the neck. The **transverse ligament of the atlas** runs horizontally from one side of the atlas to the other, and holds the odontoid process against the anterior arch of the atlas. The **anterior longitudinal ligament** attaches to the anterior surface of the intervertebral discs and vertebral bodies. The **posterior longitudinal ligament** attaches to the posterior surface of all the cervical vertebral bodies and intervertebral discs. It forms the tectorial membrane that helps keep the skull on the atlas and axis. *See also* SPINE.

NECK RIGHTING REFLEX   Rotation of the trunk in the direction in which the head of the supine infant is turned. This reflex is absent or decreased in infants with spasticity. It accounts for the tendency for a newborn to lie with one arm crooked and raised behind the head while the other is extended away from the body. It is integrated soon after birth.

NECROSIS   Cell death. **Avascular (asceptic) necrosis** is cell death as a result of inadequate blood supply. *See also* APOPTOSIS.

NEGATIVE FEEDBACK   *See under* HOMEOSTASIS.

NEGATIVE IONS   Anions. Ions formed when neutral atoms or molecules gain one or more electrons. *See under* MINERALS.

NEGATIVE WORK   Work done on a muscle that is lengthening. *See* MUSCLE ACTION; RESISTANCE TRAINING.

NEOPLASM   An aberrant new growth of abnormal cells; a tumor. It is malignant if the growing cells infiltrate surrounding tissues and are carried by blood or lymph to other parts of the body where they continue their growth. Otherwise it is benign.
    Benign prostatic hypertrophy is the non-malignant enlargement of the prostate gland from an increase in cellular growth. It is the most common benign neoplasm among men, and its incidence steadily increases with age. Up to 20% of men between 40 and 64, and 40% of men older than 65 are afflicted. *See* CANCER; NEUROMA; SARCOMA; SCHWANNOMA.

Bibliography
Wehle, M.J. and Lisson, S W. (2002). Benign prostatic hypertrophy. Which nonoperative strategies are best? *The Physician and Sportsmedicine* 30(4), 41-47.

NEOVASCULARISATION   New blood vessel formation.

NEPHRITIS   *See under* KIDNEYS.

NERVE CELL   *See* NEURON.

NERVE FIBER   *See under* NEURON.

NERVE IMPULSE   *See under* NEURON.

NERVE INJURY   Neural tissue can be injured through chemical, thermal, ischemic or mechanical means. Compressive loading may result in pressure on neural tissue. Tensile loading may result in stretch injury. Shear loading may result in friction-related injury.
    The main cause for weakness after reinnervation is a decrease in the number of functional neurons that actually grow back into the correct muscle. Even if neurons grow back, if they synapse with the wrong muscle, they will be dysfunctional. Therefore, nerve injuries that occur very close to a muscle have a better prognosis of functional recovery compared with nerve injuries that occur far away from the muscle.
    See PERIPHERAL NERVE INJURIES; SPINAL CORD INJURY; SPINAL PARALYSIS.

Bibliography
Lieber, R.L. (2002). *Skeletal muscle structure, function, and plasticity. The Physiological basis of rehabilitation*. 2nd ed. Philadelphia, PA: Lippincott Williams & Wilkins.

NERVOUS SYSTEM   A system that coordinates the various activities in the body with each other and with events in the external environment. It does this by transmitting messages from one point to another. It is faster and more flexible than the endocrine system (another coordinating system in the body).

The nervous system is comprised of the central nervous system and the peripheral nervous system. The **central nervous system** (**CNS**) in vertebrates consists of the brain and spinal cord. The **peripheral nervous system** comprises nerve tissue located outside the brain and spinal cord. The peripheral nervous system can be subdivided into sensory and motor divisions. The **motor division** can be divided into the autonomic (involuntary) nervous system and somatic (voluntary) nervous system.

About 40% of the CNS is **gray matter**, which contains the cell bodies and dendrites of neurons, as well as the axon terminals that form synapses with them. Synaptic transmission and neural integration occur in gray matter. About 60% of the CNS is **white matter**, which contains axons, most of which are myelinated. Myelinated axons are specialized for the rapid transmission of information in the form of action potentials over relatively long distances. **Glial cells** account for 90% of all cells in the nervous system, providing metabolic and structural support to the neurons.

Characteristics of a mature, intact central nervous system include reflex integration and optimal functioning of reflexes in addition to freedom from: ataxia, athetosis, spasticity, overflow, sensory input problems and other constraints. *See* NEURONS.

Chronology

•1624 • René Descartes published his first treatise on physiology, *L'homme*, in which he emphasized the role of the nervous system in human movement. Descartes believed that humans were soul-containing machines running on auto-pilot. Animals were different only in that they did not have a soul.

NEURALGIA   Pain along the course of a nerve.

NEURAL PATHWAY   A response or adaptation that involves changes in nerve activity.

NEURAL TUBE DEFECT   A birth defect that results from failure of the neural tube to develop

properly during early fetal development. Neural tube defects are the most common severely disabling birth defects in the USA, with a frequency of approximately 1 of every 2,000 births.

There are three types of neural tube defects: anencephaly, encephalocele and spina bifida. Babies born with **anencephaly** have underdeveloped brains and incomplete skulls and most do not survive more than a few hours after birth. An **encephalocele** is a sac that is formed when the bones of the skull fail to develop. It may contain cerebrospinal fluid only, but part of the brain may also be present in the sac resulting in brain damage. Encephalocele results in a hole in the skull through which brain tissue protrudes. Most babies with encephalocele do not live, or survive with severe mental retardation. Spina bifida manifesta and spinal bifida occulta are nonprogressive developmental anomalies occurring between the 4th and 6th week of pregnancy, but which can be detected. After cerebral palsy, spinal bifida is the cause of more orthopedic defects in school-age children than any other condition. In the USA, it affects approximately 1 in 1,000 newborns in the USA. More girls than boys are affected. **Spina bifida manifesta** is categorized as meningocele or myelomeningocele. **Meningocele** is herniation of the dural sac through an osseous defect. The **dural sac** contains tissue that covers the spinal cord (meninges) and cerebrospinal fluid. The nerves are not usually damaged and are able to function. Therefore, little disability is usually present. This is the least common form of spina bifida. There is usually weakness in the legs, and difficulty with bladder and bowel control. **Myelomeningocele**, the most serious and common form of spina bifida, is herniation of the meninges and spinal nerves through an osseous defect. The spinal cord is damaged or not properly developed. As a result, there is always some paralysis and loss of sensation below the damaged region. About 90% of infants with meningomyelocele have hydrocephalus. Hydrocephalus in spina bifida is associated with the Arnold-Chiari II type malformation. After surgery, meningomyelocele is managed by passive range-of-motion exercises done twice daily by the family until the child learns to creep/crawl and engages in enough activity that range-of-motion therapy is not needed. **Spina bifida occulta**, a mild and common form of spina bifida, is so named because the condition is concealed under the skin. Dimpling of the skin overlying the osseous anomaly may be observed with a patch of hair. It does not cause paralysis or muscle weakness, but it may be associated with adult back problems. Between 5% and 10% of people may have spina bifida occulta. Only about 1 in 1,000 have associated problems.

Bibliography

Association for Spina Bifida and Hydrocephalus. Http://www.ashah.org

Northrup, H. and Volcik, K.A. (2000). Spina bifida and other neural tube defects. *Current Problems in Pediatrics* 30(10), 313-332.

Spina Bifida Association. Http://www.sbaa.org

NEURITIS Inflammation of a nerve.

NEUROFIBROMATOSES A set of genetic disorders which can cause tumors to grow along various types of nerves and can also affect the development of non-nervous tissue such as bone and skin. Neurofibromatoses are the most common neurological disorders caused by a single gene. There are two types of neurofibromatoses, caused by different genes, located on different chromosomes. Both types are inherited as an autosomal dominant trait. **Type I neurofibromatosis (von Recklinghausen neurofibromatosis** or **peripheral neurofibromatosis**) affects about 1 in 4,000 births, whereas **type 2 neurofibromatosis** affects about 1 in 40,000 births. Symptoms of type I neurofibromatosis include multiple café-au-lait spots and neurofibromas on or under the skin. A **café au lait spot** is a light tan, coffee-colored, birthmark that may be normal. The presence of several of these spots larger than one inch may be seen in neurofibromatsosis. Enlargement and deformation of bones and scoliosis may also occur. Occasionally, tumors may develop in the brain, on cranial nerves, or on the spinal cord. Type 2 neurofibromatosis is characterized by multiple tumors on the cranial and spinal nerves, and by other lesions of the brain and spinal cord. It is also known as bilateral acoustic, because tumors affecting both of the auditory nerves are the hallmark. Hearing loss that starts in the teens or early twenties is generally the first symptom. About 50% of people with neurofibromatosis also have learning disabilities.

See also PROTEUS SYNDROME.

Bibliography

National Neurofibromatosis Foundation, Inc. Http://www.nf.org

NEUROLOGICAL SOFT SIGNS Behavioral, perceptual and motor indicators of central nervous system dysfunction that cannot be substantiated through hardware technology such as electroencephalography.

NEUROGENIC Pertaining to an effect attributable to the nervous system.

NEUROHORMONE A hormone secreted by a specialized neuron into the bloodstream, the cerebrospinal fluid, or the intercellular spaces of the nervous system. Neurohormones include: releasing factors (e.g. corticotropin releasing factor, gonadotropin releasing hormone, thyrotropin releasing hormone, and growth hormone releasing hormone); tropic hormones (e.g. follicle stimulating hormone, luteinizing hormone, thyroid stimulating hormone, adrenocorticotropin hormone, beta endorphin and melanocyte stimulating hormone), and effector hormones (e.g. vasopressin, oxytocin, growth hormone, prolactin, thyroid hormones, cholecystokinin, adrenaline, glucocorticoids, mineralocorticoids, estrogens, progesterone and androgens).

NEUROLEPTIC i) Any of a class of psychotropic drugs used to treat psychoses, particularly schizophrenia. ii) Pertaining to a condition similar to that produced by a neuroleptic drug.

NEUROMA A tumor composed of nerve cells.

NEUROMODULATOR *See under* NEUROTRANSMITTER.

NEUROMUSCULAR ELECTRICAL STIMULATION NMES. It involves the application of electrical stimulation to produce skeletal muscle contraction as a result of the percutaneous (through-the-skin) stimulation of peripheral nerves. NMES has a variety of uses, including maintenance of muscle mass and strength during prolonged periods of immobilization. It appears that when NMES and voluntary exercise are combined, there is no significant difference in muscle strength after training when compared to either NMES or voluntary exercise alone. There is also evidence that NMES can improve functional performance in a variety of strength tasks. Two mechanisms have been proposed to explain the training effects seen with NMES. First, augmentation of muscle strength with NMES may occur in a similar manner to augmentation of muscle strength with voluntary exercise. Second, the muscle strengthening seen following NMES training may result from a reversal of voluntary recruitment of motor units order, with a selective augmentation of those with fast-glycolytic muscle fibers.

There is some evidence to suggest that NMES is effective in selective strengthening of individual muscles within muscle groups or parts of muscles. It is unclear whether this selective strengthening is due to local changes in the muscle or muscle area stimulated, or whether it is due to a change in the relative magnitude of recruitment of the different muscles within a muscle group or of the different portions of a muscle. It is currently believed that NMES can activate muscle to a relatively low percentage of maximal voluntary contraction (MVC). It is not known whether, in generating 25% MVC, 25% of the muscle fibers are generating maximal tension, or if all the fibers are generating 25% of their maximum tension, or if some 'in-between' combination is occurring. Research evidence suggests that electrical stimulation, based on proximity to electrodes, activates only a limited portion of the muscle.

Bibliography

Lake, D.A. (1992). Neuromuscular electrical stimulation: An overview and its application in the treatment of sports injuries. *Sports Medicine* 13(5), 320-336.

NEURONS Nerve cells. These are cells that are specialized for receiving and transmitting electrical signals. As many as 10,000 different subtypes of neu-

rons have been identified, each specialized to send and receive certain types of information. Each neuron comprises a **cell body** (**soma**) with a nucleus. Axons and dendrites form extensions from the cell body. A **nerve fiber** is the **axon** (long process) of a nerve cell. Nerve fibers are classified according to fiber diameter and conduction velocity, with these being highest in A and lowest in C. **'A' fibers** (and their functions) are alpha (skeletal muscle contraction), beta (touch, pressure sensation), gamma (muscle spindle stimulation) and delta (pain, temperature sensation). **'B' fibers** are visceral afferents and autonomic preganglionics. **'C' fibers** are pain, temperature sensation and autonomic postganglionics. Sensory fibers are additionally classified as I, II, III and IV.

A **nerve impulse** is an electric discharge and associated events as the discharge is propagated along a nerve fiber. An **action potential** is a localized change of electrical potential between the inside and outside of a nerve fiber that occurs when an impulse passes any point along a neuron. When there is no impulse traveling along a neuron, the inside is electrically negative to the outside. This is the **resting potential**. When an impulse passes any point, it changes that point momentarily to positive. This is the action potential.

A **sensory (afferent) neuron** is any neuron that transmits impulses towards the central nervous system (CNS). An **efferent (motor) neuron** is any neuron that conducts impulses away from the CNS to an effector organ (muscle or gland). Sensory and motor nerves do not usually interact except via the synapses in the CNS. **Synapses** are junctions between two neurons, a neuron and a gland, or a neuron and a muscle. **Sensory receptors** include mechanical receptors (such as muscle spindles and Golgi tendon organs), baroreceptors, chemoreceptors, thermal receptors, photoreceptors and pain receptors.

Motor neurons obey the **all-or-none law**: the intensity and speed of the impulses do not depend on the amount of stimulation from the central nervous system. In other words, the motor neuron reacts either with impulses of consistent intensity or not at all. The number of impulses per second can be changed. *See also* MUSCLE SPINDLES.

NEUROPEPTIDE Y   The most abundant neuropeptide in the brain. It is involved in feeding behavior, circadian rhythms, sexual function, anxiety responses and vascular resistance.

See under INSULIN.

NEUROPRAXIA   A focal blocking along the axon of a neuron secondary to focal demyelination. It is characterized by temporary paralysis of involved muscles without muscle wasting or loss of deep tendon reflexes.

NEUROTMESIS   Discontinuity of the entire nerve including the axon and the supporting connective tissue.

NEUTRAL   i) Being neither acidic nor basic. A neutral solution is one that has a pH of 7. ii) Being neither positively nor negatively charged. A neutral atom has an equal number of protons and orbital electrons.

NEUTRALIZATION   In the immune system, it is a process that occurs when antibodies block the binding site on antigens so that they cannot bind to tissues and cause damage.

NEUTRALIZER   *See under* MUSCLE ACTION.

NEUTROPHIL   *See under* LEUKOCYTE.

NEUROTRANSMITTER   A compound, secreted by a neuron from its endings, which serves to transmit a nerve impulse. Hundreds of substances are known or suspected to be neurotransmitters. Harmful effects can occur when neurotransmitter levels are too high or too low. In the most general sense, neurotransmitters include: messengers that act directly to regulate ion channels; those that act through second messenger systems; and those that act at a distance from their site of release. Calcium ions diffuse into synaptic knobs in response to action potentials, causing release of neurotransmitter. Neurotransmitters are quickly degraded or removed from synaptic clefts.

Neurotransmitters can be classed as peptide or non-peptide. **Peptide neurotransmitters** include: adrenocorticotropic hormone, angiotensin II, bradykinin, endorphins, gastrin, glucagon, growth-hormone releasing factor, insulin, oxytocin, somatostatin, substance P and thyrotropin-releasing factor. **Non-peptide neurotransmitters** include: acetylcholine, dopamine, epinephrine, GABA, glutamate, glycine, histamine, nitric oxide, norepinephrine and serotonin.

Neuropeptides are responsible for mediating sensory and emotional responses, including hunger, thirst, sex drive, pleasure and pain. Some neuropeptides are neurotransmitters, and some are neuromodulators. Examples of neuropeptides are enkephalins, endorphins and substance P.

A **neuromodulator** is a substance other than a neurotransmitter, released by a neuron, which conveys information to adjacent or distant neurons, either enhancing or damping their activities.

See under AUTONOMIC NERVOUS SYSTEM.

NEWTON'S LAWS   Isaac Newton's three laws of motion concern inertia, acceleration and action-reaction. The **Law of Inertia (First Law)** states that every body continues in its state of rest or uniform motion in a straight line except when it is compelled by external forces to change its state. The **Law of Acceleration (Second Law)** states that the rate of momentum of a body is proportional to the applied force and takes place in the direction in which the force acts. The **Law of Action-Reaction (Third Law)** states that for every action there is an equal and opposite reaction.

Chronology

•1687 • Isaac Newton published *Philosophiae Naturalis Principia Mathematica*, which included his three laws of motion. Newton analyzed the motion of bodies in resisting and non-resisting media under the action of centripetal forces. The results were applied to orbiting bodies, projectiles, pendulums and free fall near the Earth. He demonstrated that the planets were attracted toward the Sun and generally that all heavenly bodies attract one another. Newton's Law of Universal Gravitation states that all matter attracts all other matter with a force proportional to the product of their masses and inversely proportional to the square of the distance between them. All bodies in space and on Earth are affected by a force called gravity. For Newton, the creation of the force of gravity was an act of God, since he believed that bodies do not necessarily possess that quality. Newton devoted much time in his later years to theology. Newton was elected President of the Royal Society in 1703 and was re-elected each year until his death in 1727.

NIACIN   *See under* VITAMIN B$_2$.

NICOTINAMIDE   *See* NIACIN.

NICOTINAMIDE ADENINE DINUCLEOTIDE
See NAD$^+$.

NICOTINAMIDE ADENINE DINUCLEOTIDE PHOSPHATE   *See* NADPH.

NICOTINE   An alkaloid found in the leaf of the tobacco plant. Each cigarette puff delivers a hit of nicotine to the brain within 7 seconds. Diverse effects from nicotine occur as a result of both stimulant and depressant actions on various pathways in the central nervous system (CNS) and peripheral nervous system. By mimicking the action of acetylcholine, it causes stimulation of the adrenal medulla, facilitation of transmission across sympathetic ganglia and release of norepinephrine from cardiac atria and arterioles. Larger doses of nicotine, however, may cause inhibition of catecholamine response from the adrenal medulla. Increased blood pressure and bradycardia (or occasionally tachycardia) are caused by the effect of nicotine on various cardiovascular control centers (such as carotid and aortic bodies), the sympathetic and vagal ganglia, and cardiac muscle. It may cause independent central blood pressure effects by stimulation of the ventral lateral medulla in the brain. In the CNS, norepinephrine and dopamine release occurs following nicotine administration, and acetylcholine may increase or decrease depending on dose. Large doses may produce neuromuscular blockade because of receptor desensitization.

Nicotine has small, specific, positive effects on the CNS that may facilitate cognitive processes, such as attention and memory. The effects of nicotine on attention may be explained by the mild stimulant effect that nicotine has on the CNS. In some sports, such as golf, athletes use nicotine before performance, because of its anti-anxiety effect. Wesnes and Warburton (1983) argued that it is the action of nicotine on cholinergic pathways controlling attention that decreases anxiety by enabling individuals to concentrate more efficiently. Distracting thoughts are filtered out, enabling more effective performance and increased self-confidence.

The current scientific view is that nicotine, delivered through tobacco smoke, should be regarded as an addictive drug. It meets the criteria for substance abuse stated in the *Diagnostic and Statistical Manual for Mental Disorders*. 40% of heart attack patients relapse to smoking while still in hospital. Tolerance to nicotine exposure develops within a few hours in humans (smokers and non-smokers).

Nicotine stimulates the satiety center of the brain, which may explain the weight gain associated with giving up smoking and the use of nicotine by athletes for weight control. There is a great deal of evidence to suggest that cigarette smokers weigh less than non-smokers and that smokers who quit gain weight. Acute increases in resting metabolic rate following intake of nicotine suggest an important role for metabolism in explaining the effect of smoking on bodyweight.

Nicotine causes constriction of the terminal bronchioles of the lungs. This has the following effects: i) increased resistance to air flow to and from the lungs; ii) increased fluid secretion in the bronchial tree and some swelling of epithelial linings; and iii) paralysis of cilia (tiny hairs) on the surfaces of the respiratory epithelial cells, which usually beat continuously to prevent excess fluid and foreign particles from accumulating in the respiratory passageway. Chronic effects of nicotine include chronic bronchitis, obstruction of terminal bronchioles and destruction of alveolar walls.

Alcohol seems to increase the number and frequency of cigarettes smoked. There is evidence to suggest that smoking while drinking alcohol helps to maintain the integrity of the CNS through an antagonistic action of nicotine on alcohol-related performance decrements.

Withdrawal from nicotine can produce a variety of effects, including craving for tobacco, anxiety, irritability, restlessness, difficulty concentrating, headache, drowsiness, and gastrointestinal disturbances. The acute phase of nicotine withdrawal is usually over within 2 to 4 weeks, but some withdrawal symptoms, such as the urge to smoke, can continue for months or even years.

See also CARBON MONOXIDE; MARIJUANA.

Bibliography

American Psychiatric Association (1994). *Diagnostic and Statistical Manual of Mental Disorders*. 4th ed. Washington, DC: American Psychiatric Association.

Marks, B.L. and Perkins, K.A. (1990). The effects of nicotine on metabolic rate. *Sports Medicine* 10(5), 277-285.

Sherwood, N. (1995). Effects of nicotine on human psychomotor performance. *Human Psychopharmacology* 8, 155-184.

Wesnes, K. and Warburton, D.M. (1983). Stress and drugs. In Hockey, G.R.J. (ed). *Stress and fatigue in human performance*. pp203-243. Chichester, UK: John Wiley.

NICOTINIC ACID   See NIACIN.

NIPPLE IRRITATION   See BRASSIERE; JOGGER'S NIPPLE.

NITRATES   Salts of nitric acid. Nitrates are used as vasodilators and anti-ischemic agents. Nitrates such as glyceryl trinitrate are sufficiently lipid soluble to penetrate cell membranes. Nitrates directly relax smooth muscle, and hence decrease blood pressure via their effect on the venous system and (to a lesser extent) the arterial system. Nitrate administration is of benefit to patients predisposed to angina pectoris, because of its effect of preventing, delaying or decreasing ischemia. Nitrates have no effect on the exercise capacity of patients without myocardial ischemia, angina pectoris or congestive heart failure. Nitrates can be regarded as carriers of the nitrite ion that is the precursor of nitric oxide, which can act as a free radical.

See also BETA ADRENERGIC BLOCKERS; CALCIUM-CHANNEL BLOCKERS.

NITRIC OXIDE   i) An inorganic gas that is one of the nitrogen oxides (NO_x) responsible for air pollution. ii) As a free radical, nitric oxide is inherently reactive and mediates cellular toxicity by damaging critical enzymes and by reacting with superoxide to form an even more potent oxidant, peroxynitrite. Endogenous nitric oxide is generated from arginine by a family of three distinct calmodulin-dependent nitric oxide synthase enzymes.

The highest levels of nitric oxide throughout the body are found in neurons, where it functions as a unique messenger molecule. In the autononomic nervous system, nitric oxide functions as a major non-adrenergic, non-cholinergic neurotransmitter. This neurotransmitter pathway plays a particularly important role in producing relaxation of smooth muscle in the cerebral circulation and the gastrointestinal, urogenital and respiratory tracts. Dysregulation of nitric oxide synthase activity in nerves of the autonomic nervous system plays a major role in a variety of pathophysiological conditions, including migraine headache. In the brain, nitric oxide functions as a neuromodulator and appears to mediate aspects of learning and memory. It also appears to play a major role in the pathophysiology of stroke, Parkinson's disease, Huntington's disease and amyotrophic lateral sclerosis.

Nitric oxide is important in blood pressure regulation as a vasodilator and is produced under normal physiologic conditions primarily by the endothelium lining of blood vessels. The primary stimulus for the production of nitric oxide by the constitutive endothelial nitric oxide synthase found in blood vessels is most likely the shear stress caused by blood flowing through the blood vessels. Nitric oxide appears to stimulate vasodilation in both terminal arterioles and the large feeder arteries that supply blood to muscle beds. Nitric oxide released from the endothelial cells of large feeder arteries appears to be critical for supplying the necessary blood during exercise. Exercise increases nitric oxide synthesis via increases in shear stress and pulse pressure, so it is likely that nitric oxide is an important blood flow regulatory mechanism in exercise. The vasodilatory effects of nitric oxide during exercise increase the metabolically stimulated vasodilation caused by substances such as adenosine.

Nitric oxide also plays a major role in skeletal muscle. Physiologically, muscle-derived nitric oxide regulates skeletal muscle contractility and exercise-induced glucose uptake.

In the lungs, as oxygen binds to hemoglobin's heme groups, hemoglobin undergoes shape changes that enable nitric oxide to bind with cysteine. This binding results in a sulfhydryl (thiol) group in which the nitric oxide is protected from being degraded by hemoglobin's iron. After being circulated, the hemoglobin unloads not only oxygen, but also nitric oxide, which dilates the local vessels and facilitates oxygen delivery. As deoxygenated hemoglobin picks up carbon dioxide, it also picks up any circulating nitric oxide in the area and carries these gases to the lungs where they are unloaded.

Endogenously produced nitric oxide is detectable in the exhaled air of resting humans. The amount of nitric oxide in exhaled air increases during exercise, but the mechanisms underlying this response are poorly understood.

Shear stress-mediated improvement in endothelial function provides one plausible explanation for the cardioprotective benefits of exercise training. Nitric oxide also plays a protective role in preventing atherosclerosis via superoxide anion scavenging. However, risk factors such as hypercholesterolemia decrease nitric oxide release and set the stage for endothelial dysfunction and atherosclerotic lesions. Exercise reverses this process by stimulating nitric oxide synthesis and release. Endothelial dysfunction is a trigger of myocardial ischemia. The impaired production of endothelium-derived nitric oxide in response to acetylcholine and blood flow leads to paradoxical vasoconstriction and exercise-induced ischemia. Exercise training attenuates paradoxical vasoconstriction in coronary artery disease and increases coronary blood flow in response to acetylcholine. It has been shown in animal experiments that shear stress acts as a stimulus for the endothelium to increase the transport capacity for arginine, to enhance nitric oxide synthase activity and expression, and to increase the production of extracellular superoxide dismutase (which prevents premature breakdown of nitric oxide).

Bibliography

Bredt, D.S. (1999). Endogenous nitric oxide synthesis: Biological functions and pathophysiology. *Free Radical Research* 31(6), 577-596.

Gattullo, D., Pagliaro, P., Marsh, N.A. and Losano, G. (1999). New insights into nitric oxide and coronary circulation. *Life Sciences* 65(21), 2167-2174.

Gielen, S., Schuler, G. and Hambrecht, R. (2001). Exercise training in coronary artery disease and coronary vasomotion. *Circulation* 103(1), E1-E6.

Karlsson, J. (1997). *Antioxidants and exercise*. Champaign, IL: Human Kinetics.

Maiorana, A. et al. (2003). Exercise and the nitric oxide vasodilator system. *Sports Medicine* 33(14), 1013-1035.

Sheel, A.W., Road, J. and McKenzie, D.C. (1999). Exhaled nitric oxide during exercise. *Sports Medicine* 28(2), 83-90.

Shen, W. et al. (1995). Nitric oxide production and NO synthase gene expression contribute to vascular regulation during exercise. *Medicine and Science in Sports and Exercise* 27(8), 1125-1134.

NITROGEN   A gaseous element that is the major component of the atmosphere (78%) and the element on which the human food supply is most dependent. Nitrogen is unavailable to animals or plants for amino acid synthesis until it has been 'fixed,' i.e. changed into nitrogen-containing compounds that plants can use. Animals receive nitrogen by eating plants or other animals. Fixation of nitrogen is accomplished in nature through an electrical discharge in the atmosphere (lightning), through blue-green algae or through the action of bacteria located in the root nodules of leguminous plants. Once the nitrogen of the air becomes 'fixed nitrogen' in the soil, it can then be incorporated into the amino acids, purines or other compounds in plants.

NITROGEN BALANCE   The difference between nitrogen intake and nitrogen loss. It provides an estimate of a person's protein balance. A **negative nitrogen balance** occurs when nitrogen loss is greater than intake, indicating a loss of body protein. A **positive nitrogen balance** occurs when nitrogen intake is greater than loss, which indicates an increased state of protein anabolism. A negative nitrogen balance can occur even if only one of the essential amino acids is deficient, if there is an imbalance in the proportions of essential amino acids, or if overall protein intake is not sufficient to offset a negative nitrogen balance.

NITROGEN OXIDES   *See under* AIR POLLUTION.

NOCICEPTIVE REFLEXES   Reflexes triggered by painful stimuli. *See* PAIN.

NOCTURIA   Excessive urination at night. *See under* AGING.

NOISE   Error present in data collected that is unrelated to the process being studied. For example, there is noise caused by electrical interference in electromyography or mechanical vibration in a force platform. Noise may be random or systematic. **Smoothing** refers to methods used to decrease the effects of noise. Examples are filtering and fitting of data.

NON-STEROIDAL ANTI-INFLAMMATORY DRUGS   NSAIDs. Aspirin-like drugs that were developed in an attempt to decrease the gastrointestinal and hemorrhagic side effects produced by aspirin, while maintaining their positive effects of suppressing inflammation. Examples of nonprescription NSAIDs are Ibuprofen (Advil, Motrin, Nuprin) and Naproxen Sodium (Aleve). Examples of prescription NSAIDs are Diclofenac (Voltarin) and Idomethacin (Indocin).

NSAIDs interfere with the biosynthesis of prostaglandins and other related compounds by inhibiting **cyclo-oxygenase**, an enzyme involved in the synthesis of prostaglandins. During inflammation of a soft tissue, increased prostaglandin activity seems to mediate inflammation by increasing blood flow, capillary permeability, and the permeability effects of histamine and bradykinin. With muscle strain and contusion, nonsteroidal anti-inflammatory drugs (NSAIDs) can result in a modest inhibition of the initial inflammatory response and its symptoms. However, this may be associated with some small negative effects later in the healing phase.

NSAIDs decrease pain, but are not effective for the relief of severe pain. NSAIDSs decrease the set point of the hypothalamus, thus decreasing fever. NSAIDs also have anti-platelet properties, but much lower in intensity than those of aspirin. The effect of NSAISs on delayed-onset muscle soreness appears small at best.

Alcohol should never be taken with NSAIDs as it increases the risk of gastrointestinal irritation and the development of gastric ulcers. In addition to gastrointestinal irritation, possible side effects are renal impairment and hypersensitivity reactions (e.g. urticaria).

See also CORTICOSTEROIDS.

Bibliography
Almekinders, L.C. (1999). Anti-inflammatory treatment of muscular injuries in sport. An update of recent studies. *Sports Medicine* 28(6), 383-388.

NOONAN SYNDROME   A genetic condition that affects growth and development, the heart and blood clotting. It is often associated with congenital heart disease and short stature. It is inherited as an autosomal dominant trait. Worldwide, there are an estimated 1 in 1,000 to 1 in 2,500 infants who have Noonan syndrome.

Bibliography
Noonan Support Group. Http://www.noonansyndrome.org

NORADRENALINE   *See* NOREPINEPHRINE.

NOREPINEPHRINE   Noradrenaline. It is a catecholamine hormone with some of the effects of epinephrine, but also some effects that are in the opposite direction to those of epinephrine. For example, it causes a decrease (rather than an increase) in heart rate. Other effects of norepinephrine are increased lipolysis, increased glycogenolysis, increased stroke volume, increased vascular resistance and vasoconstriction.

See under AUTONOMIC NERVOUS SYSTEM.

NORMAL DISTRIBUTION   A symmetrical, bell-shaped distribution characterized by the mean and the standard deviation. The **mean** is a measure of central tendency. The **standard deviation** is a measure of dispersion (the extent to which scores deviate from the mean) and is the square root of the **variance**. In a normal distribution, approximately 68% of the observations are within 1 standard deviation from the mean, approximately 95% are within 2 standard deviations, and approximately 99.7% are within 3 standard deviations.

NORMAL FORCE The force between two bodies in contact with each other, in a direction perpendicular to the surface of contact.

NORMOTENSIVE (i) Characterized by normal tone, tension, or pressure. (ii) A person with normal blood pressure.

NOSE The organ of the sense of smell. It also serves as a passageway for air going to and from the lungs. The nasal physiologic functions, such as warming and humidification, are vital for upper airway function. Filtration of environmental particles occurs first in the nasal cavity. Vascular mucosa increases relative humidity to 95% before air reaches the nasopharynx. It is the active process of sniffing that allows environmental particles to reach the olfactory system, which is located at the skull base. Rebreathing causes increased arterial carbon dioxide levels, which results in nasal vasoconstriction and decreased nasal resistance. Going from a supine to an upright position decreases jugulovenous distension and nasal airway resistance. Exercise causes sympathetic vasoconstriction and contraction of the alae nasi, increasing the capacity of the nasal passages. Factors increasing nasal resistance include: infective rhinitis, allergic rhinitis, vasomotor rhinitis, hyperventilation, supine posture, alcohol, aspirin and cold air.

See BREATHING; EPISTAXIS; NASAL INJURIES.

Bibliography
Lin, S.J. and Danahey, D.G. (2002). Nasal aerodynamics. Http://www.emedicine.com

NOTATIONAL ANALYSIS Statistical analyses in sport are carried out by both academic researchers and analysts employed by professional sports teams or television/media companies. Automated video-computerized match analysis systems can provide data analysis within a few hours after the game is completed. Time-motion analysis by ProZone® (Leeds, England) of England's soccer star, Wayne Rooney, during the 2004 European Cup Finals, found that during a game he covered approximately 11.8 km (4,000 m was walking, 4,800 m was jogging, 1,500 m was running, 1,000 m was light sprinting, and 500 m was sprinting). Nearly 10% of Rooney's time was spent in the defending zone, 22% in the center of the pitch and 31% of his time was spent in and around the attacking penalty area.

In a study of English Premier League soccer, there was no significant difference found between the duration of the average high-intensity bursts performed by defenders, midfielders and forwards. The amount of recovery between high-intensity bursts is influenced by playing position, with midfielders having a significantly shorter recovery between bursts than defenders.

An analysis of 129 penalties from FIFA World Cup finals and the finals of the European Champions League found that 20% of penalties were saved, 7% missed and 73% were scored. There was no difference in success ratios for left-footed versus right-footed strikers. No shots above waist height were saved, although 18% of these shots were missed. In every case, the goalkeeper moved off the line before the ball was struck. The goalkeepers who took a pace forward and stood up while the striker approached the ball had the best save-to-miss ratios.

Bibliography
Hughes, M. and Franks, I. (1997). *Notational analysis of sport*. London: E & FN Spon.
Hughes, M. and Wells, J. (2002). Analysis of penalties taken in shoot-outs. *International Journal of Performance Analysis in Sport* 2(1), 55-72.
O'Donoghue, P.G. (2002). Time-motion analysis of work-rate in English FA Premier League soccer. *International Journal of Performance Analysis in Sport* 2(1), 36-43.

NUCLEIC ACIDS Chains of nucleotides (polynucleotides) whose functions are to store and to transmit genetic information.

NUCLEOLUS *See under* CELL.

NUCLEOSIDE A purine or pyrimidine base attached to a pentose. It results from the removal of phosphate from a nucleotide. A **nucleotide** is a nucleoside phosphate. Nucleosides and nucleotides are structural components of many compounds such as DNA, RNA, ATP, NAD^+, FAD and coenzyme A.

NUCLEUS *See under* CELL.

NUTRITION The science of foods and their components, including: the relationships to performance, health and disease; physiological processes (such as ingestion, digestion, absorption, transport and excretion); and the psychological, social, economic and cultural implications of eating.

The following substances may be found in food: carbohydrates, fats, proteins, vitamins, minerals, dietary fiber, water, alcohol and other substances that may be naturally occurring in the food or added by food manufacturers, but do not have nutritional value. A food with high **nutrient density** possesses a significant amount of a specific nutrient or nutrients per serving compared to its energy value.

The classic definition of **nutrient** is a component of food that cannot be made by the body, but is required for growth and development. However, non-nutrient components such as phytochemicals in the diet may have antioxidant or immune-enhancing properties. In the context of nutrition, the National Academy of Science of the Institute of Medicine has proposed that antioxidant is defined as "a substance in foods that significantly decreases the adverse effects of reactive oxygen species (ROS), reactive nitrogen species (RNS), or both on normal physiological function in humans."

The weight of scientific evidence, according to the American Dietetic Association, indicates that the optimal approach for achieving a health benefit from the intake of nutrients and other physiologically active constituents is through the consumption of a varied diet that is rich in plant food. Each fruit or vegetable contains numerous nutrients, but also phytochemicals, which are not currently replicated in pill form. Dietary constituents appear to act synergistically to improve absorption of nutrients or physiologically active dietary components. An example is lycopene in tomatoes and the enhancement of its absorption when consumed along with fat. Concentrated amounts of single substances may also adversely affect the absorption, biological transport and metabolism of other potentially beneficial substance with similar chemical properties. Synthetic forms of some nutrients may not be as effective.

It is the position of the American Dietetic Association that "when dietary intakes do not meet science-based dietary recommendations, food fortification and dietary supplementation can make an important contribution." The International Food Information Council defines **functional foods**, including whole foods and fortified, enriched or enhanced foods, as foods that provide health benefits beyond basic nutrition. The term 'functional foods' is preferred to terms such 'nutraceuticals' or 'designer foods.' Dietary supplements, unlike drugs, are not required to have strong scientific and clinical evidence for their effectiveness before being allowed onto the market. In the USA, the Dietary Supplement Health Education Act (DSHEA) of 1994, which amended the Food, Drug and Cosmetic Act of 1938, defines **dietary supplements** as certain foods intended to supplement the diet that are not represented as conventional foods.

In the USA, the **health claims** authorized under the Nutrition Labeling and Education Act of 1990 are statements that describe a relationship between a food substance and a disease or other health-related condition. Approved health claims (specifically, decrease in total and LDL cholesterol) have been made for the following functional foods and recommended amounts (bioactive components stated in parenthesis): fortified margarines (plant sterol and stanol esters) at 1.3 g/day for sterols and 1.7 g/day for stanols; psyllium (soluble fiber) at 1 g/day; soy (protein) at 25 g/day; and whole oat products (soluble fiber) at 3 g/day.

See DIET; ENERGY YIELD OF NUTRIENTS.

Bibliography

American Dietetic Association (2001). Position of the American Dietetic Association: Food fortification and dietary supplements. *Journal of the American Dietetic Association* 101, 115-125.

American Dietetic Association (2004). Position of the American Dietetic Association: Functional Foods. *Journal of the American Dietetic Association* 104, 814-826.

Garrow, J.S., James, W.P.T. and Ralph, A. (2000, eds). *Human nutrition and dietetics*. 10th ed. Edinburgh: Churchill Livingstone.

Insel, P., Turner, R.E. and Ross, D. (2004). *Nutrition*. 2nd ed. Sudbury, MA: Jones and Bartlett.

Wardlaw, G.M. (2002). *Perspectives in nutrition*. 5th ed. Boston, MA: WCB McGraw-Hill.

NUTRITIONAL ERGOGENIC AID To be effective as ergogenic aids, dietary supplements must either provide a nutrient that is normally undersupplied to cells or exert a pharmacological effect on cellular processes. A supplement has benefit only when the normal intake of a bioavailable form of a nutrient is lower than the amount that would provide maximum benefit as judged from all biological perspectives. In order to market products with little or no scientific evidence for their ergogenic potential, companies take advantage of theoretical effects based on animal studies, or even *in vitro* experiments.

Bibliography

Antonio, J. and Stout, J.R. (2001). *Sports supplements*. Philadelphia, PA: Lippincott Williams & Wilkins.

Bucci, L. (1993). *Nutrients as ergogenic aids for sports and exercise*. Boca Raton, FL: CRC Press.

Butterfield, G. (1996). Ergogenic aids: Evaluating sport nutrition products. *International Journal of Sport Nutrition* 6, 191-197.

Clarkson, P.M. (1996). Nutrition for improved sports performance. Current issues on ergogenic aids. *Sports Medicine* 21(6), 393-401.

Maughan, R.J., King, D.S. and Lea, T. (2004). Dietary supplements. *Journal of Sports Sciences* 22, 95-113.

Williams, M.H. (1993). Nutritional supplements for strength-trained athletes. *Gatorade Sports Science Exchange* 6(6).

Williams, M.H. (1999). *Nutrition for fitness and sport*. 5th ed. Boston, MA: McGraw-Hill.

Zeisel, S.H. (2000). Is there a metabolic basis for dietary supplementation? *American Journal of Clinical Nutrition* 72(2), S507-S511.

NYSTAGMUS Involuntary movement of the eyes around their natural position. This can be horizontal, vertical, circular or mixed. It causes difficulty in maintaining fixation on objects, resulting in decreased visual acuity and fatigue.

O

OBESITY The presence of excess body fat in the body. It is associated with an imbalance between energy input and energy expenditure, such that the former is greater. When humans eat high-fat diets, excess body fat is formed more easily than it is with a high carbohydrate, high fiber diet. Fats eaten above the day's nutritional requirements are nearly all stored in the body.

More than 50% of adult Americans have body mass indices of at least 25, the criterion for overweight in the USA. Moderate obesity is defined as having a body mass index of 30 to 39.9, with 40 indicating severe obesity. In the USA, the prevalence of obesity was 30.5% in 1999-2000 compared with 22.9% between 1988 and 1994. The prevalence of overweightness also increased during this period from 55.9% to 64.5%. The prevalence of overweight among US adolescents aged 12 to 19 years increased from 5% in 1980 to 15% in 2000. Median values for body mass index in the USA were 11.6 in 1990 and 22.1 in 2002. The use of body mass index is controversial, because it does not distinguish between fat mass and fat-free mass.

In the majority of cases, resting metabolic rate is greater in obese individuals. This is thought to be due to the greater fat-free mass of the obese state. Prior to adulthood, body fat increases through enlargement (hypertrophy) of individual adipocytes and increase in total cell number (hyperplasia). In extreme cases in adults, adipocyte number may possibly increase once cell size reaches the hypertrophic limit. Adipocyte size varies with weight gain or loss. There is also speculation that 'yo-yo' dieting may cause an increase in the number of adipocytes. Factors determining the amount of fat carried in adipocytes include energy intake, energy expenditure, hormones, somatotype and genes. During pregnancy, estrogen encourages fat deposition in preparation for breastfeeding. It seems likely that fat cells may increase in number during pregnancy, probably during the third trimester.

The **Pima paradox** is the fact that the American Pima Indians are the most obese population in the USA, but their genetically similar sister tribe that moved down to Mexico suffers from no obesity at all. The Mexican Pimas eat a high carbohydrate, low fat diet, and they have no cars or other modern conveniences. Physical activity is higher in Mexican Pima Indians than American Pima Indians.

Obesity is associated with increased mortality and morbidity at all ages, particularly in young people. It is associated with a worsening of several risk factors for cardiovascular disease, e.g. high blood pressure, raised serum cholesterol and triglyceride, decreased HDL cholesterol and diabetes. Obesity is associated with an increased prevalence of osteoarthritis and decreased lung function. It is also associated with increased risk of colonic, rectal and prostatic cancer (males), in addition to breast and cervical cancer (females).

Physical activity appears to lower the health risks associated with being overweight and obesity. Furthermore, active obese individuals actually have lower morbidity and mortality than normal weight individuals who are sedentary. Inactivity and low cardiorespiratory fitness are as important as overweight and obesity as mortality predictors.

Drugs to treat obesity can be divided into three groups: drugs that decrease food intake; those that alter metabolism; and those that increase thermogenesis. The inhibition of feeding by activating the sympathetic nervous system is an important satiety system that helps regulate body fat stores. Both serotonin and norepinephrine decrease food intake and augment sympathetic activity. **Phentermine (Adipex, Ionamin)**, a serotonergic drug, is an appetite suppressant used for the short-term treatment of obesity. It is contraindicated for patients with heart disease, high blood pressure, glaucoma, thyroid problems, anxiety disorder, diabetes or any seizure disorder. Phentermine and fenfluramine are the active ingredients of the notorious '**Phen-Fen**' agent, which has been associated with cardiac valvular disease and banned by the Federal Drug Agency (FDA) in 1997. **Fenfluramine (Pondimin)**, a noradrenergic drug, was removed from the market, but cardiac valvular disease does not appear to be a risk with the use of phentermine alone.

Sibutramine (Meridia) is an appetite suppressant that is used for long-term treatment of obesity. It is contraindicated for patients who have high blood pressure or a history of heart problems. Modest weight loss is achieved with sibutramine, but weight gain is significant after discontinuation. Sibutramine is a combination serotonin and norepinephrine and dopamine reuptake inhibitor whose appetite-suppressive effects appear to be related to its noradrenergic action. When its noradrenergic activity is blocked, the appetite suppression is lost.

Orlistat (Xenical) has been shown to decrease body weight by pancreatic lipase and can block 30% of the triglyceride hydrolysis in subjects eating a 30% fat diet. Due to its ability to block fat absorption, Orlistat also has the capability to inhibit absorption of fat-soluble vitamins. The unabsorbed fat can produce diarrhea and flatulence. In 1999, the FDA approved Orlistat for long-term use.

See also ABDOMINAL OBESITY; DIETING; LEPTIN.

Chronology
•1998 • In the USA, the first Federal guidelines for the treatment of overweight and obesity in adults were released by the National Heart, Lung and Blood Institute (NHLBI) as a part of its nationwide Obesity Education Initiative. It recommended a 500 to 1000 kcal per day negative energy balance; 1 to 2 lb weight loss per week for a period of 6 months.

Bibliography
American Obesity Association. Http://www.obesity.org

Andersen, R.E. (2003, ed). *Obesity. Etiology, assessment, treatment and prevention.* Champaign, IL: Human Kinetics.

Blair, S.N. and Brodney, S. (1999). Effects of physical inactivity and obesity on morbidity and mortality: Current evidence and research issues. *Medicine and Science in Sports and Exercise* 31(11), S646-S662.

Bouchard, C. (2000, ed). *Physical activity and obesity.* Champaign, IL: Human Kinetics.

Bray, G.A. (2000). Reciprocal relation of food intake and sympathetic activity: experimental observations and clinical implications Metab. *International Journal of Obesity Related Disorders* 24 S2, 8-17.

Bray, G.A. (2000). A concise review on the therapeutics of obesity. *Nutrition* 16(10), 953-960.

Carek, P.J. and Dickerson, L.M. (1999). Current concepts in the pharmacological management of obesity. *Drugs* 57(6), 883-

904.

Clark, N. (1994). Separating fat from fiction. *The Physician and Sportsmedicine* 22(3), 35-36.

Divadeenam, K. (2002). Stimulants. Http://www.emedicine.com

Esparza, J. et al. (2000). Daily energy expenditure in Mexican and USA Pima Indians: Low physical activity as a possible cause of obesity. *International Journal of Obesity-Related Metabolic Disorders* 24(1), 55-59.

Halpern, A. and Mancini, M.C. (2003). Treatment of obesity: An update on anti-obesity medications. *Obesity Review* 4(1), 25-42.

Hill, J.O. and Melanson, E.L. (1999). Overview of the determinants of overweight and obesity: Current evidence and research issues. *Medicine and Science in Sports and Exercise*, 31(11), S515-S521.

Jebb, S.A. and Moore, M.S. (1999). Contribution of sedentary lifestyle and inactivity to the etiology of overweight and obesity: Current evidence and research issues. *Medicine and Science in Sports and Exercise* 31(11), S534-S541.

Lucas, K.H. and Kaplan-Machlis, B. (2001). Orlistat - a novel weight loss therapy. *Annals of Pharmacotherapy* 35(3), 314-328.

Office of the Surgeon General (2001). *The Surgeon General's call to action to prevent overweight and obesity.* Rockville, Maryland: US Department Health and Human Services.

Ogden, C.L. et al. (2002). Prevalence and trends in overweight among US children and adolescents, 1999-2000. *Journal of the American Medical Association* 288, 1728-1732.

Pi-Sunyer, F.X. (1999). Comorbidities of overweight and obesity: Current evidence and research issues. *Medicine and Science in Sports and Exercise* 31(11), S602-S608.

Prentice, A.M. and Jebb, S.A. (1995). Obesity in Britain: Gluttony or sloth? *British Medical Journal* 311, 12 August.

Riley, R.E. (1999). Popular weight loss diets: Health and exercise implications. *Clinics in Sports Medicine* 18(3), 691-701.

Stamford, B. (1988). Creeping obesity. *The Physician and Sportsmedicine* 16(1), 143.

OBSESSIVE COMPULSIVE DISORDER *See under* ANXIETY DISORDERS.

OBTURATOR NERVE *See under* HIP JOINT, DISLOCATION.

OCCIPITO-ATLANTAL JOINT A double condyloid joint between the occipital bone of the skull and the atlas (the first cervical vertebra). Flexion, extension and lateral movement are permitted. *See* SPINE.

OCCIPITO-AXIAL JOINT A joint formed where the occipital bone of the skull is joined to the axis (the second cervical vertebra) by four ligaments, three of which (the odontoid ligaments) act to limit the extent of rotation of the cranium (skull). *See* SPINE.

OCULAR MOTOR IMPAIRMENT   Difficulties with the motor control in the eye.

O'DONOGHUE'S TRIAD   *See under* KNEE MENISCI.

OEDEMA   *See* EDEMA.

OESTROGENS   *See* ESTROGENS.

OLECRANON   The proximal bony projection of the ulna at the elbow; its anterior surface forms part of the trochlear notch.

OLECRANON APOPHYSITIS   A traction apophysitis at the olecranon. Repetitive microtrauma causes progressive fragmentation, irregular ossification and widening of the physis. It occurs when repetitive stresses are applied to the developing olecranon apophysis through the pull of the triceps muscle. It occurs especially in throwing sports, but also in other sports such as gymnastics. The olecranon apophysis ossifies around the age of 8 years in girls and 10 years in boys, and fuses at ages of 14 years and 16 years, respectively.

OLECRANON BURSITIS   'Student's elbow.' It is inflammation of the subcutaneous bursa overlying the olecranon process. It may be either an acute or chronic injury. **Acute bursitis** usually results from a direct blow to the elbow joint, e.g. a fall. **Chronic bursitis** develops from repeated trauma. Non-traumatic causes of olecranon bursitis are gout and rheumatoid arthritis. Olecranon bursitis may be aseptic or septic. The olecranon bursa does not develop before the age of 7 years. Elbow guards may help prevent olecranon bursitis.

OLECRANON FRACTURES   *See under* ELBOW JOINT COMPLEX, FRACTURES.

OLFACTION   The sense of smell. Smells are sensed by olfactory epithelium located in the nose and processed by the olfactory system.

OLIGOMENORRHEA   *See under* MENSTRUAL CYCLE.

OLIGOSACCHARIDES   *See under* CARBOHYDRATES.

OLYMPIC IDEOLOGY   Originating from the Ancient Greeks, it has generally been assumed that Olympic ideology emphasizes the following: harmonious development of the athlete's physical and intellectual development, health, beauty and all-round athletic competition rather than specialization. Lammer (1992) argues that this assumption is the product of a nineteenth century idealization of Greek antiquity. The elite athlete of the classical period was physically trained for the most part and specialized early in his career. The body was not the goal of his efforts, but rather a means to achieve honor and recognition, thus determining his social prestige and status among his peers. In the *Odyssey*, Homer stated that, "...there is no greater glory for a man while he yet lives than that which he achieves by hand or foot." The noble warrior-athlete would be presented with a crown as a sign of victory. The artists, however, were usually of lower birth and would receive money and material prizes. This shows that the two groups cannot have been fulfilling the same educational ideal with their participation in public competition. There does not seem to have been any athlete from 600 to 400 BC who also gained victory in artistic competition or vice versa.

See also AMATEURISM; CHARACTER BUILDING; COMMERCIALISM; DRUG; GENDER; SOCIOLOGY OF SPORT.

Chronology

•776 BC • Anthropologists and archaeologists believe that Olympic festivals took place long before 776 BC, but this is the first clear record of the Ancient Olympic Games, which subsequently took place at four yearly intervals. Homer claimed that Pelops, the god of affluence, founded the Olympics in 1370 BC. Another theory is that Achilles staged an Olympic Games (c. 1250 BC) in honor of Patroclus, one of his generals, after he had won the Trojan War. There was only one event: the stade race, a sprint of about 180 to 185 meters. During the Ancient Olympics, a truce was declared throughout the Greek world and all wars had to stop. No one was allowed to carry weapons into Olympia.

Women were excluded from the Ancient Olympic Games, but had their own Games every four years in honor of Hera, the wife of Zeus. According to Pausanias, a 2nd century AD Greek traveller, the Heraea Games were administered by a committee of 16 women from the city of Elis and other married women for unmarried (maiden) competitors. The maidens competed in footraces in the Olympic stadium itself, but "the course of the stadium is shortened for them by about one sixth of its length." There were three age groups. The winning maidens received crowns of olive and a portion of a cow sacrificed to Hera. There is some evidence that the Heraean Games predated the Olympic Games.

•576 BC • Until this time, half the Olympic champions were from Sparta. After this date, there were few Spartan victories. In the 7th century BC, Tyraeus voiced the official policy of Sparta when he stated in a poem that excellence in athletics was not to be compared with excellence in military matters. Nevertheless, Sparta had long taken pride in her victories at the Ancient Olympic Games. In Sparta, women received military training, owned property and ran the country when the men were away fighting wars.

•393 AD • Thirteen years after he made Christianity the official faith of the Roman Empire, Emperor Theodosius I issued a decree in Milan that prohibited the Olympic Games. He branded them pagan rituals.

•1850 • Inspired by the Ancient Olympic Games, physician William Penney Brookes founded the Wenlock Olympian Class in order to "promote the moral, physical and intellectual improvement of the inhabitants of the town and neighborhood of Wenlock, and especially of the working classes." Sports ranged from cricket to athletics. Banners with Greek inscriptions were paraded and winners were honoured with laurel branches and medals bearing a representation of Nike - the Greek goddess of victory. In 1860, this organization became known as the Wenlock Olympian Society.

•1881 • William Brooks had begun writing to government officials in Greece in an effort to convince the Greeks to revive the Olympic Games on an international scale.

•1889 • The first International Congress of Physical Education was held in conjunction with the Universal Exposition in Paris - a meeting organized by Baron Pierre de Coubertin, who had been commissioned by the French Government to make a study of modern physical culture methods.

•1890 • Baron Pierre de Coubertin dined with William Brooks at the Gaskell Arms in Much Wenlock. It is said that this is where the modern Olympics were started.

•1893 • Baron Pierre de Coubertin made his second visit to the USA, where he generated interest in his plans for the Olympic Games. He visited the universities of California, Stanford, Tulane and Princeton. At the University Club in New York City, there were representatives of Harvard, Yale, Princeton and Columbia. Coubertin attempted to convince the Americans that the idea of the Olympic Games was not a dream, but was he concerned that the concept of an international Olympic festival was still foreign to their way of thinking.

•1894 • The International Olympic Committee (IOC) was founded by Baron Pierre de Coubertin, with the goal being to contribute to a peaceful future for humankind through the educational value of sport. Olympism is based on the love of athletic training and competition displayed by the pre-Hellenistic Greeks, and that artistic beauty was epitomized in the essential beauty of man's body, mind and spirit. The hope for world peace through international Olympic competition was also central to Olympism.

•1896 • The first modern Olympic Games were held in Athens. It involved about 300 competitors from 13 countries. Only five sports have been on the program of every modern Games: cycling, fencing, gymnastics, swimming and track-and-field athletics. American James Connolly was the first champion. In winning the triple jump, Connolly received a laurel wreath, an olive branch and a certificate.

•1908 • Ethelbert Talbot, of Pennsylvania, an Anglican bishop, addressed athletes of the 4th Modern Olympic Games: "The important thing in these Olympics is not so much winning as taking part, just as the most important thing in life is not the triumph but the struggle. The essential thing is not to have conquered but to have fought well."

•1912 • The modern pentathlon was introduced to the Olympic Games and comprised riding, fencing, shooting, swimming and cross-country running. It was modelled on the ancient Greek pentathlon that had been designed to test the skills of the athlete solider.

•1921 • The motto 'citius, altius, fortius' ('faster, higher, stronger') was adopted as the motto of the modern Olympic movement. It was originally composed by Father Henri Didon of the Catholic Dominican order, a prefect of the Arcueil Parisien College, teacher and friend of Baron Pierre de Coubertin. In 1895, Father Didon stated, "You who wish to surpass yourself, fashion your body and spirit to discover the best of yourself, strive always to go one step further than that you were aiming for: Faster. Higher. Stronger."

•1940 • The Olympic Games were cancelled because of the outbreak of World War II.

Bibliography

Athens Environmental Foundation. Http://www.athensenvironmental.org

Ferenc, T. (1992). Ethos and Olympism: The ethic principles of Olympism. *International Review for the Sociology of Sport* 27(3), 223-234.

Gardiner, E.N. (1910). *Greek athletic sports and festivals*. London: MacMillan & Co.

Lammer, M. (1992). Myth or reality: The classical Olympic athlete. *International Review for the Sociology of Sport* 27(2), 107-118.

OMENTUM A double-layered sheet or fold of peritoneum. The lesser and greater omentum attach the stomach to the body wall or to other abdominal organs. The **greater omentum** is a thin and transparent membranous sac (peritoneum) that houses enlarged adipocytes within its membranous pockets. This is a fat-laden fold of peritoneum that hangs down from the greater curvature of the stomach and connects the stomach with the diaphragm, spleen, and transverse colon. The greater omentum always contains some adipose tissue, but in obese people it accumulates in substantial quantity. The **lesser (smaller) omentum** joins the stomach and the first part of the duodenum with the liver, and also contains adipose tissue. Omental fat can be excessive in persons with diabetes, severe obesity, and in HIV patients who use protease inhibitors. *See under* ABDOMINAL OBESITY.

OMPHALION An anatomical landmark that is the midpoint of the navel (umbilicus).

OPEN-LOOP CONTROL *See under* MOTOR LEARNING.

OPEN WOUNDS Injuries that are exposed to the external environment, e.g. abrasions and lacerations

OPERANT CONDITIONING Instrumental conditioning. It is a type of learning in which the probability of a behavior recurring is increased or decreased by the consequences that follow. Whereas classical conditioning forms an association between two stimuli, operant conditioning forms an association between a behavior and a consequence. A **stimulus** is anything that causes some kind of behavioral response. Behavior may be followed by consequences that increase or decrease the probability of response in that particular situation. Thorndike's (1927) **Law of Effect** is that actions followed by pleasant or rewarding consequences tend to be repeated, whereas actions followed by unpleasant or punishing consequences tend not be repeated.

Operant conditioning is exemplified by the experiments by B.F. Skinner where he trained rats and pigeons to press a lever in order to obtain a food reward. A **reward** is a return for a correct response to a stimulus.

Reinforcement is the key to Skinner's theory. A reinforcer is anything that strengthens the desired response. A **primary reinforcer** is a stimulus, such as food, that is inherently reinforcing and typically satisfies a physiological need. A **secondary reinforcer** is a stimulus that has acquired reinforcing properties through association with other reinforcers. Money and praise are common secondary reinforcers. **Positive reinforcement** is an increase in the frequency of a behavior when followed by an event or stimulus the student finds pleasurable. Although a reward is pleasurable, it does not necessarily increase behavior. **Negative reinforcement** is an increase in the frequency of behavior as a result of removal or avoidance of aversive stimuli (removing or terminating something the person perceives as unpleasant, such as being ignored). Negative reinforcement is when a person exhibits good behavior because they are intimidated or frightened by the consequences. In contrast, positive reinforcement is when people exhibit good behavior because they look forward to the consequences.

Extinction is designed to withhold or cease reinforcement of a previously reinforced response (using either positive or negative reinforcement). It results in the weakening of the frequency of the response. **Shaping** is the consistent reinforcement of successive approximations (small steps) to the target behavior until the target (terminal) behavior is achieved. A **token economy** is a reinforcement system in which tokens (e.g. 'points') are earned when a specific target behavior is achieved. **Differential reinforcement** is reinforcement of behavior by consistently praising correct performance and selectively ignoring errors. **Contingency contracting** is based on the premise that a behavior performed at high frequency can be used to increase one having a low frequency. **Fading** is a procedure that ensures the persistence of desired behaviors after reinforcement is ended, e.g. the gradual removal of the physical guidance as the person learns to perform the skill unassisted. It can be gradual decrease in any reinforcement that is designed to help the student become increasingly independent. **Conditioned reinforcement** is reinforcement that occurs when a previously neutral stimulus that has been paired with a primary reinforcer elicits the same response as the primary reinforcer. **Chaining** is a specialized application of conditioned reinforcement requiring that several behaviors must be completed before a reward is given. In the **total chain**, all behaviors are to be completed at once. In the **forward chain**, behaviors are mastered step-by-step in a forward direction. In a **backward chain**, behaviors are mastered step-by-step in a backward direction. The **Premack Principle** states that any behavior that is independently more probable than some other behavior can be used as a reward to strengthen the lower-probability response, such as the promise of free playtime when structured instruction is completed. **Response cost** is a procedure whereby undesirable behaviors are penalized by taking away a reward object already in the possession of the person. **Superstitious behavior** is an undesired behavior that is unrelated to the desired behavior, but is accidentally reinforced and then becomes fixed in the subject's mind as necessary for reinforcement. (*See also under* RITUALS.)

Punishment is the opposite of both positive and negative reinforcement. It is any unpleasant action that decreases the frequency of a behavior. **Negative punishment** is the removal of a positive stimulus. **Positive punishment** is the addition of an aversive stimulus, something the subject seeks to avoid. Punishment decreases the likelihood of behavior; negative reinforcement (like positive reinforcement) increases the likelihood of a behavior.

Punishment should be an unpleasant experience that is understood to be a direct consequence of the inappropriate behavior. It should not involve physical abuse. Children who are physically or harshly punished by their parents are more likely to be aggressive with others outside of the home. Sometimes punishment is effective, but it is generally a poor way to eliminate unwanted behavior in most situations. Reasons for punishment failing are: people often administer punishment inappropriately or mindlessly; the recipient of punishment often responds with anxiety, fear or rage; the effectiveness of punishment is often temporary, depending heavily on the presence of the punishing person or circumstances; most misbehavior is hard to punish immediately; punishment conveys little information; and an action intended to punish may instead be reinforcing because it brings attention. The Australian Sports Commission states, "Punishment may or may not be an effective deterrent to undesirable behavior, but it does nothing to indicate to young people what alternative behavior is acceptable, nor how they can modify their behavior. The threat of punishment can also increase the amount of pressure under which a young person performs, often leading to a mistake as a result of the fear of the consequences of making an error." Many coaches use running or other forms of physical activity as a punishment. However, athletes should not be taught to associate physical activity with punishment. John Wooden, legendary basketball coach of UCLA, has noted that punishment leads to antagonism and that it should be used rarely. Nonparticipation in competition would probably be a more effective form of punishment for those who have failed to train appropriately. Wooden (1997) states that the worst punishment he could give his basketball team was to deny them the privilege of practicing together.

A good alternative to punishment is extinction of undesired behaviors combined with reinforcement of alternative ones. Another alternative to punishment is the use of a **time-out**, which involves withholding positive reinforcers and removing the individual from a reinforcing environment for a specific period of time. The individual should be made aware of the behaviors that are targeted for decrease and these behaviors should be concretely defined. With children, short periods of time-out are generally more effective than longer periods (as a general guide: 2 to 5 minutes for 2 to 5 year-olds; 5 minutes for 6 to 8 year-olds; 10 minutes for 8 to 10 year-olds; and 10 to 20 minutes for 10 to 14 year-olds). *See* CLASSICAL CONDITIONING; PSYCHOLOGICAL SKILLS TRAINING; COACHING.

Bibliography

Anshel, M.H. (2003). *Sport psychology: From theory to practice*. 4th ed. San Francisco: Benjamin Cummings.

Australian Sports Commission. Junior sport. Factsheet. Http://www.ausport.gov.au

Guidelines for using time out with children and preteens. Http://www.childdevelopmentinfo.com

Hull, C. (1943). *Principles of behavior*. New York: Appleton-

Century-Crofts.

Premack, D. (1962). Reversibility of reinforcement relations. *Science* 36, 255-257.

Skinner, B.F. (1950). Are theories of learning necessary? *Psychological Review* 57(4), 193-216.

Skinner, B.F. (1953). *Science and human behavior*. New York: MacMillan.

Thorndike, E.L. (1927). The law of effect. *American Journal of Psychology* 39, 212-222.

Thorndike, E. (1932). *The fundamentals of learning*. New York: Teachers College Press.

Wade, C. and Tavris, C. (2003). *Psychology*. 7th ed. Upper Saddle River, NJ: Prentice Hall.

Wooden, J.R. with Jamison, S. (1997). *Wooden: A lifetime of observations and reflections on and off the court*. Lincolnwood, IL: Contemporary Books.

OPIATE   i) A sleep-inducing drug. ii) Any narcotic. iii) An opium preparation. iv) Any tranquilizing agent. A **narcotic** is a drug that diminishes the brain's awareness of sensory impulses, especially pain. An **analgesic** is a drug that induces pain relief. An opiate is a drug derived from **opium** (the dried latex from unripe seed heads of the oriental poppy *papaver somniferum*). Opium is a naturally occurring mixture of morphine and codeine. **Morphine** is an exogenous substance that is extracted from opium. **Heroin (diamorphine)** is a synthetic opiate. Morphine and heroin are both prohibited by the World Anti-Doping Agency (WADA).

Chronology

•1993 • The International Olympic Committee (IOC) removed codeine from its narcotic analgesic class of banned substances. Previously, many athletes who tested positive for codeine claimed to be unaware that they had taken the drug.

Bibliography

World Anti-Doping Agency. Http://www.wada-ama.org

OPIOIDS   Opioid peptides. It is a class of endogenously produced compounds that interact with receptors in both the central nervous system and the peripheral nervous system, thus constituting a widespread neuroendocrine system. See ENDORPHINS.

OPPOSITIONAL DEFIANT DISORDER   A recurrent pattern of hostile and disobedient behavior toward authority figures, typically seen in children below the age of 9 or 10 years, which is manifested by at least four of the following behaviors: losing one's temper; arguing with adults; actively defying the requests or rules of adults; deliberately annoying others; blaming others for one's own misbehavior or mistakes; being touchy or easily annoyed by others; being angry and resentful; and being spiteful and vindictive. One of these criteria is met only if the behavior occurs more frequently than is typically observed in individuals of comparable age and developmental level. The disturbance in behavior causes clinically significant impairment in social, academic or occupational functioning. Oppositional defiant behavior must be present for six months or more and the individual should not meet the criteria for a conduct disorder and, if the individual is age 18 years or older, criteria are not met for Antisocial Personality Disorder. In general, the disruptive behaviors associated with oppositional defiant disorder are less serious that those exhibited in conduct disorder.

Before puberty, oppositional defiant disorder occurs more frequently in males than in females; thereafter it affects the sexes equally. The overall prevalence rate ranges from 2 to 16%.

Many authorities consider oppositional defiant disorder to be a less severe type of conduct disorder, rather than a qualitatively different type of disorder. What distinguishes oppositional defiant disorder from other types of conduct disorder is that it does not include more severe antisocial or aggressive acts that violate the law or the rights of others. The majority of children with oppositional defiant disorder do not develop conduct disorder.

Bibliography

American Psychiatric Association. (1994). *Diagnostic and statistical manual of mental disorders*. 4th ed. Washington, DC: American Psychiatric Association.

OPSINIZATION   A process in the immune system that involves coating the membrane of an antigen, making it easier for phagocytes to adhere to and engulf the antigen.

OPTICAL FLOW   *See under* TIMING ACCURACY.

OPTICAL RIGHTING REFLEX   *See under* LABYRINTHINE REFLEX.

OPTIC NERVE The nerve that carries visual signals from the retina to the brain. **Optic nerve atrophy** is damage or degeneration to the optic nerve. Vision loss will be dependent on the amount of damage, but may include blurred vision, poor color and night vision, and light sensitivity. **Optic nerve hypoplasia** is underdevelopment of the optic nerve *in utero*, resulting in a small optic nerve and visual impairment. The degree of visual impairment varies significantly, but there is usually an acuity loss.

ORAL CONTRACEPTIVES Commonly known as 'the pill,' these drugs contain steroid hormones and inhibit ovulation by preventing the normal gonadotropic effects of the hypothalamus. The primary effect is to suppress secretion of luteinizing hormone, and hence ovulation by mimicking the rise in plasma progesterone that occurs in the luteal phase. If ovulation does occur, then oral contraceptives will interfere with implantation and sperm migration, because they promote secretory-phase uterine conditions.

The **combined estrogen and progesterone pill** is more popular than the progesterone-only pill. The normal menstrual cycle ceases and there is no ovulation (except in rare cases when other mechanisms function to prevent pregnancy). The most common system of combined pill is the 21-day system, in which the pill is taken for 21 consecutive days followed by 7 days without. During the 7-day break from taking the pill, 'hormone withdrawal bleeding' will occur, which is usually much lighter than normal periods. The combined pill also thickens the cervical mucus, which acts as a barrier to sperm. The lining of the uterus (womb) is thinner, thus making it less suitable for implantation of a fertilized egg. Common side effects are nausea, headaches, breast tenderness, lethargy, weight gain, higher blood pressure and depression. Many combined preparations use phasic preparations in which the dosage of each hormone varies. There is a stepwise increase in progesterone at each phase change (2 or 3 changes, depending on the type of pill). With combined pills, contraceptive failure may occur with concomitant antibiotic therapy. Spotting and breakthrough bleeding are possible signs of diminished contraceptive effectiveness.

The combined pill containing ethinylestradiol and the selective progestogen, desogestrel, in a phasic regimen (DSG, Tri-merci) has been shown to decrease facial seborrhea (oiliness). The desogestrel (50/100/150 micrograms) and ethinylestradiol (35/30/30 micrograms) were taken for three phases of 7 days, followed by a 7-day pill-free interval, for six cycles. In women with facial seborrhea and mild or moderate acne, the use of desogestrel appears to improve seborrhea after only a single cycle and acne grades after 3 cycles. These improvements are accompanied by increases in self-esteem and self-confidence.

The **progesterone-only pill**, formerly known as the mini-pill, is not as effective as the combined pill. Unlike the combined pill, it does not cause a cessation of ovulation. In some women, it will stop ovulation half of the time. It works mainly by thickening the mucus at the entrance of the uterus (the cervix), thus providing an effective barrier to sperm. Most suitable for women over the age of 30 years and smokers, it must be taken at the same time every day and may cause menstrual irregularities.

Most female athletes use oral contraceptives for contraceptive purposes, but cycle manipulation and control of premenstrual symptoms are secondary advantages of its use. It is possible for athletes to manipulate their menstrual cycles around competitive events. Typically, the oral contraceptives would be taken daily for the first 21 days after completion of menstruation, but not for the next seven days. The resultant decrease in blood estrogen and progesterone levels allows menstruation to occur.

The belief that the pill negatively affects health and athletic performance may be explained by the fact that the first oral contraceptive preparations contained 100 to 175 micrograms of estrogen and 10 mg of progesterone. At this dose, significant adverse effects were seen, including increased risk of venous thromboembolism. However, the modern pill contains only 30 to 50 micrograms of estrogen and 0.3 to 1 mg of progesterone. At this lower dose, many of the concerns about adverse effects have been allayed.

Modern oral contraceptives can decrease the amount of bleeding, risk of iron deficiency and frequency of cramps. Combined pills increase cardiac output more than progesterone-only pills, implying that the estrogen effect dominates. An increased stroke volume may potentially increase oxygen delivery to the tissues and the decrease in menstrual blood loss may also be beneficial for performance. It is thus possible that oral contraceptives may improve athletic performance. The most important variable may simply be the decrease in pain. There is evidence that female soccer players using oral contraceptives suffer less traumatic sports injuries than those not using oral contraceptives. A possible explanation for this finding is that (as a group) females using oral contraceptives have better neuromuscular coordination due to alleviation of certain premenstrual symptoms.

The main side effect of oral contraceptives is increased risk of cardiovascular disease. This risk can be minimized if the pill contains the lowest possible dose of estrogen. Low-dose oral contraceptives (typically less than 35 micrograms of estrogen and less than 1 microgram of progesterone) provide effective fertility control, while minimizing risk of cardiovascular disease.

Oral contraceptives may have negative effects on lipid metabolism, but these are likely to be offset by the positive effects of exercise training. The effects of oral contraceptives on growth hormone, which is also a potent stimulator of lipolysis, depend on the relative concentrations of estrogen and progesterone, which increase and decrease growth hormone levels, respectively. The stimulation of lipolysis in adipose tissue leads to an increase in the availability of free fatty acids in skeletal muscle. The decrease in insulin sensitivity associated with oral contraceptive use decreases both the blood glucose uptake and carbohydrate utilization in skeletal muscle. Mild hyperinsulinemia and decreased insulin sensitivity are still evident with modern oral contraceptives.

Scientific evidence does not support the belief that use of oral contraceptives is associated with weight gain. Overall, the advantages of oral contraceptives for female athletes appear to outweigh potential disadvantages. Nevertheless, there is individual variation in response to oral contraceptives and these should be clinically monitored.

Chronology

•1960 • In the USA, the Food and Drug Administration (FDA) approved the first oral contraceptive. Within 2 years of its initial distribution, 1.2 million American women were using oral contraceptives.

Bibliography

Bemben, D.A. (1993). Metabolic effects of oral contraceptives. Implications for exercise response of premenopausal women. *Sports Medicine* 16(5), 295-304.

Bennell, K., White, S. and Crossley, K. (1999). The oral contraceptive pill: A revolution for sportswomen? *British Journal of Sports Medicine* 33(4), 231-238.

Lebrun, C.M. (1993). Effect of the different phases of the menstrual cycle and oral contraceptives on athletic performance. *Sports Medicine* 16(5), 295-304.

Nielsen, J.M. and Hammar, M. (1991). Sports injuries and oral contraceptive use. Is there a relationship? *Sports Medicine* 12(3), 152-160.

Prilepskaya, V.N. et al. (2003). Effects of phasic oral contraceptive containing desogestrel on facial seborrhea and acne. *Contraception* 68(4), 239-245.

ORAL INJURIES   *See under* TEETH.

ORBITALE   An anatomical landmark that is the lower or most inferior position on the margin of the eye socket.

ORBITAL FRACTURE   *See under* EYE INJURIES.

ORGAN   A member of a system (e.g. nervous system) composed of cells and tissues associated in performing some special function for which it is especially adapted. The organs of the body are composed of four primary tissues: epithelial, connective, muscle and nervous tissue.

ORGANELLE   A membrane-bound structure that forms part of the cytoplasm of a cell and has a specialized function, e.g. a mitochondrion. An organelle in a cell is analogous to an organ in an organism. Examples are lysosomes, mitochondria and plasma membranes. *See also* BACTERIA.

ORGANIC   Pertaining to a chemical compound that contains carbon. Carbohydrates, lipids, proteins and vitamins are all organic. Minerals and water are inorganic because they contain no carbon.

ORIENTING REFLEX Orienting response. It is the response of an animal to an unexpected or novel stimulus or alteration of a stimulus. It involves adjustments of head, body or sensory organs to pay close attention to the stimulus. In higher vertebrates including humans, it is mediated at the brain stem level.

ORIGIN *See under* MUSCLE ATTACHMENTS.

ORLISTAT *See under* OBESITY.

ORNITHINE *See under* GROWTH HORMONE.

OROPHARYNX *See under* PHARYNX.

ORTHOPEDIC IMPAIRMENT As defined by the Federal Register (1999) in the USA, a term that refers to severe orthopedic impairment that adversely affects a child's educational performance. The term includes impairments caused by congenital anomaly (e.g. clubfoot), disease (e.g. poliomyelitis) and other causes (e.g. cerebral palsy).

Orthopedic impairments should be distinguished from physical impairments that are covered solely under Section 504 of the Rehabilitation Act of 1973. Under the Individuals with Disabilities Education Act (IDEA), the orthopedic impairment must adversely affect the student's educational performance. Section 504, however, requires only that the impairment substantially limit one or more of a student's major life activities.

ORTHOSIS The straightening of a deformity.

ORTHOSTASIS Standing upright.

ORTHOSTATIC TOLERANCE The ability to regulate blood pressure while upright. The gravitational stress of sudden standing normally causes pooling of blood in the venous capacitance vessels of the legs and trunks. The subsequent, transient decrease in venous return and cardiac output results in decreased blood pressure (hypotension). Baroreceptors in the aortic arch and carotid bodies activate autonomic reflexes that rapidly normalize blood pressure by causing a transient tachycardia.

Orthostatic intolerance encompasses disorders of blood flow, heart rate and blood pressure regulation that are most easily demonstrable during orthostatic stress, yet are present in all postures. A distinction can be made between acute and chronic orthostatic intolerance. **Acute orthostatic intolerance** usually manifests as presyncope or syncope. Presyncopal patients remain conscious during their transient loss of postural tone. These conditions are caused by cerebral malperfusion, usually resulting from a large and abrupt fall in blood pressure. Vasovagal syncope (classic simple faint) is an instance of acute orthostatic intolerance. The most popular theory of vasovagal syncope attributes fainting to a stretch reflex of the left ventricle. This reflex is presumably activated when decreased venous return underfills the left ventricle. Other theories of fainting include epinephrine or renin surges and vasopressin decreases. With **chronic orthostatic intolerance**, there is a high incidence of blurred vision, fatigue, nausea, neurocognitive deficits, sleep problems, heat and palpitations.

Patients with **true orthostatic hypotension** are defined by the American Autonomic Society as those with a persistent fall in systolic/diastolic blood pressure of more than 20/10 mm Hg within 3 minutes of assuming the upright position. Orthostatic hypotension is accentuated in the early morning due to overnight natriuresis and may also be more prominent after eating a meal and after exercise. Blood pressure falls during exercise, even though the effect of gravity is eliminated when the patient is recumbent. This is due to a lack of vasoconstriction, which normally occurs in other vascular beds during exercise that compensate for the vasodilation in exercising muscles. In the elderly, decreased baroreceptor responsiveness, coupled with decreased arterial compliance, accounts for frequent orthostatic hypotension.

Hypovolemia, often induced by abuse of diuretics, is the most common cause of symptomatic orthostatic hypotension. Cardiac causes of sudden-onset postural hypotension include cardiac arrhythmia. Orthostatic hypotension is more frequent in diabetic than nondiabetic patients treated with anti-hypertensive drugs. Acute or subacute severe hypovolemia caused by disease may produce ortho-static hypotension due to a decrease in cardiac output, despite intact autonomic reflexes. Hypokalemia impairs the reactivity of vascular smooth muscle and may limit the increases in peripheral vascular resistance on standing. The adrenocortical hypofunction of Addison's disease may lead to hypovolemic orthostatic hypotension in the absence of adequate salt intake. Shy-Drager syndrome and idiopathic orthostatic hypotension are two, possibly related, primary neuropathic disorders commonly associated with severe orthostatic hypotension. In patients with Shy-Drager syndrome, plasma norepinephrine does not increase on stand-ing; in those with idiopathic orthostatic hypotension, norepinephrine appears to be depleted from the sympathetic nerve endings.

Humans counteract orthostatic tolerance by the muscle pump, neurovascular compensation and neu-rohumoral effects. The muscle pump is the primary defense against pooling. It is partially neutralized during quiet standing and is nearly inconsequential while standing without motion. Weakened muscle pump ability is a key reason that astronauts are so vulnerable to orthostatic stress. During exposure to low gravity, astronauts develop rapid leg muscle atrophy and refractory lower limb pooling.

Neurovascular compensation is the second line of defense against orthostatic intolerance. Rapid changes in arterial resistance vessel tone (vasoconstriction) limit flow to the extremities and to the sphlanchnic vascular bed, while promoting passive emptying. Arterial resistance increases because of vasoconstric-tion. Limb venoconstriction is not an important aspect of the orthostatic response, but veins and venules do contribute to the regulation of venous return to the heart by passive elastic properties.

Neurohumoral effects provide the third line of defense. Once upright posture has been established, secretion of epinephrine and vasopressin as well as the activation of the renin-angiotensin-aldosterone system cause sodium and water retention, as well as expansion of the circulating blood volume.

Endurance training decreases orthostatic toler-ance, possibly because of a decreased capacity for reflex vasoconstriction or because increased total blood volume may attenuate mechanoreceptor responsiveness. Whole body resistance training increases orthostatic tolerance, possibly mediated by alterations in vascular compliance.

Fighter pilots become exposed to negative pres-sure in the lower body during aerial maneuvers that increase the gravitational forces on the body. To decrease the risk of syncope, pilots wear a 'g-suit,' with bladders that inflate around the legs and waist to assist in pumping blood to the heart. Pilots also utilize breathing techniques that invoke the Valsalva maneuver to improve venous return. The higher a pilot's 'g-tolerance,' the more extreme are the air-craft maneuvers that can be performed.

Orthostatic tolerance is compromised after space flight and this can severely inhibit the functional cerebral capacity of astronauts during re entry and landing.

See BED REST; MICROGRAVITY.

Bibliography
Lightfoot, J.T. et al. (1994). Resistance training increases lower body negative pressure tolerance. *Medicine and Science in Sports and Exercise* 26(8), 1003-1011.

Stewart, J.M. (2003). Orthostatic intolerance: An overview. Http://www.emedicine.com

ORTHOTIC SHOE INSERTS *See under* FOOT PRONATION.

ORYZANOLES   Plant sterols isolated from the processing of rice brain oil that occur as esters of ferulic acid. Oryzanoles and ferulic acid function as antioxidants, but have been promoted by sellers of dietary supplements as growth-hormone releasers. There is no scientific evidence of any anabolic effects. Animal research has shown that it may actually create a catabolic or anti-anabolic state.

Bibliography
Wheeler, K.B. and Garleb, K.A. (1991). Gamma oryzanol-plant sterol supplementation: Metabolic, endocrine, and physiolog-ic effects. *International Journal of Sport Nutrition* 1(2): 170-7.

OSGOOD-SCHLATTER'S DISEASE   A traction apophysitis of the tibial tuberosity. It is a mechanical disorder involving microavulsion of the patellar tendon at the anterior portion of the developing ossification center of the tibial tuberosity, due to repeated traction injuries. It is the most common apophyseal overuse injury, and it primarily affects boys of age 10 to 16 years. Most cases occur in association with rapid growth when bone is growing fast and muscles become tight. It occurs in kicking sports, mountain biking and deceleration sports such as squash. It is almost always a self-limiting condition, with symptoms abating upon maturity of the tibial tubercle apophysis.

OS MAGNUM *See* CAPITATE BONE.

OSMOLALITY The concentration of particles in solution. To express the concentration of a solution in terms of particles, the unit called the osmole is used in place of the gram. 1 **osmole** is 1 g molecular weight of undissociated solute, i.e. it is 1 mole (6.02×10^{23}) of solute particles. 1 g molecular weight of glucose (i.e. 180 g) is equal to 1 osmole of glucose, because glucose does not dissociate into ions. A solution containing 1 mole of glucose in each liter has a concentration of 1 osmole per liter. If a solute dissociates into 2 ions, 1 g molecular weight of the solute equals 2 osmoles, because the number of osmotically active particles is twice as great as in the case of the undissociated solute. 1 g molecular weight of sodium chloride, for example, is equal to 58.8 g or 2 osmoles. A solution that has 1 osmole of solute dissolved in each kilogram of water is said to have an osmolality of 1 osmole per kilogram.

Osmosis is the transport of a solvent, through a selectively permeable membrane (such as a cell membrane) that separates two solutions of different solute concentration, from the solution that is dilute in solute to the solution that is concentrated. Osmosis is a spontaneous process, so it must be the result of a downhill energy system. This energy system is water potential. When there is a net movement of water across the cell membrane, the cell will either swell or shrink depending on the direction of the net movement. Selectively permeable membranes surround all cells. They are permeable to water, but not larger molecules such as proteins.

Osmosis distributes water throughout the fluid containing intracellular, extracellular and plasma components of the body. The major absorption of ingested water and water contained in foods occurs by osmosis in the small intestine.

Osmotic pressure (**osmotic gradient**) is the physical pressure on one side of a membrane required to compress a fluid and to prevent the osmotic movement of water from the other side. The physical pressure involved is the sum of all the forces of the different molecules striking a unit surface area at a given instant.

The normal osmolality of the extra-cellular fluid and intra-cellular fluid is about 300 milliosomoles per kilogram of water. At normal body temperature, 37 degrees Celsius, a concentration of 1 osmole per liter will cause 19,300 mm Hg osmotic pressure in the solution. The 300 milliosmolar concentration of the body fluids gives a total calculated osmotic pressure of the body fluids of 5,790 mm Hg. The measured value for this, however, averages only about 5,500 mm Hg, because many of the ions in the body fluids, such as sodium and chloride ions, are highly attracted to one another; consequently, they cannot move entirely unrestrained in the fluids and create their full osmotic potential.

It is difficult to measure kilograms of water in a solution, which is required to determine 'osmolality.' Therefore physiologists usually use '**osmolarity**,' which is the osmolar concentration expressed as osmoles per liter of solution rather than per kilogram of water (osmolality). Strictly speaking, it is osmoles per kilogram of water (osmolality) that determine osmotic pressure. For dilute solutions, such as those in the body, however, the quantitative difference between osmolarity and osmolality is less than 1%.

If a cell is placed in a solution of impermeant solutes having an osmolarity of 282 mOsm/l, the cells will not shrink, because the water concentrations in the intra-cellular fluid and extra-cellular fluid are equal and the solutes cannot enter or leave the cell. Such a solution is said to be **isotonic**, because it neither shrinks nor swells the cells. An isotonic solution has the same solute concentration as that found in the intracellular and extracellular fluid.

The osmolality of an isotonic enteral product is about 300 mOsm/kg. Examples of isotonic solutions are a 0.9% solution of sodium chloride or a 5% solution of glucose. If a cell is placed into a **hypotonic** solution that has a lower concentration of impermeant solutes (less than 282 mOsm/l), water will diffuse into the cell, causing it to swell. Water will continue to diffuse into the cell, diluting the intracellular fluid while also concentrating the extracellular fluid until both solutions have about the same osmolarity. If a cell is placed in a **hypertonic** solution having a higher concentration of impermeant solutes (greater than 282 mOsm/l), water will flow out of the cell into the extra-cellular fluid, concentrating the intra-cellular fluid and diluting the extra-cellular fluid. The cell will shrink until the two concentrations become equal.

Bibliography

Guyton, A.C. and Hall, J.E. (2000). *Textbook of medical physiology*. 10th ed. Philadelphia, PA. W.B. Saunders Co.

OSMOMETER A device for measuring molecular weights by measuring the osmotic pressure exerted by solvent molecules diffusing through a semi-permeable membrane.

OSMORECEPTOR A cell that can generate an action potential in response to changes in the blood's osmolality.

OSMOSIS *See under* OSMOLALITY.

OSMOTIC POTENTIAL A component of water potential; it is a measure of the effect of solute particles on a substance's ability to absorb or release water.

OSMOTIC PRESSURE *See under* OSMOLALITY.

OSSICLES Sesamoid bones and accessory bones. **Sesamoid bones** are small bones that develop inside a tendon where the tendon passes over a bony prominence, such as the two sesamoid bones of the 1st metatarsophalangeal joints. The other metatarsophalanageal joints occasionally have sesamoid bones. Sesamoid bones are also found in other locations of the body, such as the *peroneus longus* tendon. The sesamoids are important for bearing weight, protecting tendons and decreasing friction. **Sesamoiditis** is an acute or chronic inflammation of the sesamoids. Weight-bearing activities, climbing stairs or wearing high-heeled shoes will aggravate sesamoiditis. A fracture of the sesamoid can occur from an axial load such as a fall, or it can manifest as a stress fracture with an insidious onset. Fracture most commonly involves the medial sesamoid.

Accessory bones are formed when complete ossification does not occur and the secondary center of ossification remains separate from the rest of the bone. An example is the *os trigonum* that arises as a secondary ossification center in the posterior process of the talus. About 50% of individuals have an *os trigonum*, which is known as the trigonal (Stieda's) process when it is fused to the talus. In either case, its inferior surface typically articulates with the calcaneus.

See also FABELLA.

OSSIFICATION The primary center of ossification is an area of hyaline cartilage in the center of the shaft of a long bone where ossification typically begins. As bone increases in size, the primary center of ossification expands toward the ends of bone as adjacent cartilage regions become osteogenic. The epiphysis at each end continue interstitial production of cartilage, but the epiphyseal regions do not expand because cartilage is replaced on the diaphyseal side by bone at the same rate as it is produced. The epiphyseal plate extends horizontally across bone and is the region where cartilage replacement during expansion occurs. The secondary center of ossification develops, about the time of birth, in the epiphyses of long bones. The cartilage between the primary and secondary ossification centers is called the epiphyseal plate. The point of union of the primary and secondary ossification centers is called the **epiphyseal line**.

OSTEITIS PUBIS A self-limiting osteonecrosis of the pubis and synchondrosis. It occurs commonly from repetitive shear stress across the pubic symphysis in running, jumping and kicking. It is thought that the pathogenesis includes subacute periostitis. Inflammation is not a histological finding. It is associated with sports hernia.

OSTEOARTHRITIS *See under* ARTHRITIS.

OSTEOBLASTS *See under* BONE.

OSTEOCHONDRAL FRACTURE *See under* FRACTURE.

OSTEOCHONDRAL INJURIES *See* KNEE, OSTEOCHONDRAL INJURIES.

OSTEOCHONDRITIS Inflammation of bone and cartilage.

OSTEOCHONDRITIS DISSECANS A disease process that causes subchondral bone to lose its blood supply as a result of a form of osteonecrosis. Subsequently, the overlying articular cartilage becomes damaged secondary to loss of support from the avascular subchondral bone. Articular cartilage and fragments of the subchondral bone may become detached and form a loose body in the joint. Possible causes are ischemia, abnormal ossification in the epiphysis, genetic abnormalities and trauma.

In the knee, osteochondritis dissecans is mainly found on the posterolateral aspect of the medial femoral condyle. It is common in the 12 to 16 years age group, and is generally thought to be the result of cumulative stress to the subchondral bone, resulting in subchondral stress fractures. In throwing athletes, osteochondritis dissecans is the most common cause of irreversible elbow damage. It is thought that spontaneous necrosis and fragmentation of the capitellar ossific nucleus results from compression forces at the radio-capitellar joint. It tends to occur in 10 to 16 year olds.

OSTEOCHONDROSES Epiphyseal growth plate disorders. *See* BLOUNT'S DISEASE; FRIEBERG'S DISEASE; KIENBÖCK'S DISEASE; KOHLER'S DISEASE; OSGOOD-SCHLATTER'S DISEASE; OSTEOCHONDRITIS DISSECANS; PANNER'S DISEASE; PERTHES' DISEASE; SCHEURMANN'S DISEASE; SINDING-LARSEN-JOHANSSON'S DISEASE.

OSTEOCHONDROSIS DEFORMANS TIBIAE *See* BLOUNT'S DISEASE.

OSTEOCLASTS Cells responsible for bone destruction by resorbing the calcium from bone.

OSTEOGENESIS IMPERFECTA FOUNDATION A group of hereditary disorders, characterized by fragile bones and multiple fractures at birth or during childhood. A person may have just a few or as many as several hundred fractures in a lifetime. Fractures peak between 2 and 15 years of age, after which the incidence of fractures decreases. Most cases of osteogenesis imperfecta inherited as an autosomal dominant trait. The genetic defect affects the quantity or quality of the body's production of collagen. In the USA, there are between 20,000 and 50,000 persons with osteogenesis imperfecta.

There are four recognized types of osteogenesis imperfecta. Type I is the most common and mildest type of osteogenesis imperfecta. Type II is the most severe form and is frequently lethal at or shortly after birth. In Type III, there are often fractures present at birth and X-rays may reveal healed fractures that occurred before birth. Type IV is between Type I and Type III in severity.

Indicators of osteogenesis imperfecta are short stature and small limbs that are bowed in various distortions from repetitive fractures. Joints are hyperextensible, with predisposition for dislocation. Chest defects (barrel and pigeon shapes) limit respiratory capacity and aerobic endurance, and spinal defects are common. These are partly from osteoporosis caused by lack of exercise. Most persons with osteogenesis imperfecta use wheelchairs. However, one person with severe osteogenesis imperfecta may use a walker, while another person may use a wheelchair.

There is no cure for it, so treatment is aimed at preventing or controlling symptoms, maximizing independent mobility, and developing optimal bone mass and muscle strength. **Rodding** is a surgical procedure in which a metal rod is implanted within a bone (usually the long bones of the thigh and leg). This is done when bowing or repeated fractures of these bones has interfered with a child's ability to being to walk. Despite numerous fractures, restricted activity and short stature, most children and adults with osteogenesis imperfecta lead productive and successful lives. Exercise, especially aquatics, is recommended for people with osteogenesis imperfecta because it promotes strength of muscle and bone, which can help prevent fractures.

See also EHLERS-DANLOS SYNDROME.

Bibliography

Osteogenesis Foundation. Http://oif.org

Osteoporosis and Related Bone Diseases National Resource Center. Http://www.osteo.org

Sherill, C. (1998). *Adapted physical activity, recreation and sport. Cross disciplinary and lifespan.* 5th ed. Boston, MA: McGraw-Hill.

Winnick, J.P. (2000, ed). *Adapted physical education and sport.* 3rd ed. Champaign, IL: Human Kinetics.

OSTEOGENIC   Bone forming.

OSTEOLYSIS   Bone resorption.

OSTEONECROSIS   Avascular necrosis in bone. Death of bone cells resulting from a cessation of blood flow necessary for normal cellular function. *See* OSTEOCHONDRITIS DISSECANS.

OSTEOPENIA   *See under* OSTEOPOROSIS.

OSTEOPOROSIS   A metabolic disease characterized by a decrease in the total amount of bone and microarchitectural deterioration of bone tissue. The decrease in bone mass is due to excessive resorption of bone, rather than decreased bone synthesis. It mostly affects trabecular bone and the endosteal surface of cortical bone. Dual-energy x-ray absorptiometry (DEXA) is an accepted clinical tool for assessing bone disorders such as osteoporosis. It uses low energy x-ray to measure the quantity of bone. Osteoporosis is estimated to cause 1.5 million fractures per annum in the USA, in people of 50 years and older.

Primary osteoporosis may occur in two types:

Type I osteoporosis (post-menopausal), which is the accelerated decrease in bone mass that occurs when estrogen levels fall after menopause; and **Type II osteoporosis (age-related)**, which is the inevitable loss of bone with age that occurs in both men and women. **Secondary osteoporosis** may develop at any age as a consequence of hormonal, digestive and metabolic disorders, as well as prolonged bed rest and weightlessness (space flight) that result in loss of bone mineral mass.

Osteopenia is a condition of decreased bone mineralization. It occurs when the formation of bone (osteod synthesis) is insufficient to offset normal bone loss (bone lysis). It is generally considered to be the first step in the development of osteoporosis. The World Health Organization (WHO) recognizes osteopenia, for people 50 years and older with lower than average bone density who do not have osteoporosis. WHO defines osteopenia as a bone density between one standard deviation (SD) and 2.5 SD below the mean bone density of a normal young adult. Osteoporosis is defined as 2.5 SD or more below that reference point. With athletes, these results should be interpreted carefully, because young athletes have not reached their peak bone density, and standards for bone mineral density are not well established for women younger than 30 years. Osteopenia is a risk factor for injuries to the spine, such as a burst fracture in which a vertebral body is crushed in all directions.

Osteoporosis is associated with a greater risk of fractures, vertebral instability and abnormal spinal curvature. It is more common in females. Risk factors for osteoporosis in female athletes include low levels of estrogens, delayed puberty, amenorrhea, low use of oral contraceptives, anovulation (absence of ovulation) or a short luteal phase, low androgen levels, high cortisol levels, low bodyweight, low percentage body fat, eating disorders, low energy intake, low calcium intake, high protein intake, high fiber intake, family history of osteoporosis and lack of mechanical load on the bones.

The decreased bone mass in amenorrheic athletes can reflect both inadequate acquisition of peak bone mass during adolescence and excessive bone loss in later years. Physically active individuals generally have greater bone mass than more sedentary individuals. Resistance training may have a more profound site-specific effect than aerobic exercise. There is currently no evidence that exercise alone, or exercise and calcium supplementation, can prevent the rapid decrease in bone mass in the immediate post-menopausal years.

A position stand by the American College of Sports Medicine states: i) weight-bearing exercise is essential for the normal development and maintenance of a healthy skeleton, and activities that focus on increasing muscle strength may also be beneficial, particularly for non-weight bearing bones; ii) sedentary women may increase bone mass slightly by becoming more active but the primary benefit may be in avoiding the further loss of bone that occurs with inactivity; iii) exercise cannot be recommended as a substitute for hormone replacement therapy at the time of menopause; and iv) the optimal program for older women would include activities that improve strength, flexibility and coordination that may indirectly, but effectively, decrease the incidence of osteoporotic fractures by lessening the likelihood of falling.

Ideal treatment for osteoporosis consists of decreasing training volume, increasing body weight and maintaining adequate energy intake to re-establish normal menses (Harmon, 2002). The next best option is hormone replacement therapy. Low-dose contraceptives contain 8 times the estrogen (0.020 mg ethinyl estradiol) necessary to preserve bone mass. **Biphosphonates** (such as alendronate sodium and risedronate sodium) significantly increase bone density and subsequently decrease fracture rates in postmenopausal women. Biphosphonates are not recommended for premenopausal women, because research on rats has shown that pregnancies were adversely affected.

Bibliography

American College of Sports Medicine (1995). Position stand on osteoporosis and exercise. *Medicine and Science in Sports and Exercise* 27(4), i-vii.

Ernst, E. (1994). Can exercise prevent post menopausal osteoporosis? *British Journal of Sports Medicine* 28(1), 5-6.

Ernst, E. (1998). Exercise for female osteoporosis. A systematic review of randomised clinical trials. *Sports Medicine* 25(6), 359-368.

Harmon, K.G. (2002). Evaluating and treating exercise-related menstrual irregularities. *The Physician and Sportsmedicine* 30(3), 29-35.

Khan, K. et al. (2001, eds). *Physical activity and bone health.* Champaign, IL: Human Kinetics.

Layne, J.E. and Nelson, M.E. (1999). The effects of progressive resistance training on bone density: A review. *Medicine and Science in Sports and Exercise* 31(1), 25-30.

Munnings, F. (1992). Osteoporosis: What is the role of exercise? *The Physician and Sportsmedicine* 20(6), 127-138.

Otis, C.L. and Lynch, L. (1994). How to keep your bones healthy. *The Physician and Sportsmedicine* 22(1), 71-72.

OSTEOTOMY   A surgical procedure that involves cutting a bone, using an instrument such as a saw.

OS TRIGONUM   *See under* OSSICLES.

OTHER HEALTH IMPAIRMENTS   As defined by the federal government in the USA, a term that refers to a person having limited strength, vitality or alertness to environmental stimuli that results in limited alertness with respect to the educational environment, that is due to chronic or acute health problems such as asthma, attention-deficit hyperactivity disorder, diabetes, epilepsy, a heart condition, hemophilia, lead poisoning, leukemia, nephritis, rheumatic fever or sickle cell anemia; and adversely affects a child's educational performance.

OTITIS EXTERNA   *See* SWIMMER'S EAR.

OTITIS MEDIA   Inflammation of the middle ear. It accounts for more conductive disorders than any other condition. It prevents the Eustachian tubes from ventilating and keeping dry the middle ear cavity, and from equalizing air pressure on the two sides of the eardrum. It may occur secondary to upper respiratory tract infection. When Eustachian tubes are clogged, activities that involve changes in altitude and pressure, such as flying or diving, should be avoided.

OVERFLOW   i) A term used to describe the persistence of a training response from a specific type of training to an additional parameter or variable that was not trained or specifically emphasized. ii) The inability to move one part of the body without associated movements of other parts. It is a common indicator of clumsiness. Examples of overflow are facial grimaces when concentrating on a hand-eye or hand-foot motor task, and an increase in muscle tone or a mirroring action on the noninvolved side when trying to perform one-arm or one-leg movements. Overflow may be caused by poorly integrated reflexes, and can be considered to be remnants of the mass flexor and extensor patterns present at birth, when body parts cannot move independently of one another. Overflow is normal in early childhood, diminishes by ages 6 to 8 years, and generally disappears by adolescence. *See under* MOTOR DEVELOPMENT.

OVERLOAD   *See under* TRAINING.

OVERTRAINING   Imbalance between training and recovery. It appears to be caused by too much high-intensity training and/or too little recovery time. Overtraining indicates that an individual has been subjected to training and extraneous stressors to the extent that he cannot perform at an optimal level following an appropriate regeneration period. **Overreaching** follows the induction of short-term overtraining. The symptoms of overreaching can be reversed by a longer-than-normal regeneration period. **Chronic overtraining (overtraining syndrome; staleness)** is a dysfunction of the neuroendocrine system, localized at the hypothalamic level. It is characterized by fatigue, poor performance, a weakening of immunity and depression. Unlike overreaching, which is reversible within days to weeks, complete recovery from chronic overtraining may take weeks to months. A distinction can be made between staleness and burnout. Loss of motivation is the central feature of burnout, but stale athletes are often found to be highly motivated.

Signs and symptoms of overtraining include: apathy; lethargy; sleep disturbance; lowered self-esteem; mood changes; feelings of depression; difficulty in concentrating; fear of competition; decreased performance; lack of desire to train; inability to meet previously attained performance; chronic fatigue; increased heart rate and rating of perceived exertion (RPE) at set workload, decreased

strength; decreased tolerance of pain during training; prolonged recovery following training; immune suppression with increased rates of infection; decreased muscle glycogen; decreased body iron stores; increased cortisol; decreased testosterone; loss of appetite and decreased body weight; amenorrhea or oligomenorrhea; and gastrointestinal disturbances.

Overtraining appears as a disturbance of either the sympathetic or parasympathetic nervous system. It has been proposed that **parasympathetic overtraining** may be a reflection of an advanced state of overtraining closely associated with exhaustion of the neuroendocrine system, while **sympathetic overtraining** may reflect a prolonged stress response preceding exhaustion. Alternatively, sympathetic overtraining may predominantly affect speed and power athletes, while endurance athletes are more prone to parasympathetic overtraining. There is evidence that overtraining may be associated with Addison's disease. Parasympathetic overtraining is characterized by diminished maximal secretion of catecholamines, combined with an impaired full mobilization of the lactic acid system.

Both high-intensity aerobic exercise and heavy resistance exercise are associated with significant increases in cortisol. Cortisol induces the breakdown of cellular proteins, thereby liberating amino acids for gluconeogenesis. It also increases levels of proteolytic enzymes (enzymes that break down proteins) and inhibits protein synthesis. It has a greater catabolic effect in fast-twitch than slow-twitch muscle fibers. In muscle, the catabolic effects of cortisol are countered by the anabolic effects of testosterone and insulin. If a greater number of receptors are bound with insulin, or if testosterone blocks the genetic element in the DNA for cortisol, protein is conserved or increased. If a greater number of receptors are bound to cortisol, then protein is degraded and lost. It has been postulated that elevated resting serum cortisol and/or diminished testosterone-to-cortisol ratios are indicative of not only the anabolic/catabolic balance, but also overtraining. It seems more likely, however, that the testosterone-to-cortisol ratio indicates the actual physiological strain in training, rather than overtraining syndrome.

Bibliography

Deschenes, M.R. et al (1991). Exercise induced hormonal changes and their effects upon skeletal muscle. *Sports Medicine* 12(2), 80-93.

Fry, R.W., Norton, A.R. and Keast, D. (1991). Overtraining in athletes. An update. *Sports Medicine* 12(1), 32-65.

Kellman, M. (2002, ed). *Enhancing recovery. Preventing underperformance in athletes*. Champaign, IL: Human Kinetics.

Kellman, M. and Kallus, K.W. (2001). *Recovery-stress questionnaire for athletes*. Champaign, IL: Human Kinetics.

Kibler, W.B., Chandler, T.J. and Stracener, E.S. (1992). Musculoskeletal adaptations and injuries due to overtraining. *Exercise and Sport Sciences Reviews* 20, 99-126.

Kreider, R.B., Fry, A.C. and O'Toole, M.L. (1998, eds). *Overtraining in sport*. Champaign, IL: Human Kinetics.

Kuipers, H. and Keizer, H.A. (1988). Overtraining in elite athletes. *Sports Medicine* 6, 79-92.

Lehman, M. et al (1993). Overtraining in endurance athletes: A brief review. *Medicine and Science in Sports and Exercise* 25(7), 854-862.

Noakes, T. (1989). *Lore of running*. 3rd ed. Champaign, IL: Leisure Press.

Urhausen, A., Gabriel, H. and Kindermann, W. (1995). Blood hormones as markers of training stress and overtraining. *Sports Medicine* 20(4), 251-276.

Urhausen, A. and Kindermann, W. (2002). Diagnosis of overtraining: What tools do we have? *Sports Medicine* 32(2), 95-102.

OVERUSE INJURIES   Injuries that occur from repetitive loading rather than traumatic loading. **Traumatic loading** is the application of a single force of sufficient magnitude to cause injury to a biological tissue. **Repetitive loading** is the repeated application of a non-traumatic load that is usually of relatively low magnitude.

Tissue overuse injury occurs when loss of tissue homeostasis and degeneration results in loss of cell matrix integrity. This may be either symptomatic or asymptomatic. **Clinical sports overuse injury** occurs when tissue damage, resulting from an overuse or abusive exercise pattern, becomes symptomatic to the athlete or produces loss of function. Intrinsic factors relating to overuse injuries in sport include misalignments, leg length discrepancy, muscular imbalance and muscular insufficiency. Extrinsic factors include training errors, surfaces, environmental conditions and footwear. Overuse injuries are classified as follows: pain after the activity only (Grade I); pain after the activity that does not restrict, but may affect performance (Grade II); pain with activity that restricts and moderately-to-severely affects performance (Grade III); and pain occurring with activity and at rest (Grade IV). *See also under* TENDON.

Bibliography

Krivickas, L.S. (1997). Anatomical factors associated with overuse sports injuries. *Sports Medicine* 24(2), 132-146.

Renstrom, P. and Johnson, R.J. (1985). Overuse injuries in sport. A Review. *Sports Medicine* 2, 316-333.

OXALOACETATE   *See under* KREBS CYCLE.

OXIDASE   A type of dehydrogenase enzyme, which catalyses the oxidation of a substrate by removal of hydrogen, which combines with molecular oxygen.

OXIDATION   *See under* REDOX REACTIONS.

OXIDATIVE DEAMINATION   *See under* AMINO ACID DEGRADATION.

OXIDATIVE PHOSPHORYLATION   *See under* AEROBIC ENERGY SYSTEMS; PHOSPHORYLATION.

OXIDATIVE STRESS   *See under* FREE RADICALS.

OXIDOREDUCTASES   *See under* ENZYME.

OXYGEN   A gaseous element that is essential for the support of life. With the normal oxygen content of air (20.93%) and at a sea-level atmospheric pressure of 760 mm Hg, partial pressure of oxygen is 20.93 multiplied by 760. This equals 159 mm Hg.

The partial pressure of oxygen in inspired air is lowered by water vapor in the respiratory passages. There is a further decrease in the partial pressure of oxygen when the inspired air mixes with the expiratory reserve volume, residual volume and air in the anatomic dead space. As a result, alveolar partial pressure of oxygen (103 mm Hg) is considerably lower than ambient partial pressure of oxygen. Partial pressure of oxygen in the pulmonary arteries and systemic veins is greater than in the pulmonary veins and systemic arteries. Expired air has a greater partial pressure of oxygen than alveolar air, because of the mixing of alveolar air with dead space air during expiration. Changes in partial pressure of oxygen from rest to maximal exercise are gradual and related to the intensity of the exercise.

Oxygen is carried in the blood to the tissues chemically bound to hemoglobin. About 98.5% of the total oxygen in the arterial blood is carried in this way. The remainder is physically dissolved and carried in the blood plasma.

Partial pressure of oxygen is decreased with increasing altitude. When the oxygen concentration in the alveoli becomes too low for oxygen to be adequately supplied to the hemoglobin, as can occur at high altitude, chemoreceptors found in the aortic and carotid bodies are stimulated to transmit impulses along the vagus and glossopharyngeal nerves to the medulla of the brain. This causes the respiratory center in the brain to increase alveolar ventilation. A similar process takes place when alveolar oxygen content increases above normal.

The ability of the pulmonary system to maintain arterial oxygen pressure is very rarely a threat to oxygen transport during prolonged heavy exercise in healthy persons at sea level.

See also ALVEOLAR-ARTERIAL PARTIAL PRESSURE OF OXYGEN DIFFERENCE; ARTERIAL-MIXED VENOUS OXYGEN CONTENT DIFFERENCE; END-TIDAL PARTIAL PRESSURE OF OXYGEN; RESPIRATORY CONTROL.

Bibliography

Dempsey, J.A. and Manohar, M. (1992). The pulmonary system and endurance. In: Shephard, R.J. and Astrand, P.O. (eds). *Endurance in sport*. pp61-71. Oxford: Blackwell Scientific Publications.

Powers, S.K. and Beadle, R.E. (1985). Control of ventilation during submaximal exercise: A brief review. *Journal of Sports Sciences* 3, 51-65.

OXYGEN CONSUMPTION

The amount of oxygen utilized by the body's metabolic processes in a given period of time. It is measured using calorimetry. The processes involved in oxygen consumption are oxidation and phosphorylation. The two processes are usually linked in that oxidation provides the energy for phosphorylation. *See also* OXYGEN UPTAKE.

OXYGEN DEBT

The original 'oxygen debt' concept was that the lactic acid produced in contracting muscle, as a result of insufficient oxygen supply during exercise, was converted back to glycogen by the 'Cori cycle' in the liver during recovery. Although a large amount of lactate may be oxidized after exercise, lactic acid cannot be said to cause the oxygen debt, because oxidation of lactic acid does not lead to additional oxygen consumption. In fact, lactate is converted to pyruvate, which in effect substitutes for pyruvate that would otherwise have been supplied by glucose or glycogen. The total oxygen debt is the total amount of oxygen consumed during recovery, and is now more commonly known as **post-exercise oxygen consumption**. It has a rapid and a prolonged component. Some of the mechanisms underlying the rapid component of post-exercise oxygen consumption are well known, e.g. replenishment of oxygen stores, resynthesis of creatine phosphate, lactate removal; and increased body temperature, circulation and ventilation. Elevated temperatures of the magnitude experienced in heavy exercise have the effect of loosening the coupling or linkage between oxidation and phosphorylation. Less is known about the mechanisms underlying the prolonged component of post-exercise oxygen consumption. A sustained increased circulation, ventilation and body temperature may contribute, but the cost of this is low. An increased rate of triglyceride / fatty acid cycling and a shift from carbohydrate to fat as substrate source are of importance for the prolonged component after exhaustive aerobic exercise. There seems to be an absence of sustained post-exercise oxygen consumption when the intensity or duration of exercise is low. A more prolonged and substantial post-exercise oxygen consumption has been found after hard- versus moderate-resistance exercise.

There is a strong relationship between aerobic fitness and the aerobic response to repeated sessions of high-intensity exercise. Theoretically, an increase in aerobic fitness could enhance recovery from anaerobic performance, both by supplementing anaerobic energy during the exercise and by providing aerobically derived energy at a faster rate during the recovery period. Additionally, any improvements that aid in transport to and from the muscle, such as increased blood flow, could enhance the removal of lactate, hydrogen ions and heat.

See also under ANAEROBIC CAPACITY; GROWTH.

Bibliography
Børsheim, E. and Bahr, R. (2003). Effect of exercise intensity, duration and mode on post-exercise oxygen consumption. *Sports Medicine* 33(14), 1037-1060.

Tomlin, D.L. and Wenger, H.A. (2001). The relationship between aerobic fitness and recovery from high intensity intermittent exercise. *Sports Medicine* 31(1), 1-11.

OXYGEN DEFICIT   The difference between the theoretical requirement of oxygen in a period of exercise and the amount of oxygen actually used. Oxygen deficit is due to limited cellular utilization of oxygen as a result of metabolic adjustments. The oxygen deficit at the onset of activity is smaller, but not eliminated, in a trained individual, because oxidative phosphorylation is activated sooner due to increased number of mitochondria that are sensitive to low levels of ADP and phosphate. *See under* ANAEROBIC CAPACITY; GROWTH.

OXYGEN DRIFT   The increase in oxygen consumption during 'steady state' exercise, when it is performed for extended periods. Sustained cycle-pedaling for 45 to 60 minutes at an intensity of 60% maximal oxygen uptake, for example, typically produces a progressive rise in metabolic rate, manifest as a 10 to 15% increase in oxygen uptake. It is termed the **slow component of oxygen uptake kinetics**. This increase in oxygen uptake is most evident at exercise intensities above the lactate threshold. This phenomenon is poorly understood, but it seems that a combination of increased muscle temperature and circulating catecholamine hormones may contribute to the oxygen drift during running on level ground. Larger oxygen drift during downhill running seems to be due to greater increases in muscle temperature during negative work. Magnitude of oxygen drift is lower after training. This may be due to concomitant decreases in catecholamine hormones, lactate and body temperature rise during any given submaximal workload. *See also under* INTERVAL TRAINING.

Bibliography
Robergs, R.A. and Roberts, S.O. (2000). *Fundamental principles of exercise physiology*. Boston, MA: McGraw-Hill.

OXYGEN INHALATION   Use of oxygen as an ergogenic aid. There is evidence that oxygen inhalation (breathing 100% oxygen) during submaximal and maximal exercise leads to an increase in aerobic performance, an increase in maximal oxygen uptake, a decrease in lactate and a decrease in pulmonary ventilation. The decrease in pulmonary ventilation would decrease the oxygen cost of breathing and theoretically liberate significant oxygen for use by working muscles. Oxygen inhalation during sports performance is usually either impractical or forbidden by the rules. There is no ergogenic effect derived from breathing oxygen-enriched gas before exercise or during recovery.

Chronology
•1932 • Japanese swimmers won every swimming event except one in the Olympic Games. The Japanese, who had never won an individual medal in Olympic swimming, made pioneering use of slow-motion underwater movies to closely analyze Johnny Weissmuller's style. Weissmuller had won nearly all the sprint-swimming events at the 1928 Olympics. The Japanese swimmers attributed their Olympic victories to breathing in pure oxygen before competing.

•1954 • Roger Bannister published one of the first studies on the use of oxygen as an ergogenic aid. His paper, "The effects on the respiration and performance of adding oxygen to the inspired air" was published in *Journal of Applied Physiology*. (In the same year, Bannister ran the first sub-four minute mile (3:59.4), around the University of Oxford's Iffley Road track.)

OXYGEN PULSE   Oxygen uptake divided by the heart rate. It is thus the amount of oxygen extracted by body tissues over a single heartbeat or single stroke volume.

OXYGEN TRANSPORT   *See under* OXYGEN.

OXYGEN UPTAKE   The amount of oxygen extracted from inspired gas in a given period of time. It depends on the ability of the heart to pump oxygenated blood to the working muscles (cardiac output) and the ability of the working muscles to extract oxygen from the blood (arterial-mixed venous oxygen difference). This is expressed in the

Fick relationship, i.e. oxygen uptake equals cardiac output multiplied by arterial-mixed venous oxygen difference.

In the steady state, oxygen uptake equals the oxygen consumption. Oxygen uptake may differ from oxygen consumption under conditions in which oxygen is being utilized from the body's stores. After the start of constant load exercise, oxygen uptake usually reaches its steady state faster than carbon dioxide output. After the start of exercise, there is a period of time (usually about 15 seconds) in which the mixed venous blood entering the pulmonary capillaries bed has not changed its composition. During this time, any increase in oxygen uptake reflects increased blood flow through the lungs and not an increased arterial-mixed venous oxygen difference across the lungs. Before a steady state phase of gas exchange is reached, there is a period of time in which the mixed venous blood gas concentrations are changing. When the steady state is attained, mixed venous blood gas concentrations become constant.

During unsteady states, the respiratory quotient does not truly reflect the proportions of substrates being used to produce energy. Oxygen uptake does not reflect oxygen consumption if an oxygen debt is being incurred or paid off, and carbon dioxide output does not reflect carbon dioxide production if the body carbon dioxide stores are changing. In such unsteady states, the ratio of carbon dioxide output to oxygen uptake, as determined by analysis of mixed expired gas, is known as the respiratory exchange ratio. In a steady state, the respiratory quotient is equal to the respiratory exchange ratio. During exercise, the change in respiratory exchange ratio is a combination of changes in respiratory quotient and changes in the oxygen and carbon dioxide stores of the body. The carbon dioxide stores are large compared to the oxygen stores. The carbon dioxide stores are nearly all in the blood and change quickly, whereas the oxygen stores are largely in body tissues and change slowly.

See also under GROWTH; OXYGEN UPTAKE, MAXIMAL.

OXYGEN UPTAKE, KINETICS   Characteristics

of oxygen uptake differ with exercise intensity. Oxygen uptake rises exponentially during the first minutes of low-intensity, constant-load exercise (the **'fast component' of oxygen uptake**) and reaches a steady state after approximately three minutes. Neither the slope of the increase in oxygen uptake with respect to work rate, nor the time constant of oxygen uptake responses, has been found to be a function of work rate within this domain, indicating a linear dynamic relationship between the oxygen uptake and the work rate. There are some factors, however, such as physical training and pathological conditions, which can alter the oxygen uptake kinetic responses at the onset of exercise.

When exercise is performed at a work rate above the lactate threshold, the oxygen uptake kinetics become more complex. An additional component, termed the **'slow component' of oxygen uptake** by Whipp and Wasserman (1972), is developed after a few minutes of exercise. The slow component either delays the attainment of the steady-state oxygen uptake or drives the oxygen uptake to the maximum level, depending on exercise intensity. The magnitude of this slow component also depends on the duration of the exercise. Possible causes for the slow component of oxygen during heavy exercise include increases in blood lactate levels, increases in plasma epinephrine levels, increased ventilatory work, elevation of body temperature and a progressive recruitment of less efficient motor units (made up of type IIb fibers).

The slow component has been shown to be significantly lower in the second of two bouts of heavy constant-load cycling exercise, possibly because the first bout may act as a 'warm up' or 'conditioning' exercise that facilitates a more rapid establishment of intracellular homeostasis during the second bout (i.e. greater oxygen availability partly due to increased vasodilation), leading to the recruitment of fewer type II muscle fibers (Burnley et al, 2000).

Bibliography
Burnley, M. et al. (2000). Effects of prior heavy exercise on phase II pulmonary oxygen uptake kinetics during heavy exercise. *Journal of Applied Physiology* 89, 1387-1396.

Gaesser, G.A. and Poole, D.C. (1996). The slow component of oxygen uptake kinetics in humans. *Exercise and Sport Sciences*

Reviews 24, 35-70.

Xu, F. and Rhodes, E.C. (1999). Oxygen uptake kinetics during exercise. *Sports Medicine* 27(5), 313-327.

Zoladz, J.A. and Korzeniewski, B. (2001). Physiological background of the change point in VO_2 and the slow component of oxygen uptake kinetics. *Journal of Physiological Pharmacology* 52(2), 167-184.

OXYGEN UPTAKE, MAXIMAL

The point at which there is no further increase in oxygen uptake despite increases in workload. Because the anaerobic energy systems are very limited, maximal oxygen uptake is directly related to maximal work capacity.

It is not clearly understood whether maximal oxygen uptake is limited by **central factors** (oxygen transport system) or **peripheral factors** (ability of skeletal muscle to use oxygen). Noakes (1997) maintains that the absence of an oxygen uptake plateau in some subjects is proof that oxygen transport is not a limiting factor for maximal oxygen uptake, and proposes instead that endurance performance is limited by peripheral factors. The consensus of scientific opinion, however, is in favor of the limitation being due to central factors. It seems that peripheral changes account for the majority of the improvement in maximal oxygen uptake, because of the increase in capillary surface area for oxygen diffusion resulting from new capillary formation. This allows an increased diffuse flux of oxygen, both by increasing the capillary wall area available for diffusion and by decreasing the mean intercapillary distance over which oxygen must diffuse. An increased mitochondrial density further contributes to a decrease in the mean distance over which oxygen must travel from red blood cells to cytochromes. There is a corresponding increase in the concentration of Krebs cycle enzymes. An increased oxidative capacity will allow for an increased utilization of fat as a metabolic fuel during exercise. At maximal exercise, the capacity of the muscle capillary network is never reached.

The following ergogenic aids have been used to improve oxygen uptake: blood doping, altitude training, erythropoietin, oxygen inhalation and phosphate loading.

Bibliography

Bassett, D.R. and Howley, E.T. (1997). Maximal oxygen uptake: 'Classical' versus 'contemporary' viewpoints. *Medicine and Science in Sports and Exercise* 29(5), 591-603.

Dempsey, J.A. and Manohar, M. (1992). The pulmonary system and endurance. In: Shephard, R.J. and Astrand, P.O. (eds). *Endurance in sport*. pp61-71. Oxford: Blackwell Scientific Publications.

Hartley, L.H. (1992). Cardiac function and endurance. In: Shephard, R.J. and Astrand, P.O. (eds). *Endurance in sport*. pp72-79. Oxford: Blackwell Scientific Publications.

Maughan, R.J. (1992). Aerobic function. *Sport Science Review* 1(1), 28-42.

Noakes, T.D. (1997). Challenging belief: Ex Africa semper aliquid novi. *Medicine and Science in Sports and Exercise* 29(5), 571-590.

Powers, S.K. and Williams, J. (1987). Exercise-induced hypoxaemia in highly trained athletes. *Sports Medicine* 4, 46-53.

Saltin, B. and Strange, S. (1992). Maximal oxygen uptake: 'Old' and 'new' arguments for a cardiovascular limitation. *Medicine and Science in Sports and Exercise* 24(1), 30-37.

Sutton, J.R. (1992). Limitations to maximal oxygen uptake. *Sports Medicine* 13(2), 127-133.

Wagner, P.D. (1991). Central and peripheral aspects of oxygen transport and adaptations with exercise. *Sports Medicine* 11(3), 133-142.

Wagner, P.D. (1995). Muscle oxygen transport and oxygen-dependent control of metabolism. *Medicine and Science in Sports and Exercise* 27(1), 47-53.

OXYGEN UPTAKE, MEASUREMENT OF

Oxygen uptake is most commonly measured using open-circuit spirometry. This involves measuring the quantity and quality of expired air. It seems that 90% of the total variability of a physiological measurement, such as maximum oxygen uptake, is accounted for by biological variability, with only 10% of the variability accounted for by technical problems associated with measurement (Macfarlane, 2001).

Up until the mid 1970s, traditional measurements of metabolic and respiratory variables during exercise required a Tissot-type spirometer or a Douglas bag plus a gas meter to collect and measure the volume of the expirate. A **Tissot spirometer** is a large water-sealed spirometer designed for accumulating expired gas over a long period of time; the counterbalancing of the bell is compensated for the bell's change in buoyancy as it emerges from the water, keeping the contained gas precisely at ambient atmospheric pressure. **Douglas bags** (rubber or plastic bags) or meteorological balloons are used to collect expired gas over a specified time period.

Diffusion of gases through the walls of early fabric/rubber Douglas bags affected validity. If a Douglas bag is only acting as a reservoir to sample mixed expired air, then a mixing chamber can be used instead. A **mixing chamber** usually consists of a chamber containing baffles (physical obstructions to flow) that mix the dead space and alveolar gases expired by the subject. It enables an average value of the mixed expired gas to be estimated. Mixing chambers are best suited to situations where the gas concentrations do not change rapidly. A small aliquot of expired gas was taken for analysis using chemical absorption methods, such as the Lloyd-Haldane or Scholander apparatus, in which oxygen and carbon dioxide are absorbed by chemicals, to provide the fractional concentrations of oxygen and carbon dioxide. **Aliquot sampling techniques** involve continuous sampling of a portion of expired air that has been collected in a small rubber bag (aliquot).

Over the last 40 years, more than 20 different automated systems have been commercially produced. The validity and reliability of all these different systems is not well know, with relatively few independent studies having been published in this area. One of the first automated systems was the Metabolic Measuring Cart developed by Beckman Instruments. It measured ventilation with a turbine volume transducer and had a mixing chamber. Gas analysis involved measurement of mixed expired gas fractions with oxygen and carbon dioxide electronic analysers. Macfarlane (2001) concluded that, even under ideal conditions, it is unlikely that the accuracy of modern automated systems can surpass the accuracy of a skilled operator using traditional methods involving Douglas bags and chemical analysis of oxygen and carbon dioxide via Haldane or Scholander analysis. This is caused, in part, by the potential nonlinearity of the many transducers used, but also by the problem that automated systems have of temporally matching gas flows and fractions. Nevertheless, many of the modern laboratory-based and portable systems produce acceptably valid and reliable data.

A pneumotachometer can be used to measure the gas volume collected in the Douglas bags or meteo-rological balloons. A **pneumotachometer (flow meter)** is a device that measures instantaneous gas flow rates during breathing by recording the pressure difference across a device of fixed flow resistance. The flow signal from the pneumotachometer is integrated and multiplied by respiratory frequency to determine pulmonary ventilation. Pneumotachometers are typically used in computerized exercise testing systems. A spirometer can also be used directly to measure the volume of expired air, and for calibrating pneumotachometers. Electronic gas analyzers or mass spectrometers are used for gas analysis.

Breathing valves separate inspired from expired gas flows, so that expired gas can be collected and analyzed. Ideally, a breathing valve should prevent contamination of either gas flow by the other, have resistance to both inspiration and expiration, and have a low re-breathed volume (dead space). In exercise testing, valve dead space is often incorporated into calculations of gas exchange. The volume of the breathing valve and mouthpiece apparatus is considered to be in series with the anatomic dead space.

Gas analysis is a procedure for determining the concentration of gases. In exercise testing, **carbon dioxide fraction** is often measured using an analyser based on absorption of infra-red light. **Oxygen fraction** is often measured using either a paramagnetic or an electrochemical analyser. The **paramagnetic type** is based on measuring changes in oxygen quantity in a chamber located in a magnetic field. The **electrochemical type** depends on chemical reactions between oxygen and a reusable substrate that results in the generation of an electric current. This current is proportional to the quantity of oxygen molecules reacting with the substrate. **Mass spectrometers** can be used to measure oxygen, carbon dioxide and nitrogen fractions. In the fixed-collector type, sample gases are ionised, accelerated by an electric field and subjected to a magnetic field. Because the direction taken in this field by the different ions depends on their mass, the fraction of each gas can be measured.

Ignoring the effects of water vapor pressure can lead to errors of up to 25% in the measurement of the fractional concentration of oxygen in expired air. Mass spectrometers can be adjusted automatically to ignore the contribution of water vapor (i.e. effectively measuring dry air), but most oxygen and carbon dioxide analyzers are sensitive to the presence of water vapor.

Various criteria are used to determine maximal oxygen uptake. The most widely accepted criterion for the achievement of maximal oxygen uptake during a graded exercise test is a plateau in oxygen uptake as the work rate continues to increase. Less than 50% of subjects tested actually demonstrate a plateau. Other criteria include: i) blood lactate concentration in the first five minutes of recovery greater than 8 mmol/L; ii) respiratory exchange ratio at completion of test greater than one; and iii) heart rate at completion of test greater than 85% of age-predicted maximum.

Compared to an intermediate-speed protocol, fast protocols (large work-rate increments per minute) and slow protocols (small work rate increments per minute) have been found to cause underestimation of true maximal oxygen uptake. Fast protocols may cause subjects to end the graded exercise test early because of insufficient muscle strength to accommodate large work rate increases during the final stages of the test. Slow protocols require high motivation to deal with the high levels of lactate associated with heavy, prolonged exercise and involve a significant increase in core temperature which would result in a redistribution of the cardiac output. Less blood, and therefore less oxygen, would be going to the working muscles and more blood would be going to the cutaneous circulation in an effort to dissipate heat.

The exercise modalities that are most commonly used for exercise testing are running on a treadmill or cycling on a bicycle ergometer. The most widely used protocol for bicycle ergometer graded exercise tests has a warm up period of about 4 minutes. The work rate during the warm up period is typically unloaded or a light work rate such as 15 watts. Immediately after the 4 minute warm up, the work rate is increased incrementally by a certain power each minute until the subject reaches his or her limit of tolerance. The increment size is that predicted to produce a test duration of 8 to 12 minutes from the time the work-rate increment started.

Common treadmill protocols include: **Naughton** (2-minute exercise periods of increasing intensity, alternating with 3 minutes of rest with exercise periods varying in % grade and speed); **Astrand** (constant speed at 5 mph and, after 3 minutes at 0% grade, the grade increases 2.5% every 2 minutes); **Bruce** (grade and/or speed change every 3 minutes, but the 0% and 5% grades are omitted for healthy subjects); **Balke** (after 1 minute at 2% grade, grade increases 1% per minute and the speed is maintained at 3.3 mph); **Ellestad** (initial grade at 10% and later grade of 15%, while speed increases every 2 or 3 minutes); and **Harbor** (after 3 minutes of walking at a comfortable speed, the grade increases at a constant pre-selected amount each minute, so that the subject achieves maximal oxygen uptake in approximately 10 minutes).

Breath-by-breath measurement is the expression of a physiological variable averaged over one respiratory cycle. It is a method for measurement of respiratory gas exchange in which the product of respired gas volume and simultaneously measured expired gas concentration is mathematically integrated using a computer. It may involve measuring the quantity and quality of both inspired gas and expired gas in order to estimate alveolar transport of oxygen and carbon dioxide. Measurement of end-tidal oxygen and end-tidal carbon dioxide may be used for estimating alveolar gas concentrations and sampled from the mouthpiece or facemask.

With breath-by-breath systems, errors in the delay time between gas flows and gas analysis can alone cause up to a 30% error in oxygen uptake at high breathing frequencies.

Alveolar gas exchange differs from total lung gas exchange measured at the mouth, because of significant breath-to-breath changes in the amounts of oxygen and carbon dioxide that are stored in the lungs. In the long term, these amounts fluctuate with differing breathing patterns, and total lung gas exchange averages to the same value as alveolar gas exchange. However, in breath-to-breath measurements, discrepancies arise between the two methods especially when the subject is not in a steady state.

Alveolar gas exchange is obtained by subtracting expired from inspired gas quantities for a particular breath, and making corrections for breath-to-breath changes in alveolar gas concentration and functional residual capacity. It has been shown that the corrections for changes in functional residual capacity provide a more precise description of breath-to-breath oxygen uptake and carbon dioxide output.

Chronology

•1790 • Antoine Lavoisier measured oxygen consumption of his assistant Armand Seguin during rest and exercise. Gas metabolism was measured using a facemask. The expired carbon dioxide was absorbed with a solution of alkali hydroxides; the oxygen content of the inhaled air was presumably measured by leading the oxygen into a water-soluble compound. This was the first attempt to measure human gas metabolism during quantified exercise.

•1911 • Scottish physiologist C.J. Douglas introduced a bag for collection of exhaled air, which was later analyzed for its content. Douglas developed his bag in preparation for the Anglo-American expedition to Pike's Peak in Colorado. The bag was later named after him and is still widely used in exercise physiology.

Bibliography

American College of Sports Medicine (2000). *ACSM's guidelines for exercise testing and prescription.* 6th ed. Philadelphia, PA: Lippincott Williams and Wilkins.

Beaver, W.L., Lamarra, N. and Wasserman, K. (1981). Breath-by-breath measurement of true alveolar gas exchange. *Journal of Applied Physiology* 51(6), 1662-1675.

Bradley, P.W. and Younes, M. (1980). Relation between respiratory valve dead space and tidal volume. *Journal of Applied Physiology* 49, 528-532.

Davis, J.A. (1995). Direct determination of aerobic power. In:

Maud, P.J. and Foster, C. (1995). *Physiological assessment of human fitness.* pp9-17. Champaign, IL: Human Kinetics.

Fawkner, S. and Armstrong, N. (2003). Oxygen uptake kinetic response to exercise in children. *Sports Medicine* 33(9), 651-669.

MacDougall, J.D., Wenger, H.A. and Green, H.J. (1991, eds). *Physiological testing of the high-performance athlete.* 2nd ed. Champaign, IL: Human Kinetics.

Macfarlane, D.J. (2001). Automated metabolic gas analysis systems: A review. *Sports Medicine* 31(12), 841-861.

Maiolo, C. et al. (2003). Physical activity energy expenditure measured using a portable telemetric device in comparison with a mass spectrometer. *British Journal of Sports Medicine* 37(5), 445-457.

McConnell, T.R. (1988). Practical considerations in the testing of maximal oxygen uptake in runners. *Sports Medicine* 5, 57-68.

Porcari, J.P. et al. (1989). Walking for exercise testing and training. *Sports Medicine* 8(4), 189-200.

Skinner, J.S. (1993). *Exercise testing and exercise prescription in special cases: Theoretical basis and clinical application.* 2nd ed. Philadelphia, PA: Lea and Febiger.

Wasserman, K., Hansen, J.E., Sue, D.Y. and Whipp, B.J. (1999). *Principles of exercise testing and interpretation.* 3rd ed. Philadelphia, PA: Lippincott Williams & Wilkins.

OXYHEMOGLOBIN   *See under* HEMOGLOBIN.

OXYTOCIN   A hormone secreted by the posterior pituitary gland. It stimulates muscles of the uterus and breasts and is important during birth and lactation.

OZONE   See under AIR POLLUTION.

P

PACINIAN CORPUSCLE *See under* MECHANORECEPTORS.

PADDING The use of any material with impact absorption qualities that is applied to vulnerable body parts to minimize the effects of direct contact. There is little evidence to show that shoulder pads decrease the incidence of severe shoulder injuries in contact sports. However, well-fitting shoulder pads constructed of materials that effectively disperse the force of impact appear to decrease the direct contact and decrease the potential for soft tissue damage.

Bibliography
Gerrard, D.F. (1998). The use of padding in rugby union. An overview. *Sports Medicine* 25(5), 329-332.

PAGET-SCHROETTER SYDNROME *See under* THROMBOSIS.

PAIN An unpleasant sensory and emotional experience associated with actual or potential tissue damage, or described in terms of such damage.

A **noxious stimulus** is one that is damaging to normal tissues. In addition to the informational content, the input from **nociceptors** (receptors for pain) strongly affects emotions. **Nociception** is the detection of tissue damage by specialized transducers attached to A delta and C fibers. The stimuli for pain are physical agents (thermal/mechanical) and chemical agents (extrinsic substances, such as acids; and intrinsic substances such as histamine that are released from damaged tissues by proteolytic enzymes).

According to the original Gate Control theory, pain impulses must get past a 'gate' in the spinal cord. The gate is a pattern of neural activity that either blocks pain messages coming from the skin, muscles and internal organs or lets those signals through. Normally the gate is kept shut, either by impulses coming into the spinal cord from large fibers that respond to pressure and other kinds of stimulation or by signals coming down from the brain itself. When body tissue is injured, the large fibers are damaged and smaller fibers open the gate, allowing pain messages to reach the brain unchecked. Gate Control theory does not fully explain the many instances of severe, chronic pain that occur without any sign of injury or disease. With phantom pain, for example, a person continues to feel pain that seemingly comes from an amputated limb or from an organ that has been surgically removed. The revised Gate Control theory takes into account the effects of memories, emotions, expectations, or signals from various brain centers. Pain comes in different varieties. These different types of pain involve different chemical changes and changes in the activity of neurons at the site of injury or disease and in the spinal cord and brain.

Pain thresholds and pain tolerance levels have been found to increase following exercise. **Pain threshold** refers to the least experience of pain that a subject can recognize. **Pain tolerance level** is the greatest level of pain that a subject is prepared to tolerate. Diminished sensitivity to pain (**hypoalgesia**) may occur during and following exercise. It is not known whether there is a specific intensity of exercise that is required to produce the hypoalgesia response. **Analgesia** is the absence of pain in response to stimulation that would normally be painful. **Exercise-induced analgesia** is poorly understood, but it seems that there are multiple analgesia systems including opioid and non-opioid systems. An **analgesic drug** such as aspirin is used to provide pain relief.

Anesthesia is the loss of sensation resulting from pharmacological depression of nerve function or from neurological dysfunction. The use of local anesthetic painkilling injections in professional football can counter the negative effects on performance of injury and lower the rate of players missing matches through injury. In the majority of cases in professional American football, these injections are probably safe, especially in those areas that are most commonly injected (acromioclavicular joint sprains, finger and rib injuries, and iliac crest hematomas).

Intra-articular injections to the knee, ankle, wrist, joints of the foot, and to the pubic symphysis and major tendons of the lower limb are best avoided in most circumstances.

See ENDORPHINS; PERCEIVED EXERTION.

Bibliography

International Society for the Study of Pain. Http://www.issp-pain.org

Koltyn, K.F. (2000). Analgesia following exercise: A review. *Sports Medicine* 29(2), 85-98.

Koltyn, K.F. (2002). Exercise-induced hypoalgesia and intensity of exercise. *Sports Medicine* 32(8), 477-487.

Melzack, R. and Wall, P.D. (1965). Pain mechanisms: A new theory. *Science* 150, 971-979.

Melzack, R. and Wall, P.D. (1988). *The challenge of pain.* 2nd ed. London: Penguin Books.

Melzack, R. (1990). Phantom limbs and the concept of a neuromatrix. *Trends in Neuroscience* 13, 88-92.

Orchard, J.W. (2004). Is it safe to use local anesthetic painkilling injections in professional football? *Sports Medicine* 34(4), 209-219.

PALLOR   Paleness.

PALMAR GRASP REFLEX   A primitive reflex that is present at birth and normally persists through the 4th month of age. It is elicited by tactile stimulation of the palm of the hand with the response that all four fingers of the stimulated hand flex or close. It marks the beginning of eye-hand coordination and visual body awareness. The palmar reflex allows the infant to practice grasping and letting go of objects. Failure of this reflex to become integrated interferes with the development of the voluntary grasp and release mechanism.

PALMAR MANDIBULAR REFLEX   Babkin reflex. A primitive reflex that is normally present at birth and lasts until around 3 months. It is elicited by applying pressure simultaneously to the palm of each hand. As a result, one or more of the following responses occur: the mouth opens, eyes close, neck flexes and head tilts forward.

PALSY   *See* PARALYSIS.

PANCREAS   A gland, located near the duodenum and below the stomach, which is both an endocrine gland and an exocrine gland. The **islets of Langerhans** are endocrine tissues with two types of cells: **alpha cells**, which secrete glucagon; and **beta cells**, which secrete insulin. The exocrine part of the pancreas secretes digestive enzymes.

PANGAMIC ACID   Also known as vitamin B_{15}, although it is not actually a vitamin. There does not appear to be a physiological basis to ingestion of pangamic acid as an ergogenic aid. Synthetic mixtures that are sold as pangamic acid can be harmful.

PANIC ATTACK   *See under* ANXIETY DISORDERS; HYPERVENTILATION.

PANNER'S DISEASE   Osteonecrosis of the capitellum of the distal humerus at the elbow during primary ossification. It occurs as a result of repeated compressive forces to the lateral side of the elbow during sports such as gymnastics. It usually occurs between the ages of 5 and 10 years. In adults, such forces may cause osteochondral dissecans and osteochondral defects of the capitellum and radial head, loose bodies and degenerative changes.

PANTOTHENIC ACID   A vitamin of the B_2 group. It is a constituent of co-enzyme A.

PAP SMEAR   A test for cancer, especially of the female genital tract, in which a smear of exfoliated cells and secretions are specially stained and examined under a microscope for pathological changes.

PARACHUTE REFLEXES   Parachute reactions. Propping reflexes. Postural reflexes that are protective extension movements of the limbs used to break or prevent a fall and appear to be related to the attainment of upright posture. There are four such reflexes, named for the direction in which the body is falling (downward, sideward, forward and backward). The downward parachute, which refers to being dropped or falling feet first, develops first (at about 4 months of age) and is the only one that involves the legs. The other three reactions are the natural propping responses of both arms (falling forward or backward) or one arm (falling sideward).

The sideward parachute develops next, at 6 to 8 months, then the forward parachute at 7 to 8 months, and the backward parachute at 9 to 10 months. All of the parachute reflexes remain throughout the lifespan. These reactions are often delayed or absent in persons with severe disability.

It has been found that when the parachute reflexes appear by the age of 10 months in late-sitting infants, most of those infants would achieve independent walking by 15 months. A delay in the parachute reflexes predicts a delay in walking.

Bibliography

Jaffe, M. et al. (1996). The parachute reactions in normal and late walkers. *Pediatric Neurology* 14(1), 46-48.

PARACRINE *See under* EICOSANOIDS.

PARALYMPICS *See under* ADAPTED PHYSICAL ACTIVITY.

PARALYSIS Palsy. It is the loss of the ability to move a body part. It involves complete loss of strength in an affected limb or muscle group. A condition causing weakness (**paresis**) may progress to paralysis. Strength may, however, be restored to a paralyzed limb.

PARAPLEGIC *See under* SPINAL PARALYSIS.

PARASITE It is an organism that lives on, or in, another organism and draws its nourishment from that organism.

PARASYMPATHETIC NERVOUS SYSTEM *See under* AUTONOMIC NERVOUS SYSTEM.

PARATENON *See under* TENDON.

PARATHYROID HORMONE *See under* CALCIUM.

PARENTS Guidelines for how parents can support their children in sport include: emphasize performance rather than competitive outcome; decrease the pressure to win by putting sport in the context of life as a whole; believe that sport's primary value is the opportunity for self-development; understand the risk of failure; communicate true concerns directly with the coach; understand and respect the differences between parental roles and coaching roles, avoiding coaching 'over the shoulder' of the coach and/or public questioning the coach's decisions; control negative emotions and think positively; avoid using punishment and withdrawal of love; provide critical emotional support rather than constant nagging; recognize and understand expressions of insecurity and anxiety; show empathy, i.e. an understanding of what the child is feeling and an awareness of the pressures and demands that the sport places on the athlete; and avoid the use of guilt, such as "We've done so much for you... ."

Parents communicate their value for a given area of achievement and their belief about their child's likelihood of success in that area. Parents facilitate their children's understanding of information about their ability. Hellstedt (1987) distinguished between parents who are under-involved (a relative lack of emotional, financial, or functional investment), moderately involved (firm parental direction, but with enough flexibility that the athlete is allowed significant involvement in decision making) and over-involved parents (who yell during competition, disagree with the coach about their child's amount of playing time, consistently asking their child to try harder and provide 'unsolicited coaching'). When the degree of identification with their children becomes excessive, parents begin to define their own self-worth in terms of their son's or daughter's successes or failures (Smith and Smoll, 1996). The term '**vicarious motivation**' can be used to refer to the parent who seeks to experience, through his son or daughter, the success he or she never knew as an athlete.

Bibliography

Feigley, D.A. Guidelines for supportive parents. Youth Sports Research Council. Http://youthsports.rutgers.edu

Hellstedt, J.C. (1995). Invisible players: A family systems model. In Murphy, S.H. (ed.). *Sport psychology interventions.* pp117-146. Champaign, IL: Human Kinetics.

PARESIS Muscle weakness that is associated with incomplete paralysis.

PARESTHESIA   Abnormal burning, tingling, numbness or prickling feeling in any part of the body, such as the hands, arms, legs or feet.

PARKINSON'S DISEASE   A progressive disorder of the central nervous system that affects more than 1.5 million persons in the USA. It affects 1 to 2% of people over the age of 60 years, with the chance of developing the disease increasing with age. Cholinergic activity is unaffected in Parkinson's disease, but the decrease in dopamine content of the substantia nigra and its terminal fields in the putamen disturb the balance between cholinergic and dopaminergic systems in the striatum. The striatum (putamen and caudate nucleus) is involved in the control of movement and balance. It connects to and receives impulses from the substantia nigra. Parkinson's disease results when more than 80% of the dopaminergic neurons in the substantial nigra have been lost.

Symptoms of Parkinson's disease include: tremor at rest due to high muscle tone in both flexors and extensors through the range of passive movements; an inability to initiate normal movements; a mask-like face with little blinking of the eyes; a forward posture with shuffling gait and no arm swinging; poor balance; and stiff falling. There may be dementia and/or cognitive disturbances.

Approximately 5 to 15% of Parkinson's patients have familial Parkinsonism and a genetic history consistent with autosomal dominant pattern of inheritance. When three or more people are affected in a family, especially if they are under 50 years of age, it is suspected that there may be a gene making this family more likely to develop the disease. There is some evidence that the mutation in the gene that codes for a protein called human alpha-synuclein on chromosome 4 is associated with development of early-onset Parkinson's disease and that this single gene deficit may be sufficient to account for the Parkinson's disease phenotype. It is inherited as an autosomal dominant trait. However, it has been found that there is a large amount of alpha-synuclein protein in accumulations of protein called Lewy bodies in people who have non-inherited Parkinson's as well as in the brains of people who have inherited

Parkinson's. Thus alpha-synuclein seems to play an important role in all forms of Parkinson's disease. The parkin, DJ1 and PINK1 genes have all been found in Parkinson's patients who had siblings with the condition, but whose parents did not have the disease (recessive inheritance). There is some evidence to suggest that these genes may also be involved in early-onset Parkinson's (diagnosed before the age of 30 years).

Levodopa is the most common drug therapy in Parkinson's disease. It is a precursor of dopamine that is capable of crossing the blood-brain barrier, and thus it is used to treat the dopamine deficit. Levodopa is converted to dopamine in the brain, and 'charges up' the remaining dopaminergic neurons. It is effective against bradycardia and rigidity in many (but not all) cases. Tremor and balance may not be helped. **Sinemet** is a drug used in Parkinson's disease that is a mixture of levodopa and carbidopa. **Carbidopa** blocks the breakdown of dopamine.

Pallidotomy is surgery in which the globus pallidus is lesioned. By interrupting the neural pathway between the globus pallidus and the striatum or thalamus, it may improve symptoms of tremor, rigidity and bradycardia.

Bibliography
American Parkinson Disease Association, Inc. Http://www.apda-parkinson.org
National   Human   Genome   Research   Institute. Http://www.genome.gov

PARONYCHIA   Infection of the folds of the skin surrounding a finger nail.

PARS INTERARTICULARIS   *See under* SPINE; SPONDYLOLYSIS.

PARTIAL PRESSURE OF GASES   *See under* GAS.

PARTURITION   The process of giving birth.

PASSIVE TRANSPORT   A passive transport process requires no energy. Simple diffusion, facilitated diffusion, filtration and osmosis are forms of passive transport.
See also ACTIVE TRANSPORT.

PATELLA   *See under* PATELLOFEMORAL JOINT.

PATELLAR REFLEX   *See under* STRETCH REFLEX.

PATELLAR TENDINOSIS   Jumper's knee. Localized collagen degeneration and subsequent fibrosis at the bone-tendon junction of the inferior patellar pole (rather than inflammation; hence it is not tendinitis). The spectrum can be divided into four stages: (i) pain occurs only after activity; (ii) pain starts at the beginning of activity, dissipates after warm-up, and recurs with fatigue; (iii) pain occurs at rest and with activity and affects performance; and (iv) the patellar ligament completely ruptures. It occurs most often from an eccentric action of the *quadriceps femoris* when landing from a jump in sports such as basketball and volleyball, but it also occurs in other sports (e.g. tennis). Approximately 60% of the landing force is absorbed distal to the knee. A wide range of hip or knee flexion combined with forefoot landing can further decrease landing forces by another 25%.

Anatomic characteristics that may be associated with patellar tendinosis include: patella alta, poor patellofemoral tracking, patellar instability, malalignment, and leg-length discrepancy. Pes planus, decreased ankle dorsal flexion, coxa vara and femoral anteversion may also contribute.

Bibliography
Cook, J.L. et al. (2000). Overuse tendinosis, not tendinitis. Part 2. *The Physician and Sportsmedicine* 28(6), 31-46.

DePalma, M.J. and Perkins, R.H. (2004). Patellar tendinosis. Acute patellar tendon rupture and jumper's knee. *The Physician and Sportsmedicine* 32(5).

PATELLOADDUCTOR REFLEX   *See* CROSSED ADDUCTOR REFLEX.

PATELLOFEMORAL JOINT   The articulation of the patella with the trochlea of the femur. The **trochlea** is the groove into which the patella fits. The **patella** (knee cap) is a sesamoid bone in the quadriceps tendon. It improves the efficiency of the quadriceps muscles (see below), decreases friction, improves stability and protects the anterior aspect of the knee joint. Stability of the patella is provided by the anatomy of the trochlea and patella, static tension in the medial and lateral retinaculum, and by the dynamic control of the *quadriceps femoris* muscles. The **lateral retinaculum** connects the patella to the iliotibial band on the lateral side of the knee. The **medial retinaculum** supports the patella and helps prevent lateral dislocation. The **quadriceps tendon** provides proximal support to the patella. The *vastus medialis obliquus* is a smaller component of the *vastus medialis* muscle; it is the lower, horizontal portion. It is especially important in maintaining patellofemoral joint balance and normal tracking of the patella. The **patellar tendon** runs between the patella and the tibial tuberosity. Force created by the quadriceps is transmitted through the quadriceps tendon and patellar tendon (also patellar ligament) to the tibial tuberosity. The patella effectively moves the tendon line of action away from the knee joint instantaneous center, increasing the moment arm of the *quadriceps femoris* muscles, thus increasing its mechanical advantage.

The patellofemoral joint is subjected to large forces, because the tibia and femur act as long levers. During running, the retropatellar surface is subject to forces approximately five-times body weight.

Acute injuries to the patellofemoral joint include direct trauma, dislocation, subluxation, patellar fracture, quadriceps tendon rupture and patellar ligament rupture.

Patellar dislocation can be acute, recurrent or permanent. The patella is dislocated if it is displaced completely out of the trochlea. Most dislocations are lateral dislocations. Acute dislocation of the patella may occur as a result of violent impact on a normal patella or from an external rotation and a valgus load with the knee in extension. Chronic dislocation of the patella should be considered as a separate entity, in that the patella never actually engages the sulcus through its range of motion. The **sulcus** is the femoral groove that accommodates patella motion. It can be of developmental origin due to excessive external rotation of the *quadriceps femoris* muscle group in relation to the femur, or it can be acquired through fibrosis and contracture of the *vastus lateralis* muscle.

Subluxation of the patella is a transient displacement of the patella from its normal location within the trochlea. Subluxation of the patella can be minor, major or recurrent. It can occur with or without tilt. **Patellar tilt** is a functional lateralization of the patella due to excessive lateral ligamentous tension. It is thought that patients with subluxation of the patella are unlikely to develop cartilage damage unless they have the feature of tilt.

Patellofemoral dysplasia is a term that refers to both subluxation and dislocation of the patella to varying degrees. **Lateral patellar compression syndrome** presents with the same symptoms as patellofemoral dysplasia, but axial radiographs taken at 30 degrees of knee flexion do not exhibit subluxation of the patella.

Bipartite patella arises when there are two separate centers of bone formation (ossification centers). If these two ossification centers do not eventually fuse, an accessory bone arises from the second center that is attached to the patella by fibrous or cartilage tissue. This is often on the superiolateral corner of the patella. See also PLICA.

PATELLOFEMORAL STRESS SYNDROME

Patellofemoral pain syndrome. Anterior knee syndrome. Excessive lateral pressure syndrome. Patellofemoral stress syndrome is a broad term describing and inclusive of all chronic pathology related to the anterior knee. All of these conditions tend to be grouped together, due to the common symptoms of classic insidious onset of diffuse knee pain made worse by squatting, kneeling, sitting with knees in flexion and rising after long periods of sitting. It accounts for up to 50% of all overuse injuries, and is the most common knee problem encountered in clinical practice.

The pathology responsible for the patellofemoral stress syndrome is unclear. It was frequently called chondromalacia patellae in the past, implying articular cartilage destruction as a source of pathology. Arthroscopic studies have not revealed true chondromalacia, other than slight softening of the patellar articular cartilage, in most cases. Therefore, the term chondromalacia patellae has been abandoned in favor of terms, such as patellofemoral stress syndrome, which do not imply etiology.

The '**miserable malalignment syndrome**,'

consisting of increased femoral anteversion, tibia varus, external (lateral) tibial torsion and excessive pronation of the feet, is frequently blamed for patellofemoral stress syndrome. Individuals with this anatomical configuration have an increased Q angle that encourages lateral tracking of the patella. The increased pelvic width of women further increases the Q angle and may explain the increased frequency of patellofemoral stress syndrome in female athletes. The combination of increased femoral anteversion and external tibial torsion disrupts normal patellofemoral mechanics, thus predisposing athletes to develop the syndrome. Genu varus and tibial varus have been implicated because they require excess pronation in order for the foot to achieve a plantigrade position. Internal rotation of the tibia may promote further internal rotation of the femur simulating increased femoral anteversion. Other risk factors include: patellar abnormalities, low lateral femoral condyle, shallow trochlea, fracture of the patella, incorrect functioning of the extensor mechanism of the knee joint, weak *vastus medialis obliquus* muscle, overdeveloped *vastus lateralis* muscle and tight lateral retinaculum. A patella with a flat under-surface is more likely to move laterally than one with a deep central ridge. With **patella alta**, a mobile small patella sits high above the joint line and the patella tendon is one and a half times longer than the length of the patella. Consequently, the *vastus medialis obliquus* loses some of its effect in stabilizing the patella. A low lateral femoral condyle allows the patella to shift laterally more easily than a high lateral condyle. A laterally positioned tibial tubercle increases the Q angle, as does a wide pelvis or external tibial torsion. A weak *vastus medialis obliquus* tends to cause the patella to be pulled laterally. A tight lateral retinaculum may cause high lateral pressure syndrome; the patella is pulled laterally during flexion in spite of an adequate *vastus medialis obliquus*.

See also under GENDER DIFFERENCES.

Bibliography

LaBrier, K. and O'Neill, D.B. (1993). Patellofemoral stress syndrome. Current concepts. *Sports Medicine* 16(6), 449-459.

PATHOGENIC Capable of causing disease. A **pathogen** is an organism that causes disease.

PATRIARCHY *See under* GENDER.

PCL Posterior cruciate ligament. *See under* KNEE LIGAMENTS.

PEAK EXPERIENCE An altered state of consciousness that is associated with peak performance. The concept of peak experience was introduced to describe those moments when a person experiences feelings of total unity, inner strength and wholeness of being, as well as loss of fears, inhibitions and insecurities. Athletes may be in a state of flow during their peak performances. Peak experiences are limited to peak performance, but flow states are not limited to peak experiences.

Bibliography

Maslow, A. H. (1968). *Motivation and personality*. 2nd ed. New York: Harper and Row.
McInman, A.D. and Grove, J.R. (1991). Peak moments in sport: A literature review. *Quest* 13, 333-351.

PECTUS DEFORMITIES As a result of excessive growth of the costal cartilages, the ribs and cartilages 'buckle' and push the sternum either inward or outward. In **pectus excavatum** (funnel chest) the sternum is depressed in a concave shape and in **pectus carinatum** (pigeon chest), the sternum is protruded in a convex shape. Pectus deformities affect about1% of the population, more commonly in boys than girls.

Pectus deformities are often noticeable at birth, but become more apparent during the period of rapid skeletal growth in early adolescence. From around the age of 18 years, the deformity remains the same. Weight gain and chest hair (in men) usually decreases the appearance of the deformity. Physiological disturbance is uncommon, despite a subjective decrease in exercise tolerance. Musculoskeletal abnormalities associated with pectus deformities include scoliosis, Marfan's syndrome and Poland's syndrome.

Poland's syndrome is a group of unilateral congenital abnormalities of the chest wall with or without involvement of the arm on the same side. The most common abnormality is absence of the *pectoralis major* and *pectoralis minor* muscles. Syndactylism with absence of the sternal head of the *pectoralis major* can occur. *See also* BARREL CHEST; FLAIL CHEST.

Bibliography

Poland's Syndrome. Http://www.polands-syndrome.com
UK Pectus Excavatum and Pectus Carinatum Information Site. Http: www.pectus.org
Williams, A.M. and Crabbe, D.C. (2003). Pectus deformities of the anterior chest wall. *Paediatric Respiratory Reviews* 4(3), 237-242.

PEDOMETERS These are simple, inexpensive body-worn motion sensors that are used to assess and motivate physical activity behaviors. A value of 10,000 steps per day appears to be a reasonable estimate of daily activity required for healthy adults to gain health benefits. However, such a value may not be sustainable for some groups, such as older adults and individuals with chronic disease.

The following indices be used to classify pedometer-determined physical activity in healthy adults: less than 5,000 steps per day may be used as a 'sedentary lifestyle index;' 5,000 to 7,499 steps per day is typical of daily activity excluding sport/exercise and might be considered 'low active;' 7,500 to 9,999 is 'somewhat active;' 10,000 steps per day is the threshold for individuals to be classified as 'active;' and individuals who take more than 12,500 steps per day are likely to be classified as 'highly active.'

Construct validity is the extent to which a measurement corresponds with other measures of theoretically-related parameters. Positive relationships regarding indicators of fitness and pedometers range from weak to moderate depending on the fitness measure utilized.

Chronology

•490 • Leonardo da Vinci designed what was probably the first pedometer. It involved a lever arm attached to the thigh. When the thigh moved back and forth with each step, gears were rotated and the steps counted.

Bibliography

Tudor-Locke, C. and Bassett Jr., D.R. (2004). How many steps/day are enough? Preliminary pedometer indices for public health. *Sports Medicine* 34(1), 1-8.

Tudor-Locke, C. et al. (2004). Utility of pedometers for assessing physical activity: Construct validity. *Sports Medicine* 34(5), 282-291.

PEER RELATIONSHIPS   *See under* SELF EFFICACY.

PELVIC GIRDLE   Pelvis. The **innominate bone** forms one half of the pelvic girdle and arises from a fusion of the ilium, ischium and pubis. The pelvic girdle also includes the sacrum and coccyx. It connects the trunk to the lower extremities for weight bearing purposes, supports the abdominal contents and allows passage of the excretory canals. There is little motion across the joints of the pelvic girdle. The **acetabulum** is contained within two columns of innominate bone and it forms the socket in which the head of the femur articulates forming the hip joint. Whereas movements of the shoulder girdle take place in its own joints, the pelvic girdle is dependent on the lumbosacral and other lumbar joints, as well as the hip joints, for its movements.

The pelvis may tilt forwards, backwards and sideways. These movements take place in the sagittal plane around a coronal axis. During **forward (anterior) tilting**, the lower part of the pelvis, at the pubic symphysis, turns downward and the posterior surface of the sacrum turns upwards. It is accompanied by hip flexion and compensated by lumbar extension. During **backward (posterior) tilting**, the pubic symphysis moves forwards and upwards, while the posterior surface of the sacrum turns downwards. It is accompanied by hip extension and compensated by lumbar flexion. The hamstrings are involved in control of the pelvis by pulling down on the ischial tuberosity, creating posterior tilt of the pelvis. Tightness in the hamstrings can cause significant postural problems by flattening the low back and producing a chronic posterior tilt of the pelvis.

Lateral pelvic tilt is a frontal plane motion around an anteroposterior axis. One joint serves as the axis (pivot) and the opposite iliac crest elevates (**pelvic hike**) or drops (**pelvic drop**) around the axis. Pelvic hike on the left side, while standing on the right leg, results in abduction of the right hip. It is compensated by left lateral flexion. Pelvic drop on the left side, while standing on the right leg, results in adduction of the right hip. It is compensated by right lateral flexion.

Pelvic rotation occurs in the horizontal (transverse) plane about a vertical axis, and is described as being in a forward or backward direction. Although pelvic rotation can occur through the middle of the pelvis, it most commonly occurs in single-leg support around the axis of the supporting hip joint. When the right leg is supporting, **forward rotation** of the pelvis occurs when the left side of the pelvis moves anteriorly (the motion of the pelvis produces medial rotation of the right hip joint). It is compensated by lumbar rotation to the left. When the right leg is supporting, **backward rotation** of the pelvis occurs when the left side of the pelvis moves posteriorly (the motion of the pelvis produces lateral rotation of the right hip joint). It is compensated by lumbar rotation to the right.

The muscles within the pelvis may be divided into two groups: i) the *obturator internus* and the *piriformis*; and ii) the *levator ani* and the *coccygei*. The *levator ani* is a broad, thin muscle that forms most of the pelvic floor. It has two parts: the *pubococcygeus* and *iliococcygeus*. The *levatores ani* constricts the lower end of the rectum and (in females) the vagina, and is also involved in forced expiration. The *coccygei* pull forward and support the coccyx, after it has been pressed backward during defecation or parturition. Together, the *levatores ani* and *coccygei* form the **pelvic diaphragm** that supports the pelvic viscera. The pelvic diaphragm stretches across the floor of the pelvic cavity like a hammock and separates the pelvis from the perineum. It is reinforced in the perineum by muscles and fasciae of the urogenital diaphragm.

See also LUMBAR-PELVIC RHYTHM; PUBIC SYMPHYSIS; SACRO-ILIAC JOINT.

Bibliography

Bartlett, R. (1997). *Introduction to sports biomechanics*. London: E & FN Spon.

Levangie, P.K. and Norkin, C.C. (2001). *Joint structure and function: A comprehensive analysis*. 3rd ed. Philadelphia, PA: F.A.

Davis Company.

Norris, C.M. (2000). *Back stability*. Champaign, IL: Human Kinetics.

PENTOSE Any of a class of carbohydrates containing five carbons. Pentoses are present in foods in only small quantities; they are essential components of nucleic acids.

PENTOSE PHOSPHATE PATHWAY A side branch of glycolysis using glucose 6-phosphate as a substrate in order to produce NADPH and ribose 5-phosphate.

PEPSIN *See under* GASTROINTESTINAL SYSTEM.

PEPTIDE Two or more amino acids bonded together. A peptide bond unites the alpha-carboxyl group of one amino acid to the alpha-amino group of another amino acid to form a dipeptide with the loss of a water molecule.

PEPTIDE HORMONES The following substances are prohibited by the World Anti-Doping Agency (WADA), including their mimetics, analogues and releasing factors: erythropoietin; growth hormone and insulin-like growth factor (IGF-1); chorionic gonadotrophin; pituitary and synthetic gonadotrophins; and insulin and corticotrophins.

Chronology
•1988 • Peptide hormones were added to the International Olympic Committee (IOC)'s list of banned substances.

Bibliography
World Anti-Doping Agency. Http://www.wada-ama.org

PERCEIVED EXERTION The feeling of how heavy and strenuous a physical task is. Perceived exertion depends on many factors, including sensory cues, somatic symptoms and emotional factors. The **Borg RPE scale** is used for rating of perceived exertion. The scale is constructed so that certain psychophysical functions can be assessed according to the basic assumption that physiological strain grows linearly with exercise intensity and that

perception should follow the same linear increase. It is a numerical scale of 6 to 20 that relates closely to the heart rates from rest to maximal exercise when multiplied by a factor of 10. It provides a fairly accurate measure of how the subject feels in relation to the level of exertion, and it also allows the experimenter to know when the subject is near the point of exhaustion. A revised scale has recently been adapted that attempts to provide a ratio scale of RPE values (ranging from 0 to 10).

Bibliography
Borg, G. (1998). *Borg's perceived exertion and pain scales*. Champaign, IL: Human Kinetics.
Noble, B.J. and Robertson, R.J. (1996). *Perceived exertion*. Champaign, IL: Human Kinetics.

PERCEPTION In cognitive psychology, a process or set of processes that primarily depends on sensory input but also depends on past experience. Whereas perception may be defined as a cognitive process, **sensation** is concerned with sensory processes only. **Perceptual-motor skill** is a term used to emphasize the relationship between input from the environment and the selection and control of movement.

Perceptual constancies allow us to perceive objects as stable, despite changes in the sensory patterns they produce. **Perceptual illusions** occur when sensory cues are misleading or when we misinterpret cues.

There is some evidence to suggest that visual abilities can be developed with training. However, experts do not possess superior visual systems compared to less skilled performers. The visual hardware does not appear to limit performance at the elite level in sport. Eye movement recording techniques have generally not been able to distinguish between what experts and novices fixate in a visual display. Sport-specific training programs that develop the knowledge base underlying skilled perception are likely to be more effective than the generalized visual training programs proposed by sports optometrists.

Compared to novices, experts are faster and more accurate in recognizing and recalling patterns of play, are able to quickly and accurately detect objects of relevance such as the ball from background distractions, are superior in anticipating the actions of opponents and are more accurate in event prediction given a particular set of circumstances. In snooker, for example, experts demonstrate superior recall of ball positions from an actual match but not when the balls are scattered randomly on the table. *See* GESTALT PSYCHOLOGY; VISION.

Bibliography

Abernethy, B. (1993). Searching for the minimum essential information for skilled perception and action. *Psychological Research* 55, 131-138.

Abernethy, B., Wann, J. and Parks, S. (1998). Training perceptual-motor skills for sport. In: Elliott, B. (ed). *Training in sport.* pp1-68. Chichester, UK: John Wiley & Sons.

Abernethy, B., Neal, R.J. and Konig, P. (1994). Visual-perceptual and cognitive differences between expert, intermediate, and novice snooker players. *Applied Cognitive Psychology* 8, 185-211.

Williams, A.M. and Grant, A. (1999). Training perceptual skill in sport. *International Journal of Sport Psychology* 30(2), 194-220.

Williams, A.M., Davids, K. and Williams, J.G. (1999). *Visual perception and action in sport.* London: E & FN Spon.

PERFECTIONISM *See under* COGNITIVE INTERVENTIONS; GOALS.

PERFUSION The passage of a fluid through the vessels of an organ.

PERICARDIAL TAMPONADE *See under* HEART INJURY.

PERINEUM In males, it is the region between the anus and the scrotum. In females, it is the region between the vagina and the anus.

PERIODIZATION The subdivision of the training year into a number of periods. The intensity of training varies because, despite the overload principle of training, athletes cannot train continuously at a high intensity. A **macrocycle** (generally a year's training) is divided into two or more **mesocycles** (parts of a year's training) that revolve around dates of major competitions.

For a distance runner, a typical periodization program involves dividing the year into six-week periods. Each period emphasizes one particular type of training, while putting less emphasis on the others. In each period, 15 days would be quality sessions and 27 days would be easy or recovery.

For weightlifting sports, a typical periodization program consists of two phases: preparation and competition. In the preparation phase there is high volume (many repetitions) and low intensity (low average weight lifted relative to the weight at which only one repetition can be done). As weeks pass, volume decreases and intensity increases, thus leading to the competition phase. Two or more complete cycles may fit into a training year.

Bibliography

Bompa, T.O. (1999). *Periodization. Theory and methodology of training.* 4th ed. Champaign, IL: Human Kinetics.

Bompa, T.O. (1999). *Periodization training for sports.* Champaign, IL: Human Kinetics.

Daniels, J. (1989). Training distance runners: A primer. *Gatorade Sports Science Exchange* 1(11).

Garhammer, J. and Takano, B. (1992). Training for weightlifting. In: Komi, PV (ed). *Strength and power in sport.* pp357-369. Oxford: Blackwell Scientific Publications.

PERIORBITAL HEMATOMA Periorbital ecchymosis. Black eye. Impact forces can cause significant swelling and hemorrhage into the surrounding eyelids and hence discoloration. **Bilateral deep periorbital hematoma** ('raccoon eyes') may be the only sign of a basilar skull fracture, especially if caused by head trauma remote to the eye.

PERIOSTEUM Specialized connective tissue covering all bones of the body. The periosteum is secured to the underlying bone by **Sharpey's fibers**, which are extremely dense where the periosteum provides anchoring points for tendons and ligaments.

PERIOSTITIS Inflammation of the periosteum. *See* FOOTBALLER'S ANKLE; LATERAL EPICONDYLITIS; MEDIAL EPICONDYLITIS.

PERIPHERAL ARTERIAL DISEASE It is chronic obstruction of the arteries supplying blood to the lower extremities, and is marked by symptoms, such as **intermittent claudication,**

which is discomfort in the leg muscles brought on by walking and relieved by rest. Pain typically occurs in the calf and disappears quickly. The usual cause of intermittent claudication is decreased circulation of the femoral artery, because of atherosclerotic changes. Most patients with intermittent claudication improve with a regimen that includes aggressive risk-factor modification (especially cessation of smoking), exercise, platelet inhibition and drug therapy to improve walking distance. Vasoactive drugs such as **Cilostazol**, an anti-platelet, antithrombotic agent have been shown to cause significantly positive effects on walking distance. Cilostazol decreases symptoms of intermittent claudication, and has been shown to improve walking distance by about 40 to 60%.

Critical limb ischemia is a severe obstruction of the arteries, which seriously decreases blood flow to the extremities and has progressed to the point of severe pain and even skin ulcers or sores. The pain caused by critical limb ischemia can wake an individual at night. Amputation occurs in about 25% of all patients with critical limb ischemia. Interventions such as balloon angioplasty will be considered for patients with critical limb ischemia.

Since persons with peripheral arterial disease have systemic atherosclerosis, there is an associated increase in morbidity and mortality from other cardiovascular diseases. The risk factors that contribute to peripheral artery disease are similar to those associated with other forms of atherosclerosis, with diabetes and cigarette smoking posing the greatest risk. Peripheral arterial disease affects 8 to 10 million people in the USA, of which one-third to one-half are symptomatic. *See also under* ILIAC ARTERY.

Bibliography

Clement, D.L. (2000). Medical treatment of peripheral artery occlusive disease (PAOD). *Acta Chirurgica Belgica* 100(5), 190-193.

Comerota, A.J. (2001). Endovascular and surgical revascularization for patients with intermittent claudication. *American Journal of Cardiology* 87(12A), 34D-43D.

Creager, M.A. (2001). Medical management of peripheral arterial disease. *Cardiology Review* 9(4), 238-245.

Curci, J.A. and Sanchez, L.A. (2003). Medical treatment of peripheral arterial disease. *Current Opinion in Cardiology* 18(6), 425-430.

Dawson, D.L. et al. (2000). A comparison of cilostazol and pentoxifylline for treating intermittent claudication. *American Journal of Medicine* 109, 523-530.

Ouriel, K. (2001). Peripheral arterial disease. *Lancet* 358 (9289), 1257-1264.

Regensteiner, J.G. and Hiatt, W.R. (1995). Exercise rehabilitation for patients with peripheral arterial disease. *Exercise and Sport Sciences Reviews* 23, 1-24.

Schainfeld, R.M. (2001). Management of peripheral arterial disease and intermittent claudication. *Journal of the American Board of Family Practitioners* 14(6), 443-450.

PERIPHERAL NERVES   Nerves that are composed of nerve fibers, layers of connective tissue and blood vessels. Peripheral nerves are surrounded by a supporting structure of fibroblasts and collagen fibrils (the **epineurium**). Within the epineurium, there are bundles of individual nerve axons (**fasciculi**) surrounded by fine collagen fibrils and lamellated sheaths of perineural cells (the **perineurium**). The perineurium provides tensile strength and elasticity to the nerve and serves as a diffusion barrier to regulate the intrafascicular fluid. The individual axons are bound together by a connective tissue matrix consisting of collagen tissue, elastic fibers and fatty tissue (the **endoneurium**). Functionally, the elasticity of the fibers of the epineurium contributes to the slack within the nerve by maintaining undulations in the nerve. This permits lengthening of the nerve without nerve fibers being strained. The epineurium also provides protection to the nerve fibers, while the loose packing around the fasciculi protects the nerve from compressive forces. The epineurium has a low capacity for resistance to traction forces. Once slack is removed, continued elongation will cause nerve injury. The blood supply within the peripheral nerve is vital to the survival and functional integrity of the axons. Peripheral nerve roots receive contributions from the dorsal and ventral rami exiting the spinal cord.

Peripheral nerves are susceptible to injury in the athlete, because of the excessive physiological demands that are made on both the neurological structures and the soft tissues that protect them. Spinal nerve roots are more susceptible than peripheral nerves to mechanical deformation, mainly because of the lack of protective connective tissue layers in nerve roots.

During sport, peripheral nerves may be damaged by compression, tension (traction), ischemia and laceration. Compression of a nerve can cause injury to both nerve fibers and blood vessels in the nerve, mainly at the edges of the compressed nerve segment, but also by ischemic mechanisms. Compression injury occurs when nerves lie superficially (e.g. ulnar nerve at medial epicondyle) or where excessive pressure can arise (e.g. median nerve at carpal tunnel). The endoneurium resists nerve compression by dissipating pressure and functioning as a shock absorber. Nerves composed of large, closely packed fasciculi with little endoneurium are most susceptible to injury. Tension induces changes in intraneural blood flow and nerve fiber structure before the nerve trunk ruptures. Tension injury occurs when the stretch applied to the nerve exceeds the elastic and deforming capacity of the nerve and surrounding tissues. Inversion injury to the ankle, causing injury of the peroneal nerve, is an example of the mechanism of traction injury. Ischemia is the least commonly encountered mechanism of nerve injury in sport. The vascular anastomoses on the nerve surface and within the perineurium of the peripheral nerve help to protect the nerve against ischemia. Ischemic nerve injury occurs in athletes who suffer arterial compromise from entrapment, fracture or dislocation. It also occurs in those who develop a compartment syndrome. Laceration of a peripheral nerve is also an unusual cause of injury, but can occasionally be seen in high velocity contact sports such as ice hockey, where equipment and playing surface are the usual factors. The most common peripheral nerve injury in the athlete is the burner.

See also BOWLER'S THUMB; BRACHIAL PLEXOPATHIES; FEMORAL NERVE PALSY; GUYTON'S TUNNEL SYNDROME; HIP JOINT, NERVES; LATERAL FEMORAL CUTANEOUS NERVE; MEDIAN NERVE; MORTON'S NEUROMA; OBTURATOR NERVE ENTRAPMENT; PERONEAL NERVE; PIRIFORMIS SYNDROME; POSTERIOR INTEROSSEUS NERVE SYNDROME; PUDENTAL NERVE; RADIAL NERVE; SCIATIC NERVE; SUPRASCAPULAR NERVE; SURAL NERVE; TARSAL TUNNEL SYNDROME; TIBIAL NERVE; ULNAR NERVE, WARTENBERG'S SYNDROME.

Bibliography
Feinberg, J.H., Nadler, S.F. and Krivickas, L.S. (1997). Peripheral nerve injuries in the athlete. *Sports Medicine* 24(6), 385-408.
Feinberg, J. and Spielholz, N.I. (2002, eds). *Peripheral nerve injuries in the athlete*. Champaign, IL: Human Kinetics.

PERIPHERAL NERVOUS SYSTEM Nerve tissue located outside the brain and spinal cord. *See under* NERVOUS SYSTEM.

PERIPHERAL VISION The visual field that can be seen without a change in fixation of the eyes. Peripheral vision is involved in visual attention in motor skill performance, as shown by javelin throwers being unable to throw properly if they wear blinkers.

PERISTALSIS The movement of a tubular structure such as the intestine, characterized by waves or alternate circular contraction and relaxation of the tube by which the contents are propelled onward.

PERITONEUM The membrane enveloping the abdominal viscera and lining the abdominal cavity. The **parietal peritoneum** is part of the membrane that lines the abdominal cavity. The **visceral peritoneum** is the portion that covers the internal organs (viscera) and forms the outer layer (serosa) of most of the intestinal tract. The **peritoneal cavity** is the space enclosed by the peritoneum. It is divided into two portions, the peritoneal (greater) sac and the omental (lesser) sac. Under normal conditions, the peritoneal cavity is a potential cavity, since the parietal and visceral layers are in contact. The two sacs are connected by the **foramen of Winslow (epiploic foramen)**. It is the neck of communication between the cavity and the omental sac. In females, the uterine tubes open directly into the peritoneal cavity.

Acute peritonitis is either primary (a rare disease in which the peritoneum is infected via the bloodstream) or secondary to many causes, the most common of which is perforation of the gastrointestinal tract. One cause in sexually active women is pelvic inflammatory disease that results from infection by bacteria such as chlamydia.

See also MESENTERY; SEXUALLY TRANSMITTED DISEASES.

PERMEABILITY A property that relates a flow of something (the flux) to a driving force (the concentration gradient). *See* ACTIVE TRANSPORT; PASSIVE TRANSPORT.

PERMEASE A membrane-associated protein that allows a specific small molecule to enter the cell.

PERONEAL Pertaining to the outer (fibular) side of the lower leg.

PERONEAL NERVE The **common peroneal nerve** is a continuation of the sciatic nerve and is derived from the 4th lumbar to 2nd sacral (L4-S2) nerve roots. After passing through the lateral aspect of the popliteal fossa, the common peroneal nerve passes behind the fibular head, winds around the neck of the fibula and descends the leg superficially in close proximity to the fibula. It then passes through the *peroneus longus* muscle and divides into the superficial and deep peroneal branches. The **superficial peroneal nerve** innervates the *peroneus longus* and *peroneus brevis* and supplies sensation to the dorsum of the foot. The **deep peroneal nerve** innervates the *tibialis anterior*, *peroneus tertius* and all the toe extensor muscles. It supplies sensation to the first web space of the foot. The common peroneal nerve is injured more frequently than either of its branches in isolation. It can be injured by a stretch injury or by direct compression, usually from a blow to the lateral aspect of the leg near the fibular head, but occasionally by a fascial band. Such injuries are associated with inversion injuries at the ankle joint, and also knee injuries. Hockey pucks, soccer kicks and American football helmets may deliver direct blows to the fibular head. The peroneal nerve can also be compressed by repetitive microtrauma. This type of injury has been reported most frequently in runners. Runners with peroneal nerve compression tend to have a tight fascial band at the edge of the *peroneus longus* muscle. Bungee jumping

may cause a peroneal nerve injury, most likely as a result of repeated tension and shear forces on the nerve. The deep peroneal nerve can be compressed at the ankle by tight ski boots, ice skates or roller blades. These mild neuropraxic injuries can be prevented readily by modification of footwear.

PEROXISOMES Small spherical organelles surrounded by a single membrane that contain a variety of enzymes such as oxidases and catalases that function in the degradation of amino acids, fatty acids and other substances. *See under* FREE RADICALS.

PERSONALITY A person's characteristic patterns of behavior that contribute to his or her uniqueness. The study of personality is concerned with the description and explanation of individual differences and consistencies. In Ancient Greece, Hippocrates suggested that there were four basic personality types, associated with the four bodily humors: melancholic (depressed; produced by an excess of black bile), choleric (irritable; produced by excess of yellow bile), sanguine (optimistic; produced by blood) and phlegmatic (calm; produced by phlegm). Sheldon et al (1954) investigated the link between temperament and body type. Endomorphs tend to be sociable, relaxed and even tempered. Mesomorphs tend to be noisy, callous and fond of physical activity. Ectomorphs tend to be restrained, self-conscious and fond of solitude. There does seem to be some relationship between body type and personality.

Sport psychology has been largely concerned with trait theories, with personality being viewed as a collection of traits. Eysenck identified the following personality types (dimensions): extravert vs. intravert; neurotic vs. stable; and intelligence vs. psychoticism. Catell (1965) proposed that personality could be expressed in terms of 16 "source traits," expressed as opposites, which make up the 16-PF questionnaire: reserved vs. outgoing; less intelligent vs. more intelligent; affected by feelings vs. emotionally stable; submissive vs. dominant; serious vs. happy-go-lucky; expedient vs. conscientious; shy vs. venturesome; tough minded vs. tender minded; trusting vs. suspicious; forthright vs. shrewd; self assured vs. apprehensive; conservative vs.

experimenting; group dependent vs. self sufficient; undisciplined self conflict vs. controlled; and relaxed vs. tense. Catell also identified eight "surface traits," such as exvia (like extraversion), anxiety, depression, arousal and fatigue. Similar to Eysenck's personality types, these surface traits are produced through combinations of source traits and represent more general mood. Extraversion refers to sociable and outgoing behavior, while intraversion refers to shy, cautious and inwardly reflective behavior. Eysenck proposed that extraverts have lower cortical arousal than intraverts and therefore they need greater external stimulation to experience the same excitement as intraverts. Athletes tend to be high in extraversion and low in anxiety. This may be due to assertiveness, sensation seeking, competitiveness, and a lack of inhibition of on-going behavior and immediate reactions. Long-distance runners tend to be more introverted than most other athletes. Sensation seeking has been regarded as part of a broader impulsive-sensation-seeking trait that represents the optimistic tendency to approach novel stimuli and explore the environment. It may have a high biological or genetic basis, with certain hormones such as testosterone playing an important role.

One of the most popular personality inventories, The Myers-Briggs Type Indicator, measures four dimensions of personality: extraversion vs. intraversion; sensing vs. intuition; thinking vs. feeling; and judging vs. perceiving.

Most contemporary researchers of personality accept the 'Big Five model' with its five major factors: Neuroticism (e.g. calm vs. worrying, hardy vs. vulnerable, secure vs. insecure); Extraversion (e.g. retiring vs. sociable, quiet vs. talkative, inhibited vs. spontaneous); Openness (e.g. conventional vs. original, unadventurous vs. daring, conservative vs. liberal); Agreeableness (e.g. irritable vs. good-natured, ruthlessness vs. soft-hearted, selfish vs. selfless); and Conscientiousness (careless vs. careful, undependable vs. reliable, negligent vs. conscientious). Proponents of trait theories argue that such theories can integrate much human behavior into meaningful wholes. Critics of this view argue that the interaction of situations and personality traits

need to be considered.

Kelly's (1955) Personal Construct theory is based on the premise that individuals strive to make sense of the world and themselves by constructing personal theories. Hypotheses (expectations) derived from these theories are tested and modified. Personality is viewed as a set of constructs, which are represented as bipolar dimensions such as open-minded vs. dogmatic. Based on Personal Construct theory, Butler (1991) designed the "performance profile" as a means of enabling an athlete to present a self-concept as a visual display that supplies information to both the athlete and the coach. It can be used to identify areas of perceived need for improvement, the athlete's beliefs as to what constitutes peak performance, areas where the athlete might resist improvement, the discrepancy between the athlete's and coach's beliefs, post-performance analysis and monitoring progress. *See also* PSYCHOLOGICAL SKILLS TRAINING.

Bibliography

Butler, R.J. (1991). *The performance profile: Developing elite performance*. London: British Olympic Association Publications.

Butler, R.J. and Hardy, L. (1992). The performance profile: Theory and application. *The Sport Psychologist* 6, 253-264.

Eysenck, H.J. (1991). Dimensions of personality: 16, 5 or 3? Criteria for a taxonomic paradigm. *Personality and Individual Differences* 12, 773-790.

Eysenck, H.J., Nias, D.K. and Cox, D.N. (1982). Sport and personality. *Advances in Behavior Research and Therapy* 4(1), 1-56.

Fisher, A.C. (l984). New directions in sport personality research. In: Silva, J.M. and Weinberg, R.S. (eds). *Psychological foundations of sport*. pp70-80. Champaign, IL: Human Kinetics.

Goldberg, L.R. (1993). The structure of phenotypic personality traits. *American Psychologist* 48, 26-34.

Kelly, G.A. (1955). *The psychology of personal constructs*. Vols. I and II. New York: Norton.

McCrae, R.R. and Costa, P.T. Jr. (1989). The structure of interpersonal traits: Wiggins' circumplex and the five-factor model. *Journal of Personality and Social Psychology* 56, 586-595.

Sheldon, W.H. (1954). *Atlas of men: A guide for somatotyping the adult male of all ages*. New York: Harper.

Silva, J.M. (1984). Personality and sport performance: Controversy and challenge. In: Silva, J.M. and Weinberg, R.S. (eds). *Psychological Foundations of Sport*. pp59-69. Champaign, IL: Human Kinetics.

Zuckerman, M.(1994). *Behavioral expressions and biosocial bases of sensation seeking*. New York: Cambridge University Press.

PERSPIRATION *See* SWEAT.

PERTHES' DISEASE   Legg-Calvé-Perthes' disease. It involves avascular necrosis of the femoral head. The exact cause is unknown. The changes in blood supply to the developing femoral head of the young child, between the ages of 2 and 8 years, increase the potential for development of this disease following injury.

PERVASIVE DEVELOPMENTAL DISORDERS
It is a broad diagnostic category for severe impairment in reciprocal social interaction or communication skills and/or the presence of stereotyped behavior, interests and activities. This category includes conditions such as autism, Asperger's disorder and Rett's disorder. A diagnosis of Pervasive Development Disorder Not Otherwise Specified may be made when a child does not meet the criteria for a specific diagnosis, but there is a severe and pervasive impairment in specified behaviors. Despite the concept of Autistic Disorder and Pervasive Developmental Disorder Not Otherwise Specified being two distinct types of pervasive developmental disorder, there is clinical evidence suggesting that Autistic Disorder and Pervasive Developmental Disorder Not Otherwise Specified are on a continuum.

Federal law in the USA does not yet distinguish between autistic disorder and other forms of pervasive developmental disorders. Autistic disorder is one of the disabilities specifically defined in the Individuals with Disabilities Act (IDEA), the federal legislation under which children and youth with disabilities receive special education and related services. IDEA, which uses the term "autism," defines the disorder as "a developmental disability significantly affecting verbal and nonverbal communication and social interaction, usually evident before the age of 3 years, which adversely affects a child's educational performance. Other characteristics often associated with autism are engagement in repetitive activities and stereotyped movements, resistance to environmental change or change in daily routines, and unusual responses to sensory experiences."

In each type of pervasive developmental disorder, infants develop normally for several months, after which delays or abnormal function become **pervasive**, affecting every aspect of life and seriously limiting the children's ability to learn in the same ways as their peers.

Bibliography

American Psychiatric Association (1994). *Diagnostic and Statistical Manual of Mental Disorders*. 4th ed. Washington, DC: American Psychiatric Association.

PES ANSERINUS   The tendinous insertion of the *sartorius*, *gracilis* and *semitendinosus* muscles onto the anteriomedial aspect of the proximal tibia. The **pes anserinus bursa** is located between the medial collateral ligament and the three *pes* tendons about 2 cm distal to the anteriomedial joint line. **Pes anserinus syndrome** is a tendinitis/bursitis that is found most commonly in long distance runners, but may also occur in sports that involve pivoting, cutting, jumping and deceleration. It is usually caused by overuse, friction or by a direct contusion. Risk factors include tight hamstrings.

PES CAVUS   Claw foot. It is a foot with a high longitudinal arch. It is usually a congenital deformity. The pes cavus is relatively inflexible as it is combined with tight calf musculature and tight plantar aponeurosis. If the cavus is significant, then a varus heel and clawing of the toes may also be present. There is decreased mobility in the subtalar joint and decreased internal rotation of the tibia during locomotion. After the foot strikes the ground, the heel remains everted, the longitudinal arch remains high and rigid, and the mid-tarsal joint does not unlock. With a relatively small weight-bearing surface, there is increased risk of pressure concentration and incorrect load distribution. As a result, there is increased risk of injuries such as stress fractures of the foot, plantar fasciitis and Achilles paratenonitis. Hammer toe may develop. Pes cavus can be treated with orthopedic shoes and, in severe cases, with surgery.

PES PLANUS   *See under* FLAT FEET.

PHAGOCYTES   *See under* LEUKOCYTE.

PHAGOCYTOSIS   *See under* ACTIVE TRANSPORT; IMMUNITY.

PHALANGES   Bones making up the skeleton of the fingers or toes. *See* SAND TOE.

PHARYNX   A musculomembranous sac between the mouth and nares (of the nose) and the esophagus (throat). The part of the pharynx above the level of the soft palate is the **nasopharynx**, which connects the posterior nares and the eustachian tube. The **oropharynx** is the portion of the pharynx that lies posterior to the mouth. It is continuous above with the nasopharynx and below with the laryngopharynx. *See also* LARYNX.

PHASIC   Intermittent.

PHENOMENOLOGY   A school of thought in psychology that regards the behavior of a person at any given moment as being primarily determined by that person's perception of the world. Each person has a unique view of the world's phenomena. A **phenomenon** is anything that is capable of being perceived. Thus, to understand another person's behavior, it is necessary to understand how he or she perceives the world.

PHENOTYPE   *See under* HEREDITY.

PHENYLALANINE   An essential, 9-carbon amino acid. When degraded, 4 of the carbons of phenylalanine enter the Krebs cycle at the fumarate stage and 4 enter through acetoacetyl CoA; therefore it is both ketogenic and glucogenic (glycogenic). The 9th carbon is lost as carbon dioxide.

PHENYLKETONURIA   An inherited condition caused by a disturbance in amino acid metabolism such that the production of the liver enzyme phenylalanine hydroxylase, which converts dietary L-phenylalanine to tyrosine, is inhibited. It is inherited as an autosomal recessive trait

Dangerous levels of L-phenylalanine can cause irreversible damage to the central nervous system. It is the only gene-based disorder that is completely treatable if detected early enough, but left untreatable phenylketonuria will result in severe mental retardation. Treatment involves following a scientifically controlled diet that eliminates foods containing phenylalanine, such as diet cola.

In the USA, 1 in 10,000 to 1 in 25,000 is born with phenylketonuria. In the USA, newborns are routinely screened for phenylketonuria. The American Academy of Pediatrics recommends that infants whose initial test was taken within the first 24 hours of life should be tested again at one to two weeks of age.

Maternal phenylketonuria occurs in women with successfully treated phenylketonuria, but who discontinued their special diet that eliminates all high protein foods. During pregnancy, high blood levels of phenylalanine in the mother damage the fetus. In up to 90% of such cases, the babies will have mental retardation and/or a small head size (microcephaly). Most of these babies do not inherit phenylketonuria, but are suffering from brain damage caused by high levels of phenylalanine during pregnancy. Maternal phenylketonuria can be prevented if these women resume their special diet prior to pregnancy and continue with it throughout the pregnancy, thus controlling blood phenylalanine levels.

Bibliography
National Organization for Rare Disorders. Http://www.rarediseases.org
National PKU News. Http://www.pkunews.org

PHILOSOPHY   (i) See under SPORTS PHILOSOPHY. (ii) A set of values and principles that guide work in a professional field. *See* HUMAN MOVEMENT; PHYSICAL EDUCATION.

Bibliography
Siedentop, D. (2004). *Introduction to physical education, fitness and sport.* 5th ed. Boston, MA: McGraw-Hill.

PHLEBITIS   *See under* VARICOSE VEINS.

PHOBIA   *See under* ANXIETY DISORDERS.

PHOSPHATE BUFFER   *See under* BUFFERING.

PHOSPHATE LOADING   *See under* PHOSPHORUS.

PHOSPHATIDATE A salt or ester of phosphatidic acid. **Phosphatidate phosphatase** is an enzyme that catalyses the hydrolysis of phosphatidate producing inorganic phosphate and 1, 2-diacylglycerol. *See under* LIPIDS.

PHOSPHATIDYLSERINE A naturally occurring, phospholipid nutrient that is required for the functioning of all cells of the body, but is most concentrated in the brain. It is used in the treatment of Alzheimer's disease and attention-deficit disorder. It attenuates cortisol during endurance and weight-training exercise, which may help speed recovery from intense training.

PHOSPHOCREATINE *See* CREATINE PHOSPHATE.

PHOSPHOFRUCTOKINASE PFK. An enzyme that exists in two forms: PFK-1 for glycolysis and PFK-2 for gluconeogenesis. In muscle, PFK-1 dominates.
 See also under ENZYME.

PHOSPHOFRUCTOKINASE DEFICIENCY Glycogenosis type 7. Tarui's disease. It is a carbohydrate processing disorder that is inherited as an autosomal recessive trait. It causes exercise intolerance, with pain, cramps and, occasionally, myoglobinuria. Onset is typically during childhood, and progression varies widely.

PHOSPHOGLYCERATE KINASE DEFICIENCY Glycogenosis type 9. It is a carbohydrate processing disorder that is inherited as an X-linked recessive trait. It may cause anemia, enlargement of the spleen, mental retardation and epilepsy. More rarely, it may cause weakness, exercise intolerance, muscle cramps and episodes of myoglobinuria.

PHOSPHOGLYCERATE MUTASE DEFICIENCY Glycogenosis type 10. It is a carbohydrate processing disorder that is inherited as an autosomal recessive trait. It causes exercise intolerance, cramps, muscle pain and, sometimes, myoglobinuria. Permanent weakness is rare.

PHOSPHOLIPIDS *See under* LIPIDS.

PHOSPHORUS An element, which, in its ionic form, is the most abundant mineral in the human body after calcium. About 85% of the phosphate is located in bone as calcium salts. It is important for bone and teeth formation, as a component of the high-energy compounds ATP and creatine phosphate, and in buffering of acidic end products of energy metabolism. Increased plasma levels of phosphorus have been found in highly trained runners after exercise. There is some evidence that acute 'phosphate loading' will enhance performance. Phosphorus supplementation over an extended period of time, however, can result in lowered blood calcium. Nutritional deficiencies are rare. When phosphate depletion has been observed, the concentrations of ATP and 2,3 diphosphoglycerate in red blood cells are decreased.

Dairy products, meat and fish are rich sources of phosphorus. 8 oz of yogurt (plain, non-fat) contains 383 mg of phosphorus. 3 oz of salmon (cooked) contains 252 mg of phosphorus. The phosphorus in bean, peas, cereals and nuts is present in a storage form of phosphate called phytic acid (phytate). Only about 50% of the phosphorus from phytate is available to humans due lack of phytases, which are enzymes that are involved in the breakdown of phytates.

The recommended dietary allowance (RDA) for phosphorus is based on the maintenance of normal serum phosphate levels in adults. In adults, the RDA is 700 mg/day.

Bibliography
Oregon State University. The Linus Pauling Institute. Micronutrient Information Center. Http://lpi.oregonstate.edu/infocenter

PHOSPHORYLASE *See under* AMP; LACTIC ACID.

PHOSPHORYLASE DEFICIENCY *See under* LACTIC ACID.

PHOSPHORYLATION The transfer of energy in the form of phosphate bonds. **Substrate-level**

phosphorylation is the transfer of phosphate ions directly from a phosphorylated intermediate or substrates to ADP without any oxidation occurring. It involves free energy coupling (i.e. combining an exergonic reaction with an endergonic reaction) so that the overall reaction is exergonic. **Oxidative phosphorylation** involves transport of electrons to oxygen via the electron transport chain, the generation of a proton gradient in the intermembranous space of the mitochondria, the ability to regulate the movement of hydrogen ions down this gradient, and the harnessing of the free energy generated from the movement of the hydrogen ions down the gradient of ADP phosphorylation to form ATP. In certain situations (e.g. heat build-up in muscles from prolonged work), the linkage between oxidation and phosphorylation can be loosened or uncoupled.

PHOSPHORYLASE *See under* ENZYME.

PHOTOSYNTHESIS The process by which plants, algae and photosynthetic bacteria use energy from sunlight to combine carbon dioxide from the atmosphere with water from the earth to form carbohydrate (usually glucose) and oxygen. In the glucose molecule, the chemical bonds between carbon and hydrogen hold energy from the sun. The energy originates from the center of the sun, where it is converted to heat by the fusion of hydrogen.

PHYSICAL ACTIVITY Bodily movement that is produced by the contraction of skeletal muscles and that substantially increases energy expenditure above resting level.
  See also EXERCISE.

PHYSICAL CULTURE *See under* RESISTANCE TRAINING.

PHYSICAL EDUCATION To pursue a lifetime of healthful physical activity, a physically educated person: has learned skills necessary to perform a variety of physical activities; knows the implications of and the benefits from involvement in physical activities; does participate regularly in physical activity; is physically fit; and values physical activity and

its contribution to a healthful lifestyle (National Association for Sport and Physical Education, 1986). A high-quality physical education program includes: opportunity to learn, meaningful content, and appropriate instruction. Instructional periods should total a minimum of 150 minutes per week (elementary) and 225 minutes per week (middle and secondary school). Qualified physical education specialists should provide a developmentally appropriate program. All students should be included, and physical activity should not be used as punishment. In the USA, data from the Centers for Disease Control and Prevention (CDC)'s School Health Policies and Programs Study (2000) found that required physical education is taught only by physical education teachers in 69.8% of elementary schools that require physical education, in 64.2% of middle/junior high schools that require physical education, and in 61.2% of senior high schools that require physical education. 94.5% of schools have students with permanent physical or cognitive disabilities who participate in required physical education. The percentage of states with policies requiring schools to implement measures to meet the physical education needs of students with disabilities varies according to the policy: mainstreaming students into regular physical education as appropriate (80.0%); providing adapted physical education as appropriate (82.2%); using modified equipment in regular physical education (59.1%); using modified facilities in regular physical education (56.8%); using teaching assistants in regular physical education (55.8%); and including physical education in individualized education plans (81.8%).
  See also DISABILITY; HEALTH; KINESIOLOGY; PHYSICAL FITNESS; PLAY.

Chronology
•c. 380 BC • Plato stated, "Gymnastics as well as music should receive careful attention in childhood and continue through life. … Now my belief is not that the good body improves the soul, but that the good soul improves the body…" (*Republic*, Book III).
•335 BC • Aristotle opened his Lyceum (also known as the Peripatic School of Philosophy). Aristotle believed that education of the body must precede that of the intellect.
•1265 • St. Thomas Aquinas sought to apply the insights of Aristotelian philosophy to medieval ecclesiastical thought. Aquinas was a Dominican friar who tried to resolve the tension

between the conflicting claims of reason (or philosophy) and faith (or theology) in his great works *Summa Theologica*. Between the 11th to 15th centuries, Crusaders brought back to Europe new religious views and concepts of Artistotle's science and dialectics. This stimulated a new skepticism in the Christian world. Aquinas was critical of the Platonic conception of humans as rational souls inhabiting powerless, material bodies. Like Aristotle, he saw the human being as a complete union of soul and body. He embraced the idea of physical fitness and recreation as a positive force in promoting social and moral well-being.

•1582 • Richard Mulcaster, headmaster at Merchant Taylors' School, and one of the most famous teachers of his time, believed that "exercise of the body should always accompany and assist the exercise of the mind."

•1693 • John Locke published *Some Thoughts Concerning Education*, which started as follows; "A sound mind in a sound body, is a short, but full description of a happy state in this world." Locke followed Cartesian (from Descartes) dualistic philosophy that the mind and body are distinct, and (in opposition to what Plato believed) that all ideas came from experience rather than being brought into the world with the soul. Education was therefore important.

•1762 • Jean Jacques Rousseau's novel *Emile* was based on the belief that the body and the intellect should develop in harmony. Rousseau believed that children should live an active outdoor life and thereby develop their senses. Rousseau depicted movement and sport as an ideal form of human activity and fulfillment.

•1774 • Johann B. Basedow's Philanthropinum was founded at Dessau in Germany, providing for the first time a gymnastic system suitable for school children. Basedow combined the educational ideas of Jean Jacques Rousseau with those of Francis Bacon and John Comenius. Emile was more influential in Germany than it was in France. In the Philanthropinum, physical activities comprised recreational activities like fencing, manual labor such as carpentry, martial arts, and summer outdoor activities such as hunting and fishing. The Philanthropinum closed in 1793.

•1786 • Johann Christoph GuthsMuths became leader of the Schnepfenthal Educational Institute. GuthsMuths' program included gymnastic skills such as exercises on the climbing mast, horizontal bar, vaulting apparatus, balance beam and rope ladders, and stunts in tumbling. GuthsMuths' manuals were the first published by a practical physical educator. His book *Gymnastics for Youth* (1793) was translated into English in 1800. Like Rousseau, GutsMuths believed that the development of the body should precede development of the mind and that girls and women should not engage in heavy physical activity.

•1804 • In Sweden, Pehr Henrik Ling was appointed to the University of Lund, where he went on to study anatomy and physiology, applying his knowledge to gymnastics. Ling believed that body movements should not be determined by apparatus, as in the German system, but that the apparatus should be designed so as to secure the desired results, whether they were military, educational or rehabilitational. He insisted that medicine and physical education must be allies and that teachers of physical education must have theoretical knowledge as well as practical ability.

•1804 • At Yverdon in Switzerland, Johann Heinrich Pestalozzi founded what Gerber (1971) describes as the "most celebrated institute in the history of education." It attracted students from all over the world. Pestalozzi, who was influenced by Jean Jacques Rousseau, believed that moral education was the foundation of the other two basic aspects of education: intellectual and practical education. He promoted development of the physical capacities of man through physical labor, but also believed in the importance of gymnastics and games. Pestalozzi influenced subsequent educational reformers such as Friedrich Froebel and Friedrich Jahn and John Dewey.

•1816 • Friedrich Ludwig Jahn of Prussia, published *Die Deutsche Turnkunst* (German Gymnastics), expressing a dislike for artificial exercises. Jahn's close friends and disciples, Charles Follen, Charles Beck and Frances Lieber, brought the Turner movement to America.

•1823 • The Round Hill School at Northampton, Massachusetts was founded by Joseph G. Cogswell and George Bancroft as a private school for boys. It was based on the philosophy of two Swiss Educators, Heinrich Pestalozzi, who was influenced by Rousseau and laid the foundations for modern pedagogy, and Phillip Emenuel von Fellenberg, who used Pestalozzi's theories.

•1825 • Charles Follen established a program of German gymnastics at Harvard and the first college gymnasium in America. The following year he established a similar program at the Boston Gymnasium, which was the first public outdoor gymnasium to be built in the nation. Under Follen's direction, students constructed equipment such as wooden horses and laid out areas for running and jumping. Gymnastics was not recognized as part of the educational program.

•1826 • Under the leadership of German immigrants, gymnastics was introduced to four of the leading men's colleges in America: Yale, Harvard, Amherst and Dartmouth.

•1827 • The Round Hill School became the first secondary school in the America to make physical education (gymnastics) a part of the regular course of instruction and Charles Beck became the first recognized teacher of physical education in America.

•1831 • Catherine Beecher's *A Course of Calisthenics for Young Ladies* was the first manual of physical education in America. Beecher was a pioneer who promoted physical education for women.

•1840 • Per H. Ling's *The General Basis of Gymnastics* was published, a year after his death. Exercises were classified into four groups: educational, aesthetic, military and medical. Ling visited Nachtegall's private gymnasium in Copenhagen 1799 – 1804 and probably read GutsMuths's *Gymnastics for the Young* that was popular in Denmark at that time. Ling believed that German gymnastics were too complicated. Ling's [Swedish] gymnastics emphasized body position rather than movement sequences, and involved spending a long time in artificial and strained postures.

•1848 • Adolph Spiess introduced his gymnastics system into the school of the Grand Duchy of Hesse. Acquainted with Jahn, GuthsMuths and other leaders of the time, Spiess was responsible for the successful development and organization of school gymnastics in Germany. Unlike Jahn, Spiess conceived of gymnastics as a pedagogical rather than a political process, part of the school life rather than the political process.

•1853 • Mathias D. Roth founded a private institution of medical gymnastics in England, published a book on Ling's free exercises, and unsuccessfully campaigned to the British Government for introduction of Swedish gymnastics into English elementary schools.

•1860 • In Belgium, Jacob Happel introduced the Belgian system of gymnastics and established an institute to prepare teachers in this system. A year later, A.S. Ulrich inaugurated the Swedish system in opposition to the Belgian system.

•1861 • Dioclesian Lewis founded the Normal Institute for Physical Education in Boston. It was the first training institute for gymnastic instructors in the USA and stayed open until 1868. Four physicians were employed from the Harvard Medical School to teach courses in anatomy, physiology and hygiene. Lewis was heavily influenced by the philosophy of Catherine Beecher. He developed a system of light gymnastics, called the 'new gymnastics,' based on the use of hand apparatus (such as light dumb bells) and set to music. It emphasized agility, grace of movement, flexibility and posture. It was popular in the 1850s through the 1870s. Lewis' system of gymnastics was the favored form for women's colleges in the 1860s.

•1861 • Matthew Vassar established Vassar Female College, based on the belief that good health was essential for the development of women's mental and moral powers. Vassar was influenced by the Swedish system of gymnastics and the works of Dioclesian Lewis.

•1864 • Catherine Beecher joined the staff of Dioclesian Lewis' new school for girls in Lexington, Massachusetts but the two had philosophical differences on calisthenics. Beecher could be regarded as the originator of the first American system of gymnastics and the first woman physical education leader in America. In the late nineteenth century, the calisthenics of Beecher and Lewis lost popularity, as most women's colleges changed to the Dudley A. Sargent's system.

•1864 • Hjalmar F. Ling, son of Per H. Ling was placed in charge of school gymnastics at the Royal Gymnastics Central Institute in Stockholm. Like his father, Hjalmar especially emphasized breathing and style. According to Gerber (1971), "were it not for the work of his son Hjalmar Ling [Swedish gymnastics] would never have been incorporated into the schools of Sweden or any of the many other countries (e.g. Denmark) which adopted it."

•1865 • The North American Gymnastics Association was established. One of its main aims was concerned with the introduction of physical education into American schools.

•1866 • The Normal School of the North American Gymnastic Union was established in New York City in order to meet the need for trained instructors in the German system of gymnastics. Its graduates became instructors in Turnvereins and public schools throughout America. They objected to the emphasis placed on games and sports in American society.

•1866 • The Calisthenium and Riding Academy at Vassar College was the first gymnasium at a woman's college in the USA.

•1868 • Vassar College became the first college in the USA that required all students to take physical education classes.

•1874 • Henry Fowle Durant founded Wellesley College. Like Matthew Vassar, Durant included sport and physical education in his plan for a women's college.

•1881 • Dudley A. Sargent founded a gymnastic training institution, the Sargent Normal School, for individuals (mainly young women attending the Harvard Annex) who were interested in becoming teachers of physical training. It later became Radcliffe College.

•1882 • The London School Board extended the Swedish system of gymnastics to boys' schools. It was not popular, and in 1893 the Board officially discontinued it for boys.

•1883 • Hartvig Nissen introduced the Swedish system of gymnastics to America, at the Swedish Health Institute in Washington, DC. He came to Washington as Vice-Consul for Norway and Sweden. Mary Hemenway, widow of Boston's prosperous shipping merchant, provided funding for teacher training in Swedish gymnastics. The teachers were trained by Baron Nils Posse. By 1890, more than 400 had been thus trained.

•1884 • N.H. Rasmussen introduced Swedish gymnastics in Denmark. When the Danish Government published a new official handbook on gymnastics, it was based primarily on the Swedish system.

•1885 • Baron Nils Posse, a graduate of the Central Institute of Gymnastics (CIG), began introducing Swedish gymnastics (medical and educational) into the Boston public schools and hospitals.

•1885 • Oberlin was the first college to organize a department of physical education for women and Blacks. It was also the first to have a woman as the head of physical education for women. Delphine Hanna established the first 4-year curriculum for a Bachelor's degree in PE for women.

•1885 • Bergman Österberg, while continuing to work for the London School Board, started a Training College for Teachers of Physical Education at Hampstead. It was the first institution to train physical education teachers in England. In 1895, it moved location and became known as Dartford College and was the first residential college for training specialist teachers in physical education. Österberg based her training on Ling's Gymnastics and, in 1887, she published a pamphlet advocating the use of the Swedish system of gymnastics for young working class women who had no access to apparatus or facilities. She did not neglect team games, however.

•1887 • Dudley A. Sargent instituted the Harvard Summer School of Physical Education, which was to prove a successful venture over a number of years. With the exception of President Eliot, the Harvard authorities were not pleased at having such an "unacademic" venture on the campus (Gerber, 1971).

•1889 • A conference at Massachusetts Institute of Technology in Boston, Massachusetts, attended by leading physical educators, had presentations from proponents of both the German and Swedish systems with the purpose being to decide what method of exercise would be most suitable for educational institutions. Funded by philanthropist Mrs. Mary Hemenway, it was called "A Conference in the Interest of Physical Training." Dudley A. Sargent stated; "What America needs is the happy combination which the European nations are trying to effect; the strength-giving qualities of the German Gymnasium, the active and energetic properties of the English sports, the grace and suppleness acquired from French calisthenics, and the beautiful poise and mechanical precision of the Swedish free movements, all regulated, systematized, and adapted to our peculiar needs and institutions."

•1889 • Mary Hemenway founded the Boston Normal School of Gymnastics (not to be confused with the Boston Normal School) that emphasized the Swedish system of gymnastics. Like the Sargent School, although it was originally open to both women and men, it became a school for women only. In 1909, Hemenway's Boston Normal School of Gymnastics became the Department of Hygiene and Physical Education of Wellesley College. It offered a 5-year course for the bachelor's degree. Boston Normal School of Gymnastics was the first of the private schools to seek collegiate affiliation. The Department was closed in 1953 when Wellesley College returned to the status of a pure liberal arts college.

•1891 • In the USA, the office of the Commissioner of Education reported on the status of physical training in the schools of 272 leading cities across the nation. 83 schools had a special director of physical education for the entire school system. Another 81 schools required that exercises must be taught by the classroom teacher. 10% of schools had established exercise programs before 1887, and of those offering physical education 41% used the German system, 29% the Swedish system, 12% Delsarte system and 18% a combination of these.

•1895 • In Britain, the Education Department gave official approval to the Swedish system of gymnastics and stated, "the higher grant for Discipline and Organization will not be paid to any school in which provision is not made for instruction in Swedish or other drill or suitable physical exercises."

•1897 • The University of Nebraska established the first major in physical education leading to a bachelor's degree.

•1899 • Thirty-one alumni of Bergman Österberg's [Dartford] College met and formed an association that came to be known as the Ling Association.

•1901 • The Teachers College of Columbia University, inspired by Thomas D. Wood, became the first institution to offer a masters degree with specialization in physical education. Wellesley College was the first to set up a graduate curriculum in physical education that was open only to persons who had completed a major in physical education at undergraduate level.

•1902 • Mills College was the first women's college in the USA to adopt the German system of gymnastics.

•1905 • The following organizations unsuccessfully sought amalgamation with the Ling Association in order to gain more recognition from the Board of Education: the British College of Physical Education (founded in 1891), the Gymnastics Teachers Institute (1897) and the National Society for Physical Education (1897). The latter three organizations advocated German gymnastics, whereas the Ling Association advocated the Swedish system.

•1907 • Under the leadership of Wilbur P. Bowen, Ypsilanti in Michigan was the first public normal school to offer specialization in physical education. Many public normal schools went on to provide specialization in physical education.

•1909 • In Britain, physical training was made a compulsory and

examinable subject in all teacher-training colleges. The Board of Education produced a new *Syllabus of Physical Training* that was largely based on Swedish gymnastics.

•1910 • A committee of the National Society for the Study of Education investigated the school health program in the USA. It defined the function of physical education as the supervision of fundamental motor activities expressed in play, games, dancing, swimming, gymnastics and athletics. It concluded that, "progress in physical education must be away from all formal, artificial kinds of movements."

•1911 • The Fédération Internationalè D'Education Physique (International Institution of Physical Education) was established by followers of the Ling system of gymnastics at an international congress in Denmark. The delegates were sympathetic to Swedish gymnastics. In 1923, it was revived as the International Federation of Educational Gymnastics. In 1930, it became the International Federation of Ling Gymnastics.

•1912 • In Britain, the Board of Education used the term 'physical education' rather than 'physical training' for the first time.

•1913 • In Japan, a physical education syllabus was published. It was based largely on Swedish gymnastics.

•1913 • Charles H. McCloy left the USA to spend thirteen years working in China. He promoted physical education through his work as a staff member of the Chinese National Council of the Young Man's Christian Association (YMCA), as director of a physical education school in Nanking (1921-1924) and as an author of several books that were published in Chinese. China had been established as a republic in 1911.

•1914 • The Ollerup Gymnastic High School was founded by Niels Bukh on the island in Denmark that was the birthplace of Hans Christian Anderson. Bukh had led a team of Danish gymnasts on an exhibition tour in 1912 through Europe including the UK. Bukh developed a Danish system of gymnastics that emphasized the development of mobility, strength and agility. It was introduced to the USA in 1925, with his exercises being taught at colleges such as Goucher, Mount Holyoke, Smith, Radcliffe and Wellesley.

•1916 • The British College of Physical Education (1891), the Gymnastic Teachers' Institute (1897) and the National Society of Physical Education (1897) amalgamated to form the British Association for Physical Training.

•1916 • John Dewey's *Democracy and Education* was published. Dewey believed in teaching the whole child and that the physical and mental could not be separated. He was convinced that play was important in education because if a child enjoyed an activity, then he or she would become more involved which would lead to greater learning. At this time, Dewey was a professor of philosophy at Columbia University and America's greatest philosopher. His ideas have become the basic educational tenets of the educational philosophy of pragmatism. In emphasizing that the curriculum is best learned by doing rather than by theorizing, Dewey's concepts were not new. Charles Pierce was the founder of pragmatism and Froebel had used many of them in his kindergarten, but Dewey extended these principles to all grades. The psychologists G. Stanley Hall, William James and Edward L. Thorndike were also important pragmatic or Progressive education movement.

•1917 • California voted in compulsory physical education for all lower schools and normal schools. In 1918 Clark Hetherington became California's first state physical education supervisor; the second of its kind in the country following New York State.

•1919 • In Austria, Karl Gaulhofer was appointed head of the department of physical education at the Federal Ministry of Education. With Margarete Streicher, Gaulhofer developed Natürliches Turnen ('natural' physical education) that emphasized outdoor activities that differed greatly from the artificial exercises of German and Swedish gymnastics.

•1919 • In Britain, the Board of Education produced a new Syllabus of Physical Education; it was still largely based of the Swedish system.

•1922 • Clark W. Hetherington published *School Program in Physical Education* in which he stated that both the German and Swedish systems of gymnastics had contributed generously to the American program, but that, "A system which has drawn its breath of life from a foreign culture radically different in its purpose from American life cannot be transplanted." He argued that America required a physical education program that would help educate children for the free and self-directing responsibilities of a democratic society. Hetherington was the foremost scholar and philosopher of physical education of his day. Along with Thomas D. Wood and Rosalind Cassidy, Hetherington was one of the architects of the 'new physical education.' Based on John Dewey's pragmatic philosophy, the 'new physical education' focused on the individual and on the development of democratic values. It moved away from the formal gymnastic systems of the late 1800s and stressed the need to include exercise, games, sports, and free play in the program. By the mid-1920s the 'new physical education' had become firmly established in the elementary and secondary schools as America's system of physical education.

•1923 • The new Soviet Government showed its regard for physical education by appointing the Supreme Council of Physical Culture. The theory of Soviet physical education was based in large part on the teachings of P.F. Lesgaft and I. Pavlov. Lesgaft stated that all life phenomena can be explained in environmental terms and that heredity was unimportant. He believed that physical exercise improved the intellectual processes and felt that people should be able to isolate and consciously control specific body movements and then apply them to any practical activity. Lesgaft was critical of foreign systems of gymnastics. Pavlov, a physiologist, declared that exercise was important for improving the functioning of the central nervous system and the body as a whole.

•1924 • The National Institute of Health and Physical Education was founded in Tokyo and in 1941 it was reorganized to become the Tokyo College of Physical Education.

•1924 • The first Ph.D. programs in education with a major in physical education were initiated at New York University and Teachers College, Columbia University.

•1927 • Thomas D. Wood and Rosalind Cassidy published *The New Physical Education: A Program of Naturalized Activities of Education Toward Citizenship*. It became one of the leading texts in physical education training programs.

•1929 • A compulsory physical education law was passed in China, following earlier influences from the West (including the introduction of gymnastics by the YMCA).

•1930 • In the USA, 39 states had enacted some form of legislation requiring physical education to be delivered in public schools.

•1933 • The Carnegie College of Physical Education became the first college in England where men could obtain specialist training. The course differed from that offered in women's colleges in that it was open only to teachers who were already qualified to teach other subjects and it had to include a general training. Two years later, Loughborough College introduced one-year courses in physical education.

•1987 • In the USA, House Congressional Resolution 97 was introduced in the Senate to encourage state and local governments to provide a high quality, daily physical-education program for children and youths from kindergarten through the twelfth grade.

•2000 • The Physical Education for Progress Act was approved by Congress, making available $375 million over the following five years. The Secretary of Education was authorized to award grants to help initiate, expand, and improve physical education programs for kindergarten through grade-12 students. Funds could be used to purchase equipment, develop curriculum, hire and/or train PE staff, and support other initiatives designed to enable students to participate in physical education activities.

•2001 • The National Association for Sport and Physical Education (NASPE) reported that states in the USA vary widely in the degree to which they mandate physical education as part of the state education system. Although states typically set minimum standards, there is wide variance in the way that individual school districts interpret those standards.

Bibliography

Gallahue, D. and Cleland, F. (2003). *Developmental physical education for all children*. Champaign, IL: Human Kinetics.

Gerber, E.W. (1971). *Innovators and institutions in physical education*. Philadelphia: Lea & Febiger.

Hackensmith, C.W. (1966). *History of Physical Education*. New York: Harper and Row.

McIntosh, P.C. (1968). *Physical Education in England since 1800*. London: Bell and Hyman.

McIntosh, P.C. et al. (1981). *Landmarks in the history of physical education*. London: Routledge and Kegan Paul.

Mechikoff, R.A. and Estes, S.G. (2002). *A history and philosophy of sport and physical education. From ancient civilization to the modern world*. 3rd ed Boston, MA: McGraw-Hill.

National Association for Sport and Physical Education (1992). *Outcomes of quality physical education programs*. Reston, VA: National Association for Sport and Physical Education.

National Association for Sport and Physical Education (1995). *Moving into the future: National Standards for Physical Education*. Reston, VA: National Association for Sport and Physical Education.

National Association for Sport and Physical Education (2002). *Active start: A statement of physical activity guidelines for children birth to five years.* Reston, VA: National Association for Sport and Physical Education.

National Association for Sport and Physical Education (2003). *Concepts and principles of physical education: What every student needs to know.* Reston, VA: National Association for Sport and Physical Education.

National Association for Sport and Physical Education (2004). *Physical activity for children: A statement of guidelines.* Reston, VA: National Association for Sport and Physical Education.

National Association for Sport and Physical Education (2004). *Moving into the future: National Standards for Physical Education* 2nd ed. Reston, VA: National Association for Sport and Physical Education.

Rice, E.A., Hutchinson, J.L. and Lee, M. (1958). *A brief history of physical education.* 4th ed. New York: The Ronald Press Company.

Swanson, R.A. and Spears, B. (1995). *History of sport and physical education in the United States.* 4th ed. Boston, MA: WCB/McGraw-Hill.

Van Dalen, D.B. and Bennett, B.L. (1973). *A world history of physical education.* 2nd ed. Englewood Cliffs, NJ: Prentice Hall.

Zeigler, E.F. (1979). *History of physical education and sport.* Englewood Cliffs, NJ: Prentice Hall.

PHYSICAL FITNESS A set of attributes that people have or achieve relating to the ability to perform physical activity. A distinction can be made between health-related fitness and skill-related fitness. The distinction is couched in terms of what the fitness is required for. **Health-related fitness** involves exercise undertaken for reasons related to maintaining or improving health, and emphasizes cardiovascular fitness, flexibility, strength and muscular endurance. **Skill-related fitness** involves exercise undertaken for reasons of maintaining or improving skill in sport and emphasizes cardiovascular fitness, flexibility, strength, muscular endurance, and also speed, power, agility, balance and coordination. Historically, physical fitness for military purposes has been important. *See also* TRAINING.

Chronology

•380 BC • Plato, a pupil of Socrates, held that gymnastics should not be promoted as end in itself, but rather as a means of developing military fitness and healthy bodies to house healthy minds. Plato proposed a plan in which children would play childhood games until they were 6 years of age, from when they would begin a more systematic study of dancing, riding, archery and javelin throwing.

•264 BC • The first gladiatorial games were offered in Rome by the sons of Junus Brutus Pera in their father's honor after he had died. Professional gladiators were mainly condemned criminals,

prisoners of war and slaves. They fought either animals or each other, generally until death. Blood as a form of entertainment had a political purpose: to teach the local Romans how to fight in preparation for visits outside their empire and to display the strength and courage of the Roman citizen to unemployed visitors to the city of Rome.

•170 AD • Claudius Galen, a Greek, became physician to the son of Emperor Marcus Aurelius. He had studied in Asia Minor before practicing in Alexandria and Rome, and developed systematic descriptions of the human body. He also became a physician for gladiators. Galen was critical of the excessive and brutish training program for professional athletes and gladiators. He believed that physical education should enable men to enjoy the glowing health of harmoniously proportioned bodies and should make them alert and physically fit for civil and martial duties.

•326 AD • Emperor Constantine, who had legalized the practice of Christianity in 313 AD, issued a decree forbidding the condemnation of criminals to the beasts. This effectively dried up the main supply of gladiators. In 312 AD, Emperor Constantine was converted to Christianity.

•404 AD • Telemachus, a Christian monk, jumped into a gladiatorial arena and tried to separate the two gladiators. The crowd climbed into the arena and killed the monk. Emperor Honorius issued an edict forbidding gladiatorial fights, but animal combats continued for another century. In 476 AD, the Roman Empire collapsed in the West.

•1095 • The first Crusade was called by Pope Urban II in an effort to rescue Jerusalem from Muslim Turks who were threatening the Byzantine Empire and denying Christian pilgrims access to the Holy Land. The period of the Crusaders lasted until 1291, failing in their original purpose of halting the advance of Islam.

•1179 • Pope Alexander III forbade the holding of tournaments (contests of armed horsemen) and refused Christian burial to those who died in them. In England, tournaments were introduced in the twelfth century by King Richard I, who attributed the courage and skill of the French in battle to their practical experience in tournaments. The tournament was the favorite peacetime amusement of the people. Chivalric education involved training young men to observe the social and moral customs of war, religion and gallantry that had been formulated by feudal society. Acceptance of the code of behavior was one of the requirements of knighthood. It was strong through to 1350, but declined through to the sixteenth century.

•1365 • King Edward III, in view of war with the French, proclaimed that men must focus on their bow and arrow shooting skills rather than engage in activities such as football or cockfighting "with no profit in them."

•1423 • La Giocosa, one of the court schools of the Renaissance, under the mastership of Vittorino da Feltre, was established by Gianfrancesco Gonzaga, the Lord of Mantua. At La Giocosa, there was a program of physical education that included games, riding, running, leaping, fencing and ball games, led by specialist teachers. Exercise was deemed necessary for a number of reasons including good health, training in the martial arts and development of a rugged spirit.

•1457 • James II, the King of Scotland, attempted to ban golf, because many of the populace were playing golf rather than preparing for war against the English.

•1804 • Christian VII, the King of Denmark appointed Franz Nachtegall professor of gymnastics at the University and director of the Military Gymnastic Institute. Nachtegall was appointed superintendent of civilian and military gymnastics in 1821. He advocated and taught the gymnastics of Johann Christoph GuthsMuths.

•1816 • Friedrich Ludwig Jahn of Prussia, published *Die Deutsche Turnkunst* (German Gymnastics), expressing a dislike for artificial exercises. To Jahn, gymnastics were a tool for achieving political goals. His methods were not based on anatomy and physiology. The supreme aim of physical education was to develop sturdy citizens possessing a love for their homeland and to win the War of Liberation against the French, which had begun three years earlier.

•1858 • In England, Archibald MacLaren opened a gymnasium in Oxford. Gymnasia with equipment similar to MacLaren's were built at public schools such as Wellington and Winchester, but gymnastics never posed a threat to the standing of team games because gymnastics was run by non-commissioned army officers, who were regarded as being of inferior social status. MacLaren's system had come to be used in the military and naval schools to supplement games and sports to improve the physical fitness of soldiers and sailors. In 1861, the British Government built a gymnasium for the army at Aldershot modeled after MacLaren's Oxford Gymnasium.

•1870 • At a time when the House of Commons in Britain received the Education Bill, Mathias D. Roth approached influential members of the House with the argument that sports and games were inadequate exercise for elementary school children and that only gymnastics would prepare them properly for industrial work and as candidates for the army and navy. Despite Roth's lobbying, the Education Bill was passed without including compulsory gymnastics for elementary school children.

•1902 • In Britain, the Board of Education, in consultation with the War Office, published *A Model Course of Physical Training*. It mainly comprised military drill and encouraged schools to appoint Army instructors. It was not well received by the National Union of Teachers. A Government Interdepartmental Committee later found it unsatisfactory and in 1904 produced its own *Syllabus of Physical Exercises*. Another Interdepartmental Committee, on Physical Deterioration, could not prevent a decline in support for military drill over the next decade and an increase in support for Swedish drill.

•1904 • In Denmark, four years after educational gymnastics was demilitarized, school gymnastics was separated from military gymnastics in every way.

•1905 • President Theodore Roosevelt ordered that all classes at West Point participate in the gymnastics program of Colonel Koehler, who in 1892 had added to his calisthenics requirement riding, fencing, boxing, wrestling, and swimming.

•1915 • At a time when the majority position in the education press seemed to favor physical education over military drill, the Massachusetts Commission on Military Education issued a report that opposed military training for boys between the ages of 14 and 21 years, because it created an aversion to military life. Dudley A. Sargent led the battle for gymnastics against the principals of the Boston schools who held out for military drill. At Bowdoin College, students voted between gymnastics and military drill for a requirement. The result was unanimously in favor of gymnastics.

•1916 • The American Physical Education Association (APEA) officially approved Dudley A. Sargent's opposition to military training substituting physical education in Massachusetts schools.

•1916 • In New York State, the Welsh Bill prescribed mandatory physical training (a minimum of 20 minutes per day) for all students above the age of 8 years. A companion law, the Slater Bill, set up a Military Training Commission whose purpose was to establish and oversee military training for young men between the ages of 16 and 19 years. The Commission could legally compel military training for a maximum of three hours per week on top of what was provided by the Welsh Bill.

•1917 • In the USA, the National Education Association's Committee on Military Training in the Public Schools issued a report in which it argued against the use of military drill in elementary and secondary schools. It recommended that schools institute compulsory physical education as part of a comprehensive drive for national unity and security.

•1918 • In the Soviet Union, a year after the October (Bolshevik) Revolution in the Soviet Union in which the monarchy was overturned and communism came to rule, Lenin established Vsevobuch, an organization that trained individuals in several military disciplines including physical training. The previous year he signed a decree for the establishment of regular physical activity in the school system.

•1923 • When Joseph H. Pilates, who was born near Dusseldorf in 1880, was asked to teach his fitness system to the Germany army he decided to emigrate to the USA where he opened a studio in New York. His exercise method emphasizes pelvic, core and thoracic stabilization, breathing, posture, and mind-body harmony. Influenced by Eastern philosophy, his method was embraced by popular dance instructors and choreographers such as Martha Graham (the 'mother of modern dance'), George Balanchine (artistic director of the New York Ballet) and Jerome Robbins. As a child, Pilates overcame physical limitations such as rickets and asthma to become an accomplished in many sports.

•1931 • The Soviet government launched an awards system to encourage the masses to develop their physical fitness under the title "Ready for Labor and Defense."

•1935 • The City of Santa Monica hired UCLA coach Cecil Hollingsworth to teach gymnastics at Muscle Beach. By the late 1930s there were around 50 regulars and thousands of spectators came to watch them. Harold Zinkin has described Muscle Beach as the "birth place of the physical-fitness boom in America." Hollywood celebrities, such as Mae West and Kirk Douglas, frequented Muscle Beach along with many athletes, circus performers, wrestlers, college gymnasts and movie stuntmen. Former Muscle Beach regulars were employed by the military to train new recruits during World War II. Muscle Beach in Santa Monica was closed in 1959, after five Muscle Beach users who lived in a board-walk apartment were allegedly found partying with two underage girls. The City bulldozed Muscle Beach and turned it into Beach Park 4. About the same time, a small group of weightlifters was using less prominent facility called 'The Pen' that was owned and operated by the City of Los Angeles. It is now known as 'Muscle Beach Venice.'

•1936 • Jack LaLanne opened America's first health club, in Oakland, California. It included a health-food store and a juice bar.

•1940 • Victor Tanny and his brother Armand opened a gym on Second Street in Santa Monica. They opened another gym the following year in Long Beach. Coastal blackouts during World War II forced the Tanny's gyms to close. By 1947, Vic Tanny had opened several gyms around Los Angeles, and by 1960 he owned 84 gyms throughout the country. In developing lavish facilities, Tanny and his brother helped to create the modern health club and inspired many others to build gyms. Tanny sold his clubs in 1963. Joe Gold, a close friend of the Tannys, opened the first Gold's Gym in 1964 about two blocks from Muscle Beach. Gold, served in the Coast Guard and suffered spinal injuries that later made it necessary for him to use a wheelchair.

•1942 • In the USA, President Franklin Roosevelt established in the Office of Defense, Health and Welfare Services, a Division of Physical Fitness to promote interest in health and physical fitness among all age groups.

•1943 • Out of 9 million registrants examined for the armed services of the USA, almost 3 million were found to be unfit for any form of military duty. At the War Conference, the Chief of Athletics and Recreation of the Services Division of the US Army stated: "Our physical programs in high schools have been a miserable failure. Physical Education through play must be discarded and a more rugged program substituted."

•1956 • In the USA, a special White House Conference on the fitness of school children was held in response to the Minimum Muscular Fitness Test of Hans Kraus and Sonya Weber in 1953 that involved 4,264 US school children and 2,870 European school children from comparable urban and suburban communities. 57.9% of US children failed; but only 8.7% of the Europeans failed. Later in the same year, the American Association for Health, Physical Education and Recreation (AAHPER) held a Fitness Conference in Washington and President Dwight Eisenhower established a President's Council on Youth Fitness and a President's Citizens Advisory Committee on the Fitness of American Youth.

•1958 • Operation Fitness was launched by the American Association for Health, Physical Education and Recreation (AAHPER) to stimulate fitness nationally in the USA.

•1958 • The Jack LaLanne Show was syndicated on national television in America. It had begun as a local program in San Francisco in 1951 and was on air until 1984. LaLanne offered motivational talks, nutritional advice and exercises that people could be performed at home.

•1962 • In an article entitled "The Vigor We Need" published in *Sports Illustrated* (16 July), President John F. Kennedy emphasized the importance of physical fitness for guaranteeing peace and also the "physical hardihood" that enabled Americans to overcome "tenacious foes" in the two World Wars. In the same year, an article told to W. Gill for a newspaper by R.M. Marshall, entitled "Toughening Our Soft Generation," stated that 40% of men called under military draft between 1948 and 1962 had been declared ineligible (most for physical defects). Marshall also pointed to the Soviet Union's "trouncing" of the USA in the Summer Olympics of 1956 and 1960.

•1967 • Bill Bowerman, the University of Oregon track coach, published a book called *Jogging*, which became an instant best seller and inspired America's jogging craze.

•1968 • Kenneth Cooper, a medical doctor for the US Air Force, published *Aerobics*, followed two years later by *The New Aerobics*. These two popular books established a physiological rationale for using exercise to promote a healthy lifestyle.

•1969 • Jackie Sorenson started 'Aerobic Dance,' which was a choreographed set of dance patterns set to music with the goal of improving cardiovascular fitness.

•1969 • Judi Sheppard Missett created 'Jazzercise,' which combined jazz dance with cardiovascular exercise.

•1970 • Ron Fletcher, a Martha Graham dancer who had consulted with Pilates in the 1940s, opened a studio in Beverley Hills that attracted many Hollywood celebrities. In the 1990s, Pilates' techniques became popular in the field of rehabilitation, where most Pilates exercises are performed using apparatus.

•1972 • Mildred Cooper, Kenneth Cooper's wife, published *Aerobics for Women*.

•1982 • Jane Fonda, a Hollywood actress, released her first fitness video, following the best-selling *Jane Fonda's Workout Book* (1981).

•1984 • In the USA, the National Children and Youth Fitness Study (NCYFS I) showed that 61.7% of students in grades 10 to 12 participated in vigorous physical activity for 20 or more minutes 3 or more days a week.

•1984 • In *The Exercise Myth*, H.A. Solomon, a physician, stated, "The ideal exercise in virtually every respect is walking. Certainly nothing could be more convenient."

•1985 • President Ronald Reagan established the President's Commission on Americans Outdoors. It was found that Americans look to mountains, seaside, lakes and playgrounds for exercise and healthy leisure. 48% of Americans identified themselves as "outdoor people." It was also found that 155 million people walk for pleasure, 93 million people use bicycles, 50 million hike on trails, 11 million ski on trails, 10 million ride horses on trails and 5 million go backpacking.

•1985 • The President's Council on Physical Fitness and the Sports School Population Fitness Survey found that 70% of all girls (aged 6 to 17 years) tested could not do more than one pull up, with 55% not being able to do even one. 40% of boys, ages 6 to 12 years, could not do more than one pull up and 25% could not do any.

•1986 • The Young Men's Christian Association (YMCA) of the USA introduced the YMCA Fitness Leaders course, a standard program for training and certifying leaders of fitness classes.

•1988 • Physical Best was introduced by the American Alliance for

Health, Physical Education, Recreation and Dance (AAHPERD) to replace the Health-Related Physical Fitness Test. Designed to help students meet its National Association for Sport and Physical Education (NASPE)'s health-related standards, it involved cardiovascular endurance, body composition, flexibility, and upper-body and abdominal strength and endurance.

•1990 • The Youth Risk Behavior Survey, a component of the Youth Risk Behavior Surveillance System, asked a representative sample of 11,631 students in grades 9 to 12 in the 50 states, the District of Columbia, Puerto Rico and the Virgin Islands to report how many of the 14 days preceding the survey they had been vigorously active (i.e. "at least 20 minutes of hard exercise that made you breathe heavily and made your heart beat fast"). It was found that 37% of students reported being vigorously active three or more times a week, but it was less among female students (24.8%) than male students (49.6%).

•1998 • The National Association for Sport and Physical Education introduced the first-ever physical activity guidelines for children 5 to 12 years of age, calling for a minimum of 30 minutes of physical activity per day. This recommendation was revised in 2004 to include a minimum of 60 minutes and up to several hours of physical activity per day.

Bibliography

American College of Sports Medicine (2000). *ACSM's guidelines for exercise testing and prescription.* 6th ed. Philadelphia, PA: Lippincott Williams and Wilkins.

American College of Sports Medicine (2001). *ACSM's resource manual for Guidelines for Exercise Testing & Prescription.* 4th ed. Philadelphia, PA: Lippincott Williams & Wilkins.

American College of Sports Medicine (2003). *ACSM fitness book.* 3rd ed. Champaign, IL: Human Kinetics.

Balanced Body, Inc; Http://www.pilates.com

Brooks, D.S. (2004). *The complete book of personal training.* Champaign, IL: Human Kinetics.

Corbin, C.B. et al. (2005). *Concepts of physical fitness: Active lifestyles for wellness.* 12th ed. Boston, MA: McGraw-Hill.

Durstine, J.L. and Moore, G.E. (2003). *ACSM's Exercise management for persons with chronic diseases and disabilities.* 2nd ed. Champaign, IL: Human Kinetics.

Earle, R.W. and Baechle, T.R. (2004). *NSCA's Essentials of personal training.* Champaign, IL: Human Kinetics.

Fahey, T.D., Insel, P.M. and Roth, W.T. (2005). *Fit and well: Core concepts and labs in physical fitness and wellness.* 6th ed. Boston, MA: McGraw-Hill.

Green, J. (1986). *Fit for America. Health, fitness, sport and American society.* New York: Pantheon Books.

Greenberg, J.S., Dintiman, G.B. and Oakes, B.M. (2004). *Physical fitness and wellness. Changing the way you look, feel and perform.* 3rd ed. Champaign, IL: Human Kinetics.

Griffin, J.C. (1998). *Client-centered exercise prescription.* Champaign, IL: Human Kinetics.

Hardman, A.E. and Stensel, D.J. (2004). *Physical activity and health. The evidence explained.* London: Routledge.

Heyward, V.H. (2002). *Advanced fitness assessment and exercise prescription.* 4th ed. Champaign, IL: Human Kinetics.

Howley, E.T. and Franks, B.D. (2003). *Health fitness instructor's handbook.* 4th ed. Champaign, IL: Human Kinetics.

Isaacs, L.D. and Pohlman, R.L. (2004). *Preparing for the ACSM Health/Fitness Instructor Certification examination.* 2nd ed. Champaign, IL: Human Kinetics.

Jackson, A.W. et al. (2004). *Physical activity for health and fitness.* Champaign, IL: Human Kinetics.

Mackinnon, L. et al. (2003). *Exercise management: Concepts and professional practice.* Champaign, IL: Human Kinetics.

Nieman, D.C. (2003). *Exercise testing and prescription.* 5th ed. Boston, MA: McGraw-Hill.

O'Brien, T.S. (2003). *The personal trainer's handbook.* 2nd ed. Champaign, IL: Human Kinetics.

Powers, S.K. and Dodd, S.L. (2003). *Total fitness and wellness.* 3rd ed. San Francisco, CA: Benjamin Cummings.

Sharkey, B.J. (2002). *Fitness and health.* 5th ed. Champaign, IL: Human Kinetics.

Solomon, H.A. (1984). *The exercise myth.* Orlando, FL: Harcourt Brace Jovanovich.

Swain, D.P. and Leutholtz, B.C. (2002). *Exercise prescription: A case study approach to the ACSM guidelines.* Champaign, IL: Human Kinetics.

The official Jack La Lanne World Wide Web Site. Http://www.jacklalanne.com

YMCA (1999). *Principles of health and fitness.* 3rd ed. Champaign, IL: Human Kinetics.

Zinkin, H. and Hearn, B. (1999). *Remembering Muscle beach. Where hard bodies begun. Photographs and memories.* Santa Monica, CA: Angel City Press.

PHYSIQUE The natural constitution, or physical structure, of a person. *See under* GROWTH.

PHYSIOLOGY, HUMAN The science of the functioning of the body.

Chronology

•1757 • The first volume of lbrecht von Haller's *Elementa Physiologiae Corporis Humani* (The Elements of the Physiology of the Human Body) was published. It marked the modernization of physiology.

•1837 • German physiologist Heinrich Gustav Magnus first analyzed blood and corrected a flaw in Antoine L. Lavoisier's explanation. Lavoisier had assumed that hydrogen and carbon were oxygenated in the lungs, but Magnus argued that combustion must occur throughout the body and not just in the lungs. His experiments showed that both carbon dioxide and oxygen existed in arterial and venous blood.

Bibliography

Germann, W.J. and Stanfield, C.L. (2001). *Principles of human physiology.* San Francisco, CA: Benjamin Cummings.

Marieb, E.N. (2002). *Anatomy and physiology*. San Francisco, CA: Benjamin Cummings.

Tortora, G.J. and Grabowski, S.R. (2003). *Principles of anatomy and physiology*. 10th ed. New York: John Wiley and Sons.

Vander, A., Sherman, J. and Luciano, D. (2001). *Human physiology. The mechanisms of body function*. 8th edition. Boston, MA: McGraw-Hill.

West, J.B. (2004). *Respiratory physiology*. 7th ed. Philadelphia, PA: Lippincott Williams & Wilkins.

PHYSIS *See* EPIPHYSEAL GROWTH PLATE.

PHYTOCHEMICALS A group of thousands of chemicals found in plants that may have health protective effects for humans, but are not essential for life. One of the largest categories of phytochemicals is the flavonoids, of which more than 4,000 have been identified in plants such as herbs. Examples of herbs that provide substantial amounts of flavonoids are chamomile, onions, rosemary, sage and thyme. Research has suggested that flavonoids extend the activity of vitamin C, act as antioxidants, protect LDL cholesterol from oxidation, inhibit platelet aggregation, and act as anti-inflammatory and anti-tumor agents.

See also under FRENCH PARADOX; ZOO-CHEMICALS.

Bibliography
Craig, W.J. (1999). Health-promoting properties of common herbs. *American Journal of Clinical Nutrition* 70(3S), S491-S499.

PHYTOSTEROLS *See under* STEROIDS.

PICA An eating disorder typically defined as the persistent eating of nonnutritive substances for a period of at least one month at an age in which this behavior is developmentally inappropriate (e.g. over 18 to 24 months of age).

PICKWICKIAN SYNDROME *See under* HYPOVENTILATION; SLEEP-WAKE CYCLE.

PIGEON CHEST *See under* PECTUS DEFORMITIES.

PILATES *See under* PHYSICAL FITNESS.

PINEAL GLAND A small lobe in the forebrain that is located near to the center of brain in humans. It secretes the hormone melatonin. *See* JET LAG.

PINNA *See under* CAULIFLOWER EAR.

PINOCYTOSIS *See under* ACTIVE TRANSPORT.

PIRIFORMIS SYNDROME A rare condition that can develop due to compression of the sciatic nerve as it exits deep to the *piriformis* muscle posteriorly. The ***piriformis*** is a muscle that has its origin on the anterior aspect of the sacrum from the 2nd sacral to 4th sacral vertebrae (S2 to S4) and its insertion on the upper surface of the greater trochanter of the femur. The sciatic nerve travels underneath the *piriformis* and superior to the *gemellus superior* and *gemellus inferior* muscles in 80 to 85% of the population. In 15 to 20% of the population, the nerve passes directly through the *piriformis*, leaving it vulnerable to entrapment that may occur if the *piriformis* is irritated and goes into spasm.

PISIFORM One of the carpal bones in the proximal row.

PITUITARY GLAND An endocrine gland located beneath the base of the brain. It is subdivided into the **anterior pituitary gland** (**hypophysis**) and the **posterior pituitary gland** (**neurohypophysis**). Hormones secreted by the anterior pituitary gland are thyrotropin, corticotropin, gonadotropic hormone, prolactin and endorphins. The posterior pituitary gland does not actually synthesize its own hormones. They are produced in the hypothalamus and secreted into the posterior gland. The posterior pituitary gland secretes vasopressin and oxytocin. The release of hormones from the posterior gland is neurally controlled.

PLACENTA The organ responsible for metabolic interchange between fetus and mother.

PLANAR Confined to a single plane.

PLANE A flat surface. A surface such that a straight

line that joins any two of its points lies entirely in that surface. An **inclined plane** is a plane at an angle to some force or reference line.

Three **cardinal (primary) planes** describe position of the human body: sagittal, frontal and transverse. Each cardinal plane bisects the body and pass through the center of gravity. There are an infinite number of planes parallel to the cardinal planes.

The **sagittal (anterioposterior) plane** is a vertical plane that divides the body into right and left portions. The plane that divides the body into these equal portions is termed the **mid-sagittal plane**. The term **medial** refers to relative locations that are closer to this mid-sagittal plane, and **lateral** refers to locations that are farther from the mid-sagittal plane. The **frontal (coronal) plane** is a vertical plane that divides the body into front and rear portions. It is perpendicular to the sagittal plane. The term **anterior** refers to relative locations that are closer to the front of the body, while **posterior** means toward the rear. The **transverse plane** is a horizontal plane that divides the body into upper and lower portions. It is perpendicular to both sagittal and frontal planes. The term **superior** refers to relative locations that are toward the top of the head, while **inferior** means toward the soles of the feet.

Axes of the body are formed by the intersection of planes. The rotational movement of a body segment occurs in a plane and around an axis. The **lateral axis (x-axis)** is the intersection of the frontal and transverse planes. The **longitudinal (vertical) axis (y-axis)** is the intersection of the sagittal and frontal planes. The **sagittal axis (z-axis)** is the intersection of the sagittal and transverse planes. A **principle axis** is directed through a body's center of gravity.

PLANTAR FASCIA   Fascia that runs from the calcaneus to the heads of the metatarsals. It acts as a truss, maintaining the medial longitudinal arch of the foot and assisting with shock absorption during weight-bearing activities. In evolutionary terms, the plantar fascia is associated with the time when the Achilles tendon extended to the toes.

The most common site of heel pain is the medial calcaneal tuberosity, which is the origin of the plantar fascia and of the following muscles: *flexor digitorum brevis*, *quadratus plantae* and *abductor hallucis*. A **heel spur** ('**traction spur**') is calcification that may occur at the attachment of the plantar fascia to the medial calcaneal tuberosity.

PLANTAR FASCIITIS   Inflammation of the plantar fascia, either at its attachment to the calcaneus or more distal along the plantar fascia itself. It occurs when the plantar fascia is stretched, and is a common injury in both athletes and non-athletes. In athletes, the cause is most likely related to a single trauma (e.g. stepping on a rock in the heel region) or chronic stress of the plantar fascia (e.g. the repetitive stress of running especially when good arch support is lacking in the shoes). Anatomical factors associated with plantar fasciitis include pronation, pes cavus and leg length discrepancy. Pronation increases the tension placed on the plantar fascia during weight bearing. Achilles tendon tightness often causes compensatory pronation. Leg length discrepancy may contribute to the development of plantar fasciitis by causing pronation on the side of the short leg.

The low incidence of plantar fasciitis in barefoot populations may be accounted for by an adaptation from barefoot running that transfers the impact to the yielding musculature, sparing the plantar fascia. When running barefoot on hard surfaces, a runner compensates for the lack of cushioning underfoot by plantar flexing the foot at contact, thus giving a softer landing.

Bibliography

Frederick, E.C. (1986). Kinematically mediated effects of sports shoe design: A review. *Journal of Sports Sciences* 4, 169-184.

Warburton, M. (2001). Barefoot running. *Sportscience* 5(3). Http://www.sportsci.org

PLANTAR-FLEXED FIRST RAY A 1st metatarsal bone with a neutral position below the level of the lesser metatarsals, but can be moved back to or above that level by some force applied to its plantar aspect. Compensation takes place by dorsal flexing the first ray with subtalar joint pronation. Plantar-flexed first ray may be associated with conditions such as hammer toes, Haglund's deformity, plantar fasciitis, low back pain and lateral knee pain.

Bibliography
Clinicians Corner. Http://www.footmaxx.com/clinicians

PLANTAR GRASP REFLEX *See* BABINKSI REFLEX.

PLANTAR KERATOSIS *See under* CORN.

PLANTIGRADE A plantigrade position of the foot is characterized by walking or running on the full sole of the foot.

PLASMA i) See BLOOD PLASMA. ii) *See under* LYMPH.

PLASMA EXPANDERS Substances that are used to increase the volume of plasma in the blood and are preparations based on gelatin, polygeline and hetastarch, e.g. Gelofusine and Haemaccel.

PLASMA MEMBRANE *See under* CELL

PLASMA VOLUME *See under* BLOOD PLASMA.

PLASMINOGEN A precursor of **plasmin**, an enzyme that digests the protein fibrin. **Plasminogen activator** is an enzyme that catalyses the conversion of plasminogen to plasmin. See BLOOD CLOTTING.

PLASTIC DEFORMATION A strain in a material that is permanent and will not recover when the stress is released. Unlike an elastic material, a plastic material retains its change in size and shape when the load causing the change is removed. Deformation occurs instantly when a load is applied and continues to occur as long as the load is applied or until the material fails, and there is no dependency on the rate of loading. The **plastic range** is the strain range between the elastic limit and the failure point. A **ductile material** is one that has a large plastic deformation before it breaks. Metals are typically the most ductile materials (i.e. they can be shaped by hammering, rolling or pulling without fracturing and they can be fabricated by forging or by casting, depending on the specific metal or alloy). **Necking** is a phenomenon that occurs as a material is deformed under tension in the plastic range: the cross-sectional area of the material decreases as the material lengthens.

PLATELETS Thrombocytes. These are a type of blood cell that are the cytoplasmic fragments of megakaryocytes, circulating as small discs in the peripheral blood. They are responsible for hemostasis (the stoppage of bleeding) and maintaining the endothelial lining of the blood vessels. During hemostasis, platelets clump together and adhere to the injured vessel in this area to form a plug and further inhibit bleeding. They have a short life span. Aged platelets are removed by fixed macrophages. *See under* CARDIOVASCULAR DISEASE.

PLAY Activity that is intrinsically motivated, i.e. activity done for its own sake without extrinsic rewards. It is the primary way in which children learn about their bodies and movement capabilities. Children's free play is characterized by the absence of external controls or constraints, but it often ends up being controlled by adult intervention. While children's play tends to be romanticized, it may involve aggressive pranks, vandalism or bullying.

Piaget argued that behaviors become play when they are repeated for functional pleasure. Activities pursued for functional pleasure appear early in the sensorimotor period. An infant repeating movements such as shaking a rattle over and over, while exhibiting pleasure, is an example of early play. By $2\frac{1}{2}$ to $3\frac{1}{2}$ years of age, children may start to display an awareness of each other and even to imitate each other. Significant social interaction, however, does not occur until $3\frac{1}{2}$ to $4\frac{1}{2}$ years. Cooperative play develops at $4\frac{1}{2}$ to 5 years and involves group-oriented games. Group leadership tends to be determined by the individual who is superior at performance of physical activities such as running and throwing. A distinction can be made between developmental and nondevelopmental play apparatus. **Developmental play apparatus** fosters skill development, e.g.

jungle gym, climbing pole and chinning bar for strength development. **Nondevelopmental play apparatus** includes slides, swings, merry-go-rounds and see-saws. Performance suffers when a child is required to attempt a motor task with equipment that is not developmentally appropriate. *See also under* SPORT.

Chronology

•1826 • Friedrich Froebel, an orthodox Protestant from Germany, published *The Education of Man*. Froebel believed that "play is the highest phase of child development" and his concepts of kindergarten and education through self-activity (observing, discovering and creating) were developed on a worldwide basis (including the first private kindergarten in America at Wisconsin in 1855). In 1851, the Prussian government perceived Froebel's ideas as threatening to the nation's stability and banned kindergartens.

•1838 • In *Health and Beauty: An Explanation of the Laws of Growth and Exercise*, John Bell observed that the absence of city playgrounds, especially for girls, made necessary the establishment of methodical exercise in schools.

•1862 • John Swett became the Superintendent of Public Instruction for the State of California. Swett was an advocate of gymnastics and calisthenics rather than military drill, and emphasized the value of play in education.

•1885 • Boston Sand Garden was the first supervised American playground for children. It was built by the Boston Women's Club and provided sand piles for children to play.

•1891 • The Central Committee for the Advancement of Folk and Child Play in Germany was formed with Emil T. von Schenckdorff as chairman and with the broad aim of "embodiment of play in the life of the people." This committee advocated games and outdoor activities rather than the gymnastics of Adolf Spiess and Friedrich Jahn, and its work was strengthened in 1909 by the Prussian Government's publication of a new instruction manual that officially introduced the 'new' physical education to schools.

•1900 • Joseph Lee, a philanthropist and the 'father of the American playground,' proposed that a model playground be developed.

•1906 • The Playground Association of America was founded largely through the efforts of Luther Gulick and Henry Curtis to induce both municipal and rural communities to organize playgrounds and recreation centers. Curtis had been a student of G. Stanley Hall. With respect to the theory of play, Gulick followed the thinking of G. Stanley Hall in drawing connections between the moral and physical development of the athlete and the skills of the citizen of modern society.

•1907 • *The Normal Course in Play*, prepared by a committee under Clark Hetherington, represented the first attempt to outline a scientific, comprehensive training for recreation workers.

•1907 • John Mason Tyler, Professor of Biology at Amherst College, published *Growth and Education*. This was an influential book on the application of biological principles to child growth.

Like many of his contemporaries, Tyler saw a place for both gymnastics and natural activities. He categorized both as physical training. He believed that play and games had social value, because "the conception of fair and unfair play is almost the first genuine and spontaneous moral distinction which the child makes."

•1908 • Jane Addams, a well-known social worker who was Director of Hull House in Chicago, organized the Playground Association of America. It was the predecessor of the National Recreation and Parks Association. In 1909, Addams published *The Spirit of Youth and the City Streets*.

•1908 • The Playground Association of America set "play in institutions" as one of its objectives. This was one of the first references to recreation for people with disabilities.

•1909 • Jessie Bancroft's *Games for School, Home and Playground* was published. Bancroft had received some training as a student of Dudley A. Sargent at the Harvard Summer School of Physical Education, and she went on to become the first woman in the USA to hold the title of Director of Physical Education of Public Schools.

•1910 • A committee of the National Society for the Study of Education investigated the school health program in the USA. It defined the function of physical education as the supervision of fundamental motor activities expressed in play, games, dancing, swimming, gymnastics and athletics. It concluded that, "progress in physical education must be away from all formal, artificial kinds of movements."

•1911 • The Playground Association of America became the Playground and Recreation Association of America. This was an indication that playgrounds had become just one part of a broader movement, recreation for older children and adults.

•1913 • A study commission, headed by Carl Diem, was initiated by authorities in Germany who sought an answer to the success of American athletes – German born or otherwise. After visiting the USA and seeing the playground movement in Chicago and other cities, the commission recommended vast additional play areas in all German cities. The practices of American colleges and universities in physical education were adopted in German universities.

•1990 • The Americans with Disabilities Act (P.L. 101-336) led to a revolution in playground design to make facilities accessible to children with disabilities.

Bibliography

Payne, V.G. and Isaacs, L.D. (2005). *Human motor development. A lifespan approach*. 6th ed. Boston, MA: McGraw-Hill.

PLEGIA Total loss of voluntary control of muscle.

PLETHYSMOGRAPH A device for measuring variations in the size of bodily parts and in the flow of blood through them.

PLEURA A thin membrane enclosing the lungs and permits free movement of the lungs inside the thoracic cavity. **Pleural pressure** is the pressure within the pleural space. During quiet breathing, the pleural pressure is negative, i.e. it is below atmospheric pressure.

PLEURISY An inflammation of the pleura, the lining of the lungs, with subsequent pain.

PLICA An embryologic remnant, present in 65% of normal people that may impinge on the joint space as a fold of synovium near the underside of the quadriceps tendon or along the free edge of the medial patellofemoral joint. There are four named plicae in the knee. **Plica syndrome** involves snapping and pain in the patellofemoral joint.

PLICA PALPEBRONASALIS An epicanthal fold of skin of the upper eyelid (from the nose to the inner side of the eyebrow) that covers the inner corner (canthus) of the eye. The presence of an epicanthal fold is normal in people of Asiatic descent. It is also common in children with Down syndrome.

PLYOMETRIC TRAINING A type of training designed to increase power. It commonly takes the form of '**depth (drop) jumping**.' This typically involves the athlete jumping from a high box and rebounding off the floor onto another (usually lower) box. Schmidtbleicher (1992) recommends that drop jumps be performed in 3 to 5 sets of 10 repetitions, with rest intervals of 10 minutes between sets. In terms of vertical jumping, depth jumping can be distinguished from squat and counter-movement jumping. A **squat jump** involves no pre-stretch movement whereas a **counter-movement jump** involves the prior flexion of the ankle, knee and hip joints, which is a pre-stretch. A depth jump involves making a vertical jump after landing from a drop of a specific height and involves flexion or countering of landing.

The theory behind its use is based on the stretch-shortening cycle. Muscle contraction is much stronger, if it is immediately preceded by a rapid lengthening or pre-stretching of that muscle. This is due to the release of stored elastic energy from the recoil following passive stretching of the elastic, non-contractile components of muscle. In a depth jump, there is additional release of chemical energy through a 'pre-load effect,' which occurs when the muscle is contracted eccentrically before it is contracted concentrically. The additional time permits more coupling of cross bridges, and thus increased breakdown and ATP synthesis. If there is a delay between stretching the muscle and concentric contraction, some of the stored energy will be dissipated. During the delay, thick and thin filaments become detached and reattach under less stretch. If the stretch magnitude is too great, fewer cross bridges are able to remain attached and less elastic energy is available. A more rapid stretch creates more elastic energy.

There has not been strong empirical research evidence for the effectiveness of plyometric training in improving performance in sport. Like ballistic stretching, it can cause damage to muscle, ligaments and other tissues. Impact forces of at least three or four times body weight are not uncommon in plyometrics. There is risk of injuries such as tibial stress syndrome or even stress fractures. Athletes who attempt high depth jumps should be able to squat at least 1.5 times their body weight.

In addition to jumps, plyometric exercises for the lower extremities include bounds, hops, leaps, skips and ricochet (rapid rate of leg and foot movement). Plyometric exercises for the trunk and upper body include swings, twists, tosses, passes and throws (often using a medicine ball).

Chronology
•1972 • Valery Borzov, the Soviet sprinter won both the 100 m and 200 m at the Olympic Games. According to anecdotal evidence, the use of plyometrics was partly responsible for his success. It was originally called the 'shock method' by the Russians.

Bibliography
Bobbert, M.F. (1990). Drop jumping as a training method for jumping ability. *Sports Medicine* 9(1), 7-22.

Chu, D.A. (1996). *Explosive power and strength*. Champaign, IL: Human Kinetics.

Chu, D.A. (1998). *Jumping into plyometrics*. 2nd ed. Champaign, IL: Human Kinetics.

Duda, M. (1988). Plyometrics: A legitimate form of power training? *The Physician and Sportsmedicine* 16(3), 213-218.

Norris, C.M. (2000). *Back stability*. Champaign, IL: Human

Kinetics.

Radcliffe, J. and Farentinos, R. (1999). *High-powered plyometrics*. Champaign, IL: Human Kinetics.

Schmitbleicher, D. (1992). Training for power events. In: Komi, P.V. (ed). *Strength and power in sport*. pp381-395. Oxford: Blackwell Scientific Publishers.

Siff, M.C. (2000). Biomechanical foundations of strength and power training. In Zatsiorsky, V. (ed). *Biomechanics in sport. Performance enhancement and injury prevention. Vol. IX of the Encyclopedia of Sports Medicine*. pp103-139. Oxford: Blackwell Science.

PNEUMOTACHOMETER *See under* OXYGEN UPTAKE, MEASUREMENT OF.

PNEUMOTHORAX Air is trapped in the pleural space, causing a portion of a lung to collapse. The two most common types are traumatic and spontaneous. **Spontaneous pneumothorax** occurs unexpectedly with or without the presence of underlying disease. It may occur as a result of other pulmonary conditions such as asthma, cystic fibrosis, emphysema and pneumonia. The most generally accepted cause of spontaneous pneumothorax is rupture of subpleural blebs or bullae. A history of smoking tobacco and recent substance abuse are often associated with the condition. Spontaneous pneumothorax can be either primary (occurring in persons without clinically or radiologically apparent lung disease) or secondary (in which lung disease is present and apparent). Most individuals with primary spontaneous pneumothorax have unrecognized lung disease.

Traumatic pneuomothorax is caused by penetrating or blunt trauma to the chest, with air entering the pleural space directly through the chest wall, through visceral penetration, or through alveoloar rupture resulting from sudden compression of the chest.

Traumatic and spontaneous pneumothoraces are rare, but potentially dangerous, conditions found in athletic activity. Sports-related spontaneous pneumothorax has been described in scuba diving, weightlifting and jogging. It has been postulated that elevated intrathoracic pressure during activity, combined with mechanical factors of the underlying blebs or bullae, may lead to their eventual rupture. A 27-year old weightlifter developed mild chest pain and dysnea after 'bouncing' a 250 lb barbell off his chest. Emergency tube thoracostomy was used to treat the pneumothorax and one month later he resumed lifting without recurrence.

See also HEMOTHORAX.

Bibliography
Ciocca, M. (2000). Pneumothorax in a weightlifter: The importance of vigilance. *The Physician and Sportsmedicine* 28(4), 97-103.

Curtin, S.M., Tucker, A.M. and Gens, D.R. (2000). Pneumothorax in sports. *The Physician and Sportsmedicine* 28(8), 23-32.

POISEUILLE'S LAW *See under* CIRCULATORY SYSTEM.

POISSON'S EFFECT An applied compressive load causes tensile stress and strain perpendicular to the imposed load; or an applied tensile load results in compressive stress and strain perpendicular to the imposed load. Consider a compressive load that is imposed on a ball: it not only causes compressive stress and strain that compresses the ball in the direction of the load, but also causes tensile stress and strain (i.e. perpendicular to the imposed load) that makes the ball get wider. *See also under* SPINE.

POLAR COORDINATE SYSTEM A pair of numbers that locate a point: (i) the distance of the point from the origin; and (ii) the angle made by the radius to the point and polar axis (the fixed line through the origin). *See also* CARTESIAN COORDINATE SYSTEM.

POLARITY The property of a physical system that has two points with different (usually opposite) characteristics, such as one which has opposite charges or electrical potential.

POLARIZED LIGHT Light in which the electric and magnetic field vectors oscillate only in specific directions.

POLAR LIPIDS *See* MEMBRANE LIPIDS.

POLIOMYELITIS Polio. It is a highly infectious,

viral infection that invades the nervous system and can cause total paralysis within hours. The virus enters the body through the mouth and multiplies in the intestine. The name is derived from the part of the spine attacked by the virus. Polio means 'gray,' referring to the color of the nerve cell bodies it attacks. **Myelitis** refers to infection of the protective coating around the nerve fibers. The polio destroys only motor nerve cells, which are found in the anterior part of the spinal cord and in the brain. Because people with polio have sensation, pain is a concern. Muscle and joint pain are particularly aggravated by cold temperature and excessive exercise. It mainly affects children under five years of age. Many persons with poliomyelitis have scoliosis. There is no cure for polio, but it can be prevented through vaccination that protects an individual for life. Among those paralyzed, 5 to 10% die when their breathing muscles become immobilized. Until the 1950s, polio was the leading cause of orthopedic impairments in the USA, where there are now approximately 300,000 polio survivors with some degree of disability. In the 1980s, 25% of these persons began to experience new joint and muscle pain, muscle weakness, severe fatigue, sensitivity to cold temperature, and respiratory problems. This set of symptoms has been termed **postpolio syndrome**. The cause is not understood.

Bibliography
Global Polio Eradication Initiative. Http://www.polioeradication.org
World Health Organization. Http://www.who.int

POLITICS   *See under* SPORT.

POLYCYTHEMIA   Erythrocythemia. *See under* RED BLOOD CELL.

POLYCYSTIC OVARY SYNDROME   Women who have polycystic ovary syndrome usually have a normal uterus and fallopian tubes, but have ovaries that contain several small cysts. Polycystic ovary syndrome is associated with constant production of estrogen that causes the endometrium to become abnormally thick and to be shed spontaneously. Along with irregular or absent ovulation, this causes

intermittent bouts of amenorrhea or periods with heavy bleeding. About 50% of women with polycystic ovary syndrome are obese. Women with polycystic ovary syndrome have more resistance to the action of insulin than normal women and are at higher risk of developing diabetes. *See under* HYPERANDROGENISM.

POLYDYPSIA   Excessive thirst.

POLYGON   A flat or plane, closed figure made up of at least three lines. Triangles and rectangles are examples of polygons.

POLYMER   A substance containing giant molecules and thus a large number of atoms. Examples include polynucleotides and polypeptides. **Polymerization** is forming large molecules from small molecules.

POLYMERASE   An enzyme that catalyzes the covalent joining of nucleotides, e.g. DNA polymerase and RNA polymerase.

POLYPEPTIDES   *See under* PROTEIN SYNTHESIS.

POLYSACCHARIDES   *See under* CARBOHYDRATES.

POLYURIA   The excretion of excessive urine.

PONDERAL INDEX   *See under* SOMATOTYPING.

POPLITEAL   Pertaining to the back of the knee.

POPLITEAL ARTERY ENTRAPMENT SYNDROME   A partial or complete occlusion of the popliteal artery as a result of aberrant anatomy in the popliteal fossa, giving rise to pain in the lower leg. The **popliteal artery** is a continuation of the superficial femoral artery in the popliteal space. It supplies blood to the knee and calf. The most common cause of popliteal artery entrapment syndrome is compression of the artery below the *gastrocnemius* muscle. Popliteal artery entrapment syndrome occurs mainly in younger athletes, possibly because younger people are more often involved in vigorous training, which can lead to functional hypertrophy of the *gastrocnemius*. Hypertrophy of the *gastrocnemius* medial head may contribute to functional entrapment of the popliteal artery because of their proximity. The most common symptom is claudication, with pain provoked by some level of work. Repeated popliteal artery compression causes trauma to the artery wall, leading to premature localized atherosclerosis. As the pathology progresses, acute ischemia can occur if there is an occlusion of the artery or thrombosis within an aneurysm. Treatment of popliteal artery entrapment syndrome usually includes surgical exploration, release of the popliteal artery and a myomectomy of the medial *gastrocnemius* head.

Bibliography

Wang, D. (2002). Popliteal artery entrapment masquerading as asthma. *The Physician and Sportsmedicine* 30(8), 23-26.

POPLITEAL CYST   Baker's cyst. It is usually found in the popliteal fossa. It is a type of cyst that results from flux of fluid in association with a bursa (*semimembranosus* or medial *gastrocnemius* bursa) or may be caused by herniation of the synovial membrane through the joint capsule. Popliteal cysts usually develop following trauma, including tears of meniscal tissue that have been weakened by degeneration. The lateral central meniscus is thicker and subject to decreased peripheral vascularity, caused by its separation from the knee joint capsule by the popliteus tendon and is thus most prone to degeneration.

POPLITEAL FOSSA   A hollow area that appears on the posterior surface of the knee.

POPLITEUS TENDON INJURY   The *popliteus* muscle has its origin on the lateral condyle of the femur, and runs beneath the lateral collateral ligament before inserting onto the posterior tibia. The *popliteus* muscle and its tendon function to decelerate and internally rotate the tibia during gait. The popliteus tendon is typically injured through overuse, and is experienced as lateral knee pain, which most commonly afflicts those involved in downhill walking or running, those who run on banked terrain, and those with hyperpronation of the foot causing external rotation of the tibia. It is much more common in the female athlete.

PORPHYRIN   The heterocyclic compound, present in hemoglobin, cytochromes and other hemoproteins that has a tetrapyrrole ring structure in which iron is chelated.

PORTAL   Pertaining to a porta, or entrance, especially to the **porta hepatis (hepatic portal)**, which is the transverse fissure on the visceral surface of the liver where the portal vein and hepatic artery enter the liver and the hepatic ducts leave.

POSITION   The location of an object or a point on the object with respect to a designated reference point in the environment.

POSITIVE IONS   Cations. These are ions formed when neutral atoms or molecules lose one or more electrons.

POSITIVE PSYCHOLOGY   *See under* HUMANISTIC PSYCHOLOGY.

POSITIVE SUPPORT REFLEX   A primitive reflex that is normal between the ages of 3 to 8 months. It is elicited by the soles of the feet touching the floor with the response of increased extensor tone (plantar flexion at the ankle joint). It strengthens the hip and knee extensors needed for straight-back sitting and standing.

Failure of this reflex to become integrated prevents independent standing and walking. In non-ambulatory persons, it creates difficulty (along with the extensor thrust reflex) in wheelchair posture adjustments and/or wheelchair transfers because sensory input from footplates stimulates the soles of the feet, which, in turn, increases extensor tone. If it is only partially integrated, it affects walking by causing toe walking and contributes (with the crossed extension reflex) to scissoring, narrowing the base of support, and producing backward thrust of the trunk with compensatory lordosis using arm extension to assist with balance. It also interferes with kicking a ball.

POSTERIOR   Dorsal. Pertaining to the back (rear) of the body.

POSTERIOR CRUCIATE LIGAMENT   *See under* KNEE LIGAMENTS.

POSTERIOR INTEROSSEUS NERVE SYNDROME   Entrapment of the posterior interosseus nerve. This nerve is the major terminal branch of the radial nerve, which winds around the radius to the dorsal side of the forearm to provide motor and sensory function to the dorsal forearm and wrist. The posterior interosseus nerve can be entrapped at three sites: the fibrous bands from the radio-humeral joint, the proximal fibrous origin of the *supinator* muscle (arcade of Frohse) and the origin of the *extensor carpi radialis brevis* muscle. Posterior interosseus nerve syndrome may be caused by repetitive pronation and supination, as well as eccentric action of the forearm muscles.

POSTERIOR TIBIAL REFLEX   The tendon of the posterior tibial is tapped with a reflex hammer behind the medial malleolus, with the result that there is supination of the foot due to reflex contraction of the *tibialis posterior* muscle.

POST-TRAUMATIC STRESS DISORDER   *See under* ANXIETY DISORDERS.

POSTURAL DEVIATIONS   *See* FLAT BACK; FORWARD HEAD; KYPHOSIS; LORDOSIS; ROUND SHOULDERS; SCOLIOSIS; TORTICOLLIS; WINGED SCAPULAE.

POSTURAL HYPOTENSION   *See under* ORTHOSTATIC TOLERANCE.

POSTURAL REFLEXES   *See under* REFLEXES.

POSTURE   The position of the different segments of the body relative to each other. Good posture is both mechanically functional and economical; it implies a balance between antagonistic muscle groups. It is a convention that standing posture is accepted as the individual's basic posture from which all other postures arise. **Stance** is the posture or initial position adopted before a particular movement is taken.

The center of gravity does not remain motionless during erect standing posture. Oscillations of the center of gravity are limited by the stretch reflex, kinesthesis and vision. When involuntary swaying is prevented, there is a tendency for syncope to occur. The involuntary swaying is thought to act as a pump, assisting venous return and ensuring adequate circulation for the brain. Consumption of alcohol causes greater swaying. Postural sway is higher in women throughout adulthood, and it increases with age. In general, excessive postural sway reveals poor balance and stability.

Postural muscle tone is the tone of the postural muscles that hold the body upright against the pull of gravity. Mechanisms involved in resisting the downward pull of gravity include the extensor thrust reflex, the static type of stretch reflex in response to gravitational pull, the muscular action evoked by forward-backward swaying, visual orientation and labyrinthine reflexes. The **postural (anti-gravity) muscles** are the extensors of the head, neck, trunk and lower extremities; and the flexors of the upper extremities.

An ideal posture is one in which the body segments are aligned vertically and the line of gravity passes through all joints axes. Ideal posture is impossible to achieve, but possible to get close to. Assessment of posture can be done using a hanging plumb line (line of gravity) and observing, perpendicular to the sagittal plane, the relationship of the anatomical landmarks to the line of gravity. Observation of the alignment of the foot, ankle and knee is made from the front. Leg and foot alignment is correct when a line drawn from the anterior superior iliac spine bisects the patella, ankle joint and 2nd toe. If the lower extremities are well proportioned and correctly aligned, a person should be able to put a coin between their thighs, knees, calves and ankles; and simultaneously hold all the coins in place. The ideal foot position with normal structure of the feet and legs is one in which the toes are pointing straight ahead or only slightly abducted. When the feet are abducted to any great extent, the weight of the body is forced over the longitudinal arch instead of over the outer borders of the feet with their stable structure. Observations for lateral deviations in the spine, and unequal levels in the pelvis and shoulders, are made from the rear. If scoliosis (lateral deviation of the spine) is present, one side of the back will be more prominent when the individual is asked to flex the trunk.

Postural torques are due to: i) the spine being situated closer to the posterior surface of the body than to the anterior; ii) the supporting base (the feet) being projected forward from the lower extremities instead of centered beneath them; iii) the spinal column being curved anterioposteriorly; iv) the chest forming an anterior load upon which gravity is constantly exerting a rotational force; and v) the weight of breasts in women. During erect standing, the center of gravity for the whole body is anterior to the spinal column, placing the spine under a constant forward bending moment. To maintain body position, this torque must be counteracted by tension in the back extensor muscles. Because the spinal muscles have small moment arms, they must generate large forces to counteract the flexion torques produced by the weight of the body segments and external loads.

In chairs, the function of an arm rest is to unload the shoulder girdle that is suspended on the spine by muscles and ligaments. The weight of the arms is about 10% of body weight. Sitting far back in the chair, with the entire back resting against its contours, permits the chair to aid in holding the body. In sitting, stooped postures often occur because of the role of the eyes in combination with the work of the hands. All sedentary workers should be taught to adopt a variable posture that causes the load to transfer from tissue to tissue, decreasing the risk injury or irritation.

Warm up increases compliance of the spine, but sitting on the bench (e.g. during a volleyball match) for 20 minutes loses it. Sitting on the bench with a flexed lumbar spine creates and/or exacerbates a posterior disc bulge. Sitting in taller chairs with an angulated seat pain decreases lumbar flexion and related problems.

With regard to comfortable sleeping, a good bed should: adapt to body curvatures; be neither too soft nor too hard; have spring action; have good ventilation; and be neither too warm nor too cold.

Posture is important during weight lifting. In a squat lift, there is flexion of both the knees and the spine. In a stoop lift, the knees remain extended, but the spine flexes. In a squat lift, an object can be held closer to the body's line of gravity than with a stoop lift. This decreases the length of the lever arm from the body's line of gravity to the center of gravity of the object. During heavy weightlifting, the spine should be kept in a position of neutral lordosis (the midpoint between available anterior and posterior pelvic tilt) that provides the greatest comfort and functional stability. The spine should flatten as the weight is lifted and this should prevent hyperflexion of the spine as long as the object (e.g. barbell) is pulled towards the pelvis. The spine flattens to minimally compress the lumbar discs and to unload the facet joints. In this position, tissue recoil provides substantial extension power.

During heavy lifts by a group of power lifters, Cholewicki and McGill (1992) found that although the lifters appeared outwardly to have a very flexed spine, the lumbar joints were actually 2 to 3 degrees from full flexion. This explains how they could lift such huge loads without sustaining the injuries that are suspected to be associated with full lumbar flexion. A motor control error that results in a temporary decrease in activation to one of the inter-segmental muscles (e.g. a lamina of *longissimus*, *iliocostalis* or *multifidus*) may allow rotation at just a single joint to the point at which passive or other tissues could become irritated or injured. The risk of this occurring has been found to be greatest when high forces are developed by the large muscles and low forces are developed by the small inter-segmental muscles; or when all muscle forces were low, such as during a low-level exertion. This mechanism of motor control error, resulting in temporary inappropriate neural activation, explains how injury might occur during extremely low load situations, such as picking a pencil from the floor following a long day at work performing a very demanding job.

The 'golfer's lift' decreases spine loads for repeated lifting of light objects. The hips act as a pivot in which one leg is cantilevered behind with isometric muscle contraction, forming a counterweight to rotate the upper body back to upright.

When pushing a cart handle, directing the pushing force vector through the lumbar spine decreases the low back moment and minimizes the muscular loads (McGill, 2002). A pushing force directed through the shoulder causes a high reaction torque that is balanced by muscular force, imposing a corresponding compressive load on the spine. Redirecting the transmissible vector through the low back decreases this moment arm (and the moment), the muscle forces, and the spine compressive load. The reaction moment about the low back results from the applied force vector and the perpendicular distance from the force to the lumbar spine. A smaller reaction moment results in lower internal tissue loads necessary to support the moment; this spares the spine.

Postural deviations are classified as either structural or functional. Causes of postural deviations include injury, disease, habit and skeletal imbalance. A **structural deviation** is permanent and involves a change in the bony structure. Because of the change in the bone structure, corrective exercise is of little use. Surgery or placing the body area in a cast is required. A **functional deviation** is a condition in which only the soft tissue, such as muscle and ligaments are primarily involved. Functional disorders can largely be corrected using exercise.

See INTRA-ABDOMINAL PRESSURE; KYPHOSIS; LORDOSIS; MISALIGNMENTS; PELVIS; SCOLIOSIS; SPINE.

Chronology

•1825 • In an article entitled "Physical Education" in the *Boston Medical Intelligencer*, James Field, a medical doctor in London discussed lack of exercise in relation to curvature of the spine among girls. Field opposed the notion of female fragility and helplessness.

•1855 • In *Letters to the People on Health and Happiness*, Catherine Beecher described the distortion of women's bodies by "evil" tight dresses: "The small floating ribs are pressed unequally and lateral-

ly against the spine, because the intestines can not yield the equal support required."

•1862 • Dioclesian Lewis published *The New Gymnastics for Men, Women, and Children* that also appeared in the *American Journal of Education*. Lewis declared that even the "feeblest" of girls would need little more than an hour a day of his "new gymnastics" to be "transformed in two or three years from crooked, pale, nervous creatures, into ruddy, vigorous, sound women."

•1884 • Delphine Hanna enrolled in Dio Lewis' Summer School, but soon became disillusioned by the lack of a scientific basis to Lewis' system of physical education and transferred to Dudley A. Sargent's School before graduating in 1885. In the same year, she worked with Boston orthopedic physicians to study the treatment of spinal curvature and also studied the Delsarte School of Expression. Later, she incorporated the best of this system into her posture training work. François Delsarte was a French vocal and dramatics teacher whose system included deep breathing exercises augmented by poses to denote various emotions. The Delsarte system brought prominence to the rhythmic and aesthetic aims of exercise.

•1900 • A cross-section of physical education practice in the USA showed a conglomeration of activities drawn from German gymnastics, Swedish gymnastics, Dudley Sargent's exercises, the Young Man's Christian Association (YMCA), athletics, and the new play and recreation movement. School physical education was largely physical training with its emphasis on health, correction of physical defects such as poor posture, and mental discipline through gymnastics and calisthenics.

•1913 • Jessie H. Bancroft, Assistant Director of Physical Training in the New York City Schools, published *The Posture of Children* (1913). Her work included taking measurements of the pelvic and shoulder girdles in order to design seats.

•1933 • In Britain, the Board of Education produced a new *Syllabus of Physical Training*. It was still largely based on the Swedish system and emphasized the importance of posture. It stated, "Correct posture is necessary for good health and for complete physical development. It makes the body more useful, skilful and beautiful. It helps to produce self respect and therefore self-confidence, and thus even from the narrow utilitarian point of view it has definite value."

Bibliography

Bloomfield, J., Ackland, T.R., and Elliott, B.C. (1994). *Applied anatomy and biomechanics in sport*. Melbourne: Blackwell Scientific Publications.

Cholewicki, J. and McGill, S.M. (1992). Lumbar posterior ligament involvement during extremely heavy lifting estimated from fluoroscopic measurements. *Journal of Biomechanics* 25(1), 17-28.

Hall, S.J. (1999). *Basic biomechanics*. 3rd ed. Boston, MA: WCB McGraw-Hill.

Levangie, P.K. and Norkin, C.C. (2001). *Joint structure and function: A comprehensive analysis*. 3rd ed. Philadelphia, PA: F.A. Davis Company.

McGill, S. (2002). *Low back disorders: Evidence-based prevention and rehabilitation.* Champaign, IL: Human Kinetics.

Norris, C.M. (2000). *Back stability.* Champaign, IL: Human Kinetics.

Tinning, R. (2001). Physical Education and back health: Negotiating instrumental aims and holistic bodywork practices. *European Physical Education Review* 7(2), 191-205.

POTASSIUM A metallic element, which, as a 'macromineral' in the human body, is dissolved in the body as ions, and is therefore an electrolyte. Potassium is found almost exclusively inside the cells. Its concentration in intracellular water helps to maintain a balance between intracellular fluid and extracellular fluid. It is also involved in nerve impulse conduction and skeletal muscle contraction. There is little potassium in extracellular fluid, and therefore the potassium concentration of plasma and sweat is much lower than sodium. There is good evidence that potassium has a supporting role in the control of exercise hyperpnea, predominantly through modulation of arterial chemoreflex. Heat acclimatization has little effect on the amount of potassium lost in urine or sweat. The most likely causes of potassium depletion are through gastrointestinal loss from vomiting and diarrhea, and through the kidneys when diuretics are used. Most athletes meet their requirements for potassium in the normal diet. Fruits and vegetables are rich sources of phosphorus. Potato (medium size, baked with skin) contains 721 mg of potassium. One banana (medium size) contains 467 mg of potassium. The adequate intake for potassium in adults is in the range of 1,600 mg to 2,000 mg/day.

See also under FATIGUE; SODIUM-POTASSIUM PUMP.

Bibliography

Lindinger, M.I. and Sjogaard, G. (1991). Potassium regulation during exercise and recovery. *Sports Medicine* 11(6), 382-401.

Oregon State University. The Linus Pauling Institute. Micronutrient Information Center. Http://lpi.oregonstate.edu/infocenter

Paterson, D.J. (1997). Potassium and breathing in exercise. *Sports Medicine* 23(3), 149-163.

POTENTIAL ENERGY *See under* ENERGY.

POWER Work done per unit time. Average power is equal to the work done divided by the time during which the work is being done. The Standard International unit for power is the watt (W). A power of one **Watt** is produced when work is performed at a rate of one Joule per second. This is the same as a force of one Newton being exerted at a velocity of one metre per second; or a torque of one Newton-metre being exerted at an angular velocity of one radian per second. The US Customary unit is horsepower (hp) or foot pound force per second (ft.lbf/sec). 1 watt (W) = 1 J/s. 1 horsepower = 736 W. 1 W = 0.737 ft.lbf/sec. 1 hp = 746 W. 1 ft.lbf/sec = 1.356 W.

Angular power is the product of torque and angular velocity. **Joint power** is the product of joint angular velocity and the corresponding internal joint moment at a given point in time. It indicates the generation or absorption of mechanical energy by muscle groups or other soft tissues. **Internal joint moments** indicate the net moment of force generated by muscles, bones and passive soft tissues that counteract the tendency for joint rotation caused by gravity.

POWER, TRAINING Power is increased if either the same amount of work is accomplished in a shorter period of time, or an increased amount of work is accomplished in the same amount of time. Power may also be expressed as force multiplied by velocity. For human movement, power can be regarded as strength multiplied by speed. Power production is maximal when the muscle acts against a load that is about one-third of the maximum voluntary contraction force or when the muscle shortens at one-third of the maximum shortening velocity. **Critical power** is the maximum power that can be sustained for a set period of time.

Strength-speed (low velocity), speed-strength (intermediate velocity) and explosive strength (high velocity) are concepts of power. Maximal strength is the basic quality that influences power performance. According to Schmitbleicher (1992), an increase in maximal strength is always connected with an improvement of relative strength and therefore with improvement of power abilities.

In some sports, it is necessary to overcome resistance with the greatest possible speed of muscle action at the beginning of the movement, whereas in others the maximal acceleration should be delayed to reach a maximal velocity for the equipment or the body or parts of the body. If external loads are low, the influence of maximal strength becomes less and the rate of force development increases to become the predominating factor. '**Explosive strength**' refers to the **maximal rate of force development**. It is equal for all loads that are higher than about 25% of maximum force. '**Starting strength**' refers to the **initial rate of force development**. Ballistic movements against resistance lower than 25% of maximum force are determined from the initial rate of force development. The initial rate of force development is essential in sports where great initial speed is necessary for optimal performance (e.g. boxing, fencing). If the load to overcome is light, initial rate of force development predominates. If the load is increased (as in shot put), maximal rate of force development predominates. For movements of 250 ms or less, initial rate of force development and maximal rate of force development are the main factors. Movements of more than 250 ms are dominated by the maximal strength factor.

Training methods for the rate of force development produce a neuromuscular adaptation along with only minimal effects of muscle hypertrophy. Optimal adaptation occurs only after a training period of 6 to 8 weeks with four training units per week. These methods are characterized by short-term extremely fast maximal actions against near maximum loads, or in the case of eccentric actions, against supramaximal loads. A distinction is made between action and movement velocity. The action velocity is high, but the movement velocity from the load is very low.

For a training period of similar length, a phase of hypertrophy training followed by rate of force development training shows better results than a mixed methods training over the same period of time (Schmitbleicher, 1992). Mixed methods aim to develop maximal strength and power within a unique training program. A typical mixed program uses a pyramid approach starting with loads at 70% and then set by set with decreasing repetitions up to

100%, and vice versa. For elite athletes, there are difficulties with the mixed method. If an athlete starts with low loads and a lot of repetitions, neuronal fatigue will occur before attempting the near maximal contraction that serves for the adaptation in rate of force development. When starting with maximal contractions, high intramuscular lactate concentrations develop during consecutive sets, with lower loads and high repetitions, therefore decreasing the adaptation effects on the nervous system.

See also PLYOMETRIC TRAINING; RESISTANCE TRAINING; SPEED; STRENGTH.

Bibliography
Newton, H. (2002). *Explosive lifting for sports*. Champaign, IL: Human Kinetics.

Schmitbleicher, D. (1992). Training for power events. In: Komi, P.V. (ed). *Strength and power in sport*. pp381-395. Oxford: Blackwell Scientific Publishers.

Siff, M.C. (2000). Biomechanical foundations of strength and power training. In Zatsiorsky, V. (ed). *Biomechanics in sport. Performance enhancement and injury prevention. Vol. IX of the Encyclopedia of Sports Medicine*. pp103-139. Oxford: Blackwell Science.

Stamford, B. (1985). The difference between strength and power. *The Physician and Sportsmedicine* 13(7), 155.

POWER-VELOCITY RELATIONSHIP   Power increases as velocity increases until a peak is reached. Each muscle group has an optimum movement velocity to produce peak power, depending on its muscle fiber composition.

PRACTICE   The **power law of practice** is a mathematical law describing the change in rate of performance improvement during skill learning; large amounts of improvement occur during early practice, but smaller improvements characterize further practice. In an experiment on cigar making, Crossman (1959) found that workers still showed some performance improvement after seven years of experience, during which time they had made over 10 million cigars.

Distributed (spaced) practice is a method of learning in which the practice sessions are widely spread out over time rather than close together (**massed practice**). Research evidence suggests that distributed schedules lead to better learning than massed schedules for learning continuous motor skills and that massed practice schedules result in better learning for discrete motor skills.

Practice variability refers to the variety of movement and context characteristics the learner experiences while practicing a skill. In an experiment on free throw shooting (Schoenfelt et al., 2002), the 'constant practice' group, which practiced only from the free-throw line, improved during the three weeks of practice, but two weeks later on a retention test, returned to their pretest level of performance. Three 'variable practice' groups, only one of which included shooting from the free-throw line, improved during practice and performed on the retention test at a higher level than they had on the pretest. Increased amount of practice variability is usually associated with an increased amount of performance error during practice. When it occurs in the initial learning stage, however, more performance error can be better than less error for skill learning.

Contextual interference is the interference that results from performing variations of a skill within the context of practice. The **contextual interference effect** is the learning benefit resulting from performing multiple skills in a high contextual interference practice schedule (e.g. random practice), rather than performing the skills in a low contextual interference schedule (e.g. blocked practice). Possible explanations of the contextual interference effect include: i) learners having to use more elaborate processing strategies to keep the tasks distinct and facilitating better memory representations of the tasks; and ii) learners being forced to go through more solution generations with random practice, which ultimately leads to better retrieval. The contextual interference effect tends to be found in research involving laboratory tasks. In applied settings, higher amounts of contextual interference tend to enhance the learning of skill variations that are more similar than different. Due to their complexity, the learning of sport skills may require more practice than has been included in those studies that have not found the effect. Furthermore, the learning of sport skills may require

a progression of low to high amounts of contextual interference, rather than only a high amount. For children, practice schedules that produce lower amounts of contextual interference tend to produce better learning.

See also under EXPERTISE.

Bibiography

Battig, W.F. (1966). Facilitation and interference. In E.A. Bilodeau (Ed.). *Acquisition of skill.* pp215-244. New York: Academic Press.

Brady, F. (1998). A theoretical and empirical review of the contextual interference effect and the learning of motor skills. *Quest* 50, 266-293.

Donovan, J.J. and Radosevich, D.J. (1999). A meta-analytic review of the practice distribution effect: Now you see it, now you don't. *Journal of Applied Psychology* 84, 795-805.

Lee, T.D. and Genovese, E.D. (1988). Distribution of practice in motor skill acquisition: Learning and performance effects reconsidered. *Research Quarterly for Exercise and Sport* 59, 59-67.

Lee, T.D. and Genovese, E.D. (1989). Distribution of practice in motor skills acquisition: Difference effects for discrete and continuous tasks. *Research Quarterly for Exercise and Sport* 59, 277-287.

Lee, T.D. and Magill, R.A. (1983). The locus of contextual interference in motor skill acquisition. *Journal of Experimental Psychology: Learning, Memory and Cognition* 9, 730-746.

Lee, T.D. and Magill, R.A. (1985). Can forgetting facilitate skill acquisition? In Goodman, D., Wilbert, R.B. and Franks, I.M. (eds). *Differing perspectives in motor learning, memory and control.* pp3-22. Amsterdam: North Holland.

Magill, R.A. (2004). *Motor learning and control. Concepts and applications.* 7th ed. Boston: MA: McGraw-Hill.

Magill, R.A. and Hall, K.G. (1990). A review of the contextual interference effect in motor skill acquisition. *Human Movement Science* 9, 241-289.

Sanderson, F.H. (1983). Length and spacing of practice sessions in sport skills. *International Journal of Sport Psychology* 14(2), 116-122.

Schoenfelt, E.L. et al. (2002). Comparison of constant and variable practice conditions on free-throw shooting. *Perceptual and Motor Skills* 94, 1113-1123.

Shea, J.B. and Morgan, R.L. (1979). Contextual interference effects on the acquisition, retention, and transfer of a motor skill. *Journal of Experimental Psychology: Human Learning and Memory* 5, 179-187.

Shea, J.B. and Zimny, S.T. (1983). Context effects in memory and learning movement information. In R.A. Magill (Ed.). *Memory and control of action.* pp345-366. Amsterdam: North Holland.

Schmidt, R.A. (1975). A schema theory of discrete motor skill learning theory. *Psychological Review* 82, 225-260.

PRADER-WILLI SYNDROME A condition that is diagnosed by obesity, short stature, poor development of the genital organs, small hands and feet, and an insatiable appetite. It is sometimes associated with autism. Individuals with this syndrome often have mild mental retardation, postural defects, and motor problems such as hypotonia. Motor milestones are typically delayed one or two years. Hypotonia improves, but deficits in motor planning, strength, coordination and balance may continue. Most people with Prader-Willi syndrome are missing a small portion of chromosome 15 that appears to come from the paternal side of the family. In the USA, the prevalence is 1 in 12,000 to 1 in 15,000 people.

Bibliography
Prader Willi Syndrome Association USA. Http://www.pwsusa.org

PRASTERONE *See* ANDROGEN SUPPLEMENTS.

PRAXIS Motor planning See DYSPRAXIA.

PREECLAMPSIA *See under* PREGNANCY.

PREGNANCY Gestation. It is the period of time between conception and childbirth. In humans, it is usually about 280 days. To avoid compromising fetal growth, caloric intake must be adequate to offset the combined demands of pregnancy and exercise. Based on Hytten and Leitch's (1971) theoretical estimates, it has been recommended that pregnant women consume an additional 300 kcal/day. However, there is wide variation in energy expended by pregnant women. It has been found that energy expenditure tends to exceed energy intake. Women's bodies may compensate for increases in metabolism during pregnancy by minimizing fat deposition, or decreasing the energy requirement for activity and the thermic effect of feeding. Severe energy restriction may result in ketosis, which harms the fetus. Kopp-Hoolihan et al. (1999) concluded that well-nourished women use different strategies to meet the energy demands of pregnancy and the combination of strategies used by individual women is not entirely predictable from pre-pregnant indices. Therefore the use of a single recommendation for increased energy intake in all pregnant women does not appear justified.

Morning sickness or nausea associated with pregnancy is most common early in pregnancy as the mother's body adjusts to changes in hormone levels. Heartburn may be experienced as a result of upward displacement of the esophageal sphincter, because of increased intra-abdominal pressure. Growth of the breasts, uterus and fetus increases lumbar lordosis and shifts the center of gravity forward, putting strain on the lower back. Hormonal changes lead to increased joint laxity and mobility.

An **abortion** is termination of pregnancy before the fetus is viable (i.e. capable of survival outside of the uterus). A **spontaneous abortion (miscarriage)** is a natural loss of the fetus. 15 to 50% of pregnancies are terminated by spontaneous abortions, usually during the first trimester. Most are due to chromosomal abnormalities, the most common of which is probably Down syndrome.

Pregravid weight refers to a woman's weight status prior to conception. If a woman's pregravid weight is approximate for her height, then gestational weight gain should be 25 to 35 lb. More than 10% of women are below ideal, i.e. 28 to 40 lb. More than 20% of women are above ideal, i.e. 15 to 25 lb.

During submaximal exercise, cardiac output increases above values in non-pregnant women, except perhaps late in pregnancy. Both heart rate and stroke volume contribute to the elevated cardiac output. Exercise arterial-venous oxygen difference is lower during pregnancy, suggesting that the higher cardiac output is distributed to non-exercising vascular beds. There is some evidence to suggest that the perfusion of exercising muscle is unchanged during pregnancy. The fetus needs a constant supply of oxygen and nutrients. Uterine blood flow decreases during exercise, due largely to increased release of nor-epinephrine and epinephrine. Heat production may also decrease uterine blood flow. In pregnant women who are well trained before becoming pregnant, however, there may be a decrease in the release of norepinephrine and epinephrine, and a decrease also in heat production with exercise. The decrease in uterine blood flow is linearly correlated with the intensity and the duration of exercise. The maximal decrease averages approximately 25%. Uterine oxygen consumption is maintained due to compensation through hemoconcentration, redistribution of blood flow within the uterus, and increased oxygen extraction.

The pregnant woman tends to hyperventilate during exercise, causing an increase in pulmonary ventilation and a decrease in arterial partial pressure of carbon dioxide. This is thought to be due to the effect of progesterone on the respiratory center. The pregnant woman must work hard during inspiration to displace the enlarging uterus downward. Probably because of the combined effect of limited expansion of the diaphragm (owing to an enlarged uterus) and increased fetal oxygen demand, maximal oxygen uptake is significantly decreased in pregnant women during exercise as compared with non-pregnant women.

Weight gain, uterine contractility, duration of pregnancy and labor do not seem to be altered by sport during pregnancy. There are certain contraindications to sport during pregnancy, however, including the presence of diabetes (see below), pregnancy-induced hypertension, pre-term rupture of membrane, pre-term labor during the prior or current pregnancy, incompetent cervix, persistent second-to-third trimester bleeding and intra-uterine growth retardation.

Swimming is particularly suitable for pregnant women. Swimming strokes in the prone (face-down) position promote optimum blood flow to the uterus. A woman's core temperature does not rise so quickly when swimming, because heat loss by conduction is more efficient in water than air. The fetus thus gets an extra safeguard against overheating. The fetus' neural tube is closing during the first trimester, which makes the possibility of overheating more serious. During the third trimester, the potential conflict between the woman and her fetus for glucose and blood flow is greatest. Pressure of the water encourages water loss, making swimming a particularly appealing option for pregnant women who tend to have edema. Diving and jumping into a pool are not recommended, because of the risk of injury to the mother or fetus, particularly after the first trimester when the fetus is no longer within the pelvis.

Until 1994, the American College of Obstetricians and Gynecologists guidelines stated that a pregnant woman should not let her heart rate exceed 140 beats per minute. The new guidelines (2002) defined strenuous exercise as occurring when a person is unable to talk normally while exercising. It is recommended that there is no exercise in the supine (face-up position), such as backstroke in swimming, after the fourth or fifth month of gestation is complete. The enlarging uterus falls back onto the vena cava and may cause hypotension in the pregnant woman and a decreased blood supply to the fetus. There is concern that exercise during pregnancy places competing demands on the cardiovascular system. While exercise diverts blood flow to the exercising muscle, pregnancy diverts blood flow to the placenta. Another concern is the increase in body core temperature; core temperature must not exceed 38 degrees Celsius. Non-weight-bearing exercise (e.g. swimming) is preferable to weight-bearing exercise (e.g. jogging). Non-weight bearing, water-based exercise results in smaller fetal heart rate changes and a lower maternal heart rate than the same exercise performed on land. Exercise should be stopped and medical attention sought if any of the following symptoms occur: pain; vaginal bleeding; dizziness or feeling faint; increased shortness of breath; rapid heartbeat; difficulty walking; uterine contractions; chest pain; or fluid leaking from the vagina.

Hyperbaric environments may adversely affect fetal development in pregnant women who dive. Decompression during ascent may place a fetus at increased risk. It is the official position of major diving organizations, such as the Professional Association of Diving Instructors (PADI), that pregnant women should not dive.

Resistance training may assist in management of many of the rigors of pregnancy. Women who have never participated in resistance training, however, should not begin during pregnancy. Ballistic exercises should be avoided, since pregnancy is associated with joint and connective tissue laxity. The Valsalva maneuver, thus also heavy resistance training, should be avoided because oxygen delivery to the placenta may be decreased.

Low birth weight is 1501 to 2500 g, **very low birth weight** is less than 1501 g and **extremely low birth weight** is less than 1000 g. Low birth weight is not necessarily associated with premature birth. Low birth weight caused by intra-uterine impoverishment is associated with mental retardation. Cerebral palsy is more closely associated with prematurity than low birth weight. The incidence of prematurity and low birth weight is higher among infants born from multi-fetal pregnancies. This also leads to higher rates of perinatal mortality and morbidity. Consumption of alcohol during pregnancy not only increases the risk of low birth weight, but also miscarriage, still birth, and death in early infancy. Heavy drinkers are two to four times more likely to have a miscarriage between the fourth and sixth month of pregnancy than are nondrinkers.

Pivarnik (1998) argued that participation in moderate to vigorous activity throughout pregnancy may enhance birth weight, but more severe regimens could result in lighter offspring. Although some data suggest that strenuous exercise may lead to delivery of babies with a lower weight at birth, these deliveries are nevertheless within the normal limits and are due partly to lower body fat in the baby. No consistent differences have been reported between exercisers and non-exercisers in terms of rate of spontaneous abortion or rupture, incidence of pre-term labor, fetal distress or birth abnormalities and ability to carry to term.

Gestational diabetes mellitus is the most common complication of pregnancy, affecting 3 to 6% of pregnant Americans. It occurs mainly during the third trimester of pregnancy, and is the consequence of hormone-related insulin resistance. There are three significant factors that influence the development of gestational diabetes mellitus: a genetic predisposition, a decrease in insulin action and impaired beta-cell function. The American Diabetes Association has endorsed exercise as a helpful adjunctive therapy for gestational diabetes mellitus when euglycemia is not affected by diet alone. The effects of exercise on insulin secretion, insulin sensi-

tivity and glucose metabolism make it reasonable that regular exercise may be effective in preventing or treating gestational diabetes mellitus. Although the gestational diabetes mellitus usually resolves in the postpartum period, it is associated with a higher risk of Type-2 diabetes later in life.

Potential benefits of a properly-designed prenatal exercise program include: improved aerobic and muscular function; facilitation of recovery from labor; enhanced maternal psychological well-being that may help counter feelings of stress, anxiety and depression frequently experienced during pregnancy; more rapid return to pre-pregnancy weight, strength and flexibility level; fewer obstetric interventions; shorter active phase of labor and less pain; less weight gain; improved digestion and decreased constipation; greater energy reserves; decreased 'post-partum (after-birth) belly' and decreased back pain during pregnancy. Many of the physiologic and morphologic changes of pregnancy persist 4 to 6 weeks into the post-partum period. Thus, pre-natal exercise routines should be resumed gradually, based on a woman's physical capability.

High-risk pregnancy is one in which the expectant mother has a condition before or during pregnancy that increases her unborn child's chances of experiencing either prenatal or postnatal problems. Medical conditions that may result in high-risk pregnancies include asthma, cancer, diabetes and cardiovascular disease. **Pre-eclampsia** is a toxemia of pregnancy condition characterized by hypertension and edema later in pregnancy. It affects up to 8% of pregnancies and accounts for 15% of all deaths of women during childbirth. It appears linked to overproduction of thromboxane, a substance produced in the body's platelets. Early detection can be eased by bed rest and anti-hypertensive drugs.

In the absence of obstetric or medical complications, pregnant women can observe the same general precautions for air travel as the general population and can fly safely up to 36 weeks of gestation. In-craft environmental conditions, such as low cabin humidity and changes in cabin pressure, coupled with the physiologic changes of pregnancy, do result in maternal adaptations, which could have transient effects on the fetus. Pregnant air travelers with medical problems that may be exacerbated by a hypoxic environment, but who must travel by air, should be prescribed supplemental oxygen during air travel. Pregnant women who are at significant risk for pre-term labor or with placental abnormalities should avoid air travel.

Postpartum pelvic floor exercises, when performed with a vaginal device providing resistance or feedback, appear to decrease postpartum urinary incontinence and to increase strength.

See also DEPRESSION; HUMAN CHORIONIC GONADOTROPIN; TERATOGEN.

Bibliography

American College of Obstetricians and Gynecologists (1994). *Exercise during pregnancy and the postpartum period*. Technical Bulletin #189. Washington, DC: ACOG.

American College of Obstetricians and Gynecologists, Committee on Obstetric Practice (2002). ACOG committee opinion. Air travel during pregnancy. *International Journal of Gynecology and Obstetrics* 76(3), 338-9.

Armstrong, L.E. (2000). *Performing in extreme environments*. Champaign, IL.: Human Kinetics.

Artal, R. and Sherman, C. (1999). Exercise during pregnancy. *The Physician and Sportsmedicine* 27(8), 51-60.

Bell, R. and O'Neill, M. (1994). Exercise and pregnancy: A review. *Birth* 21(2), 85-95.

Cohen, G.C. (1991). Exercise in pregnancy. *Gatorade Sport Science Exchange* 3(31).

Dewey, K.G. and McCrory, M.A. (1994). Effects of dieting and physical activity on pregnancy and lactation. *American Journal of Clinical Nutrition* 59(2S), 446-452.

Harvey, M.A. (2003). Pelvic floor exercises during and after pregnancy: A systematic review of their role in preventing pelvic floor dysfunction. *Journal of Obstetrics and Gynaecology Canada* 25(6), 487-498.

Hytten, F.E. and Leitch, I. (1971). *The physiology of human pregnancy*. London: Blackwell Scientific Publications.

Kopp-Hoolihan, L.E. et al. (1999). Longitudinal assessment of energy balance in well-nourished, pregnant women. *American Journal of Clinical Nutrition* 69(4), 697-704.

Pitkin, R.M. (1999). Energy in pregnancy. *American Journal of Clinical Nutrition* 69: 583.

Pivarnik, J.M. (1998). Potential effects of maternal physical activity on birth weight: Brief review. *Medicine and Science in Sports and Exercise* 30(3), 400-406.

Professional Association of Diving Instructors. Http://www.padi.com

Sady, S.P. and Carpenter, M.W. (1989). Aerobic exercise during pregnancy. Special considerations. *Sports Medicine* 7, 357-375.

White, J. (1992). Exercising for two. What's safe for the active pregnant woman? *The Physician and Sportsmedicine* 20(5), 179-186.

PREHENSION The act of grasping. It is one of the major motor skills that develop during infancy. It is critical to the development of a multitude of hand movements. Motor milestones include: reflexive grasp (birth), voluntary grasp (3rd month), two-hand palmar grasp (3rd month), one-hand grasp (5th month), pincer grip (9th month), basic release (12th to 14th month), controlled grasp (14th month), eating without assistance (18th month) and controlled release (18th month).

PRELOAD *See under* CARDIAC CYCLE.

PRE-PERFORMANCE ROUTINE A sequence of task-relevant thoughts and actions that an athlete engages in systematically prior to his or her performance of a specific sport skill. There is evidence that consistency of pre-performance routines is associated with superior performance. Boutcher (1990) recommended that performers assess the consistency of their pre-performance routines by time analysis. As Jackson and Baker (2001) note, however, this recommendation is based upon a causal inference made from correlational data and rests on the assumption that performers do better because they have more consistent routines. An equally plausible interpretation is that better performers have more consistent routine time because they are performing well. Interventions aimed to increasing the consistency of pre-performance routines have not usually resulted in improved performance (e.g. Cohen et al, 1990).

In a study of the most prolific goal kicker of all time in rugby union, it was found that certain physical aspects of his routine remain consistent, but both his concentration time and physical preparation time increased with kick difficulty. With respect to the difficulty of the kick, the number of steps taken and the glances up at the posts during the concentration period remained consistent. Concentration time, physical preparation time, and the number of glances during the physical preparation period all increased as kicks became more difficult. As the angle of the kick became more acute, the kicker spent more time walking away from the ball. This appears to be due to his attempts to ensure that his position and hence angle of approach to the ball was optimal. The kicker perceived the timing of his routine to be highly consistent, but differences of approximately 60% were found in actual concentration times. Psychological skills that were reported included thought stopping, cueing and imagery, but use of these skills was not consistent. Imagery is used in competitive situations to try to mentally simulate practice conditions, thereby detaching himself from the importance of the occasion. Jackson and Baker (2001) argue that it is the successful application of coping strategies rather than the temporal consistency of his pre-performance routine that is likely the most important determinant of his kicking performance in the competitive environment.

Bibliography

Boutcher, S.H. (1990). The role of performance routines in sport. In Jones, J.G. and Hardy, L. (eds). *Stress and performance in sport*. pp231-245. Chichester, England: John Wiley & Sons.

Cohn, P.J., Rotella, R.J. and Lloyd, J.W. (1990). Effects of a cognitive-behavioral intervention on the pre-shot routine and performance in golf. *The Sport Psychologist* 4, 33-47.

Jackson, R.C. and Baker, J.S. (2001). Routines, rituals, and rugby: Case study of a world-class goal kicker. *The Sport Psychologist* 15, 48-65.

Moran, A.P. (1996). *The psychology of concentration in sport performers: A cognitive analysis*. Hove, England: Psychology Press.

Wrisberg, C.A. and Pein, R.L. (1992). The pre-shot interval and free throw shooting accuracy: An exploratory investigation. *The Sport Psychologist* 6, 14-23.

PRESBYCUSIS *See under* AGING; DEAF.

PRESBYOPIA *See under* AGING.

PRESSOR REFLEX A reflex that increases blood pressure.

PRESSURE A stress applied uniformly in all directions. The Standard International unit is the pascal (Pa). 1 pascal (Pa) = 1 N/m^2. 1 mmHg = 133.3 Pa. Pressure on a plane surface is equal to the force acting normal to the surface divided by the area of the surface. In a fluid, the concept of pressure at a point is the normal force that would be applied on a small plane of unit area placed at that point. Any change in pressure at any point within a confined fluid will be transmitted without loss to all other points of the fluid. This is Pascal's fundamental principle of the transmission of pressure in an enclosed, ideal fluid at rest. The static pressure in a fluid is referred to as **hydrostatic pressure**.

See also under MECHANORECEPTORS.

PRESSURE PAD Pressure platform. A measuring instrument consisting of a set of force transducers with a small surface contact area over which the mean pressure for the area of contact is calculated. For a small number of selected areas of the contact surface, pressures can be measured using individual sensors. Pressures acting on various anatomical regions can be measured rather than just the resultant acting on (say) the whole foot.

Plantar pressure insoles are commercially available and can be used to measure the plantar pressure between the foot and shoe. This is generally more important for the sports performer than the pressure between the shoe and the ground, measured by pressure platforms.

PRESSURE, PSYCHOLOGICAL A state that occurs when one or more factors increase the importance of performing well on a particular occasion. *See under* STRESS.

PREVALENCE *See under* EPIDEMIOLOGY.

PRIAPISM *See under* PUDENTAL NERVE.

PRINCIPLE AXIS *See under* PLANE.

PRION PROTEIN A protein that can transmit disease.

PROGESTERONE A steroid hormone secreted by the ovaries. Its secretion is controlled by the gonadotropic hormones. Progesterone promotes secretory-phase uterine conditions, suppresses uterine contractile activity during pregnancy, promotes growth of glandular tissue in breasts but suppresses milk production. It appears to decrease sodium reabsorption by blocking the effect of aldosterone on the renal tubules. Thus progesterone has a diuretic-like effect and promotes sodium and water loss.

See ESTROGENS; MENSTRUAL CYCLE; ORAL CONTRACEPTIVES.

PROGESTOGENS   A group of steroid hormones that have the effect of progesterone.

PROGRESSIVE RELAXATION   *See under* RELAXATION.

PROHORMONE   Precursor of a hormone.

PROJECTILE   A body or object launched into the air that is subject only to the forces of gravity and air resistance. The trajectory of simple projectiles, such as a ball, is determined by: gravitational acceleration, aerodynamic forces, projectile speed, projection angle and projectile height. **Projection angle** (**release angle**; **take-off angle**) is the angle between the projectile's velocity vector and the horizontal at the instant of release or take-off. In the absence of aerodynamic forces, all projectiles will follow a parabolic trajectory, determined by the magnitude of the projection angle. A **parabola** is a curve that is symmetrical along its apex. This means that the area of each side is equal.

Projection speed is the magnitude of the projectile's velocity vector at the instant of release or take-off. When the projection angle and height are held constant, the projection speed will determine the magnitude of a projectile's **apex** (maximum vertical displacement) and its **range** (maximum horizontal displacement). The greater the projection speed, the greater is the apex and range. The **horizontal component of velocity** is calculated as the projection velocity multiplied by the cosine of the projection angle. The **vertical component of velocity** is calculated as the projection velocity multiplied by the sine of the projection angle. At 45 degrees, the sine of the angle is equal to the cosine of that angle. For any given velocity, therefore, the horizontal velocity equals the vertical velocity. In general, if the maximum range of a projectile is critical, then a projection angle to optimize the horizontal velocity (i.e. less than 45 degrees) would be chosen. If height is important, an angle of greater than 45 degrees would be chosen. Increasing the velocity of projection increases the range more substantially than increasing either the angle or the height of the projection. Top shooters in basketball use many different trajectories, depending on the distance from the basket. In general, a lower trajectory should be used on shorter shots (where a large margin of error is not needed) and a higher trajectory on long shots (where a large margin of error is needed).

PROKARYOTES   Simple cells having only a single membrane. These include bacteria and blue-green algae – believed to be the first cells to arise in biological evolution. Prokaryotes have one molecule of double-helix DNA and lack the highly specialized organelles that characterize eukaryotic cells. *See also under* EUKARYOTE.

PROLACTIN   A hormone produced by the anterior pituitary gland. It increases breast milk production. Sucking of the nipple decreases the production of **prolactin-inhibiting hormone**, which is produced by the hypothalamus. Prolactin inhibits testosterone and mobilizes fatty acids. It is secreted more during exercise. There is some evidence that resting values may be lower in trained women. High levels of prolactin can result in decreased secretion of luteinizing hormone and follicle-stimulating hormone with subsequent amenorrhea.

PROLINE   A non-essential, glucogenic (glycogenic), 5-carbon amino acid. It is synthesized from glutamate.

PRONATION   *See under* ELBOW JOINT COMPLEX; FOOT PRONATION.

PRONATOR TERES SYNDROME   Compression of the median nerve at the distal arm or proximal forearm. Causes of medial nerve entrapment within the proximal forearm include thickening of the bicipital aponeurosis (lacertus fibrosus), fibrous thickening or hypertrophy of the origin of the *pronator teres*, and compression by a thickening of the *flexor digitorum superficialis* muscle (sublimes bridge).

Pronator syndrome has been reported in motor racing drivers, weightlifters and tennis players from repetitive pronation/supination or rapid eccentric muscle actions of the forearm.

PROOXIDANT   An atom or molecule that promotes oxidation of another atom or molecule by accepting electrons. *See under* FREE RADICALS.

PROPANOLOL   *See under* BETA-BLOCKERS.

PROPORTIONALITY   The ratio of the dimension of one body part to the dimension of another body part. *See* BIACROMIAL-TO-BICRISTAL RATIO; BRACHIAL INDEX; CRURAL INDEX; RELATIVE LOWER LIMB LENGTH; STATURE.

Chronology

•1509 • In *De Divina Proportione* by Luca Pacioli, Leonardo da Vinci illustrated the golden mean (golden ratio) in the make-up of the human body. In Da Vinci's "Vitruvian Man," the ratio of distance from the feet to the navel compared to height should be the golden ratio. The ancient Greeks used a different proportion than Da Vinci. Their statues show a navel closer to the center of the body's long axis. Leonardo's drawing represents his interpretations of Vitruvius' ideas. The navel divides the height of the body in a golden section (1.618:1) and is the center of a circle enclosing the outstretched arms and legs. The pubic bone divides the height exactly in half. The ratio for length to width of triangles (to three decimal places) is 1.618. It was called the golden ratio by the Greeks, because it was considered most pleasing to the eye. The Roman architect Marcus Vitruvius Pollio (or Pollo) saw the human body as the basis for architectural harmony. In his *De Architectura Libri Decem*, Pollo wrote, "A magnificent temple cannot be constructed properly, unless it is built in an orderly manner with regard to symmetry and proportion of its parts, as is the case with a well-built man. For the human body is designed by nature, put together and created so that the head from the chin to the hairline measures one tenth of the entire body. Likewise the flat or extended hand from the wrist to the tip of the middle finger is equal to the distance from the chin to the part of the hair, i.e. one eighth part. Likewise from the bottom of the neck and the high point of the chest to the hairline, one sixth; and to the top of the head..."
•1902 • The Society of Directors of Physical Education in Colleges commissioned the modeling of a statuette based on the average measurements and proportions of the best fifty men in the all-round strength test. R. Tait McKenzie used this data for sculpture such as the "Sprinter," the first bronze cast of which was presented to President Theodore Roosevelt, who kept in on his desk in the White House. McKenzie's work differed from that of the Greeks because, while mindful of aesthetic principles, he refused to sacrifice fidelity to real life for the sake of art.

PROPPING REACTIONS   *See* PARACHUTE REACTIONS.

PROPRIOCEPTION   Sense of body awareness and position. Proprioceptors are located in muscles, tendons, joint and the inner ear. They provide information about body position, muscle length and tension, position and motion of joints, and equilibrium.

PROPRIOCEPTIVE FEEDBACK   Sensory information that derives from muscles and joints (**kinesthetic feedback**) and/or from the nonauditory labyrinths of the inner ear (**vestibular feedback**). It provides information about movement and the position of the body or limbs.

PROSTACYCLIN   A substance released by endothelial cells in response to various chemical signals and mechanical signals. It has a vasodilatory effect on smooth muscle. It inhibits platelet aggregation through activation of adenylate cyclase, which leads to an increase in intracellular cyclic adenosine. As a drug, it has a number of effects on platelets, blood vessels and nerve cells, which might improve outcome after acute ischemic stroke.

PROSTAGLANDINS   *See under* EICOSANOIDS.

PROSTATE GLAND   *See under* AGING; CANCER; NEOPLASM.

PROSTHETIC GROUP   *See under* CONJUGATED PROTEIN.

PROTEASES   *See under* EMPHYSEMA.

PROTEIN   A molecule composed of one or more polypeptide chains. **Simple proteins** are classified as globular or fibrous. **Globular proteins** are albumins (e.g. serum albumin) and globulins (e.g. myosin). **Fibrous proteins** are collagens or keratins. Proteins are required for the growth and repair of tissues, such as the contractile components of skeletal muscle. About 20% of human body weight is protein. **Biological value** refers to the efficiency with which a food protein furnishes the proper proportions and amounts of the essential amino acids needed for the synthesis of body proteins in humans or animals. Egg protein has the highest biological value and is the standard against which other proteins are measured. **Complete protein** is high-quality protein; **incomplete protein** is low-quality protein. A **high-quality protein** provides all the essential amino acids in the amounts the body needs, provides enough other amino acids to serve as nitrogen sources for synthesis of nonessential amino acids, and is easy to digest. **Complementary protein** refers to two or more incomplete proteins whose assortment of amino acids make up, or complement, each other's lack of specific essential amino acids, so that the combination provides sufficient amounts of all the essential amino acids. Red meats, poultry, fish, eggs, milk and dairy products (all animal foods) contain complete protein. The protein isolated from soybeans also provides a complete, high-quality protein equal to that of animal proteins. Protein complementation is important only for people who consume little to no animal protein. A person on a diet lacking in food from animal sources must consume a suitable variety of foods to obtain all the essential amino acids.

The recommended dietary allowance (RDA) for the sedentary population (0.8 g/kg bodyweight per day) contains a safety margin (0.35 g/kg per day) to ensure adequate protein intake. Sport nutritionists have recommended amounts in the region of 1.2 to 1.6 g/kg per day for endurance athletes and 1.2 to 1.76 g/kg per day for strength athletes. Many athletes routinely consume 1.2 to 2.0 g/kg per day, due to a high total energy intake.

It is not clear whether the increased nitrogen retention associated with increased protein intake leads to muscle hypertrophy. The most commonly used definition for the nutritional requirement for protein is the minimum amount ingested that will balance all nitrogen losses and thus maintain nitrogen equilibrium. Millward (2001) uses a different definition, that protein requirement is the minimum protein intake that satisfies the metabolic demands and which maintains body composition. Tipton and Wolfe (2004) argue that neither of these definitions based on nitrogen balance is necessarily appropriate for

athletes in training, and instead emphasize the optimum protein intake for athletic success. The optimal protein intake will vary depending on the training and competition goals of the athlete.

There is evidence to suggest that protein needs are not increased by habitual exercise. It has been argued that exercise training actually increases the efficiency of protein utilization, thus making increased intake unnecessary. The extent of any increase in protein needs with exercise is also decreased by energy provision, but may be increased by habitually high protein intake. Millward's Adaptive Metabolic Demand model proposes that the body adapts to either high or low intakes, and that this adjustment to changes in intake occurs only very slowly (Millward, 2001).

Most athletes, especially those with high training volumes and concomitant high-energy intake, probably consume sufficient protein in their normal diet. Intakes of 6,400 kcal have been reported in strength athletes. Protein of only 14% of total caloric intake would be approximately 2.5 g for a large athlete (c. 90 kg) and 3.2 g for a smaller athlete (c. 70 kg). For most athletes, therefore, recommendations for increased protein do not seem necessary. Protein intakes greater than 40% of total energy intake may limit intake of fat and/or carbohydrates, partly because protein is the most satiating macronutrient, thus compromising the benefits of these nutrients (Hall et al, 2003). However, even a small female restricting energy intake and consuming only 1500 kcal would need to consume 150 g of protein to reach 40% of total energy intake.

If 2.5 to 3 g protein is consumed, and this amount of protein is more than the metabolism can process, the excess will simply be oxidized. However, individuals with a personal or family history of liver or kidney problems may suffer harmful reactions. Excess dietary protein may be converted to carbohydrate or fat, with the excess nitrogen being converted to urea for excretion from the body via the kidneys. High protein intakes may also lead to excessive production of ketones, which must be excreted from the body by the kidneys to prevent ketosis. High protein intakes may aggravate gout, a painful inflammation of the joints. This is due to the accumulation of uric acid, which is produced from the metabolism of purines. Protein is a major source of net endogenous acid production (through sulfate excretion), which can adversely influence bone mineral density unless balanced by dietary base (e.g. potassium salts of weak organic acids abundant in fruit and vegetables).

High-protein diets may result in quick weight loss, but it is seldom permanent. Initial weight loss on high-protein diets comes from loss of body fluids. Later weight loss comes from both fat and muscle tissue. Weight is usually regained when the diet is stopped. Common side effects of high-protein diets include constipation, nausea, dehydration and fatigue. In a study funded by the Atkins Center for Complementary Medicine, 70% of patients on an Atkins diet for 6 months were constipated, 65% had halitosis ('bad breath'), 54% reported headaches and 10% had hair loss. With high-protein diets, there is increased risk of negative nitrogen balance and loss of lean body mass between training periods when high intakes are decreased (Millward et al., 1994). High protein diets may cause loss of calcium and decreased levels of urinary citrate, leading to osteoporosis and kidney stones. Urinary excretions of calcium and acids are correlated positively with intakes of animal and non-dairy animal protein, but are correlated negatively with plant-protein intake. Ketone bodies formed on a high-protein diet undergo urinary excretion with a cation to maintain electrical neutrality, resulting in the loss of cations such as calcium, magnesium and potassium. High total protein intake, especially high intake of non-dairy animal protein, may accelerate decline of renal function.

Determination of protein needs may not be as straightforward as simply expressing a quantity to be ingested per day. Other factors to consider include: composition of the protein and amino acids; timing of ingestion; and other nutrients that are ingested concurrently. Net muscle protein synthesis results from ingestion of essential amino acids only. Even single amino acids may stimulate protein synthesis resulting in net muscle protein synthesis. Essential amino acids may act to stimulate muscle protein synthesis by: supplying substrate for muscle protein

synthesis and acting as a regulatory factor. The amount of essential amino acids necessary to acutely stimulate muscle protein synthesis and net muscle protein synthesis appears to be relatively small. According to Tipton and Wolfe (2004), the most important practical issue is probably that of ensuring food protein intake immediately after resistance exercise to optimize recovery/anabolism at a time when muscle protein synthesis is increased. There is evidence to suggest that energy intake is more important for maintenance of nitrogen equilibrium than protein intake. Chittenden (1907) demonstrated that athletes can gain strength and maintain mass on relatively small protein intake (0.8 g/kg), as long as sufficient energy is available. Furthermore, energy intake may be crucial for nitrogen retention and increased lean body mass. Nitrogen balance is better maintained on a hypoenergetic diet, however, if protein intake is high. As long as energy balance is sufficient on a chronic basis, other factors are responsible for the response of muscle protein synthesis and muscle protein balance.

A meta-analysis of dietary supplements and lean mass/strength gains with resistance exercise found that protein did not have a significant effect on lean mass or strength.

Chronology

•1904 • In *Physiological Economy in Nutrition*, Russell H. Chittenden showed that the average person consumed excessive protein. Chittenden's experiments, which included athletes as well as sedentary people, led to a steady lowering of the recommended intake such that it is now essentially the same as the intake he established. Chittenden, "the father of biochemistry in America," was appointed professor of physiological chemistry at Yale in 1882. He was inspired to conduct scientific investigation of protein consumption by the low protein diet of Horace Fletcher, who was a locally reknown all-round athlete during his youth in Massachusetts before becoming a successful, but overweight businessman in San Francisco. Fletcher published *The A.B.-Z. of Our Own Nutrition* (1903) and *The New Glutton* (1903). Chittenden was impressed by Fletcher's physical fitness. The 54 year-old Fletcher was subjected to four days of the demanding training regimen of the Yale University Crew by William Anderson, director of the Yale Gymnasium, who stated: "Mr. Fletcher has taken these movements with an ease that is unlooked for. He gives evidence of no soreness or lameness and the large groups of muscles respond the second day without evidence of being poisoned by carbon dioxide... . Mr. Fletcher performs this work with greater ease and with fewer noticeable bad results than any man of his age and condition I have ever worked with." Chittenden calculated that Fletcher functioned on 45 g of protein per day, with no evidence of ill effects. Chittenden therefore lowered his own protein consumption, to 35 to 40 grams per day, with the result that his own health and fitness improved.

Bibliography

Chittenden, R.H. (1907). *The nutrition of man*. London: Heinemann.

Green, J. (1986). *Fit for America. Health, fitness, sport and American society*. New York: Pantheon Books.

Hall, W.L. et al. (2003). Cassein and whey exert different effects on appetite, plasma amino acid profiles and gastrointestinal hormone secretion. *British Journal of Nutrition* 89, 239-248.

Institute of Medicine (2002). *Dietary reference intakes for energy, carbohydrate, fiber, fat, fatty acids, cholesterol, protein, and amino acids*. Washington, DC: National Academies Press.

Lemon, P.W.R., Yarasheski, K.E. and Dolny, D.G. (1984). The importance of protein for athletes. *Sports Medicine* 1, 474-484.

Lemon, P.W.R. and Proctor, D.N. (1991). Protein intake and athletic performance. *Sports Medicine* 12(5), 313-325.

Millward, D.J. (2001). Protein and amino acid requirements: Methodological considerations. *Proceedings of the Nutrition Society* 60, 3-5.

Millward, D.J. (2004). Protein and amino acid requirements of athletes. *Journal of Sports Sciences* 22, 143-144.

Millward, D.J. et al. (1994). Physical activity, protein metabolism and protein requirements. *Proceedings of the Nutrition Society* 53, 223-240.

New, S.A. and Millward, D.J. (2003). Calcium, protein, and fruit and vegetables as dietary determinants of bone health. *American Journal of Clinical Nutrition* 77, 1340-1341.

Nissen, S.L. and Sharp, R.L. (2003). Effects of dietary supplements on lean mass and strength gains with resistance exercise: A meta-analysis. *Journal of Applied Physiology* 94, 651-659.

Ornish, D. (2004). Was Dr. Atkins right? *Journal of the American Dietetic Association* 104(4), 537-542.

Paul, G.L. (1989). Dietary protein requirements of physically active individuals. *Sports Medicine* 8(3), 154-76.

Rennie, M.J. and Tipton, K.D. (2000). Protein and amino acid metabolism during and after exercise and the effects of nutrition. *Annual Review of Nutrition* 20, 457-483.

Tipton, K.D. and Wolfe, R.R. (2001). Exercise, protein metabolism, and muscle growth. *International Journal of Sport, Nutrition, Exercise and Metabolism* 11(1), 109-132.

Tipton, K.D. and Wolfe, R.R. (2004). Protein and amino acids for athletes. *Journal of Sports Sciences* 22, 65-79.

Westman, E.C. et al. (2002). Effect of 6-month adherence to a very low carbohydrate diet program. *American Journal of Medicine* 113, 30-36.

PROTEIN SYNTHESIS Anabolism of protein from amino acids. The genes contain the information that is needed to specify what amino acids are used to make a protein and in what order. The order of amino acids for a protein is determined by the order of bases in a gene. Each amino acid is denoted by a specific sequence of three base pairs. Each of these sequences is known as a **codon.** This is the basic unit of the **genetic code**, which is the set of 64 triplets of bases (codons) corresponding to the twenty amino acids in proteins and the signals for initiation and termination of polypeptide synthesis.

There are three stages to protein synthesis: transcription, activation and translation. RNA molecules are working copies of parts of DNA, thus are tools for making proteins. There are three forms of RNA: messenger RNA, transfer RNA and ribosomal RNA.

During **transcription**, the genetic code for a gene is transferred or transcribed onto messenger RNA. This occurs in the nucleus of the cell. Thus the sequence of bases in one strand of the original DNA molecule (the other strand is not used) determines the order of bases on the messenger RNA molecule. **Messenger RNA** acts as a template for protein synthesis and it must pass from the nucleus to the cytoplasm of the cell.

During **activation**, energy from ATP is used to combine **transfer RNA molecules** with amino acid molecules. There are at least 20 different kinds of transfer RNA, the important difference between them is the sequence of bases in their anti-codons. **Anti-codons** are the three bases in a transfer RNA molecule that are complementary to the three-base codon in the messenger RNA.

Translation occurs on **ribosomes**, which are structures (comprised of protein and ribosomal RNA) that hold all the components together as an amino acid chain is made. Starting at one end of a messenger RNA molecule, a ribosome works its way along, positioning the anti-codon of each transfer RNA molecule onto a complementary codon of the messenger RNA molecule. The ribosome binds the codon and anti-codon, and then moves to the next codon of the messenger RNA molecule. After the binding takes place, the next amino acid molecule is brought into position. This binding requires energy from GTP. A peptide link is formed with an amino acid called methionine and the polypeptide chain begins to take shape. As soon as an amino acid is linked to its neighbor, its transfer RNA partner is released back into the cytoplasm to pick up another molecule of the same amino acid. This process also requires energy from GTP. The ribosome continues to work its way along the messenger RNA molecule until it reaches a codon for which there is no anti-codon. This is a signal that the synthesis of a polypeptide chain is complete. Protein molecules are made up of one or more polypeptide chains. **Polypeptides** contain more than 10 amino acids. Most have more than 100 amino acids. A **monomer** is any of the individual polypeptide chains (subunits) that make up a protein composed of multiple polypeptide chains. **Elongation** is the addition of amino acids to a growing polypeptide chain or nucleotides to a growing nucleic acid chain.

The '**central dogma of genetics**' is that the DNA of a gene codes for the production of messenger RNA, which in turn, codes for the production of a polypeptide.

The majority of protein synthesis in muscle tissue is suppressed during exercise, although synthesis of certain proteins in muscle is increased or unchanged. The suppression of protein synthesis in muscle, and the breakdown of tissue proteins in various tissues (but probably not the contractile proteins in active muscle), causes an increase in the pool of free amino acids.

There is strong evidence that amino acids not only function as precursors for protein synthesis, but also act as regulatory molecules to stimulate net muscle protein synthesis (Tipton and Wolfe, 2004). Therefore, it does not necessarily follow that there is a direct relationship between protein intake and protein synthesis. The response of muscle protein synthesis and net muscle protein balance to hyper-aminoacidemia may be linked to intracellular amino acid availability. Ingestion of a nutrient that results in hyperaminoacidemia increases amino acid delivery to the muscle, transport into the muscle cell, and intracellular amino acid availability. Increased blood flow due to exercise, as well as an elevated rate of protein synthesis due to the exercise, would lead to increased amino acid delivery to the muscle and the potential for increased muscle protein synthesis after exercise. Taken together, these factors may explain the additive effect of exercise and amino acids on net muscle protein balance. Alternatively, or in addition to, there is evidence linking the stimulation of muscle protein synthesis to the change in arterial amino acid concentrations. The regulation of muscle protein synthesis and net muscle protein balance by amino acids following exercise may respond to either changes in concentrations of arterial amino acids or intracellular amino acid availability, or both.

See also INSULIN; INSULIN-RELATED GROWTH FACTOR.

Bibliography
Tipton, K.D. and Wolfe, R.R. (2004). Protein and amino acids for athletes. *Journal of Sports Sciences* 22, 65-79.

PROTEINURIA   Albuminuria. It is the presence of protein (mainly albumin) in the urine.

PROTEOGLYCANS   *See under* GLYCO-PROTEINS.

PROTEOLYSIS   Enzymatic or hydrolytic conversion of protein into smaller substances such as amino acids.

PROTEUS SYNDROME   A condition involving atypical growth of the bones, skin and head. It is characterized by the development of benign tumors. It became widely known when it was determined that Joseph Merrick (the patient depicted in the play and movie *The Elephant Man*) rather than neurofibromatosis as was initially suggested.

Bibliography
The Proteus Foundation. Http://www.proteus-syndrome.org

PROTHROMBIN   *See under* THROMBOSIS.

PROTON   *See under* ELEMENT.

PROTON PUMP   *See under* ELECTRON TRANSPORT CHAIN.

PROTOPLASM   The substance within and including the plasma membrane of a cell.

PROTOPORPHYRIN *See under* IRON.

PROTOZOAN Any minute acellular or unicellular organism (usually non-photosynthetic).

PROVITAMIN A vitamin precursor, e.g. carotene is the pro-vitamin of vitamin A.

PROXIMAL Close to the midpoint of the body. In describing limbs, proximal refers to relative locations toward the trunk. *See also* DISTAL.

PROXIMAL INTERPHALANGEAL JOINT It is a hinge joint in the hand that allows an arc of motion of 100 degrees. The collateral ligaments, accessory collateral ligaments and volar plate complex account for most of the joint's stability. These ligaments run from a broad origin to their insertion at the base of the middle phalanx.

A **sprain of the collateral ligaments of the proximal interphalangeal joint** is one of the most common athletic injuries. It is typically caused by the finger being pulled to the side, usually toward ulnar deviation, and any subluxation either decreases spontaneously or is immediately decreased by the athlete. The volar plate has additional reinforcement from 'check ligaments,' which restrict hyperextension and also prevent rupture of the volar plate from its proximal phalangeal attachment. **Dislocation of the proximal interphalangeal joint** is usually in a dorsal direction (i.e. the middle phalanx dislocates dorsally on the proximal phalanx), with the result being either a tear or an avulsion of the volar plate of the middle phalanx. A **dorsal fracture-dislocation of the proximal interphalangeal joint** can occur when a hyperextension injury is combined with a compressive force. **Volar dislocations of the proximal interphalangeal joint** occur when a violent force is applied to a flexed joint, resulting in rupture of a collateral ligament proximally. This may be followed by a **boutonnière deformity**, which is a rupture of the central slip of the extensor mechanism over the proximal interphalangeal joint at its insertion on the base of the middle phalanx. It may result from direct trauma or acute forced flexion of the proximal interphalangeal joint with opposed active extension. Boutonnière is French for buttonhole and refers to how the proximal aspect of the middle phalanx can project through the 'buttonhole' created by the disrupted central slip and intact lateral bands. A **pseudo-boutonnière deformity** is due to a hyperextension (rather than flexion) injury to the proximal interphalangeal joint, and damage to the volar plate (rather than the central slip). It may be caused by a ball striking the end of a finger, or by a fall on an outstretched finger.

Injuries to the proximal interphalangeal joint in sport are often referred to as 'coach's finger,' because such an injury is often assessed (inaccurately) by coaches on the sideline.

Bibliography
McCue, F.C. et al. (1974). The coach's finger. *Journal of Sports Medicine* 2(5), 270-275.

PROXIMO-DISTAL See under DEVELOP-MENT.

PRURITIS Itching.

PSEUDOEPHEDRINE *See under* EPHEDRINE; GINSENG.

PSOAS PARADOX Extension/flexion role reversal. Flexion of the hip by the *psoas* muscle causes hyperextension of the lumbosacral region through anterior pelvic tilt (even though the *psoas* muscle is considered a trunk flexor). This can be observed during exercises such as double-leg raises. The lumbar vertebrae are pulled anteriorly and inferiorly by the contraction of the *psoas* muscle. Simultaneous contraction of the abdominal muscles prevents the anterior tilt of the pelvis, unless the abdominal muscles are fatigued or weak, in which case the pelvis does not rotate anteriorly and the lumbar vertebrae are not hyperextended.

See also MUSCLE ATTACHMENTS.

PSYCHIATRY The branch of medicine concerned with the diagnosis and treatment of mental disorders. In general, athletes show better emotional health than nonathletes. Elite athletes show better emotional health than nonelite athletes.

According to Glick and Horsfall (2001), pampered, highly paid professional athletes, especially men, may be developmentally immature in contrast to their 'macho adult' presentations. Athletes' tendencies to deny weaknesses and assume a macho posture are part of their personalities, resulting in denial of illness and fear of social stigma. In a small percentage of athletes, constant pressure of competition and performance may lead to dysfunctional coping skills, such as reckless driving, sexual promiscuity, and use of recreational and performance-enhancing drugs. The rationale for intervention should appeal to athletes' self interest, such as increasing skills, money or quality of life, rather than focusing on a mental illness. Elite athletes usually have great resistance to accepting the diagnosis, especially in its early stages. Athletes with narcissistic, grandiose or antisocial character traits may use denial or other defense mechanisms that prevent an effective therapeutic alliance.

Narcissism is a pervasive pattern of grandiosity (in fantasy or behavior) that is indicated by five (or more) of the following: a grandiose sense of self-importance, such as exaggerating achievements and talents, and expecting to be recognized as superior without commensurate achievements; preoccupation with fantasies of unlimited success, power, brilliance, beauty or ideal love; belief that he or she is 'special' and unique and can only be understood by, or should associate with, other special or high-status people (or institutions); need for excessive admiration; sense of entitlement (i.e. unreasonable expectations of especially favorable treatment or automatic compliance with his or her expectations); interpersonal exploitation (i.e. takes advantage of others to achieve his or her own ends); lack of empathy (unwilling to recognize or identify with the feelings and needs of others); envy of others or belief that others are envious of him or her; and arrogant, haughty behaviors or attitudes. Associated features include depressed mood and dramatic, erratic or antisocial personality.

Bibliography

American Psychiatric Association. (1994). *Diagnostic and statistical manual of mental disorders*. 4th ed. Washington, DC: American Psychiatric Association.

Begel, D. (1992). An overview of sport psychiatry. *American Journal of Psychiatry* 149(5), 606-614.

Begel, D. and Burton, R. (2000, eds). *Sport psychiatry: Theory and practice*. New York: W.W. Norton & Co.

Glick, I.D. and Horsfall, J.L. (2001). Psychiatric conditions in sport. Diagnosis, treatment and quality of life. *The Physician and Sportsmedicine* 29(8), 45-55.

PSYCHING-UP *See under* PSYCHOLOGICAL SKILLS TRAINING.

PSYCHOANALYSIS The method developed by Sigmund Freud and his disciples for treating neuroses (various types of anxiety). Psychoanalysis is also the name given to the school of thought that emerged from experiences with the psychoanalytic method, which is based on psychodynamics.

PSYCHODYNAMICS It is an approach to psychology that focuses on unconscious conflicts arising in early childhood as accounting for present behavior. Freud believed that anxiety is rooted in unconscious conflicts within an individual between unacceptable 'Id' impulses (mainly sexual and aggressive) and the constraints imposed by the 'Superego' and the 'Ego.' The **Id** is the basic mass of unconscious mind, out of which the other parts develop. The **Superego** is concerned with morality. The **Ego** is the part of the mind that is concerned with cognitive processes such as analysis and perception. The Ego also defends against negative emotions (e.g. anxiety) by using defense mechanisms, such as repression, denial, projection and reaction. Threat or danger leads to anxiety, which in turn leads to defense against the anxiety. **Repression** was considered by Freud to be the most important defense mechanism and involves pushing unpleasant memories deep into the Id. The main difference between a neurotic reaction (or something more severe) and an adaptive response is that anxiety aroused by Id wishes cannot be controlled by defenses (such as denial) and so neurotic symptoms develop. **Free association** is a psychodynamic intervention that involves the subject saying whatever comes to mind. Giges (1998) argues that directly applying procedures drawn from psychodynamic psychotherapy may be inappropriate unless the practitioner has received such training and supervised experience. Sport psychology has paid little attention to psychodynamics.

Bibliography

Apitzsch, E (1995). Psychodynamic theory of personality and sport performance. In: Biddle, S.J.H. (ed). *European perspectives on exercise and sport psychology*. pp111-127. Champaign, IL: Human Kinetics.

Giges, B. (1998). Psychodynamic concepts in sport psychology: Comment on Strean and Strean (1998). *The Sport Psychologist* 12, 223-227.

Milliner, E.K. (1987). Psychodynamic sport psychiatry. *Annals of Sports Medicine* 3, 59-64.

Strachey, J. (1961, Ed and Trans). *The standard edition of the complete psychological works of Sigmund Freud*. London: Hogarth Press.

Strean, W.B. and Strean, H.S. (1998). Applying psychodynamic concepts to sport psychology practice. *The Sport Psychologist* 12, 208-222.

PSYCHOLOGICAL MOMENTUM

Being 'on a roll.' It is exemplified by the 'hot hand' phenomenon in basketball, i.e. that when a player makes a few shots in a row, he or she is more likely to continue making them. However, research on basketball has found that a player's field goal and free-throw percentage is not contingent upon recent success or failure (i.e. there are no significant differences in field goal percentages if the player was successful with his previous two attempts or had missed them).

Bibliography

Gillovich, T., Vallone, R. and Tversky, A. (1985). The hot hand in basketball: On the misperception of random sequences. *Cognitive Psychology* 17, 295-314.

Miller, S. and Weinberg, R. (1991). Perceptions of psychological momentum and their relationship to performance. *The Sport Psychologist* 5, 211-222.

PSYCHOLOGICAL REFRACTORINESS

See under REACTION TIME.

PSYCHOLOGICAL SKILLS TRAINING

Techniques and strategies designed to enhance mental skills that facilitate performance and enjoyment of sport. Assumptions of psychological skills training are: psychophysiological states characterized by excess anxiety will impair performance; psychological skills training can decrease or remove anxiety; and psychological skills training will directly or indirectly improve athletic performance.

Boutcher and Rotella's (1987) PST program for closed-skill sports such as gymnastics consists of four stages: sport analysis, individual assessment, conceptualization and motivation, and mental skills development. The sport analysis phase involves analyzing the unique characteristics and demands of a particular activity or sport. The individual assessment phase entails establishing an individual profile of the athlete's strengths and weaknesses. The conceptual and motivational phase provides information on interaction between the athlete and the situation, the kind of commitment needed to change inappropriate behaviors, and the importance of establishing an efficient goal-setting strategy. The final phase focuses on the development of general and specific mental skills.

Vealey (1988) analyzed 27 North American psychological skills training books. The most popular psychological skills were imagery, physical relaxation, thought control and goal setting. The Athletic Coping Skills Inventory-28 contains seven subscales: coping with adversity, peaking under pressure, goal setting/mental preparation, concentration, freedom from worry, confidence and achievement motivation and coachability.

Weinberg and Comar (1994) found that 38 out of 45 interventions had positive effects, but causality could be inferred in only 20 of these. One explanation for the equivocal results in sport psychology intervention research is the widespread use of non-athletes as subjects and contrived laboratory tasks as measures of performance.

Psyching-up refers to self-directed cognitive strategies used immediately prior to or during skill execution that are designed to enhance performance. There is evidence that psyching-up may enhance performance during dynamic tasks requiring strength and/or muscular endurance. The most effective strategy appears to be seeking the optimal level of arousal in preparation for performance.

Bibliography

Boutcher, S.H. and Rotella, R.J. (1987). A psychological skills education program for closed-skill performance enhancement. *The Sport Psychologist* 1(2), 127-137.

Orlick, T. (2000). *In pursuit of excellence. How to win in sport and life through mental training.* 3ʳᵈ ed. Champaign, IL: Human Kinetics.

Smith, R.E et al. (1995). Development and validation of a multi-dimensional measure of sport-specific psychological skills: The Athletic Skills Coping Skills Inventory-28. *Journal of Sport & Exercise Psychology* 17, 379-398.

Tod, D , Iredale, F. and Gill, N. (2003). 'Psyching-up' and muscular force production. *Sports Medicine* 33(1), 47-58.

Vealey, R.S. (1988). Future directions in psychological skills training. *The Sport Psychologist* 2, 318-336.

Vealey, R.S. (1994). Current status and prominent issues in sport psychology interventions. *Medicine and Science in Sports and Exercise* 26(4), 495-502.

Weinberg, R.S. and Comar, W. (1994). The effectiveness of psychological interventions in competitive sport. *Sports Medicine* 18(6), 406-418.

PSYCHOLOGY

PSYCHOLOGY The science of mind and behavior. *See* COGNITIVE PSYCHOLOGY; EXERCISE PSYCHOLOGY; GESTALT PSYCHOLOGY; HUMANISTIC PSYCHOLOGY; PSYCHIATRY; PSYCHOANALYSIS; PSYCHODYNAMICS; PSYCHOLOGICAL SKILLS TRAINING; PSYCHOPHYSIOLOGY; SPORTS PSYCHOLOGY.

Bibliography

Wade, C. and Tavris, C. (2003). *Psychology.* 7ᵗʰ ed. Upper Saddle River, NJ: Prentice Hall.

Gleitman, H., Fridlund, A.J. and Reisberg, D. (2004). *Psychology.* 6ᵗʰ ed. New York: W.W. Norton and Co.

Gross, R. (2001). *Psychology. The science of mind and behavior.* 4ᵗʰ ed. London: Hodder and Stroughton.

PSYCHOPHYSIOLOGY A branch of psychology concerned with the inference of psychological processes from physiological measurements, especially those that relate to the brain and the autonomic nervous system. The methodology involves detecting, amplifying and recording electrical signals from the skin; e.g. electroencephalography, electrocardiography and electromyography. Psychophysiology has been used to study skilled performance in sports such as shooting where there are relatively small amounts of muscle activity from large muscle groups. It has been found that expert shooters tend to pull the trigger of the gun during the stage of the cardiac cycle called diastole when the heart muscle is relaxed and the body is more stable. The shooter is not conscious of this phenomenon. *See also* ELECTROENCEPHALOGRAPHY.

Bibliography

Collins, D (1995). Psychophysiology and performance. Biddle, S.J.H. (ed). *European perspectives on exercise and sport psychology.* pp154-178. Champaign, IL: Human Kinetics.

Hatfield, B.D. and Landers, D.M. (1983). Psychophysiology. A new direction for sport psychology. *Journal of Sport Psychology* 5, 243-259.

Helin, P., Sihvonen, T. and Hanninen, O. (1987). Timing of the trigger action of shooting in relation to the cardiac cycle. *British Journal of Sports Medicine* 21(1), 33-36.

PSYCHOTIC DISORDERS A broad term that refers to manifestations of delusions, hallucinations or other serious symptoms that grossly interfere with the capacity to meet the ordinary demands of life. A psychotic episode can occur as a complication for another specific mental disorder, e.g. bipolar disorder. *See* SCHIZOPHRENIA.

PTERNION An anatomical landmark that is the most posterior point on the calcaneus (heel of the foot) when the subject is standing.

PUBERTY *See under* GROWTH.

PUBIC SYMPHYSIS A fibrocartilagenous joint that is found anteriorly between the two innominate bones. Pain may be due to adductor strain, stress fracture of the inferior ramus or osteitis pubis. *See* GRACILIS SYNDROME; RELAXIN; SPINE.

PUDENTAL NERVE The pudental nerve contains fibers from the 2ⁿᵈ to 4ᵗʰ sacral (S2 to S4) roots of the spinal cord and is the lowest branch of the sacral plexus. It supplies sensation to the anal and genital areas. In cycling, the pudental nerve may be compressed by the pressure of a badly fitting saddle, which pushes up against the perineum. It can result in a **priapism**, which is a persistent, painful erection. A priapism can be prevented by switching from a hard, narrow racing seat to one that is wider and padded.

PULLEY *See under* LEVER.

PULL-UP REFLEX A postural reflex that is normal from 3 months through the first year. It is elicited by placing the infant in a supported standing position and tipping the infant in any direction while holding her hands. The infant responds by flexing or extending the arms in an apparent effort to maintain the upright position.

PULMONARY Of, or pertaining to, the lung.

PULMONARY CAPILLARY BLOOD VOLUME The volume of blood in the lung that is in contact with the alveolar gas at any instant.

PULMONARY EMBOLISM *See under* THROMBOSIS.

PULSE *See under* HEART RATE.

PULSE PRESSURE The difference between systolic and diastolic blood pressure. Pulse pressure measured in the periphery does not always reflect the actual central pulse pressure. Pulse pressure arises from the interaction of stroke volume and the properties of the arterial circulation. *See* BLOOD VESSEL COMPLIANCE.

PUMP BUMP *See under* ACHILLES TENDON.

PUNCH DRUNK SYNDROME *See under* HEAD INJURIES.

PUNCTURE WOUND A wound resulting from a pointed object such as a splinter.

PUNISHMENT *See under* OPERANT CONDITIONING.

PUPILLARY REFLEXES Autonomic reflexes, which are elicited by covering one eye and shining a light into the other eye. These reflexes can be used to assess head trauma.

PURINE An organic base found in nucleic acids; the predominant purines are adenine and guanine.

PURINE NUCLEOTIDE CYCLE The conversion of AMP to IMP, which is reconverted to AMP during recovery. During prolonged and intermittent intense exercise, when ammonia may be produced from the purine nucleotide cycle and amino acid deamination, ammonia accumulates to small concentrations in plasma and produces a noticeable odor in sweat.

PYLORUS A muscular or myovascular device to open or close an orifice or the lumen of an organ.

PYRIMIDINE A base that occurs in nucleic acids. The pyrimidines in DNA are cytosine and thymine; in RNA, cytosine and uracil.

PYRUVATE The salt of pyruvic acid. It is produced from phosphoenolpyruvate in the end stages of glycolysis. Depending on the metabolic conditions, there are two major fates for pyruvate: i) it can be reduced to lactate by lactate dehydrogenase in the cytosol; or ii) it can be converted to oxaloacetate by pyruvate carboxylase, which is stimulated by the presence of acetyl CoA. Oxaloacetate is then converted to phosphoenolpyruvate. A third fate for pyruvate is transamination to alanine.

There is some evidence that pyruvate supplementation may benefit endurance performance. The proposed mechanism of this effect is that extracellular pyruvate augments glucose transport into contracting muscle. It is not clear whether pyruvate supplementation provides any additional ergogenic effect to that from pre-exercise carbohydrate loading or carbohydrate ingestion during exercise.

Bibliography
Sukala, W.R. (1998). Pyruvate: Beyond the marketing hype. *International Journal of Sport Nutrition* 8(3), 241-249.

Q

Q$_{10}$ VALUE *See under* ENZYME.

Q-ANGLE The angle formed between the longitudinal axis of the femur that represents the pull of the quadriceps muscle group and a line that represents the patellar tendon. A Q-angle of greater than 15 degrees is thought to be a major factor in patellofemoral disorders due to a more lateral pull on the patella by the *quadriceps femoris* muscles. Tensile stress is placed on the lateral side of the hip joint and on the medial structures of the knee joint. The hip abductor muscles, which are under tensile stress, should be strengthened. The *quadriceps femoris* should be strengthened to stabilize the knee against abduction of the leg. The hip adductors should be stretched.

QUADRICEPS FEMORIS The *rectus femoris* and *vasti* muscles. The *rectus femoris* is the most frequently injured muscle of the *quadriceps femoris* group. It is a bi-articular muscle that has a high percentage of fast-twitch muscle fibers, and acts in an eccentric manner to decelerate motions at the hip and knee joints. It is commonly injured in sports that require sprinting or kicking. A direct blow to the thigh may cause contusion in the *quadriceps femoris*, as the muscle is compressed against the femur. The most commonly afflicted area is the anterior or anterolateral aspect of the *quadriceps femoris*. Myositis ossificans may develop in 10 to 20% of *quadriceps femoris* contusions. A rupture of the *quadriceps femoris* is caused by sudden resistance to a contraction of the muscle. Risk factors of *quadriceps femoris* rupture include tightness in the muscle, bilateral strength imbalance and leg-length discrepancy.

QUADRIPLEGIC *See under* SPINAL PARALYSIS.

QUALITY OF LIFE A condition that reflects harmonious satisfaction with one's goals and desires. It emphasizes the subjective experience rather than the conditions of life. It entails a subjective well-being and a preponderance of positive emotion. *See also* MENTAL HEALTH.

Bibliography

Berger, B.G. and McInmann, A. (1993). Exercise and the quality of life. In: Singer, R. Murphy, M. and Tennant, L.K. (eds). *Handbook of research on sport psychology*. pp729-760. New York: MacMillan.

Rejeski, W.J., Brawley, L.R. and Shumaker, S.A. (1996). Physical activity and health-related quality of life. *Exercise and Sport Sciences Reviews* 24, 71-108.

R

RACE A population of people defined by society as different from others, based on hereditary traits such as skin color. Classification of race biologically is either based on phenotypes or genotypes. Neither system is exact. **Ethnicity** refers to cultural heritage. **Ethnic markers** include language, dialect, dress, religion, art, dance, games and sports.

The following categories have been used to define the population of the USA in federal reports: American Indian or Alaska Native; Asian; Black or African American; Native Hawaiian or Other Pacific Islander; White; Hispanic or Latino; and Not Hispanic or Latino (US Office of Management and Budget, 1997).

The American Sociological Association has stated that, "race is a social construct," and warned of the, "danger of contributing to the popular conception of race as biological." Davis (1990) argued that the pre-occupation with race "itself is racist, because it is founded on and naturalizes racial categories as fixed and unambiguous biological realities, thus obscuring the political processes of racial formation."

Risch et al. (2002) argue for the continued use of self-identified race and ethnicity in biomedical and genetic research, because it reflects the genetic differences that arose on each continent after the ancestral human population dispersed from its African homeland. There are racial differences in the prevalence and incidence of disease. For example, cystic fibrosis is a far more common genetic disorder in people of northern European descent than those of African descent. African Americans are more likely than Caucasians to develop obesity, diabetes mellitus and hypertension. (*See also* SICKLE CELL TRAIT). Empirical studies indicate that aerobic capacity is lower in African Americans than Caucasians. Genetically determined and race-specific skeletal properties may partially explain racial disparities in disease and physical performance. Suminski et al. (2002) concluded from their literature review that variations in skeletal muscle properties between African Americans and Caucasians may partially contribute to group differences in disease prevalence and physical performance. The assumptions stated by the authors in making this conclusion are: i) a substantial portion of the skeletal muscle properties were determined by genetics; ii) the genes coding for specific skeletal muscle properties were discrete in terms of the racial groups examined; iii) the influence of environmental factors on the skeletal muscle properties studied were small or moderate; and iv) group differences were not the result of measurement errors.

There is an average genetic variation of 5% between racial groups, and a 95% of variation that occurs within racial groups. There is evidence that genetic diversity results in a wider range of variation in abilities among those of African descent in practically any situation that responds to a genetic component. It is not understood, however, why African countries such as Ethiopia and Kenya produce great distance runners, whereas other African countries such as Ghana and Nigeria produce great sprinters.

Höberman (1997) argues that the absence of opportunities and visible achievement in economics, politics and education has encouraged many young African American males to focus on what they can achieve through physical rather than intellectual prowess. Majors (1990) argues that African American males use sport as a means of self-expression ("cool pose"). The achievements of African Americans are used by Caucasians to reaffirm racist ideas about the abilities and potential of African Americans. A number of authors have provided counterarguments to Höberman, such as overrepresentation of African Americans in major sports being due to the failure of the American political economy to provide adequate opportunities for African Americans; or that the fixation on sports derives not from the Black community, but rather American society.

Hartmann (2000) distinguishes between a cultural critique (such as Höberman, 1997), which relies essentially on African American success in sport; and an institutional one, which emphasizes racial barriers and limitations. Sport is not just a site for the reproduction of racial stereotypes and formations, but also a site of potential struggle and challenge against them. Carrington (1998) describes how a Black cricket club in the North of England is used by Black men as both a form of resistance to White racism and a symbolic marker of the local Black community. *See also* STACKING; SUBCULTURE.

Chronology

•1619 • Africans arrived in America at the colony of Jamestown in 1619. They were initially brought as indentured servants who were theoretically free at the end of their period of servitude. In practice, however, most were made slaves; initially on an informal basis, but later through legislation. Their slave labor provided manpower to work the fields as well as to work as domestic servants.

•1790 • The first census in the USA reported 757,000 Blacks – 19% of the total population.

•1807 • The legal slave trade ended, but it continued illegally until the Civil War.

•1886 • In *Nature*, Francis Galton (a cousin of Charles Darwin) described his scheme to breed human beings who were "rich in heredity gifts of ability." In 1876, Galton had suggested twin studies as a means of evaluating the role of heredity and environment. In 1883, Galton invented the term "eugenic" (from the Greek word meaning 'well born'). He defined eugenics as "the study of the agencies under social control which may improve or impair the racial qualities of future generations physically or mentally." Galton popularized a form of applied anthropology made notorious by the Nazis in the following century (Höberman, 1992). In 1908, Galton founded the Eugenics Society of Great Britain and in 1912 an international congress on eugenics was convened in London.

•1933 • Adolf Hitler came to power in Germany. The Deutsche Turnerschaft openly identified with the goals of the Nazis. Turners believed that the major purpose of German gymnastics should be to provide for the physical, social and moral training of children and youth. In the 1930s, the primary goal of the Turnenschaft was to ensure that each member was an able-bodied individual of German stock. Jewish members were expelled. The Turnenschaft movement had thus degenerated into an antidemocratic, militaristic and racist organization that served a fascist state. In 1936, the Turnerschaft even agreed to its own dissolution in order to adjust to the organizational pattern imposed by the Nazis. Following the liberation of Germany from the Nazi regime in 1945, the Allies at first did not permit the German Turners to reorganize. In 1950, the Allies agreed to the creation of a new national organization named the Deutsche Turnerbund.

•1936 • W. Montague Cobb, the only African American to hold a doctorate in physical anthropology prior to 1950, argued that there was no evidence "to indicate that Negroid physical characters are anatomically concerned with the present dominance of Negro athletes in national competition in the short dashes and the broad jump. There is not a single physical characteristic which all the Negro stars have in common which would definitely identify them as Negroes. Jesse Owens, who has run faster and leaped farther than a human being has done before, does not have what is considered the Negroid type of calf, foot, and heel bone." Cobb also stated that, "in all those characters presumptively associated with race or physical ability, Owens was Caucasoid rather than Negroid in type. Thus, his heel bone was relatively short, instead of long; his calf muscles had very long instead of short bellies; and his arches were high and strong instead of being low and weak." According to Höberman (1997), Cobb believed all his life that Black athletic achievement could be viewed in terms of the ordeal of slavery that had been a brutal, but ultimately eugenic, process of selection. Cobb's article "Race and Runners" in 1936 was published in the *Journal of Health and Physical Education* after Jesse Owens' world record feats of May 1935, but before his four gold medals at the 1936 Olympic Games.

•1941 • In the *Journal of the American Medical Association*, Ernst Jokl reported his research on tests of fitness on a racial cross-section of South African children – English, Afrikaner, Jewish, Bantu, Cape Colored, Indian and Chinese: "We were impressed with the similarity between the standards of physical performance found in the different racial groups. No more impressive evidence for the basic equality of man has ever been adduced." Jokl, who was a first-rate Jewish sprinter, emigrated to South Africa from Germany following Nazi persecution of the Jews in 1935.

•1951 • Chuck Cooper joined the Boston Celtics, becoming the first African American player in the National Basketball Association (NBA). *Encarta Africana* states, "[Basketball] was a symbolic dialogue between Blacks and Whites, constituting a small part of the larger Civil Rights Movement that was happening throughout the United States in the 1950s. Integrated competition displayed the beauty and the creativity of African American athleticism and inspired the NBA to admit Black players."

•1954 • In Brown versus Board of Education of Topeka, racial segregation became illegal in all public schools in the USA.

•1964 • Civil Rights legislation (P.L. 88-352) passed, in the year after Martin Luther King made his "I have a dream" speech. King's assassination in 1968 triggered violence in more than a hundred cities.

•1969 • Harry Edwards' *The Revolt of the Black Athlete* was the first book written about Black athletes by a sociologist.

•1994 • The American Anthropological Association (AAA) passed a resolution stating that, "differentiating species into biologically defined 'races' has proven meaningless and unscientific."

•1995 • In research that was reported in the *Scandanavian Journal of Medicine and Science in Sports*, Bengt Saltin stated, "Kenyan runners had a muscle fiber type distribution very similar to that of successful European runners." The Kenyans run faster because they have better running efficiency, but the explanation of that superior efficiency is not known.

•1997 • Tiger Woods won the US Masters. When he appeared on the Oprah Winfrey Show, he said he was a "Cablinasian," a self-crafted acronym that reflects his ancestry. His father is Black, Chinese and Native American. His mother is from Thailand.

•1998 • The American Anthropological Association (AAA) stated that, "all normal human beings have the capacity to learn any cultural behavior. The American experience with immigrants from hundreds of different language and cultural backgrounds, who have acquired some version of American culture traits and behavior, is the clearest evidence of this."

Bibliography

American Anthropological Association. Http://www.aaanet.org

American Sociological Association. Http://www.asanet.org

Andrews, D.L. (1996). The fact(s) of Michael Jordan's Blackness: Excavating a floating racial signifier. *Sociology of Sport Journal* 13(2), 125-158.

Cann, R.L., Stoneking, M. and Wilson, A.C. (1987). Mitochondrial DNA and human evolution. *Nature* 325 (6099), 31-36.

Carrington, B. (1998). Sport, masculinity, and Black cultural resistance. *Journal of Sport and Social Issues* 22(3), 275-298.

Curtis, R.L. (1998). Racism and rationales: A frame analysis of John Höberman's Darwin's Athletes. *Social Science Quarterly* 79(4), 885-891.

Coakley, J.J. (1998). *Sport in society. Issues and controversies.* 6th ed. Boston, MA: Irwin McGraw-Hill.

Davis, L.R. (1990). The articulation of difference: White preoccupation with the question of racially linked genetic differences among athletes. *Sociology of Sport Journal* 7(2), 179-187.

Encarta africana. Http://www.africana.com/research/encarta/tt_641.asp

Hartmann, D. (2000). Rethinking the relationships between sport and race in American culture: Golden ghettos and contested terrain. *Sociology of Sport Journal* 17, 229-253.

Höberman, J. (1992). *Mortal engines: The science of performance and the dehumanization of sport.* New York: Basic Books.

Höberman, J. (1997). *Darwin's athletes: How sport has damaged Black America and preserved the myth of race.* Boston: Houghton Mifflin.

Majors, R. (1990). Cool pose: Black masculinity and sports. In Messner, M. and Sabo, D. (eds). *Sport, men and the gender order.* pp109-114. Champaign, IL: Human Kinetics.

Myers, S.L. jr (1998). Höberman's fantasy: How neoconservative writing on sport reinforces perceptions of Black inferiority and preserves the myth of race. *Social Science Quarterly* 79(4), 878-897.

Risch, N. et al. (2002). Categorization of humans in biomedical research: Genes, race and disease. *Genome Biology* 3(7). Http://genomebiology.com

Rosenberg, N.A. et al. (2002). Genetic structure of human populations. *Science* 298, 2381-2385.

Saltin, B. et al. (1995). Morphology, enzyme activities and buffer capacity in leg muscles of Kenyan and Scandinavian runners. *Scandanavian Journal of Medicine and Science in Sports* 5(4), 222-230.

Shropshire, K. and Smith, E. (1998). The Tarzan syndrome: John Höberman and his quarrels with African American athletes and intellectuals. *Journal of Sport & Social Issues* 22(1), 103-112.

Suminski, R.R., Mattern, C.O. and Devor, S.T. (2002). Influence of racial origin and skeletal muscle properties on disease prevalence and physical performance. *Sports Medicine* 32(11), 667-673.

RADIAL ACCELERATION *See* CENTRIPETAL ACCELERATION.

RADIALE An anatomical landmark that is the point at the proximal and lateral border of the head of the radius. It is found at the junction between the lateral humeral epicondyle and the head of the radius.

RADIAL NERVE The continuation of the posterior cord, 5th cervical to 1st thoracic (C5 to T1) roots of the brachial plexus. The nerve emerges in the upper arm between the long and lateral heads of the *triceps brachii* muscle, in the posterior aspect of the upper arm. It wraps around the spiral groove of the humerus, traveling from medial to lateral, emerging between the *brachioradialis* and *brachialis* muscles on the lateral aspect of the elbow. A sensory branch at this point travels distally towards the radial aspect of the wrist. The main motor branch, the posterior interosseus nerve, passes under the *supinator* muscle, through the radial tunnel and travels along the interosseus membrane towards the wrist. The radial nerve is rarely a site of focal neuropathy in the athlete. *See under* AXILLARY NERVE; POSTERIOR INTEROSSEUS NERVE; RADIAL TUNNEL SYNDROME.

RADIAL TUNNEL This consists of structures surrounding the radial nerve from between the *brachioradialis* and *brachialis* muscles in the distal arm to the distal edge of the supinator muscle in the proximal forearm. In the radial tunnel, the posterior interosseus nerve passes between the two heads of the supinator muscle. **Radial tunnel syndrome** is a disorder resulting from compression of a branch of the radial nerve in the forearm or back of the arm, or at the elbow. Causes of compression of the radial nerve at the elbow include: injury, ganglia, lipomas, bone tumors, and inflammation of the surrounding bursa or muscles.

RADIATION *See under* THERMOREGULATION.

RADICAL *See* FREE RADICAL.

RADIOACTIVITY A particular type of radiation emitted by a radioactive substance such as alpha, beta or gamma radiation. A **radioactive tracer** is a radioisotope that, when attached to a chemically similar substance or injected into a biological or physical system, can be traced by radiation detection devices, permitting determination of the distribution or location of the substance to which it is attached.

RADIOACTIVE ISOTOPE Radioisotope. It is an isotope that exhibits radioactivity.

RADIOCAPITELLAR JOINT Radiohumeral joint. *See* ELBOW JOINT COMPLEX.

RADIOCARPAL JOINT *See* WRIST JOINT.

RADIOHUMERAL JOINT *See under* ELBOW JOINT COMPLEX.

RADIOULNAR JOINTS *See under* ELBOW JOINT COMPLEX.

RADIUS OF GYRATION *See under* MOMENT OF INERTIA.

RAMUS i) A branch of a structure such as a blood vessel or nerve. ii) A slender bone process branching from a larger bone.

RATE CONSTANT *See under* CHEMICAL REACTIONS.

REACTION TIME The time elapsed between the presentation of a stimulus and a subject's response to it. **Psychological refractoriness** is the delay in responding to the second of two closely spaced stimuli. The effectiveness of a dummy pass in football or rugby can be explained in terms of psychological refractoriness. Once a player commits to a certain action, he has to complete it before he can change to another action. *See* ANTICIPATION; TIMING ACCURACY.

Chronology
•1876 • Starting with a gun was first used in athletics. Previously races were started with a drum, the word 'go' or a white handkerchief.
•1929 • Starting blocks were introduced to track athletics in Chicago, having been invented two years prior. The blocks were authorized by the International Amateur Athletics Federation (IAAF) in 1937, but did not appear in major international competition until the 1948 Olympic Games in London.
•1969 • In his controversial essay in the *Harvard Education Review*, based on measurement of reaction times, "How Much Can We Boost IQ and Scholastic Achievement?" Arthur R. Jensen stated, "It is taken for granted even by many psychologists, for example, that highly skilled athletes should outperform, say, university students in all reaction time tasks. Yet Muhammad Ali, perhaps the greatest boxer of all time in his prime, was found to show a very average reaction time." As part of his racist biology, Jensen believed that White subjects were more intelligent and that this would be reflected in faster reaction times (Höberman, 1997).
•1996 • British athlete Linford Christie was disqualified from the 100 meters final at the Olympic Games after false-starting twice. According to the results of a study published in 1999 in the *Journal of Physiology*, it is possible that Christie should not have been disqualified, because human reaction times can be much faster than the 0.1 seconds set by the International Amateur Athletics Federation (IAAF). In one of the two false starts, Christie started in 0.08 seconds. While reaction time is usually regarded as 0.1 to 0.2 seconds, research led by John Rothwell from the Medical Research Council Human Movement and Balance Unit in London found that if a loud startling sound is given at the same time as a red light, then reaction time was sometimes cut in half. A possible explanation for this phenomenon is that training may help bypass the cerebral cerebral cortex in favor of the primitive startle reflex.
•2002 • Tim Montgomery set a new world record for the 100 m with a time of 9.78 seconds at the Grand Prix final in Paris. His reaction time out of the blocks was 0.104 second.

Bibliography
Höberman, J. (1997). *Darwin's athletes: How sport has damaged Black America and preserved the myth of race*. Boston: Houghton Mifflin.

REACTIVE NITROGEN SPECIES *See under* FREE RADICAL.

REACTIVE OXYGEN SPECIES *See under* FREE RADICAL.

READINESS *See under* CRITICAL PERIOD.

REAR FOOT VALGUS A rare misalignment in which the calcaneus is everted relative to the ground with the subtalar joint in a neutral position in the sagittal plane. There is tensile stress on the medial side of the ankle and subtalar joint. It is associated with severe tibial valgus and excessive subtalar pronation. Clinical observations and symptoms include: hammer toes; plantar fasciitis; and sesamoiditis. *See also* FEMORAL VALGUS; FOOT.

Bibliography

Clinicians Corner. Http://www.footmaxx.com/clinicians

REAR FOOT VARUS Subtalar varus. The calcaneus is inverted relative to the ground with the subtalar joint in a neutral position in the sagittal plane. There is a varus angle between the midline of the lower third of the leg and the bisection of the calcaneus. It is the most common foot misalignment. Three types of rearfoot varus are clinically seen: uncompensated, partially compensated, and compensated. With **uncompensated** rearfoot varus, the heel functions in an inverted position. The degree of tibial varus is greater than the amount of available calcaneal eversion through subtalar joint pronation. With **partially compensated** rearfoot varus, the heel functions in an inverted position, but to a lesser angle than uncompensated rearfoot varus. The degree of tibial varus is only slightly greater than the available calcaneal eversion. With **compensated** rearfoot varus, the heel assumes a vertical position to the ground. Tibial varus is equal to the amount of available subtalar pronation. There is tensile stress on the lateral side of the ankle and subtalar joint. There is increased risk of injury upon landing from a jump. Clinical observations and symptoms include: plantar callus on the 2nd, 3rd and 4th metatarsals; Haglund's deformity; heel spur syndrome; Tailor's bunion; leg fatigue; knee pain; and low back pain. As a corrective, the muscles that evert the subtalar joint should be strengthened. *See also* FOOT.

Bibliography

Clinicians Corner. Http://www.footmaxx.com/clinicians

RECEPTOR A sense organ. On the basis of the stimuli detected, receptors can be classified as follows: mechanoreceptors, thermoreceptors, nociceptors, photoceptors, chemoceptors and osmoceptors.

RECEPTOR SITE It is part of a cell or molecule that specifically combines with the molecule of some other substance, such as a hormone.

RECIPROCAL ACTIVATION *See under* RECIPROCAL INHIBITION.

RECIPROCAL INHIBITION Reciprocal-inhibition reflex. It is a neurophysiological process that involves the contraction of an agonist muscle to bring about a reflex relaxation of the antagonist muscle. It occurs because sensory impulses of the agonist inhibit motor impulses to the antagonist that would otherwise cause the antagonist to reflexively contract. More specifically, it involves a decrease in the excitability of motor neurons innervating an antagonist muscle due to the stretch of the agonist muscle and activation of its Group Ia afferents and the Ia inhibitory interneuron. Reciprocal inhibition operates automatically in movements elicited by the stretch reflex and also in familiar volitional movements. In complex and less familiar movements, the operation of reciprocal inhibition depends on the skill level of the performer. Reciprocal inhibition is not necessarily required. Co-contraction (coactivation) of agonists and antagonists can occur. During a sit up, for example, the abdominal muscles (spinal flexors) contract at the same time as the back muscles (spinal extensors).

See KINETIC CHAIN EXERCISE; MUSCLES, MULTI-JOINT.

Bibliography

Enoka, R.M. (2002). *Neuromechanics of human movement*. 3rd ed. Champaign, IL: Human Kinetics.

RECOMBINANT *See under* HEREDITY.

RECOMMENDED DIETARY ALLOWANCE *See under* DIETARY REFERENCE INTAKE.

RED BLOOD CELLS Erythrocytes. These are hemoglobin-containing cells in the blood. **Erythropoiesis** is the process by which red blood cells are produced. **Erythrocythemia (polycythemia)** is an increase in the total number of red blood cells. This process may be pathological, but is also stimulated by a decreased arterial oxygen partial pressure and leads to a significant increase in oxygen carrying capacity of the blood.

See also BLOOD DOPING; ERYTHROPOIETIN; HEMATOCRIT.

REDOX POTENTIAL   The ratio of NAD^+ to NADH.

REDOX REACTIONS   Oxidation-reduction reactions. These are chemical reactions in which the electron gain (**reduction**) is directly connected with the electron loss (**oxidation**). When glucose is oxidized to carbon dioxide, for example, oxygen is reduced to water. Oxidation and reduction occur simultaneously. Protons are often transferred simultaneously with electrons.

The **oxidation number (oxidation state)** is defined as the sum of negative and positive charges in an atom, which directly indicates the number of electrons it has accepted or donated. Atoms are defined as having an oxidation number of zero, i.e. they are electrically neutral. If an atom donates an electron, it has more protons than electrons and becomes positive. It has an oxidation number of $+1$. If an atom accepts an electron, it has more electrons than protons and becomes negative. It has an oxidation number of -1. An iron ion with an oxidation number of $+3$ is expressed as iron (III), whereas an iron ion with an oxidation number of $+2$ is expressed as iron (II).

REDUCED TRAINING   *See under* DETRAINING.

REDUCTION   The gain of electrons by a chemical compound. *See also* OXIDATION.

REFERENCE FRAME   A system of coordinate axes. Inertial reference frames are fixed relative to the space in which objects are moving. Moving reference frames are 'body fixed' and move with the body being studied.

REFLEX   An involuntary movement resulting from various kinds of stimuli. Reflexes provide the body with a rapid unconscious means of reacting to certain stimuli. **Simple reflexes** have sensory information entering and motor information leaving the spinal cord at the same level, creating a **monosynaptic reflex** arc, involving involve only two neurons, one sensory and one motor; e.g. myotatic (stretch) reflex, flexor reflex and cutaneous reflex. The latency of the monosynaptic stretch reflex is about 30 ms.

Autonomic reflexes affect smooth muscle, cardiac muscle and glands. There are many reflexes involved in the cardiovascular system, e.g. atrial reflex, baroreceptor reflex, carotid sinus reflex, and pressor reflex. **Somatic reflexes** affect skeletal muscle. Those somatic reflexes mediated by the spinal cord are called **spinal reflexes**. **Propriospinal reflexes** involve information that is processed through both sides, and different levels of, the spinal cord, e.g. the crossed-extensor reflex. **Supraspinal reflexes** involve sensory information being processed in the brain after it has been received in the spinal cord, e.g. labyrinthine righting reflex. **Cranial reflexes** operate at the level of the brain, e.g. papillary reflex. **Brain stem reflexes** are reflexes regulated at the level of the brain stem (e.g. cough reflex) and the control of respiration (e.g. Herring-Breuer reflex). Their prolonged absence is one criterion of brain death. Most reflexes are **polysynaptic** and involve the activity of interneurons (or association neurons) in the integration center (one or more synapses in the central nervous system).

Reflexes can be overcome, so as not to drop a hot cup of drink, for example: the brain activates inhibitory interneurons in the spinal cord that suppress activity in the neurons that control the withdrawal reflex. Post-synaptic cells (in this case the efferent neurons that control the muscles) sum information that comes from different synaptic inputs. If the inhibitory influence that descends from the brain is greater than the excitatory influence coming from the nociceptor afferents, then the withdrawal reflex will not occur.

Two main classes of reflexes are related to skeletal movements: exteroceptive and proprioceptive. **Exteroceptive reflexes** include the extensor-thrust, flexor and crossed-extensor reflexes. **Proprioceptive reflexes** occur in response to stimulation of receptors located in the skeletal muscles, tendons, joints, and labyrinths of the inner ear. Some classifications include the extensor thrust reflex as a proprioceptive reflex.

Infant reflexes are the building blocks of the sensorimotor system and are primitive reflexes or postural reflexes. **Primitive reflexes** are those that appear during gestation or at birth in order to sustain early life and are suppressed by six months of age. Newborn infants have no motor control because every position change elicits reflexes. Any movement of the head likewise causes associated movements of other body parts. Until infants are 3 or 4 months of age, they seldom initiate voluntary, purposeful movement. When in a prone position, infants are in a flexed fetal posture referred to as **flexor tone dominance**, because the anterior surface muscles contract in response to the tactile stimuli from the surface. Movement to a supine position causes the extensor muscles on the posterior surface to automatically contract. This is called **extensor tone dominance**.

Primitive reflexes are normal in newborn infants, but are pathological when they persist beyond infancy. Most primitive reflexes are integrated at about 9 months. Those that are not integrated at the developmentally appropriate times become pathological, in that involuntary shifts of muscle tone, however subtle, interfere with smooth, coordinated movement. Individual differences in reflex integration help to explain the many degrees of clumsiness seen in the normal population. Nonambulatory individuals with severe cerebral palsy, for example, exhibit many postures and patterns similar to those of infants. Examples of primitive reflexes are asymmetrical tonic neck reflex, Babinski reflex, Doll eye reflex, Moro reflex, palmar grasp reflex, palmar grasp reflex, palmar mandibular reflex, positive support reflex, search reflex, spinal gallant reflex, startle reflex, symmetrical tonic neck reflex and tonic labyrinthine reflex. The attainment of major motor milestones corresponds very closely to the chronology of reflexes (emergence through to inhibition).

Examples of reflexes that persist into adulthood include: the **gag reflex**, when a person gags when the throat or back of mouth is stimulated; blinking reflex; yawn reflex; cough reflex; and sneeze reflex.

Postural reflexes (postural reactions) resemble later movements and are used to support the body against gravity or to allow movement. Postural reflexes must be present for individuals to adjust to changing environmental conditions during locomotion. Some postural reflexes replace primitive reflexes, but others emerge to perform unique functions. Postural reflexes are usually functioning by the age of 18 months (the time when most children perform their first jumps, using two-foot takeoffs). Examples of postural reflexes are: amphibian reflex; body righting reflex; crawling reflex; equilibrium reflexes; head righting reflex; labyrinthine reflexes; Landau reflex; neck righting reflex; parachute reflexes; pull-up reflex; segmental rolling reflexes; swimming reflex; and walking reflex. With a few exceptions (e.g. Landau reflex), postural reflexes persist throughout life. *See also* OVERFLOW; STEREOTYPIES.

REGENERATION A form of repair involving the production of new tissue that is structurally and functionally identical to normal tissue. Muscle tissue has a limited capability for regeneration. When acutely injured tissue is repaired by scar formation, structural and functional deficiencies are partially compensated for by the increased volume of the scar.

REGURGITATION A backward flowing. **Mitral regurgitation** is a backflow of blood from the left ventricle to the left atrium, owing to insufficiency of the mitral valve.

REHABILITATION Restoration of an injured athlete to self-sufficiency and an appropriate level of fitness.

REINNERVATION Restoration of nerve function.

RELATIVE ANGLE *See under* ANGLE.

RELATIVE LOWER LIMB LENGTH The ratio

of lower-limb length to standing height. Middle-distance runners and jumping athletes tend to have above-average relative lower-limb length. Sprint runners, divers, gymnasts, wrestlers, weightlifters and swimmers tend to have below-average relative lower-limb lengths. *See* PROPORTIONALITY.

RELATIVE RISK *See under* EPIDEMIOLOGY.

RELATIVE VELOCITY The velocity of a body with respect to the velocity of something else, such as surrounding fluid.

RELAXATION A response that is in the opposite direction to the 'fight or flight' response of the sympathetic nervous system. The 'relaxation response' is characterized by decreases in blood pressure, muscle tension, heart rate, oxygen consumption, respiratory rate and palmar sweat rate; and increases in galvanic skin response and alpha brain waves. Relaxation techniques include progressive relaxation, autogenic training, meditation and biofeedback.

There is good evidence for the effect of relaxation techniques on the 'fight or flight' response, but less evidence for any subsequent effects on performance. Neiss (1988) reviewed four studies that compared groups that received only relaxation treatments to equivalent control groups. Of the four groups who had only relaxation treatments, three did not perform significantly better than their respective controls (the tasks were a balancing skill, a scuba diving skill and karate sparring).

Relaxation techniques are frequently used in combination with imagery in mental practice of sport skills and to overcome anxiety, using techniques such as systematic desensitization and stress management.

Progressive relaxation is a technique that involves the subject experiencing muscle tension before learning to achieve deep muscle relaxation. Modifications of Jacobsen's method have been popular in sport psychology and form the basis of a number of psychological skills, including hypnosis.

Bibliography

Jacobsen, E. (1938). *Progressive relaxation*. Chicago, IL: University of Chicago Press.

Neiss, R. (1988). Reconceptualizing arousal: Psychobiological states in motor performance. *Psychological Bulletin* 103(3), 345-366.

Wilks, B. (1990). Stress management for athletes. *Sports Medicine* 11(5), 289-299.

Williams, J.M. and Harris, D.V. (1998). Relaxation and energizing techniques for regulation of arousal. In Williams, J.M. (ed). *Applied sport psychology: Personal growth to peak performance.* 3rd ed. pp219-236. Mountain View, CA: Mayfield.

RELAXIN A hormone, the levels of which become elevated during pregnancy, especially in the last trimester. It increases the ligamentous laxity around the pelvis. The increased laxity allows excessive movement at the pubic symphysis and sacroiliac joints, making them vulnerable to injury. *See under* GENDER DIFFERENCES.

RELEASING *See under* GRASPING.

RELIGION Belief or worship (devotion) of a supernatural power(s) considered to be divine or to have control over human destiny. **Deity** is a generic term used to refer to one or more supernatural power or being. Religion often involves rituals, a code of ethics, and a philosophy of life. **Worship** is the act of expressing reverence or praise to deity. **Prayer** is a form of worship; it is the act of attempting to verbally communicate with the supernatural. It is found in almost all the religions in the world. It is sometimes communal, as during a church service; it is also sometimes done in private. Its purpose within Christianity is to assess the will of God for one's life, to praise God, to give thanks to God, to repent of sinful behavior, to ask forgiveness, or to petition God. According to a Harris Poll® in 2003, 29% of the general public in the USA believe that God controls what happens on Earth. 50% believe that God observes, but does not control events on Earth; while 6% believe God neither observes nor controls earthly events. **Cosmology** concerns beliefs about the structure of the universe. Many religious texts have a pre-scientific view of the structure of the earth, the solar system and the rest of the universe. Around 95% of scientists and most North American adults believe that the world and the rest of the universe is billions of years old, but many conservative Christians believe in a universe less than 10,000 years of age.

An estimated 35 to 40% of National Football League (NFL) players are born-again Christians and many players openly celebrate their Christian faith after scores or credit Jesus with victory. In 2004, 20 NFL teams had on-going ministry with Athletes in Action (AIA). On the AIA website, there was a quote from Trent Dilfer of the Seattle Sea Hawks: "I now see playing in the NFL as a chance for me to influence people for Him." Faith can also be motivational or a coping mechanism. Sport involves stress, because of the uncertainty about an important outcome (winning and losing). Heavy-weight boxer, Evander Holyfield's ring robe was inscribed with a Bible verse, Philippians 4:13: "I can do all things through Christ which strengthen me." Many coaches have been accused of treating religion as group bonding that has little, if anything, to do with genuine religious faith. Many coaches and athletes, who pray, believe that the use of prayer might affect the outcome of the game. See also RITUAL; SOCIOLOGY OF SPORT.

Chronology

•1500 BC • A court used for the Aztec ball game of tlachtli (which was remarked upon by Spanish conquistadors when they arrived in Mexico in 1519) was built in Paso de la Amada, near the Pacific coast. Portraying good versus evil, and light versus darkness, tlachtli was a ritual to honor Amapan and Uappatzin, the patron deities of the game, and also Huitzilopochtli, the Aztec god of war. In competition between different segments of the community who asserted a claim to power, players used only their hips, thighs and elbows to propel a solid rubber ball at speed, bouncing it off two parallel buildings that formed the court. The captain of the losing team was sacrificed, because he represented evil.

•472 BC • The Olympics were reorganized into a five-day event. About half the time was devoted to athletic competition, with the remaining time being for religious matters. This format persisted for the next 800 years. The first historical example of prayer and the direct intervention of gods in sports competition is described by Homer in the *Iliad*. Odysseus prayed for divine assistance from Athena during his footrace with Ajax.

•50 AD • St. Paul may have arrived in Corinth, 50 miles west of Athens, where he stayed for 18 months (Acts 18:11). Paul, who was the most influential of all Christian missionaries, started to compose his own letters. Paul was a Greek-educated Jew from Tarsus, a prosperous city in an eastern province of the Roman Empire (now southeast Turkey). There is evidence that the Isthmian Games were held in this year. One school of thought is

that the Games were the reason Paul chose to settle in Corinth, but another school of thought is that the Games may have been partly responsible for the crisis that caused Paul to leave Corinth. Paul appeared before Gallio, the Roman consul, in 51 AD, and it is possible that Paul's accusation from the Jews of improperly worshipping God may have arisen from the high feeling of loyalty to the Roman Emperor Poseidon that was part of the spirit of the Isthmian Games. According to McKay (1991), the fact that Isthmia contained temples and altars to pagan idols, including the Temple of Poseidon in whose honor the chief deity of the Isthmian Sanctuary of the Games were held, would provide Paul with a similar challenge to that he faced in Athens in terms of worship of the Roman emperor. In his epistle to the Corinthians, Paul asks, "Do you not know that those who run in a race, all indeed run, but one receives the prize? So run as to get the prize. Everyone who competes in the games goes into strict training. They do it to get a crown that will not last forever. Therefore I do not run like a man running aimlessly; I do not fight like a man beating the air. No, I beat my body and make it my slave so that after I have preached to others, I myself will not be disqualified for the prize (1 *Corinthians*, 9:24-27)." Like other New Testament writers, Paul often viewed Christian life as an athletic contest, requiring strict training and focus on the finish line. Unlike the athlete's short-lived material prize and fame, however, the prize for the Christian is eternal and spiritual.

•c. 570 AD • Muhammad was born. He regarded Islam as a universal faith that would serve to unite the world. The Koran is the sacred text put together by the time of Muhammad's death in 632. In 610, Muhammad experienced a spiritual revelation when a voice from heaven told him that there was but one god, Allah. Muhammad conceived of Islam as the final stage, the spiritual fulfillment, of the Jewish and Christian traditions. In 630, Muhammad had established the notion of a 'jihad,' a holy war, to convert unbelievers, in which those who die fighting for the cause win salvation.

•1555 • John Knox, the Scottish Reformer visited his friend John Calvin, the great Protestant Reformer of Geneva. There is no strong evidence to support the popular tale that when John Knox visited Calvin on the Lord's Day (the Sabbath) he found him bowling on a green. Calvin believed that sensual pleasures like sex, as well as other physical activities, would seduce an individual away from God. Calvin's ideas eventually evolved into Puritanism.

•1618 • The "Declaration of Sport," an edict issued by King James I in his *Book of Sports*, encouraged Anglicans to participate in lawful recreational activities, such as archery, even on the Sabbath, provided these activities took place after church. This edict was reissued by his son Charles I in 1633. The Puritans disagreed with this edict, believing that Sunday should be a day spent in worship. Puritanism emerged from the Anglican Church in the late sixteenth century and embraced a variety of groups including the Congregationalists and Presbyterians. The Puritans opposed all ceremonies and rituals that they believed misdirected the spiritual relationship between humankind and God. Having emerged from the lower classes, they resented the amusements of the wealthy, more leisured groups. According to Max Weber, "Sport becomes more disordered and something is catabolized. When ΔS is negative, the reaction becomes less disordered and something is anabolized. Life involves a temporary decrease in entropy, paid for by the expenditure of energy. Energy must be expended to pay the price of organization. In other words, living organisms spend energy to overcome entropy.

Enthalpy change (ΔH) is the total heat exchange in a reaction or process. Enthalpy is an expression of heat change in a constant-pressure reaction. *In vivo* chemical reactions occur under nearly constant-pressure conditions. The oxidation of a fatty substance, such as palmitic acid, occurs very differently in the human body than it does in a calorimeter. Nevertheless, the values of ΔS and ΔH for the process are exactly the same in both pathways, because a quantity like ΔS or ΔH depends only on the final and initial states. For most biochemical reactions, the distinction between ΔS and ΔH is of little consequence. Most of these reactions occur in solution and do not involve the consumption or formation of gases. ΔH can be thought of as a measure of the energy change in a process.

The **free energy change** (ΔG) is equal to enthalpy change (ΔH) minus ΔS multiplied by the absolute temperature (T), i.e. $\Delta G = \Delta H - T\Delta S$. ΔG is the part of the total energy change in a reaction or process that is capable of doing work at constant temperature and pressure. ΔG for a biochemical reaction can be defined as the difference in free energy content between the reactants and the products under standard conditions. If ΔG is zero, the reaction will be in a state of equilibrium. Every reaction has a characteristic ΔG that can be calculated by assuming standard conditions of temperature (298 degrees Kelvin), pressure (101 kPa) and pH (7).

An **exergonic reaction** or process, e.g. ATP hydrolysis, is one in which free energy is released and ΔG is negative. An **endergonic reaction** or process, e.g. protein synthesis, is one in which free energy must be added and ΔG is positive. Exergonic reactions provide the free energy to perform all the endergonic reactions that maintain the functioning of cells and tissues. Coupling of endergonic to exergonic reactions is one of the most important

principles in biochemistry. Exergonic reactions can drive endergonic reactions, provided the sum of the two is exergonic. Muscle contraction must be driven by simultaneous hydrolysis of ATP. Amino acids cannot be joined together to make a peptide unless GTP is simultaneously hydrolyzed. Glucose molecules cannot be joined together to make glycogen unless UTP is simultaneously hydrolyzed.

Exergonic reactions usually occur spontaneously since they do not require energy. They occur because the products possess less energy in the covalent bonds than the reactants had possessed. No matter how 'spontaneous' a chemical reaction is, however, some energy is required to start the reaction. The input of energy is called **activation energy**. If a large amount of activation energy is required, then the reaction will tend not to go forward (all else held constant). If a small amount of activation energy is required, then the reaction will tend to go forward very readily.

Exergonic and endergonic refer to ΔG and spontaneity, not heat released or absorbed. In exergonic reactions, ΔH may be zero or may even be positive, but ΔG is always negative. The greater the increase in ΔS, the more negative ΔG will be, i.e. the more exergonic the reaction will be. Heat released or absorbed is referred to as **exothermic** or **endothermic**, respectively. In general, an exergonic chemical reaction is also an exothermic reaction, i.e. it gives off heat and thus has a negative ΔH.

Bibliography

Bartlett, R. (1997). *Introduction to sports biomechanics*. London: E & FN Spon.

Houston, M.E. (2001). *Biochemistry primer for exercise science*. 2nd ed. Champaign, IL: Human Kinetics.

Mathews, C.K. (2000). *Biochemistry*. San Francisco, CA: Benjamin/Cummings.

THERMOGENESIS The generation of heat. Thermogenic mechanisms are classified as either obligatory or facultative (adaptive). **Obligatory thermogenesis** is the energy released as heat during cellular and organ functions in the body, and the bulk of this heat is produced by the basal metabolism. **Facultative (adaptive) thermogenesis** is heat production that does not result in mechanical

•1964 • Before his World Boxing Association title fight against Sonny Liston, Cassius Clay was told by Malcolm X that, "This fight is the truth. It's the Cross and the Crescent fighting in the prize ring – for the first time. It's a modern crusade – a Christian and a Muslim fighting each other with television to beam it off Telstar for the whole world to see what happens." After defeating Liston, Cassius Clay announced himself as a member of The Nation, the Black Muslim sect, and changed his name to Muhammad Ali.

•1967 • Muhammad Ali refused to be drafted for military service, because he had become a Muslim minister, and the World Boxing Association (WBA) stripped him of his title. In 1971, the Supreme Court reinstated Ali's boxing license.

•1971 • At the Rose Bowl Parade, evangelical protestant leader Billy Graham summarized the spirit in which many religious organizations have made use of sports: "The Bible says leisure and lying around are morally dangerous for us. Sports keep us busy; athletes, you notice, don't take drugs. There are probably more committed Christians in sports, both collegiate and professional, than in any other occupation in America."

•1988 • Before the Olympic Games, the International Sports Coalition sponsored a World Congress on Sports to train pastors from participating nations. Courses included "How to Utilize Athletes as an Effective Medium to Communicate the Gospel" and "Practical Principles on How to Evangelize and Disciple Top Athletes."

•1990 • Bill McCartney, former football coach for the University of Colorado, and Dave Wardell, Colorado State Fellowship of Christian Athletes director, organized the first of their sport stadium rallies for Christian men. This led to the formation of the Promise Keepers. Randels and Beal (2002) note that there is little insistence on the playing of sport within the Promise Keepers, but the group's leaders adopt the language and symbolism of mainstream American male-dominated sport.

•1992 • Bill McCartney was named in a wrongful dismissal lawsuit filed by a former assistant coach who alleged that McCartney told others that "God had told him to discharge" the assistant. In the same year, McCartney was charged with, but later cleared of, violating a university policy prohibiting employees from using their job titles or university affiliation in activities not related to the university's business. At a news conference, McCartney called homosexuality "a sin" and an "abomination before Almighty God" while wearing his coach's sweater and standing at a podium with the university's logo on it.

•1992 • In her autobiography, *Lady Magic*, Nancy Lieberman-Cline disclosed her relationship in the early 1980s with Martina Navratilova. In 1996, a pamphlet by Athletes in Action, produced in conjunction with its women's touring team, highlighted a testimonial from Lieberman-Cline about her conversion to Christianity. She emphasized how her life had improved since she had accepted Christ and learned how to live according to the Bible. Like the Fellowship for Christian Athletes, Athletes in Action believes that to be saved, it is necessary to develop a personal relationship with Jesus Christ, live a Christ-centered life, and accept the Bible as the literal word of a Christian God.

•2000 • In the USA, the US Supreme Court agreed that student-led prayers in public schools violated a constitutional separation of church and state.

•2004 • The Air Force Academy's longtime football coach, Fisher DeBerry, agreed to remove a Christian banner from the team's locker room after school administrators announced they would do more to fight religious intolerance. The banner displayed the "Competitor's Creed," including the lines "I am a Christian first and last...I am a member of Team Jesus Christ." DeBerry put the banner up after his team had performed poorly on the field.

Bibliography

Athletes in Action. Http://www.aia.com

Coakley, J. (2004). *Sports in society. Issues and controversies.* 8th ed. Boston, MA: McGraw-Hill.

Coldwell, C. (1998). Calvin in the hands of the Philistines: Or, did Calvin bowl on the Sabbath? *http: www.fpcr.org/blue_banner_articles/calvin_bowls.htm.*

Eitzen, D.S. and Sage, G.H. (1997). *Sociology of North American sport.* 6th ed. Madison, WI: Brown and Benchmark.

Fagles, R. (1990). *The Iliad/Homer.* New York: Penguin Books.

Ferguson, E. (1987). *Backgrounds of early Christianity.* Grand Rapids, MI: Wm.B. Eerdmans Publishing Co.

Fellowship of Christian Athletes. Http://www.fca.org

Harris, H.A. (1966). *Greek athletes and athletics.* Bloomington: Indiana University Press.

Harris, H.A. (1972). *Sport in Greece and Rome.* Ithaca, NY: Cornell University Press.

Harris, S.L. (1995). *The New Testament: A student's introduction.* 2nd ed. Mountain View, CA: Mayfield Publishing Co.

Higgs, R.J. (1995). *God in the stadium. Sport and religion in America.* Lexington: University of Kentucky Press.

Hubbard, S. (1998). *Faith in sports. Athletes and their religion on and off the field.* New York: Doubleday.

Jable, J.T. (1974). Pennsylvania's early blue laws: A Quaker experiment in the suppression of sport and amusements, 1682-1740. *Journal of Sport History* 1(2), 107-121.

McKay, J. (1991). *Archaeology and the New Testament.* Grand Rapids, MI: Baker Book House Company.

Overman, S. (1997). *The influence of the Protestant ethic on sport and recreation.* Aldershot, UK: Avebury Press.

Park, R.J. (1977). The attitudes of leading New England Transcendentalists toward healthful exercise, active recreations and proper care of the body: 1830-1860. *Journal of Sport History* 4(1), 34-50.

Randels, G.D. and Beal, B. (2002). What makes a man? Religion, sport and negotiating masculine identities in the Promise Keepers. In Magdalinski, T. and Chandler, T.J.L. (eds). *With God on their side: Sport in the service of religion.* pp160-176. London: Routledge.

Siedentop, D. (2004). *Introduction to physical education, fitness and sport.* 5th ed. Boston, MA: McGraw-Hill.

Warrington, R. (2001). The fight for Sunday baseball in Philadelphia. Philadelphia Athletics Historical Society, Inc. Http://philadelphiaathletics.org/history/sundaybaseball.html

Weber, M. (1930). *The Protestant ethic and the spirit of capitalism.* Trans: Parsons, T. and Giddens, A. London: Unwin Hyman.

RENIN   *See under* ANGIOTENSIN.

REPAIR   In soft tissue, the replacement of damaged or lost cells and extracellular matrices with new cells and extracellular matrices.

RESIDUAL VOLUME   The volume of gas remaining in the lungs at the end of a maximal expiration. It is total lung capacity minus vital capacity.

RESIDUE   The portion of a molecule included in another larger molecule.

RESILIENCE   The amount of energy returned during unloading as a percentage of the amount of energy absorbed during loading. Resilience can be described as the ability of a material to rebound to its original size and shape with vigor; it is a material property that incorporates elasticity, toughness and strength. Tendons and ligaments are highly resilient. **Damping** (**loss coefficient**) refers to a low-level of resilience. A damping material, such as foam high jump matting, returns very little energy during unloading compared to the amount of energy that it absorbs during loading. The **hysteresis loop** is the loop on a load-deformation curve defined by the loading and unloading phases. It defines the amount of strain energy dissipated between the end of the loading phase and the end of the unloading phase. The term hysteresis comes from the Greek word *husteros* meaning later or delayed. All materials exhibit hysteresis to a certain extent. *See also* SHOCK; VISCOELASTICITY.

RESISTANCE   The difficulty with which charged particles move through an object.

RESISTANCE TRAINING   A form of training that generally involves the use of weight training to improve strength, local muscle endurance, muscle hypertrophy and power.

The American College of Sports Medicine (1998) recommends that people younger than 50 years of age should work the major muscle groups 2 to 3 days a week using 8 to 10 separate exercises with loads that allow 8 to 12 repetitions to the point of volitional fatigue (those older than 50 years are advised to perform with weight loads that allow 10 to 15 repetitions). Although more frequent training and additional sets or combinations of sets and repetitions may elicit larger strength gains, the additional improvement is relatively small for previously sedentary individuals training in the typical fitness setting. Circuit resistance training at 40 to 55% of one-repetition maximum (1-RM) as many times as possible with good form for, typically, 30 seconds, with 15 seconds rest before moving onto the next exercise station. It provides a more general conditioning, including cardiovascular fitness. As strength increases, a new 1-RM is determined.

The cardiovascular benefits of resistance training are now recognized. Previously it was thought that such training produced no cardiovasular benefits. High-volume weight training can result in increases of 5 to 10% in maximal oxygen uptake in relatively short periods of time. The mechanisms by which weight training causes this increase in maximal oxygen uptake are not understood. Other cardiovascular effects of weight training include decreased heart rate for maximal work and cardiac hypertrophy. Highest blood pressures occur at (or near) exhaustion during maximum lifts. Training appears to decrease the blood pressure during submaximal lifts.

Strength training, as part of a comprehensive fitness program, may decrease the risk of coronary heart disease, Type-2 diabetes and certain types of cancer. In the elderly, strength training improves function and decreases the risk of falls.

To ensure maximal specificity of weight training to sport, exercises should be of a multi-joint nature. The exercises should be specific to competitive events, not only in terms of the movements performed, but also the work-to-rest ratios and dominant energy systems used.

Free-weight exercises permit three-dimensional movement and do not hinder the athlete's movement pattern. Machines (as in 'multi-gyms') typically provide resistance at a single joint only, rather than providing the opportunity for kinetic chain exercise. Machines apply resistance in a guided or restricted manner. Variable resistance weight training machines have an egg-shaped cam or lever that varies its length so that the effective resistance of the load can be modified through the range of motion. This helps overcome the **sticking region**, which is the region in the range of movement of the lift where the force generated by the lifter is lower than the force due to the weight of the bar. Machines with cables typically offer a fast-to-slow movement pattern, with greater resistance and slower speed toward the end of the pattern. This contrasts with the typical slow-to-fast pattern of many sport movements. Machines do not lend themselves to ballistic or explosive exercises, and do not simulate complex muscle activation patterns characteristic of real world activities. The number of muscles required to stabilize the body during free-weight exercises is greater than when the body is fixed in a weightlifting machine. During free-weight exercise, the athlete's legs are usually used to support body weight and exert force to the ground. Balance, postural adjustments, coordination and proprioceptive responses are developed to a greater extent using free-weights.

The person lifting weights should exhale through the sticking point and inhale during the less stressful phase of the movement. Prolonged breath-holding is dangerous and invokes the Valsalva maneuver. Training partners or coaches can act as 'spotters' in order to assist the person lifting weights to move through the sticking region.

A **spotter** is some who assists in the execution of an exercise to help protect the athlete from injury. The bench press with a barbell is the most dangerous resistance training exercise. Between March 1991 and April 1992, there were 12 deaths in the USA from recreational weight training. 11 cases involved males dying of asphyxia due to barbell compression of the neck or chest as they performed heavy, bench presses in their home without a spotter. When spotting over-the-face barbell exercises (e.g. bench press), the spotter should hold the bar with an alternated handgrip, usually inside the athlete's grip, standing on a higher vantage point (ideally 'spotter plates' on the bench unit). For dumbbell exercises,

spotting should be as close to the dumbbells as possible or even the dumbbells themselves. Spotting the elbows in a 'fly' exercise would not prevent the dumbbells from striking the athlete's face or chest.

Training programs that use both concentric and eccentric muscle actions produce superior strength gains compared with either mode by itself. Heavy eccentric training ('negatives') is usually performed with loads of 120 to 130% of the maximum weight that can be lifted concentrically. The loads are lowered slowly, and a spotter assists with raising the weights through the concentric phase. In general, heavy eccentric training should not be performed in exercises that involve a high degree of lower back support such as squats and dead lifts. This is because uneven assistance from spotters can result in dangerous torques on the spine.

It is not until about the age of six years that the child has the same distribution of muscle fibers and enzyme activity in muscle as adults. Muscle fiber thickness increases from birth to about 18 years of age and this is associated with increases in muscular strength. Testosterone production increases about 20-fold when a male reaches puberty and this rapidly accelerates the development of lean muscle mass. Peak strength for males is usually achieved between the ages of 20 and 30 years, while in females it is usually achieved by the age of 20 years. High-intensity resistance training appears to be effective for increasing the strength of children. Compared with adolescents and young adults, similar relative (but smaller absolute) strength gains are made by children. Because resistance training seems to have little if any effect on the size of children's muscles, these strength gains have been associated with increases in levels of neuromuscular activation, changes in intrinsic contractile characteristics of muscle and improved coordination. Cardiovascular responses to resistance exercise are similar to those in adults: both systolic and diastolic blood pressure rises, with limited changes in heart rate and cardiac output.

The American Academy of Pediatrics, the National Strength and Conditioning Association, and the American Orthopedic Society for Sports Medicine have published position stands on prepubescent strength training. In 1985, eight sports medicine groups attended the American Orthopedic Society for Sports Medicine workshop on strength training. The consensus of these groups was that: "strength training for prepubescent boys and girls is safe with proper program design, instruction and supervision." In addition, the overall groups' position was that "the benefits of prepubescent strength training do outweigh the risks." Blimkie (1993) argued that weight training is no riskier than other youth sports or recreational activities in terms of incidence and severity of musculoskeletal injury. Maximal lifts should not be attempted until Tanner stage 5 level of development has been reached, i.e. peak height velocity will have occurred and therefore less chance of injury to the epiphyseal growth plates.

Based on injury data from the British Schoolboys Weightlifting Championships, Hamill (1994) concluded that weightlifting, which involves two lifts (the clean and jerk; and the snatch) appears to be safer than both weight training and many other sports. In 18 years, and over 100,000 heavy lifts (competition and warm-up), the only serious injuries were one boy suffering a concussion when he fell onto a weight after losing control; and another boy getting bruised when he dropped a weight onto his upper back. In neither case was there any evidence of long-term consequence.

See also BODYBUILDING; CONNECTIVE TISSUES; ENDURANCE; FLEXIBILITY; GOLGI-TENDON ORGANS; ISOKINETIC MOVEMENT; ISOMETRIC EXERCISE; INTRA-ABDOMINAL PRESSURE; KINETIC CHAIN EXERCISE; MOTOR UNIT; NEUROMUSCULAR ELECTRICAL STIMULATION; PERIODIZATION; POWER; STRENGTH; TESTOSTERONE; TRAINING FOR DISTANCE RUNNING.

Chronology

•536 BC • Milo of Croton, who later became commander of the Croton army, won the junior wrestling match at Olympia. It is recorded that he trained by carrying a calf around on his shoulders. As the calf increased in weight every day, Milo could be said to be the first exponent of weight training. Milo won six Olympic crowns in wrestling in the years 540 to 520 BC. In 1910, Milo's name was adopted by one of the first large-scale barbell manufacturers in the USA.

•1859 • George B. Windship, a graduate of Harvard and an advocate of 'heavy gymnastics,' began to tour the USA and Canada lecturing on gymnastics and giving weightlifting exhibitions. His "Lecture on Physical Culture" was illustrated by "Lifting with his Hands 929 lbs." The term "physical culture" was used widely in the 1860s through to 1910, with its use peaking around 1895. He became the foremost missionary for strength of all health reformers. He spoke of theories known today as interval training and overload. In the 1860s, he combined medicine with the Windship Gymnasium in Boston, which arguably became the most famous gymnasium for strength seekers in the USA.

•1879 • Dudley A. Sargent, director of the new Hemenway Gymnasium at Harvard, used strength tests to determine the membership of athletic squads at Harvard. He also designed many pieces of equipment that were the forerunners of modern exercise machines. Sargent's ideas and programs were made famous in the USA and Europe by William Blaikie in his popular books *How to Get Strong and How to Stay So* (1879) and *Sound Bodies for Our Boys and Girls* (1884).

•1879 • In *How to Get Strong and How to Stay So* William Blaikie drew attention to "the flat and slab-sided, almost hollow, look about the upper chest and front shoulders of two professional oarsmen whose exclusive interest in rowing had caused them to neglect the 'harmonious' development of their bodies."

•1951 • *Progressive Resistance Exercise* was published by T. De Lorme and A.L. Watkins. It concerned a method of weight training devised by the authors during the Second World War to improve the strength of patients who had injured limbs. The method involves 3 sets of 10 repetitions done consecutively, without rest in between. The first set is done with 50% of the maximum weight that can be lifted ten times (ten-repetition maximum; 10-RM), the second set is done with 75% of the 10-RM, and the final set is done with 100% of the 10-RM. It was found that as the patients trained, their strength was increased and it was necessary to increase the 10-RM weight so that strength could further improve.

•1953 • T. Hettinger and E.A. Muller published their first work on isometric training. They found that 6 seconds of isometric exercise at 75% effort increased strength.

•1956 • Jim Murray and Peter Karpovich published *Weight Training in Athletics*, which directly applied a weight-training program to sports. Prior to the 1950s, coaches of nearly all sports were reluctant to use weight training because of myths such that it would make athletes 'muscle bound' and limit their flexibility.

Bibliography

Albert, M. (1998). *Eccentric muscle training in sports and orthopedics.* 2nd ed. New York: Churchill Livingstone.

American Academy of Pediatrics (1990). Strength training, weight and power lifting, and body building by children and adolescents. *Pediatrics* 86, 801-803.

American Academy of Pediatrics (2001). Strength training by children and adolescents. *Pediatrics* 107(6), 1470-1472.

Baechle, T.R. and Earle, R.W. (2000, eds). *Essentials of strength training and conditioning.* 2nd ed. National Strength and Conditioning Association. Champaign, IL: Human Kinetics.

Behm, D.G. and Sale, D.G. (1993). Velocity specificity of resistance training. *Sports Medicine* 16(6), 374-388.

Bell, G.J. and Wenger, H.A. (1992). Physiological adaptations to velocity-controlled resistance training. *Sports Medicine* 13(4), 234-244.

Blimkie, C. (1993). Resistance training during preadolescence: Issues and controversies. *Sports Medicine* 15, 389-407.

Bloomfield, J., Ackland, T.R., and Elliott, B.C. (1994). *Applied anatomy and biomechanics in sport*. Melbourne: Blackwell Scientific Publications.

De Lorme, T.L. and Watkins, A.L. (1951) *Progressive resistance exercise*. New York: Appleton-Century-Crofts.

Enoka, R.M. (1988). Muscle strength and its development. *Sports Medicine* 6, 146-168.

Faigenbaum, M. and Pollock, M.L. (1997). Strength training: Rationale for current guidelines for adult fitness programs. *The Physician & Sportsmedicine* 25(2), 44-64.

Faigenbaum, A. and Westcott, W. (2000). *Strength and power for young athletes*. Champaign, IL: Human Kinetics.

Fleck, S.J. and Falkel, J.E. (1986). Value of resistance training for the reduction of sports injuries. *Sports Medicine* 3, 61-68.

Fleck, S.J. and Kraemer, W.J. (2004). *Designing resistance training programs*. 3rd ed. Champaign, IL: Human Kinetics.

Garhammer, J. and Takano, B. (1992). Training for weightlifting. In: Komi, P.V. (ed) *Strength and power in sport*. pp357-369. Oxford: Blackwell Scientific Publications.

Haennel, R. et al. (1989). Effects of hydraulic weight training on cardiovascular function. *Medicine and Science in Sports and Exercise* 21, 605.

Haff, G.G. (2000). Roundtable discussion: Machines versus free weights. *National Strength & Conditioning Association* 22(6), 18-30.

Hamill, B.P. (1994). Relative safety of weightlifting and weight training. *Journal of Strength & Conditioning Research* 8(1), 53-57.

Harman, E. and Frykman, P. (1990). The effects of knee wraps on weightlifting performance and injury. *National Strength and Conditioning Association Journal* 12(5), 30-35.

Jones, C.S., Christensen, C. and Young, M. (2000). Weight training injury trends. A 20-year survey. *The Physician and Sportsmedicine* 28(7), 61-72.

Kraemer, W.J., Deschenes, M.R. and Fleck, S.J. (1988). Physiological adaptations to resistance exercise. Implications for athletic conditioning. *Sports Medicine* 6, 246-256.

Lefavi, R. et al. (1993). Lower cervical disc trauma in weight training: Possible causes and preventive techniques. *National Strength and Conditioning Association Journal* 15(2), 34-36.

National Strength and Conditioning Association (1996). Youth resistance training: Position statement paper and literature review. *Strength and Conditioning* 18, 62-75.

Pereira, M.I. and Gomes, P.S. (2003). Movement velocity in resistance training. *Sports Medicine* 33(6), 427-438.

Pollock, M.L. et al. (1998). The recommended quantity and quality of exercise for developing and maintaining cardiorespiratory and muscular fitness, and flexibility in healthy adults. *Medicine and Science in Sports and Exercise* 30(6), 975-991.

Sale, D.G. (1991). Testing strength and power. In: MacDougall, J.D., Wenger, H.A. and Green, H.J. (eds). *Physiological testing of the high performance athlete*. 2nd ed. pp21-106. Champaign, Illinois: Human Kinetics.

Shephard, R.J. (1992). Effectiveness of training programmes for prepubescent children. *Sports Medicine* 13(3), 194-213.

Tanner, S.M. (1993). Weighing the risks. Strength training for children and adolescents. *The Physician and Sportsmedicine* 21(6), 105-116.

RESORPTION The first step in bone remodeling or taking away bone.

RESPIRATION Internal and external respiration. **External respiration** is the exchange of oxygen and carbon dioxide between the atmosphere and the lungs. It includes breathing, the distribution of air within the lungs, and ventilation. The [external] **respiratory system (respiratory tract)** consists of the nose, nasal passages, pharynx, larynx, trachea, bronchi and lungs. In the respiratory tract, the **conducting zone** is the upper part that functions in conducting air from the larynx to the lungs. The **respiratory zone** is the lowermost part of the respiratory tract containing the sites of gas exchange, but only in spaces with sufficiently thin walls can participate in gas exchange (see under LUNGS).

Internal respiration is the exchange of oxygen and carbon dioxide between the alveoli and lung capillaries, the transportation of oxygen and carbon dioxide by the blood, and the exchange of oxygen and carbon dioxide between the blood and body cells (the chemical reactions which take place in body cells to produce energy).

Two respiratory centers are located within the medulla oblongata of the brain stem: the inspiratory center (dorsal respiratory group) and expiratory center (ventral respiratory group). The nerves in the inspiratory center depolarize spontaneously in a cyclic, rhythmical 'on-off' pattern. During the 'on' portion of the cycle, the nerve impulses traveling via motor neurons in the phrenic nerve stimulate the diaphragm and external intercostals muscles to contract. During the 'off' portion of the cycle, the nerve impulses are interrupted, the inspiratory muscles relax and exhalation occurs. Without external influence and at rest, the inspiratory cycle brings about a respiratory cycle of about 2 seconds for inspiration and 3 seconds for exhalation (for a rate of 12 to 15 breaths per minute). **Eupnea** refers to normal respiratory frequency and oscillatory rhythm.

The expiratory center maintains inspiratory muscle tone or low-level contraction, such that the inspiratory muscles never completely relax. It brings about active contraction of the expiratory muscles (internal intercostals and abdominals) when forceful breathing is required, such as during moderate to heavy exercise.

Two neural centers in the pons area of the brain stem also act as respiratory centers and seem to be important for ensuring that the transition between inhalation and exhalation is smooth.

The sympathetic nervous system centers in the hypothalamus can influence breathing when activated by pain or strong emotions. These centers send neural messages to the respiratory centers that produce effects on breathing that are either stimulatory (e.g. hyperventilation) or inhibitory (e.g. gasping in response to cold water immersion). The centers are also important in bringing about an increase in respiration upon initiation of movement and sustaining the increase throughout the duration of exercise.

Cerebral control of breathing originates in the motor cortex. During conscious anticipation of exercise, neural impulses from the motor cortex pass directly to the respiratory muscles, bypassing the respiratory control centers in the medulla. During exercise, neural inputs to the respiratory center come from the motor cortex and from peripheral mechanoreceptors and chemoreceptors. As exercise continues, humoral (chemical) factors, such as fluctuating partial pressure of oxygen and increased partial pressure of carbon dioxide and pH, are sensed in the peripheral chemoreceptors. Arterial chemoreceptors are the most important for controlling the ventilatory response to exercise. Chemoreceptors are located centrally (in the medulla oblongata, but not in respiratory control centers) and peripherally (in the large arteries, especially at the aortic body and carotid body). **Central chemoreceptors** respond directly to the concentration of hydrogen ions in the cerebrospinal fluid surrounding the medulla oblongata. **Peripheral**

chemoreceptors respond to changes in arterial partial pressure of oxygen or the concentration of hydrogen ions (which changes when the partial pressure of carbon dioxide changes).

Irritant receptors within the conduction zone respond to foreign substances such as chemicals, noxious gases, cold air, mucus, dust and other pollutant particulates. Depending on the irritating substance and the anatomical location, a reflex response is triggered that may be a cough, a sneeze, or a bronchial constriction. Stretch receptors in the lungs respond to deep, fast inflation. Increases in lung volume stimulate the stretch receptors, which send inhibitory impulses to both the apneustic center and the inspiratory center with the result that inspiration ceases.

The **Hering-Breuer reflex (inflation reflex)** prevents over-inflation of the lungs and helps maintain respiratory rhythm. Special nerve endings located throughout the lungs are stimulated when the lungs are distended. Impulses from these endings are transmitted via the vagus nerve to the medulla, where there is inhibition of the inspiratory center and stimulation of the expiratory center. The threshold for this reflex in humans is high. It does not appear to function at rest and plays a minor role in exercise. *See also* VENTILATION.

RESPIRATORY ACIDOSIS *See under* ACID-BASE BALANCE.

RESPIRATORY CHAIN   *See* ELECTRON TRANSPORT CHAIN.

RESPIRATORY ENZYMES   These are enzymes found in the mitochondria that catalyze a series of reactions involved in the cellular oxidation of substrates. The main types of respiratory enzymes are the oxidases and the dehydrogenases.

RESPIRATORY EXCHANGE RATIO The ratio of carbon dioxide output rate to oxygen uptake rate in the lungs. *See under* OXYGEN UPTAKE; RESPIRATORY QUOTIENT.

RESPIRATORY FREQUENCY   The rate of

breathing. Respiratory frequency is influenced by the concentration of hydrogen ions in the cerebrospinal fluid; with a high concentration stimulating the respiratory center of the brain to increase respiratory frequency.

RESPIRATORY PUMP *See* VENTILATORY PUMP.

RESPIRATORY QUOTIENT The ratio of carbon dioxide produced to oxygen consumed in metabolizing tissue. The respiratory quotient varies according to the substrate that is metabolized. The respiratory quotient for carbohydrates is unity (1.0), because equal numbers of carbon dioxide molecules are produced to oxygen molecules consumed. For carbohydrates, the respiratory quotient is equal to unity; for fats, it is about 0.6 to 0.73 (depending on the carbon-length of the fatty acid that is being oxidized), because relatively more oxygen is required to oxidize fats than carbohydrate. For palmitic acid (16-carbon), the respiratory quotient is 16 to 23, i.e. 0.696. It is generally assumed that the respiratory quotient for protein is 0.82. From the metabolism of a mixture of a 'mixed diet' (40% carbohydrate and 60% fat), a respiratory quotient of 0.82 is assumed (applying the caloric equivalent of 4.825 kcal per litre of oxygen for the energy transformation). Estimating energy metabolism from steady-state oxygen uptake in this way has a maximum possible error of about 4%. Early in exercise, the respiratory quotient increases with a greater proportion of carbohydrate being used as an energy substrate. After prolonged heavy exercise, high proportions of fat are oxidized and a respiratory quotient of less than 0.8 results.

The assumption of equality between the respiratory quotient and respiratory exchange ratio cannot be made under certain conditions, including metabolic acidosis, non-steady state conditions, hyperventilation and post-exercise oxygen consumption. During metabolic conditions that increase acid production (such as intense exercise), the added carbon dioxide produced from the buffering of lactic acid in the body increases carbon dioxide production independent of oxygen consumption and therefore values of the respiratory exchange ratio can exceed 1. When exercise intensity is increased, it takes time for the oxygen consumption to increase to a level that accounts for the ATP produced during metabolism. Hyperventilation increases the volume of carbon dioxide exhaled from the lung. If this phenomenon occurs without similar increases in oxygen consumption, a higher carbon dioxide production results from indirect gas analysis calorimetry, yielding an inflated value for respiratory exchange ratio. After exercise, oxygen consumption declines but remains above pre-exercise values for several minutes, whereas carbon dioxide decreases rapidly. Consequently, the respiratory exchange ratio may decline below resting values for several minutes. *See also under* OXYGEN UPTAKE.

RESTLESS LEGS SYNDROME It is a condition that is characterized by myoclonus. The primary symptoms involve an increase in the severity of sensations during rest and an irresistible urge to move the affected limbs. The symptoms of restless leg syndrome begin or become worse when the person is at rest and may persist throughout the day, making it difficult for a person to sit motionless. There are no known causes of restless leg syndrome, but likely triggers include heredity, iron and vitamin deficiencies, caffeine and alcohol. The incidence of restless leg syndrome increases with age. Chronic conditions such as diabetes, peripheral neuropathy and Parkinson's disease can worsen and prolong symptoms of restless leg syndrome.

Restless leg syndrome is estimated to affect 5% of the population. Approximately 80% of people with restless leg syndrome have periodic limb movement disorder, but most people with periodic limb movement disorder do not experience restless leg syndrome.

Periodic limb movement disorder affects people only during sleep. It is characterized by behavior ranging from shallow, continual movement of the ankle or toes, to wild and strenuous kicking and flailing of the legs and arms. Movement of the legs is more typical than movement of the arms. These movements occur for 0.5 to 10 seconds in intervals that are separated by 5 to 90 seconds.

Abdominal, oral and nasal movement sometimes accompanies periodic limb movement disorder. Incidence of periodic limb movement disorder increases with age. It is estimated to occur in 5% of people between the ages of 30 and 50 years, but in 44% of people over the age of 65 years.

Drugs used to treat restless leg syndrome and periodic limb movement disorder include dopaminergic agents, benzodiazepines, opioids and anticonvulsants. Dopaminergic agents such as L-dopa/carbidopa are particularly effective.

Bibliography

Paulson, G.W. (2000). Restless legs syndrome. How to provide symptom relief with drug and nondrug therapies. *Geriatrics* 55(4), 35-38; 43-44; 47-48.
Restless Leg Syndrome Foundation. Http://www.rls.org

RESTRICTIVE LUNG DISEASE   Diseases that are characterized by decreased lung volume, either because of an alteration in lung parenchyma or because of a disease of the pleura, chest wall or neuromuscular apparatus. Restrictive lung diseases are characterized by decreased total lung capacity, vital capacity or resting volume. Accompanying characteristics are preserved airflow and normal airway resistance, which are measured as the functional residual capacity.

In terms of etiology, a distinction can be made between intrinsic and extrinsic lung diseases. **Intrinsic lung diseases** (lung parenchyma diseases) cause inflammation or scarring of the lung tissue (interstitial lung disease) or result in filling of the air spaces with exudates and debris (pneumonitis). Intrinsic lung diseases include idiopathic fibrotic diseases, connective tissue diseases, drug-induced lung disease, and primary diseases of the lungs (e.g. sarcoidosis). Intrinsic lung diseases are accompanied by decreased gas transfer, which may be marked clinically by desaturation after exercise. **Extrinsic lung diseases** (extraparenchymal diseases) involve the chest wall, pleura and respiratory muscles. Diseases of these structures result in lung restriction, impaired ventilatory function and respiratory failure (e.g. neuromuscular disorders).

Bibliography

Sharma, S. (2003). Restrictive lung disease. Http://www.emedicine.com

RESULTANT   *See under* FORCE.

RETE   A structure composed of a fibrous network of mesh.

RETICULAR FORMATION   *See under* BRAIN.

RETICULOCYTE   An immature red blood cell.

RETINA   The retina sends visual images to the brain through the optic nerve. **Retinopathy** is non-inflammatory disease of the retina, characterized by retinal detachment. When detachment occurs, vision is blurred. **Retinopathy of prematurity** is disruption in the normal development of blood vessels of the retina in premature infants that can result in scarring and detachment of the retina. Children with retinopathy of prematurity may have decreased visual acuity and refractive errors. A **retinal detachment** occurs when the retina is pulled away from its normal position in the back of the eye. It occurs when fluid seeps into the retinal break and separates the neurosensory retina from the retinal epithelium. This can occur days or even weeks after the initial trauma. Retinal detachment may also occur in the absence of trauma. Retinal detachments may require surgery to return the retina to its proper position in the back of the eye. Detached retina almost always causes blindness unless it is treated.

Retinitis pigmentosa is a hereditary, degenerative condition of the retinal cells, which are replaced by pigmented tissue that eventually causes tunnel vision (loss of peripheral vision) and night blindness. **Diabetic retinopathy** is a complication of diabetes, caused by changes in the blood vessels of the retina. These damaged blood vessels may leak fluid or blood, and develop fragile, brush-like branches and scar tissue. **Retinoblastoma** is a cancerous tumor of the retina. Progression of retinoblastoma may result in enucleation (removal) of the eye.

RETROCALCANEAL BURSITIS *See under* ACHILLES TENDON.

RETROVERSION *See under* FEMORAL NECK.

RETT'S SYNDROME Rett's disorder. A type of pervasive developmental disorder that appears almost exclusively in females, and is found in a variety of racial and ethnic groups worldwide. Rett's syndrome can occur in males, but is usually lethal, causing miscarriage, stillbirth or early death.

The diagnostic criteria of the American Psychiatric Association are: i) all of the following: apparently normal prenatal and perinatal development; apparently normal psychomotor development through the first 5 months after birth; and normal head circumference at birth. ii) onset of all the following after the period of normal development: deceleration of head growth between the ages of 5 and 48 months; loss of previously acquired purposeful hand skills between the ages of 5 and 30 months, with the subsequent development of stereotyped hand movements (e.g. hand-wringing); loss of social engagement early in the course of development, although often social interaction develops later; appearance of poorly coordinated gait or trunk movements; and severely impaired expressive and receptive language development with severe psychomotor retardation.

The prevalence rate in various countries ranges from 1 in 10,000 to 1 in 23,000 of live female births. Often misdiagnosed as autism, cerebral palsy or non-specific developmental delay, Rett's syndrome is characterized by microcephaly (deceleration of head growth) between the ages of 5 months and 4 years, loss of previously acquired hand skills between the ages of 5 months and 2½ years, loss of interest in the social environment, appearance of stereotyped hand-wringing movements and gait and coordination problems, and subsequent development of severe impairment in language and psychomotor function. Scoliosis is a prominent feature of Rett's syndrome, and it can range from mild to severe. Other problems may include seizures and disorganized breathing patterns during wakefulness. Breathing irregularities include episodes of breath holding and hyperventilation associated with vacant spells.

Apraxia is the most fundamental and severely handicapping aspect of Rett's syndrome. It can interfere with every body movement, including eye gaze and speech, making voluntary movement difficult.

Most girls do not crawl typically, but may 'bottom scoot' or 'combat crawl' without using their hands. Many girls begin independent walking within the normal age range, while others show significant delay or inability to walk independently. Some girls begin walking and lose the ability to walk, some continue to walk throughout life, and others do not walk until late childhood or adolescence.

Barring illness or complications, persons with Rett's sydnrome can continue to learn and enjoy family and friends well into middle age and beyond.

The discovery of a genetic mutation (MECP2) on the X chromosome (Xq28) revealed significant insight into the cause of Rett syndrome. This mutation has now been found in up to 75% of typical and atypical cases of Rett's syndrome. Although active MECP2 occurs widely throughout the body, it is especially abundant in the brain. The role of MECP2 is to silence certain genes. In Rett's syndrome, the MECP2 gene is unable to perform this role. The fact that Rett's syndrome is an X-linked dominant disease helps to explain why it is usually found only in girls. If a girl carries the faulty gene for Rett's syndrome on one of her X chromosomes, the other normal X can compensate to some extent. If a boy carries the same faulty gene on his single X chromosome, he has no normal X to compensate for the fault. The gene associated with Rett's syndrome is so important in early development of the embryo that if it is not working at least partially, the pregnancy will not become established. Mutations in MECP2 are almost always sporadic, i.e. they occur spontaneously rather than through heredity. The severity of Rett's syndrome is probably not linked to the exact location of individual mutations on MECP2, but to the X inactivation patterns in each affected girl. Rett's syndrome in boys may result from nondisjunction at the paternal first meiotic division; this is consistent with the hypothesis that two X chromosomes are required for the manifestation of Rett's syndrome. In Klinefelter syndrome, boys are XXY; i.e. they have an extra X chromosome. If one of these X chromosomes has the MECP2 mutation, Rett's syndrome can occur.

Bibliography

International Rett Syndrome Association. Http://www.rettsyndrome.org

REVERSE TURF TOE   *See under* TURF TOE.

RHABDOMYOLYSIS   The degeneration of skeletal muscle caused by excessive unaccustomed exercise, especially when accompanied by heat stress and dehydration. Symptoms include muscle pain, myoglobinuria and increased levels of muscle enzymes. Rhabdomyolysis may be fulminant (sudden-onset). In rare cases, the myoglobin can precipitate in the kidneys, causing renal failure and death.

Bibliography

Clarkson, P.M. (1993). Worst case scenarios: Exertional rhabdomyolysis. *Gatorade Sports Science Exchange* 4(42).

RHEOLOGY   The study of the flow and deformation of matter including biological fluids such as blood. All body tissues have a fluid component. The components of rheological models are the linear spring, the dashpot and the frictional element. The **linear spring** represents elasticity and the **dashpot** represents viscosity. The **frictional element** is often omitted from rheological models of biological tissues because, in normal situations, internal friction is negligible compared with other forces. If the fluid's stress-to-strain rate is linear, the fluid is termed a **Newtonian fluid**. Two standard composite models are the **Kelvin-Voight model** (spring and dashboard in parallel) and the **Maxwell model** (spring and dashpot in series). Neither of these models is sufficient for modeling tissue behavior, unless they are combined with other components.

RHEUMATOID ARTHRITIS   *See under* ARTHRITIS.

RHINITIS   'Runny nose.' It is inflammation of the mucus membrane within the nose resulting in an increased secretion of mucus. Rhinitis may be caused by infection or allergy. **Hay fever** is a form of seasonal allergic rhinitis caused by pollens that are generally wind borne, but may be fungal spores. The nose, roof of the mouth, pharynx and eyes begin to itch gradually or abruptly after the pollen season begins. These symptoms are followed by lacrimation, sneezing and clear, watery nasal discharge. **Perennial rhinitis** is nonseasonal rhinitis, which may or may not be allergic, sometimes complicated by sinusitis, nasal polyps, or sensitivity to aspirin and other non-steroidal anti-inflammatory drugs. In contrast to hay fever, symptoms of perennial rhinitis vary in severity (often unpredictably) throughout the year.

See also UPPER RESPIRATORY TRACT INFECTION.

RIBOFLAVIN   *See under* VITAMIN B_2.

RIBOSE   A pentose (5-carbon) sugar that is important as a component of ribonucleic acid (RNA). See also under PENTOSE PHOSPHATE PATHWAY.

RIBOSOMES   Complexes of rRNA and proteins that function in protein synthesis.

RIBS   The rib cage consists of 12 ribs (costae). The superior 10 ribs are attached directly (first 7), or indirectly (next 3), to the body of the sternum via costal cartilages. A rib is a **sternal** ('**true**') rib if it attaches to the sternum. Ribs that do not connect directly with the sternum are known as **false ribs**. Ribs 11 and 12 are '**floating ribs**,' because they have no anterior attachment to the sternum. The rib cage stabilizes and limits motion of the thoracic spine. Most fractures are minor and undisplaced. The 4th to 9th ribs are most commonly fractured.

See BREATHING MUSCLES; COSTOCHONDRAL INJURY; FLAIL CHEST; STERNUM

RIGID BODY   It is a body whose size and shape are not affected by the external forces acting on it. It is a theoretical (hypothetical) construct and an approximation, because all materials deform by some amount when subjected to force. In mechanics, the term '**body**' is used to represent any object, animate or inanimate. A **linked system** is a system that is represented as a series of rigid links. In biomechanical analysis, the human body is regarded as a linked system. A **body link** is a representation of a body segment in which a central straight line extends longitudinally through the body segment and terminates at both ends in axes about which the adjacent members rotate. A **body segment** is a part of the body considered separately from the adjacent parts. **Energy transfer** is redistribution of kinetic energy among body links. One link loses energy and the second gains energy in the same amount.

Bibliography

Zatsiorsky, V.M. (2002). *Kinetics of human motion*. Champaign, IL: Human Kinetics.

RIGIDITY It is the physical property of resisting change of form. It is opposed to flexibility, ductility, malleability and softness. The **modulus of rigidity** is the coefficient of elasticity for a shearing force. It is the ratio of shear stress to shear strain.

RIGOR MORTIS *See under* ATP.

RISK FACTOR *See under* EPIDEMIOLOGY; HEREDITY.

RITUALS Physical actions that are performed to symbolically express some experience or value that is held deeply by a particular group. Malinowski (1927) argued that ritual or magical behavior is associated with situations of uncertainty and threat, with risk being expressed in terms of physical danger to the participants or possibility of failure. Malinowski compared two forms of fishing among natives of the Trobriand Islands of Melanesia: lagoon and open-sea fishing. In lagoon fishing, in which man can rely upon knowledge and skill, magic does not exist. In open-sea fishing, full of danger and uncertainty, there is extensive magic and ritual.

Extending Malinowski's thesis to Western sport, Womack (1992) argues that athletes, coaches, spectators and officials turn to rituals because: i) it helps the player focus his attention on the task at hand; ii) it can be used to intimidate the other team; iii) it provides a means of coping with high-risk or high-stress situations; iv) it helps establish a rank order among team members and facilitates team communication; v) it helps in dealing with ambiguity in interpersonal relationships; vi) it can be used to reinforce a sense of individual worth under pressure for group conformity; and vii) it directs individual motivation toward achieving group goals. When a team has a losing streak, or when the athlete goes into a slump, ritual may be renegotiated.

Black magic, witchcraft and sorcery involve magical practices that are intended to bring misfortune on others. In Kenya, soccer teams have hired witch doctors to help them win.

Superstition is a set of behaviors by which a person believes that the future, or outcome of certain events, can be influenced. Superstition may be related to religion or magical thinking. Many superstitions are formed through misunderstanding of statistics or causality. Research by Skinner (1947) found 'superstition' in pigeons. Hungry pigeons in a cage were attached to an automatic mechanism that delivered food to the pigeon at regular intervals, but in no relation to the pigeon's behavior. The pigeons associated the delivery of the food with whatever chance actions they had been performing as it was delivered, and they then continued to perform the same actions. Skinner likened the 'superstitious' behavior of the pigeons to the behavior of the bowler, "who has released a ball down the alley, but continues to behave as if he were controlling it by twisting and turning his arm and shoulder."

Chronology

•2004 • The Boston Red Sox won the 100th World Series, overcoming the "Curse of the Bambino." In 1918, the Red Sox won their fifth World Series - a record at the time. George Herman ("Babe") Ruth was one of the stars of the championship-winning Red Sox team, but was sold to the New York Yankees in 1920. The Yankees, who had never won a World Series, went on to claim 26 championships after Ruth's arrival. Following their victory in 1918, the Red Sox appeared in only four World Series and lost each time.

Bibliography

Coakley, J.J. (2004). *Sport in society. Issues and controversies.* 8th ed. Boston, MA: Irwin McGraw-Hill.
Hoffman, S.J. and Harris, J.C. (2000). *Introduction to kinesiology:*

Studying physical activity. Champaign, IL: Human Kinetics.

Malinowski, B. (1948). *Magic, science and religion and other essays*. Glencoe, IL: Free Press.

Malinowski, B. (1927). *Coral gardens and their magic*. London: Routledge and Kegan Paul.

Skinner, B.F. (1947). 'Superstition' in the pigeon. *Journal of Experimental Psychology* 38, 168-172.

Womack, M. (1992). Why athletes need ritual: A study of magic among professional athletes. In Hoffman, S. (ed) *Sport and religion*. pp191-202. Champaign, IL: Human Kinetics.

RNA   Ribonucleic acid. It is a nucleic acid in which the sugar constituent is ribose. Typically, RNA is single-stranded and contains the four bases adenine, cytosine, guanine and uracil.

ROOTING REFLEX   *See* SEARCH REFLEX.

ROTATION   The movement of a body, or part of a body, around an axis. An axis is the intersection of two planes. It is movement in the transverse plane for the cervical and thoracic spine, pelvis (right and left rotation), shoulders and hips (internal and external rotation). *See* ANGLE.

ROTATOR CUFF INJURIES   Injuries to the rotator cuff may result from either macrotrauma or repetitive microtrauma (overuse). In macrotrauma, one or more of the rotator cuff tendons (usually of the *supraspinatus* muscle) are torn when they are stretched as the humerus is pulled away from the glenoid fossa. Repetitive microtrauma occurs in throwing sports when the *supraspinatus* muscle and external rotator muscles (*infraspinatus* and *teres minor*) undergo repetitive eccentric contractions, and thus generate tremendous force (up to 80% body weight) on the tendons, as they decelerate the arm. Rotator cuff tears are associated with impingement in 95% of cases. With respect to the glenohumeral joint, impingement is caused by the trapping of soft tissues between the head of the humerus and the vault formed by the acromion process of the scapula and the coraco-acromial ligament. The following soft tissues are trapped: the tendons of the *supraspinatus*, *infraspinatus*, *teres minor* and *subscapularis* muscles, the long tendon of the *biceps brachii*, and the subacromial bursa that overlies the supraspinatus tendon. Any condition that causes a narrowing of the subacromial

space may lead to impingement. Structural abnormalities include calcium deposits, a hooked acromion, and a thickened acromioclavicular joint. Functional abnormalities include overuse of the rotator cuff muscles, which results in partial tears. Rotator cuff impingement is manifest in the demonstration of a '**painful arc**.' When the upper arm is moved forwards and upwards to an angle of 90 degrees to the body and is then internally rotated, the soft tissues are compressed against the sharp edge of the coraco-acromial ligament. The mechanical irritation gives rise to painful inflammation, accompanied by edema, which further decreases the subacromial space and thus exacerbates the impingement syndrome. Rotator cuff tears are most common in people over the age of 40 years. It is thought that the rotator cuff is degenerated through chronic impingement, predisposing it to acute, complete tears.

ROTATOR INTERVAL   A triangular portion of the shoulder capsule that is located between the supraspinatus and subscapularis tendons.

ROUND SHOULDERS   Abducted scapulae. Protracted scapulae. Separated scapulae. A forward deviation of the shoulder girdle that brings the acromion processes in front of the normal gravitational line. It is usually accompanied by increased convexity in the thoracic spine, but is a distinct condition from kyphosis. Round shoulders occur when the strength of the shoulder girdle abductors (*pectoralis minor* and *serratus anterior*) becomes greater than that of the adductors (*rhomboid major*, *rhomboid minor* and *trapezius III*).

The incidence of round shoulders is high among persons who work at desk jobs and who thus spend much of their time with shoulders abducted. Athletes often exhibit round shoulders, because of overdevelopment of the anterior arm, shoulder and chest muscles resulting from sports and aquatics activities that stress forward movements of the arms. Exercises to correct round shoulders should simultaneously stretch the tightened anterior muscles and strengthen the *trapezius III* and *rhomboid* muscles.

ROYAL JELLY A milky-white substance produced by worker bees and fed to the queen bee. It has a high concentration of nutrients, especially of vitamin B complex. There is no scientific evidence that royal jelly has an ergogenic effect on athletic performance.

RUBELLA German measles. A disease caused by the rubella virus. It is a highly contagious viral infection that is characterized by a rash, swollen glands and joint pain. Regular measles is called **rubeola**. **Congenital rubella syndrome** occurs in about 25% of babies whose mothers contract rubella during the first trimester are born with one or more birth defects such as eye defects, hearing loss, heart defects, mental retardation and (less frequently) cerebral palsy. *See also* DEAFNESS.

RUFFINI CORPUSCLES *See under* MECHANORECEPTORS.

RUFFINI ENDINGS *See under* MECHANORE-CEPTORS.

RUMINATION DISORDER Repeated regurgitation and rechewing of food for a period of at least one month following a period of normal eating habits.

RUNNER'S BLADDER *See under* BLADDER.

RUNNER'S HIGH *See under* ENDORPHINS.

RUNNER'S KNEE *See* ILIOTIBIAL BAND SYNDROME.

RUNNING A form of locomotion in which there is a momentary phase of suspension during which neither foot is in contact with the ground. Most children exhibit minimal running from 18 to 24 months. Children start to run between 2 and 3 years. The skill of running becomes more efficient between the age of 4 and 5 years. Around 5 years of age, the speed of the run increases.

See also GALLOPING; SKIPPING; SLIDING; WALKING.

RUNNING ECONOMY The oxygen cost of submaximal running. It is a good predictor of endurance performance in highly trained runners who have comparable values of maximal oxygen uptake. The maximal oxygen uptake data for elite Kenyan runners, expressed as ml/kg/min, is similar to those of European and American runners. Elite African runners, such as Kenyans, have superior running economy.

An elite, female distance runner, who underwent physiological assessment during the period 1991 to 1995, improved her 3000 m race performance improved by 8% from 1991 to 1993 after which it stabilized. In contrast, maximal oxygen uptake fell from 73 ml/kg/min in 1991 to 66 ml/kg/min in 1993. Submaximal physiological variables, such as lactate threshold and running economy, improved over the course of the study. The decreased oxygen cost of submaximal running caused the estimated running speed at maximal oxygen uptake to increase from 19 km/h in 1991 to 20.4 km/h in 1995. The extensive training program adopted, together perhaps with physical maturation, resulted in improvements in submaximal fitness factors such as running economy and lactate threshold.

Oxygen consumption during running at 12 km/h has been found to be 4.7% higher in shoes of mass 700 g than in bare feet. Possible explanations for this finding include the energy cost of continually accelerating and decelerating the mass of the shoe with each stride, and the external work done in compressing and flexing the sole and in rotating the sole against the ground. Furthermore, shoes probably compromise the ability of the lower limb to act like a spring. Concern about puncture wounds, bruising, thermal injury and overuse injury during the adaptation period are possible explanations as to why runners choose not to run barefoot.

Other factors affecting running economy include: anthropometric traits (e.g. leg length); neuromuscular skill; storage of elastic energy; physiological efficiency (e.g. oxygen cost of breathing); and volume of endurance training. Larger individuals tend to be more economical per unit of body mass than smaller individuals. However, heavier runners produce and store more heat at a given submaximal running velocity (Berg. 2003). Runners with low body mass would therefore be less heat-challenged. There is evidence that flexibility is negatively related to running economy. It is possible that stiffer muscles and tendons are better able to store elastic energy during the eccentric phase of the stretch-shortening activities and that this stored energy can be released during the concentric phase of the action, thus lowering the oxygen cost of the exercise. Alternatively, inflexibility in the trunk and hip may stabilize the pelvis during the stance phase and limit the requirement for stabilizing muscular activity.

Strength training has been found to improve running economy. It probably allows muscles to utilize more elastic energy, makes the runner more stable, improves neuromuscular coordination, increases forward propulsion, and decreases the amount of energy wasted in braking forces.

Running economy may be related to the total volume of endurance training performed, since the best economy values are often found in older or more experienced athletes, or those who complete a large weekly mileage. Furthermore, athletes' most economical velocities or power outputs tend to be those at which they habitually train. Marathon runners are 5 to 10% more economical than other distance runners in terms of the amount of oxygen required for covering a given distance. The decrease in running economy during a triathlon and/or marathon could be largely linked to physiological factors, such as the enhancement of core temperature and a lack of fluid balance. At speeds exceeding 8 km/hour, running is more economical than walking. Generally, less energy is required to shorten the running stride and increase stride frequency to maintain a constant running speed than to lengthen the stride and decrease its frequency. An individual tends to use the combination of stride length and cadence that favors optimal economy. Depending on speed, overcoming air resistance can require 3 to 9% of the total energy cost of running in calm air. The energy of cutting through a headwind is significantly greater than the corresponding decrease in oxygen uptake resulting from a tail wind.

In general, children are less economical runners than adults, requiring 20 to 30% more oxygen per unit of body mass to run at a particular speed. Oxygen uptake at a given submaximal workload decreases during the years of growth. Improvement in running economy may explain parallel advances in endurance performance. The explanation for greater running economy with growth is uncertain but lower step rate, improved running mechanics and changes in the ratio of body mass to surface area may play a role. The aerobic cost of weight-bearing exercise, measured as oxygen uptake per kg, steadily declines with age. The improvements in economy are not related to the energy efficiency of muscle contraction itself, which is age-independent. Submaximal oxygen uptake per stride does not change with age, suggesting that greater stride frequency is associated with poor economy in smaller children. At the same speed, children exercise at a progressively lower intensity (% of maximal oxygen uptake) as they grow.

Berg (2003) argues that using oxygen cost to assess running economy may not be entirely sound, because neither mechanical work nor energy substrate utilization is accounted for. A higher, rather than lower, submaximal oxygen uptake may be beneficial in long duration events such as the marathon if it is associated with greater utilization of fat as a substrate, thus sparing muscle and liver glycogen stores. *See also* EFFICIENCY; GROWTH.

Bibliography

Anderson, T. (1996). Biomechanics and running economy. *Sports Medicine* 22(2), 76-89.

Bangsbo, J. (1996). Physiological factors associated with efficiency in high-intensity exercise. *Sports Medicine* 22(5), 299-305.

Berg, K. (2003). Endurance training and performance in runners. Research limitations and unanswered questions. *Sports Medicine* 33(1), 59-73.

Flaherty, R.F. (1994). Running economy and kinematic differences among running with the foot shod, with the foot bare and with the foot equated for weight. Eugene, OR: *Microform Publications. International Institute for Sport and Human Performance, University of Oregon.* Cited in Warburton (2001).

Hausswirth, C. and Lehenaff, D. (2001). Physiological demands of running during long distance runs and triathlons. *Sports Medicine* 31(9), 679-689.

Jones, A.M. (1998). A 5-year physiological case study of an Olympic runner. *British Journal of Sports Medicine* 32, 39-43.

Jones, A.M. and Carter, H. (2000). The effect of endurance training on parameters of aerobic fitness. *Sports Medicine* 29(6),

373-386.

Martin, P.E. and Morgan, D.W. (1992). Biomechanical considerations for economical walking and running. *Medicine and Science in Sports and Exercise* 24, 467-474.

Morgan, D.W., Martin, P.E., and Krahenbuhl, G.S. (1989). Factors affecting running economy. *Sports Medicine* 7, 310-330.

Morgan, D.W. and Craib, M. (1992). Physiological aspects of running economy. *Medicine and Science in Sports and Exercise* 24, 456-461.

Paavolainen, L. (1999). Explosive-strength training improves 5 km running time by improving running economy and muscle power. *Journal of Applied Physiology* 86(5), 1527-1533.

Rowland, T.W. (1996). *Developmental exercise physiology*. Champaign, IL: Human Kinetics.

Saunders, P.U. et al. (2004). Factors affecting running economy in trained distance runners. *Sports Medicine* 34(7), 465-485.

Warburton, M. (2001). Barefoot running. *Sportscience* 5(3). Http://www.sportsci.org

Weston, A., Mhambo, Z and Myburgh, K. (2000). Running economy of African and Caucasian runners. *Medicine and Science in Sports and Exercise* 32, 1130-1134.

RUNNING INJURIES

About 50 to 70% of all running injuries appear to be overuse injuries due to the constant repetition of the same movement. Recurrence of running injuries is reported in 20 to 70% of all cases. The most common running injuries are patellofemoral stress syndrome, iliotibial band friction, medial tibial stress syndrome, plantar fasciitis, Achilles paratenonitis and patellar tendon injury. The knee is the most frequent site of injury in runners. Tight hip flexors cause forward lean, anterior pelvic tilt and hyperlordosis of the lumbar spine. This puts the lumbar muscles at risk of strain.

The most important risk factor for incurring an overuse injury is a training error, such as excessive mileage, sudden change in training distance or intensity, too much hard interval training and improper footwear. Training errors are present in 60 to 80% of reported injuries to runners. In recreational runners, running distance is strongly associated with an increased risk of injury. A risk factor in road running is leg-length discrepancy caused by the pitch (camber) of the road surface (that is commonly 4 to 9 degrees). Preventive measures include limitation or decrease of weekly running distance and complete rehabilitation from injury.

Athletes in running sports have a high incidence of Achilles tendon overuse injuries. Common errors responsible for Achilles tendon injury include too rapid a return to training after a layoff and a significant increase in training (especially total distance, hill running and interval work).

At least 75% of tendon ruptures are related to sports activities involving abrupt repetitive jumping and sprinting movements. High-top shoes help prevent ankle sprains, because of their ability to limit extreme ranges of motion, provide additional proprioceptive input and decrease external joint stress. To prevent ankle sprains, shoes must also be designed to limit inversion and eversion stresses at the ankle. These stresses are greatest when the foot is in plantar flexion because the distance from the ankle joint to the ground contact point is maximized. Furthermore, the ankle joint itself is less stable during plantar flexion due to a slight degree of lateral mobility. Achilles tendon overuse injuries occur at a higher rate in older athletes than most other typical overuse injuries.

During running, ground reaction forces of 2 to 5 times normal body weight are generated. These impact forces must be dissipated by the body and may contribute to the etiology of injury. According to Nigg and Segesser (1992), a sports shoe should limit impact forces during landing, support the foot during the stance phase of the running cycle and guide the foot during the final phase of ground contact. Nigg found that fast runners land with two or three times the force of slower runners and yet are injured no more frequently. In fact, the runners who experienced the highest impact forces had fewer injuries than the lowest impact runners did. Running on hard surfaces produces no more injuries than running on soft surfaces.

Running barefoot is associated with a substantially lower prevalence of acute injuries of the ankle and chronic injuries of the lower leg in developing countries. Barefoot-adapted individuals have well-developed intrinsic foot musculature and a supple plantar fascia. In barefoot running, rigidity of the foot is supplied by the windlass mechanism, a tightening of the bands of connective tissue that run between the heel and the base of the toes. When the toes bend back during toe-off, the bands become taut, locking the long bones of the foot, deepening the arch and causing a slight resupination that centers the foot for push off. A foot that is both rigid and resupinated provides the safest and most efficient propulsion. It seems better to let the foot stabilize itself rather than to impose stability through rigid elements in the shoe.

Footwear increases the risk of ankle sprains, either by decreasing awareness of foot position provided by feedback from cutaneous mechano-receptors in direct contact with the ground or by increasing the leverage arm and consequently the twisting torque around the subtalar joint during a stumble. Behaviors induced by plantar tactile sensations offer improved balance during movement, which may explain the preference of many gymnasts and dancers for performing barefoot. Impact during running is at its highest when runners use the softest soled shoes and impact is invariably 20 to 25% greater when gymnasts land on thick soft mats when compared with hard surfaces.

Athletic shoes and mats are support surface interfaces composed of relatively soft compressible materials designed to protect against injuries occurring in sports through force of vertical impact. Impact remains high with their use, because humans land harder with them. This hard-landing strategy may be an attempt by the user to improve stability, by compressing the material to a less destabilizing thinner-stiff variety. In a study of ethyl-vinyl acetate (EVA) foams of varying stiffness, identical to that found in soles of athletic footwear, it was found that steady state vertical impact was a negative function of interface stiffness, with the softest interface producing the greatest vertical impact, and the stiffest interface the least vertical impact. It can thus be argued that currently available sports shoes and mats are too soft and thick, and should be redesigned to protect the persons using them.

Using a balance beam task, midsole hardness in men's athletic footwear was positively related to stability, and midsole thickness was negatively related. Since most types of athletic footwear and many other shoes incorporate midsoles with hardness and thickness associated with poor stability, it can be argued that both athletic performance and public safety could be enhanced through stability-optimized footwear.

Expensive athletic shoes account for 123% greater injury than the cheapest ones. From a study in which a force platform was covered by identical shoe sole material made to appear divergent and advertised divergently, it was found that impact varied as a function of advertising message. It was concluded that there is a tendency for humans to be less cautious when using new devices of unknown benefit, because of overly positive attitudes associated with new technology and novel devices.

It has been proposed that that impact forces during running are input signals that produce muscle tuning shortly before the next contact with the ground to minimize soft tissue vibration and/or decrease joint and tendon loading. There is a natural frequency at which each individual's soft tissue tends to vibrate. Soft tissue vibrations seem to be minimal during running. Just before ground contact, muscles throughout the body tense up in order to counter soft-tissue vibrations. This natural frequency of a runner's body depends mostly on weight and muscle tone. The cushioning in running shoes can amplify or damp soft-tissue resonance by shifting impact frequencies toward or away from a runner's natural frequency. Fatigue and injury may result when the muscles expend too much energy countering soft-tissue resonance.

See also under GASTROINTESTINAL SYSTEM.

Chronology

•1960 • Abebe Bikila of Ethiopa won the marathon at the Olympic Games running barefoot over the streets of Rome, which included stretches of cobblestone, in a time of 2 hours 15 minutes and 16.2 seconds. He also won the marathon in the next Olympics, running with shoes in a time of 2 hours 12 minutes and 11.2 seconds. His famous Swedish trainer, Onni Niskanene, compared Bikila's times with and without running shoes, and found that he ran faster bare foot. In 1969, a car crash left Bikila paralyzed from the waist down. The last four years of his life were spent in a wheelchair. He took up archery and became involved in disability sports. In 1973, he died of a brain hemorrhage at the age of 41 years.

•1968 • Nike, Inc. was created, following a successful venture between Bill Bowerman and his student, Phil Knight, in which they sold athletic shoes directly to athletes at track meets. According to legend, Bowerman used his wife's waffle iron to mold rubber soles in 1972. The improved traction of these soles led to the creation of Nike shoes with waffle soles.

•1984 • Zola Budd, running barefoot, broke Mary Decker's word record in the 5,000 m.

•1985 • Zola Budd ran barefoot to win the World Cross Country Championships. She later changed to running shoes to cope with muddy cross-country courses.

Bibliography

Barrett, J. and Bilisko, T. (1995). The role of shoes in the prevention of ankle sprains. *Sports Medicine* 20(4), 277-280.

Brill, P.A. and Macera, C.A. (1995). The influence of running patterns on running injuries. *Sports Medicine* 20(6), 365-368.

Frederick, E.C. and Cavanagh, P.R. (1992). Correspondence. *Medicine and Science in Sport* 24(1), 144-145.

Gross, M.L. and Napoli, R.C. (1993). Treatment of lower extremity injuries with orthotic shoe inserts. An overview. *Sports Medicine* 15(1), 66-70.

van Mechelen, W. (1992). Running injuries. A review of the epidemiological literature. *Sports Medicine* 14(5), 320-335.

van Mechelen, W. (1995). Can running injuries be effectively prevented? *Sports Medicine* 19(3), 161-165.

Nigg, B.M. (1997). Impact forces in running. *Current Opinion in Orthopaedics* 8(6), 43-47.

Nigg, B.M. and Segesser, B. (1992). Biomechanical and orthopedic concepts in sport shoe construction. *Medicine and Science in Sports and Exercise* 24(5), 595-602.

Nigg, B.M. and Wakeling, J.M. (2001). Impact forces and muscle tuning: A new paradigm. *Exercise and Sport Sciences Reviews* 29(1), 37-41.

O'Toole, M.L. (1992). Prevention and treatment of injuries to runners. *Medicine and Science in Sports and Exercise* 24(9), S360-S363.

Robbins, S.E., Gouw, G.J. and Hanna, A.M. (1989). Running related injury prevention through innate impact-moderating behavior. *Medicine and Science in Sports and Exercise* 21, 130-139.

Robbins, S.E. and Gouw, G.J. (1990). Athletic footwear and chronic overloading: A brief review. *Sports Medicine* 9(2), 76-85.

Robbins, S.E. and Gouw, G.J. (1991). Athletic footwear: Unsafe due to perceptual illusions. *Medicine and Science in Sports and Exercise* 23(2), 217-224.

Robbins, S.E. and Gouw, G.J. (1992). Correspondence. *Medicine and Science in Sports and Exercise* 24(1), 145-146.

Robbins, S. et al. (1994). Athletic footwear affects balance in men. *British Journal of Sports Medicine* 28(20), 117-122.

Robbins, S. and Waked, E. (1997). Hazards of deceptive advertising of athletic footwear. *British Journal of Sports Medicine* 31(4), 299-303.

Robbins, S. and Waked, E. (1997). Balance and vertical impact: Role of shoe sole materials. *Archives of Physical Medicine and Rehabilitation* 78(5), 463-467.

Stacoff, A. et al. (1996). Lateral stability in sideward cutting movements. *Medicine and Science in Sports and Exercise* 28, 350-358.

Wakeling, J.M. and Nigg, B.M. (2001). Modification of soft tissue vibrations in the leg by muscular activity. *Journal of Applied Physiology* 90(2), 412-420.

Wakeling, J.M., Nigg, B.M. and Rozitis, A.I. (2002). Muscle activity dampens the soft tissue resonance that occurs in response to pulsed and continuous vibrations. *Journal of Applied Physiology* 93(3), 1093-1103.

Warburton, M. (2001). Barefoot running. *Sportscience* 5(3). Http://www.sportsci.org

Wright, K. (2000). Watching your steps. A new appreciation of the diversity of running style may eventually yield shoes custom-fit to their wearers. *Scientific American Presents: Building the Elite Athlete* 52-57.

S

SACRO-ILIAC JOINT   The articulation between the sacrum and the two ilia (singular, illium). Anterior stability is provided by the *iliopsoas* muscle. Posterior stability is provided by the dorsal sacro-iliac ligaments, along with the thoraco-lumbar fascia and its attachments to the *latissimus dorsi*, *gluteus maximus*, *transversus abdominis* and *obliquus internus* muscles. A wide number of axes and motions are possible at the sacro-iliac joint, with the most common being anterior and posterior rotation of the ilia on the sacrum during flexion and extension, vertical upslips and downslips of the sacrum between the ilia, and rotation of the sacrum between the ilia. **Sacral flexion (nutation)** occurs when the base of the sacrum moves anteriorly. **Sacral extension (counternutation)** occurs when the base moves posteriorly with trunk flexion or thigh extension. With right rotation of the sacrum, the anterior surface of the sacrum faces to the right. With left rotation of the sacrum, the anterior surface of the sacrum faces to the left.

The concept of the sacro-iliac joint causing chronic low back pain is not generally accepted in orthopedic science. Pain in the region of the sacro-iliac joint may be associated with groin pain. There is some evidence that a stress fracture within the sacro-iliac joint may cause pain in some athletes.

The sacro-iliac joint is less stable in females because: the menstrual cycle and pregnancy cause lax ligaments; and the center of gravity being is in the same place as the sacrum, whereas in males it is more anterior. *See also* RELAXIN.

SACRUM   *See under* PELVIC GIRDLE.

SAGITTAL PLANE   *See under* PLANES.

SALIVA   There are three pairs of salivary glands (parotid, sublingual and submandibular) located in or near the mouth. They secrete saliva into the oral cavity in order to moisten food, lubricating it for easy swallowing. Enzymes in saliva begin the process of chemical digestion.

A dry mouth during exercise is most likely due to increased sympathetic activity, which decreases salivary flow and increases protein secretion.

SALT   i) Sodium chloride. ii) Any substance formed from a chemical reaction when a metal displaces the hydrogen from an acid.

SAND TOE   *See under* TURF TOE.

SAPONINS   *See under* PHYTOCHEMICALS.

SARCOMA   A connective tissue neoplasm that is usually highly malignant. It is formed by proliferation of mesodermal cells.

SARCOMERE   *See under* MUSCLE.

SARCOPENIA   *See under* AGING.

SATIETY   The sense of feeling full. The hypothalamus is involved in the regulation of satiety. *See also* ANOREXIA; APPETITE; HUNGER; LEPTIN.

SAVANTISM   The ability to perform skills in sport or other domains at exceptional levels, without benefit of instruction or practice. The most common are calendar, mathematical and music savants. Calendar savants have the ability to reveal the day of the week and the date of any holiday, whether it is in the past or future. Savants typically lack an understanding of what they are doing. An analogy can be made to a parrot that is able to mimic a human's voice, but has no understanding of what is being said. No single theory can explain the syndrome. For example, eidetic imagery ('photographic memory') could account for many, but not all, cases. Theories based on social isolation or sensory deprivation can be rejected by way of the fact that many savants have very stimulating environments and personal attention.

The term 'idiot savant' has been replaced by the terms, 'savant with autism' or 'savant with mental retardation.' The incidence of savantism in autism (about 10%) is about 200 times its incidence in the population with mental retardation and thousands of times its incidence in the population at large.

Bibliography
Treffert, D.A. (1988). The idiot savant: A review of the syndrome. *American Journal of Psychiatry* 145, 563-572.

SCALAR   *See under* VECTOR.

SCAPHOID   i) One of the carpal bones in the proximal row. *See under* INTERCARPAL JOINTS; WRIST JOINT, FRACTURES.   ii) A tarsal bone in the wrist or the tarsals in the foot.

SCAPHOID IMPACTION SYNDROME Impingement of the scaphoid against the radius, giving rise to dorsal wrist pain. It is seen in weightlifters and gymnasts.

SCAPULA   The shoulder blade. Fractures of the scapula are not common, because of its well-protected position, but may occur in sports such as American football, rugby, ice hockey and equestrianism.

Scapula winging (winged scapulae; projected scapulae) is characterized by prominence or protrusion of the inferior angles of the scapulae. The scapulae are pulled away from the rib cage, and vertebral borders are lifted. The *serratus anterior* muscle is an accessory inspiratory muscle, which is innervated by the long thoracic nerve. The primary function of the *serratus anterior* is to hold the inferior angle of the scapula close to the rib cage when the upper limbs are thrust forward. Scapular winging is caused by weakness of the *serratus anterior* from a long thoracic nerve injury, or by weakness of the *trapezius* muscle from an accessory nerve injury (cranial nerve XI). It may also result from rotator cuff disease, capsulitis or glenohumeral pathology, acromioclavicular injuries or scoliosis. Scapular winging is normal until adolescence, because the *serratus anterior*, a prime mover for upward rotation and abduction, is slower in developing than its antagonists. Scapular winging may be accompanied by round shoulders and thoracic kyphosis, and is also associated with congenital anomalies and postural conditions in which the ribs protrude.

See SCAPULOTHORACIC JOINT; SHOULDER GIRDLE; STERNOCLAVICULAR JOINT.

Bibliography
Reeves, R.K., Laskowski, E.R. and Smith, J. (1998). Weight training injuries: Part 2: Diagnosing and managing chronic conditions. *The Physician and Sportsmedicine* 26(3), 54-73.

SCAPULOHUMERAL RHYTHM   The coordinated action of the shoulder girdle and shoulder joints. As the arms move through a wide range of movements, the scapula cooperates by placing the glenoid fossa in the most favorable position for the head of the humerus, e.g. when the arm is abducted, the scapula rotates upward. When the arm is flexed, the scapula rotates upward and tends to slide partially around the rib cage; it abducts. Scapulohumeral rhythm varies between individuals. Within the same individual, it varies with the phase of the movement.

SCAPULOTHORACIC JOINT   A physiological joint, because of the lack of connection between the two bones. The scapula moves on the thorax.

SCAR TISSUE   Fibrous tissue that is formed by the healing process of a wound or diseased tissue. The fibrous tissue is produced by the connective tissue that migrates to the wound in the course of its repair. This fibrous tissue gradually contracts, becomes denser, and loses its blood vessels, leaving a hard white scar. In the case of scars on the surface of the skin, it is covered by an imperfect formation of epidermis. If scar tissue causes chronic problems, it may be necessary to remove it surgically. Scar tissue is an inevitable outcome of severe burns. Each year in the USA about 300,000 people suffer disfiguring injuries from fires. Another 12,000 people die each year from fires.

SCAVENGER   It is a cell that engulfs and digests debris and invading microorganisms.

SCHEURMANN'S DISEASE   Juvenile kyphosis. Dorsal epiphysitis. Scheurmann's osteochondritis. It is the most common cause of structural kyphosis of the thoracic and thoracolumbar spine. It results from epiphysitis and/or osteochondritis, either of which may cause fragmentation of vertebral bodies. One or several vertebrae are usually involved. The etiology is generally unknown. It is twice as common in girls than boys. It is frequently accompanied by a compensatory lordortic curve. Early detection and treatment through bracing can correct structural kyphosis. A variety of braces and orthotic jackets have been developed; the Milwaukee brace is considered one of the most effective for treating structural kyphosis.

Atypical Scheurmann's disease (lumbar Scheurmann's apophysitis) is a distinct entity from classic Scheurmann's disease. It is a self-limiting condition that produces pain, but not deformity or predisposition to chronic back syndromes. Athletes at risk include American footballers, gymnasts and weightlifters.

SCHIZOPHRENIA A chronic, severe and disabling brain disease. Under the diagnostic criteria of the American Psychiatric Association (APA), it involves psychotic disturbance that lasts for at least six months and includes at least one month of two or more of the following: delusions, hallucinations, disorganized speech, grossly disorganized or catatonic behavior and negative symptoms. **Negative symptoms** include flat affect (immobile and unresponsive face, poor eye contact and decreased body language), alogia (brief, empty replies during speech) and avolition (inability to initiate and persist in goal-directed activities). **Catatonia** refers to motor extremes, either purposeless hyperactivity or stupor-like hypoactivity. **Positive (psychotic) symptoms** of schizophrenia include delusions and hallucinations. By positive is meant having overt symptoms that should not be present. **Hallucinations** are false perceptions and involve seeing, feeling, tasting, hearing, or smelling something that doesn't really exist. The most common type of hallucination in schizophrenia is hearing voices. **Delusions** are false personal beliefs and involve interpreting ideas and events in unrealistic, inappropriate ways. People with schizophrenia often have delusions of persecution, or false and irrational

beliefs that they are being cheated, harassed, poisoned or conspired against. **Disorganized symptoms** include confused thinking and speech, and behaviors that do not make sense.

One out of every 1,000 persons in the world has schizophrenia at some time or another. In the USA about 2.5 million people have schizophrenia. It tends to run in families, with a person inheriting a tendency to develop the disease. It may be triggered by environmental events such as infections or highly stressful situations, or a combination of both. The onset of schizophrenia is usually during adolescence or adulthood, often appearing earlier in males than females. Schizophrenia in children is rare. Of the mental conditions that require hospitalization, schizophrenic disorders are the most common. Half of all mental patients are schizophrenic.

There are different types of schizophrenia, including paranoid, disorganized, catatonic and residual schizophrenia. In **paranoid schizophrenia**, a person feels extremely suspicious, persecuted, or grandiose, or experiences a combination of these emotions. In **disorganized schizophrenia**, a person is often incoherent in speech and thought, but may not have delusions. With **catatonic schizophrenia**, a person is withdrawn, mute, negative, and often assumes very unusual body positions. In **residual schizophrenia**, a person is no longer experiencing delusions or hallucinations, but has no motivation or interest in life. In **schizoaffective disorder**, a person has symptoms of both schizophrenia and a major mood disorder such as depression.

There are two major types of anti-psychotic medication. **Conventional anti-psychotics** (e.g. chlorpromazine; Thorazine) effectively control the 'positive' symptoms such as hallucinations, delusions and the confusion of schizophrenia. Long-term side effects include tardive dyskinesia, Parkinsonism (tremor, slowed movement and 'mask-like' facial expressions) and acute dystonic reactions (grimacing, upward gazing of the eyes, eylid tics, and unusual movements). **Tardive dyskinesia** is the presence of involuntary movements of the tongue, jaw, trunk or extremities (e.g. tongue thrusting, clicking and grunting). These involuntary movements may occur in any of the following patterns: choreiform (rapid, jerky, nonrepetitive), athetoid (slow, continual) or rhythmic (various stereotypies). Tardive dyskinesia is usually mild. **New generation (atypical) anti-psychotics** (e.g. risperidone; Risperdal) treat both the positive and negative symptoms of schizophrenia, often with fewer side effects. Anti-psychotic medications do not work immediately. Treatment success rate for schizophrenia is about 60%.

From observing and interviewing patients with schizophrenia on 10-week exercise program of twice-weekly sessions, Faulkner and Sparkes (1999) concluded that exercise has the potential to help decrease patients' perceptions of auditory hallucinations, raise self-esteem, and improve sleep patterns and general behavior. These effects may occur via the provision of distraction and social interaction rather than the exercise itself.

Bibliography

Faulkner, G. and Sparkes, A. (1999). Exercise as therapy for schizophrenia. *Journal of Sport and Exercise Psychology* 21(1), 52-69.
World Fellowship for Schizophrenia and Allied Disorders. Http://www.world-schizophrenia.org

SCHWANNOMA   A tumor that grows from **Schwann cells**, which protect nerves and provide them with the insulation they need to conduct impulses to and from the brain.

SCIATIC NERVE   The anterior and posterior ventral rami from the 4th lumbar to 2nd sacral (L4-S2) vertebrae and the anterior ventral ramus of S3 combine to form the sciatic nerve. The anterior rami contribute the fibers that become the tibial nerve, and the posterior rami contribute the peroneal fibers. The peroneal fibers are found lateral to the tibial fibers, are arranged in fewer, larger funiculi and are tethered at the knee. All these factors predispose the peroneal fibers to more severe damage when the sciatic nerve is injured. The sciatic nerve is rarely injured in sports, because major trauma, such as a fall on the buttocks, is necessary.

Sciatica is irritation or inflammation of the sciatic nerve. It is often caused by a herniated disc in the lumbar spine (especially at L4-L5 or L5-S1) that exerts pressure on one of the sciatic nerve roots. Other causes include a herniated disc, annular tear, myogenic disease, spinal stenosis, facet joint arthropathy, or compression of the nerve between the *piriformis* muscle.

See also under HAMSTRINGS.

SCOLIOSIS   Lateral curvature of the spine to the right or left in the frontal plane. Scoliosis may be classified as either structural or nonstructural (functional).

There are many causes of **structural scoliosis**, the two most common of which are idiopathic and neuromuscular. **Idiopathic scoliosis** is a structural spinal curvature for which cause has not been established. It is characterized by an S-shaped curve, usually composed of a major curve and one or two minor curves. The **major curve** is the one causing the deformity. The **minor curves**, also referred to as secondary or compensatory curves, usually occur above and/or below the major curve and are the result of the body's attempt to adjust for the major curve. A **double major curve** describes a scoliosis in which there are two structural curves that are usually of equal size. **Adolescent idiopathic scoliosis** occurs between the ages of 10 and 18 years. Structural idiopathic scoliosis occurs in 2% of all school-age children. Children with severe curvatures (20 to 40 degrees) are usually treated by means of braces or orthotics, which force the spine into better alignment and/or prevent it from deviating further. The Charleston Bending and Milwaukee braces are the two most effective, commonly used braces for the treatment of scoliosis. The treatment of scoliosis in persons who are wheelchair bound may also involve modifying the chair to improve alignment and to equalize seating pressures. In extreme cases of scoliosis, where the curve is greater than 40 degrees or does not respond to bracing, surgery is employed. This usually involves fusing the vertebrae in the affected area by means of bone grafts and implanting a metal rod. Following surgery, a brace must be worn for about a year until the fusion has solidified.

Nonstructural (functional) scoliosis has a number of known causes, primarily skeletal (e.g. leg-length discrepancy) or muscular (e.g. muscle imbalance). It can be characterized by either an S- or a C-curve. Nonstructural scoliosis can usually be effectively treated by correcting the imbalance. Once a structural, rather than functional, curve is established, corrective exercises may produce a compensatory curve rather than an abolition of the primary curve.

Chronology

•1974 • Lamar Gant set his first world record, a dead lift of 524.5 lb in the 123 lb class at the Flint Olympic Games and went on to be world champion 15 times in the sport of powerlifting. In 1985, he lifted 661 lb when weighing 132 lb. Gant had scoliosis with a curvature of between 74 and 80 degrees. During his world-record dead lifts, it has been estimated that his curvature was 100 degrees. Because of his scoliosis, Gant's trunk was shortened in relation to his height. This meant he had a shorter shoulder-to-hip lever to work, which lowered the 'sticking point' from knee height to shin height. Also he had arms that were longer than normal, and this meant he did not have to lift the bar as high. Gant finished with the bar just above his knee rather than about mid-thigh height.

Bibliography

Great Flint Afro-American Hall of Fame. Http://flint.lib.mi.us/hallfame/99/gant99.html
National Scoliosis Foundation. Http://www.scoliosis.org
Zumerchik, J. (1997, ed). *Encyclopedia of sports science*. New York: Macmillan Library Reference.

SCRATCH REFLEX

SCRATCH REFLEX   A spinal reflex by which an itch or other irritation of the skin causes a nearby body part to move over and briskly rub the affected area.

SEARCH REFLEX   Rooting reflex. A primitive reflex that is present at birth and persists until 3 to 4 months. It is also known as the **cardinal reflex**, because stimulation of the cardinal points (the four quadrants of the mouth) elicits a searching response. It helps the infant locate the source of nourishment such as the nipple of the mother's breast and then the sucking reflex enables the baby to ingest the food. The **sucking reflex** is characterized by an oral sucking action when the lips are stimulated.

SEASONAL AFFECTIVE DISORDER   'Winter blues.' A mood disorder associated with depression episodes and related to seasonal variations of light.

Symptoms of depression occur regularly during the fall or winter months, and include a loss of physical capacity and energy, increased appetite, decreased libido, hypersomnia (excessive sleep or drowsiness), anhedonia (lack of interest in normally pleasurable activities) and impaired social activity. Young people and women are at the highest risk for seasonal affective disorder. Melatonin has been linked to seasonal affective disorder. Regular exercise, especially outdoors, may help in treating seasonal affective disorder, because exercise can relieve depression. Phototherapy or bright light therapy has been shown to suppress the brain's secretion of melatonin.

Bibliography

National Mental Health Association. Http://www.nmha.org

SECOND IMPACT INJURY   *See under* HEAD INJURIES.

SECOND WIND   A phenomenon, experienced especially by endurance athletes, which is associated with the transition from dyspnea to eupnea. It occurs earlier during vigorous exercise than moderate exercise. It is more likely to occur during hot weather.
   See also BREATHING.

SECRETION   A form of active transport whereby the cell does work in passing substance through its plasma membrane.

SEDENTARY DEATH SYNDROME   A collection of disorders that may be worsened by, or directly caused by, physical inactivity and may result in death. **Sedentary people** can be defined as those who undertake no leisure-time physical activity (28% of adults in the USA) and those who undertake less than 30 minutes of moderate physical activity each day (42% of adults in the USA). Physical inactivity increases the incidence of a number of conditions, e.g. coronary heart disease, stroke, hypertension, breast cancer, colon cancer, osteoporosis and obesity. Hahn et al. (1990) reported that 256,686 deaths in the USA were attributed to being either sedentary or irregularly physically active in 1986.

Chronology
•2000 • An organization called Researchers Against Inactivity-related Disorders was formed in order to advocate support for research into the disorders associated with sedentary human lifestyle.

Bibliography
Booth, F.W. et al. (2000). Waging war on modern chronic diseases: Primary prevention through exercise biology. *Journal of Applied Physiology* 88, 774-787.

Hahn, R.A. et al. (1990). Excess deaths from nine chronic diseases in the United States, 1986. *Journal of the American Medical Association* 264, 2654-2659.

Sedentary Death Syndrome. Http://www.endseds.org

SEGMENTAL ANALYSIS *See under* CENTER OF GRAVITY.

SEGMENTAL ROLLING REFLEXES Postural reflexes that emerge 6 to 10 months after birth and persist throughout life. These reflexes are essential for the integration of cross lateral movements, such as walking, running, jumping and swimming. They allow the baby to roll over; when lying on the tummy, for example, the baby first begins to learn to hold the head up, then to raise the upper torso, and eventually to roll over and up into a sitting position. In either prone or supine posture, the segmental rolling reflexes are triggered when the shoulder or knee is raised and moved across the midline towards the other side of the body. When raising the shoulder, the knee on the same side should begin to bend. When raising the knee, the shoulder and arm should begin to roll also. Until the age of 4 months, the infant does not have these reflexes, and the body moves as a rigid unit in a 'logroll' pattern. Abnormal retention of the asymmetric tonic neck reflex delays segmental rolling, because the extended arm is stiff and will not get out of the way. Many children with coordination problems and dyspraxia do not have the segmental rolling reflexes. *See also* AMPHIBIAN REFLEX.

SEIZURE *See under* EPILEPSY.

SELENIUM An element, which as a 'trace element' in the human body, is a co-factor of glutathione peroxidase, an antioxidant enzyme that catalyses the breakdown of hydrogen peroxides and is thus important for the protection of red blood cell membranes and other tissues from damage by peroxides. The selenium contained in the enzymes acts as the reactive center, carrying reactive electrons from the peroxide to the glutathione. It is the glutathione that is the antioxidant in the reaction, not the selenium. Selenium by itself is a potent oxidant that can be very toxic if taken in excess. **Selenocysteine** is a selenium-containing amino acid that is the biologically active form of selenium.

Meat and seafood are rich sources of selenium. In plants and grains, there is wide variation in selenium content because plants do not appear to require selenium and the incorporation of selenium into plant proteins is dependent only on the amount of selenium in soil. Brazil nuts from selenium-rich soil may contain more than 100 mcg in one nut, while those grown in selenium-poor soil may provide ten times less. Salmon (3oz, cooked) contains 40 mcg of selenium. Pork (3 oz, cooked) contains 33 mcg of selenium.

The recommended dietary allowance (RDA) is based on the amount of dietary selenium required to maximize the activity of the antioxidant enzyme glutathione peroxidase in blood plasma. The RDA for adults is 55 mcg/day. *See under* FREE RADICALS.

Bibliography
Oregon State University. The Linus Pauling Institute. Micronutrient Information Center. Http://lpi.oregonstate.edu/infocenter

SELF CONCEPT It is a psychological construct involving **self-image** (the kind of person that one thinks one is) and **self esteem** (how worthy one feels one is). A distinction can be made between self-image and **ideal self** (the kind of person one would like to be). Self-concept can be considered to be multidimensional, i.e. a person has a number of situational-specific self-concepts. Physical self-concept may be different from academic self-concept, for example. Four major factors influencing the development of the self-concept are the reaction of others, comparison with others, social roles, and identification with role models. Cooley's (1902) notion of the 'looking-glass self' was that one's sense of self is derived from an appraisal of others' attitudes toward the self. Mead (1934) argued that the self-concept is a social construction; it is developed through interaction and communication with significant other people.

Body image development in early childhood is synonymous with sensorimotor development. **Body schema** is the diagram of the body that evolves in the brain in response to sensorimotor input. The body schema enables the infant to feel body boundaries, identify body parts, plan and execute movements, and know where the body is in space. During the sensorimotor period (ages 0 to 2 years), children learn to imitate facial expressions, limb movements and body positions. Motor planning (praxis) also emerges during the sensorimotor period as cognition develops and the child wants to manipulate objects/toys and to move from place to place. Language development affects learning to move and concurrent development of body image and self-concept.

Positive body image involves a clear, true perception of body shape and body parts as they really are. **Negative body image** involves a distorted perception of body shape and perception of body parts unlike what they really are. People with negative body image are at greater risk of developing an eating disorder and are more likely to suffer from feelings of depression, isolation, low self-esteem, and obsessions with weight loss. The key to developing a positive body image is to recognize and respect one's natural shape and learn to overpower negative thoughts and feelings about the body with positive, affirming, and accepting ones. Research has found that athletes have a more positive body image compared to nonathletes.

There is a sociocultural pressure for females to meet an aesthetic standard of a thin and toned physique and for males to be lean and muscular. Exposure to photographs of ultra-thin models has been associated with short-term decreases in self-esteem, distortions in body-size estimation, greater depressed modes, and increased use of pathogenic dieting. These effects appear to be particularly strong in young women who perceive the women in the photographic images as role models or as appropri-

ate sources for upward comparisons.

In a study of 41 junior volleyball club players (aged 14 to 18 years) playing in regional play, Thomsen et al. (2004) found that there is pressure from coaches to look like the ideal volleyball player with large thighs. Players are asked to develop a part of their body that they greatly fear will become too big because they believe that their nonathletic friends and peers will confuse the muscle for fat. Body image is heavily influenced by social comparison and organized around an integration of four self-evaluative physical dimensions involving: overall size, arms, abdomen and thighs. Evaluations of body image are frequently negative and appear to be exacerbated by photographic poses that emphasize an athlete's aesthetic beauty rather than her athletic prowess.

Self-presentation processes occur when a person selectively presents aspects of his or her self and/or omits self-relevant information in order to maximize the likelihood that favorable social impression will be generated and an undesired impression will be avoided. **Self-enhancement** (amplifying positive aspects) and **self-protection** (damping negative aspects) are two mechanisms by which a positive image of the self is sometimes maintained. **Self-handicapping** refers to strategies that people use to protect their self-esteem by providing excuses before events occur and explaining reasons for the anticipated lack of team success. People who self handicap do not associate failure with their low ability following failure, thereby protecting their self-esteem. The same strategies used to protect and/or enhance self-perceptions of competence and control might also be used as impression management strategies to protect and/or enhance one's public image.

Self-esteem is positively related to choice, persistence and success in a broad range of achievement and health-related behaviors. It is also related to emotional stability, adjustment to life demands, resilience to stress, and happiness. Research has shown a stronger effect of exercise on physical self-perceptions than on self esteem. The greatest improvements in self-esteem are likely in those who are initially low in self-esteem, and those who have the most to gain from exercise participation (i.e. those who are in poor physical condition).

Although the research evidence is equivocal, it seems that habitual exercisers tend to have more positive self-concepts and higher self-esteem than sedentary individuals. It should be noted, however, that 'habitual' does not imply 'addictive,' which may be negative and associated with low self-concept. There is evidence that athletes suffering 'female athlete triad' may have low self-concept associated with eating disorder. Low self-esteem is generally associated with poor performance; an expectation to perform poorly might operate in a self-fulfilling manner to cause failure.

Athletic identity is the degree to which an individual identifies with the athletic role and looks to others for acknowledgement of that role. A personal identity (self-concept) that is largely dominated by athletic identity may predispose an athlete to emotional problems during abstention from sport and during athletic career termination. *See* BIGOREXIA; BODY DYSMORPHIA; CAREER TERMINATION; EATING DISORDERS; EXERCISE DEPENDENCE.

Bibliography

Berger, B.G. and McInmann, A. (1993). Exercise and the quality of life. In: Singer, R. Murphy, M. and Tennant, L.K. (eds). *Handbook of research on sport psychology*. pp729-760. New York: MacMillan.

Brewer, B.W., Van Raalte, J.L. and Linder, D. (1993). Athletic identity: Hercules' muscles or Achilles heel? *International Journal of Sport Psychology* 24, 237-254.

Cooley, C.H. (1902). *Human nature and the social order*. New York: Scribner.

Estes, S.G. and Mechikoff, R.A. (1999). *Knowing human movement*. Boston, MA: Allyn & Bacon.

Fox, K.R. (1997, ed). *The physical self*. Champaign, IL: Human Kinetics.

Fox, K.R. (2000). Self esteem, self perceptions and exercise. *International Journal of Sport Psychology* 31(2), 228-240.

Hausenblas, H.A. and Symons Downs, D. (2001). Comparison of body image between athletes and nonathletes: A meta-analytic review. *Journal of Applied Sport Psychology* 13, 323-339.

Jones, E.E. and Berglas, S. (1978). Control of attributions about the self through self-handicapping strategies: The appeal of alcohol and the role of underachievement. *Personality and Social Psychology Bulletin* 4, 200-206.

Leary, M.R. (1992). Self-presentation processes in exercise and sport. *Journal of Sport & Exercise Psychology* 14, 339-351.

Mead, G.H. (1934). *Mind, self and society*. Chicago: University of Chicago Press.

National Eating Disorders Association. Http://www.NationalEatingDisorders.org

Payne, V.G. and Isaacs, L.D. (2001). *Human motor development. A lifespan approach*. 5th ed. Boston, MA: McGraw-Hill.

Prapavessis, H., Grove, J.R. and Eklund, R.C. (2004). Self-presentational issues in competition and sport. *Journal of Applied Sport Psychology* 16, 19-40.

Thomsen, S.R., Bower, D.W. and Barnes, M.D. (2004). Photographic images in women's health, fitness, and sports magazines and the physical self-concept of a group of adolescent female volleyball players. *Journal of Sport & Social Issues* 28(3), 266-283.

SELF CONFIDENCE   *See under* ANXIETY; SELF EFFICACY.

SELF EFFICACY   The strength of a person's conviction that he or she can successfully execute a behavior required to produce a certain outcome. Bandura's (1977) **Self-Efficacy theory** is based on the premise that behavior is determined primarily by judgments and expectations concerning the capacity of an individual to cope with environmental demands. These expectations determine the choice of goals and goal-directed actions. Self-efficacy determines the choice of activities that a person attempts, the effort expended and persistence at the activity. Self-efficacy is influenced by personal experiences, vicarious experiences, persuasion and arousal. Personal experiences repeatedly perceived as a success will enhance efficacy expectations, whereas repeated experience perceived as failure will have a negative effect on efficacy expectations. Efficacy information can be provided through observing another person performing a task. Persuasion may be verbal or non-verbal. Arousal affects behavior via the cognitive appraisal of the information conveyed by arousal.

Self-efficacy is a similar construct to self-confidence, but also includes the level of perceived competence. Bandura (1977) proposed that successful performance and low anxiety are determined by high self-efficacy. An alternative hypothesis is that successful performance and high self- efficacy are determined by low anxiety. The research evidence suggests that self-efficacy is neither just an effect nor the only significant predictor of performance.

Harter's **Competence Motivation theory** is based on the premise that motivation is determined by a person's need to feel worthy or competent. Perceived control combines with evaluations of self worth and competence to influence motivation. These feelings influence emotional states such as enjoyment that in turn influence motivation. Harter (1990) argues that children as young as 4 to 7 years make reliable judgments about cognitive competence, physical competence, social acceptance and behavioral conduct, but they are not able to make overall judgments about their global self worth. Between the ages of 8 and 12 years, children are able to differentiate between scholastic competence, social acceptance, athletic competence, physical appearance and behavioral conduct. They are also able to make an overall judgment of their global self-worth. Further developmental changes occur from youth to old adulthood. Incompetence in a domain of highly perceived importance can profoundly affect one's self-esteem.

Weiss and Duncan (1992) found that a child's actual and perceived physical competence is strongly associated with peer acceptance in sport. **Peers** are individuals who are similar in age and/or developmental level and who do not share kinship or reside within the same family. In depth interviews with 8 to 16 year-olds identified positive and negative dimensions of peer relationships (Weiss, Smith and Theeboom, 1996). Positive dimensions of peer relationships include: companionship ('hanging out together'); positive value associated with being together; reinforcement of each other's perceived competence and self esteem; instrumental assistance and tangible support; prosocial behavior emphasizing the cooperative aspects of sport; intimacy (self disclosure); loyalty (sense of commitment toward one another); things in common (interests, activities and values inside and outside of the sport context); attractive personal qualities; emotional support (feelings or expressions of concern for one another); and conflict resolution (constructive resolution of arguments, flights or conflicts). Negative dimensions include: negative conflict (verbal insults); unattractive personal qualities (self centeredness); disloyalty or insensitivity toward others; and lack of opportunities to interact (by missing practices).

See also INTRINSIC MOTIVATION; PARENTS.

Bibliography

Bandura, A. (1977). Self efficacy: Toward a unifying theory of behavioral change. *Psychological Review* 84, 191-215.

Bandura, A. (1977). *Social learning theory*. Englewood Cliffs, New Jersey: Prentice Hall.

Bandura, A. (1990). Perceived self efficacy in the exercise of personal agency. *Journal of Applied Sport Psychology* 2, 128-163.

Harter, S. (1990). Causes, correlates and the functional role of global self-worth: A life-span perspective. In Sternberg, R.J. and Kolligan, J. (eds). *Competence considered*. pp67-97. New Haven, CT: Yale University Press.

Weiss, M.R. and Chaumeton, N. (1992). Motivational orientations in sport. In Horn, T.S. (ed). *Advances in sport psychology*. pp61-99. Champaign, IL: Human Kinetics.

Weiss, M.R. and Duncan, S.C. (1992). The relationship between physical competence and peer acceptance in the context of children's sports participation. *Journal of Sport and Exercise psychology* 14, 177-191.

Weiss, M.R. (1993). Psychological effects of intensive sport participation on children and youth: Self esteem and motivation. In Cahill, B.R. and Pearl, A.J (eds). *Intensive participation in children's sports*. pp39-69. Champaign, IL: Human Kinetics.

Weiss, M.R., Smith, A.L. and Theeboom, M. (1999). "That's what friends are for:" Children's and teenagers' perceptions of peer relationships in the sport domain. *Journal of Sport and Exercise Psychology* 18, 347-379.

SELF-TALK Verbal thought. Self-talk can be used to correct bad habits, focus attention, increase or decrease level of arousal, provide self-motivation, build self-confidence, and increase self-efficacy. Self-talk modification techniques include thought stopping, changing negative to positive thoughts, using reason to challenge negative thoughts, reframing a situation using a different worldview and cognitive restructuring.

Olympic wrestlers have been found to have more positive expectations and task-specific self-talk prior to their best as opposed to worst performances. Landin and Hebert (1999) had female varsity tennis players use self-cueing to help them improve their volleying skills. *See* COGNITIVE INTERVENTIONS.

Bibliography

Gould, D., Eklund, R.C. and Jackson, S.A. (1992). 1988 US Olympic wrestling excellence: I Mental preparation, precompetitive cognition, and affect. *The Sport Psychologist* 6, 358-382.

Gould, D., Eklund, R.C. and Jackson, S.A. (1992). 1988 US Olympic wrestling excellence: II Thoughts and affect occurring during competition. The *Sport Psychologist* 6, 383-402.

Landin, D.L. and Hebert, E.P. (1999). The influence of self-talk on the performance of skilled female tennis players. *Journal of Applied Sport Psychology* 11, 263-282.

Williams, J.M. and Leffingwell, T.R. (1996). Cognitive strategies in sport and exercise psychology. In Van Raalte, J.L. and Brewer, B.W. (eds). *Exploring sport and exercise psychology*. pp51-73. Washington, DC: American Psychological Association.

Zinsser, N., Bunker, L. and Williams, J.M. (1998). Cognitive techniques for building confidence and enhancing performance. In Williams, J.M. (ed). *Applied sport psychology: Personal growth to peak performance*. 3rd ed. pp 270-295. Mountain View, CA: Mayfield.

SEMILUNAR BONE Os lunatum. It is one of the carpal bones in the proximal row.

SEMINIFEROUS TUBULES The canals through which the testicular spermatozoa are conveyed to the **rete testis**, which is a network of tubules carrying sperm from the seminiferous tubules to the **vasa efferentia** (minute ducts of the testes).

SENSATION *See under* PERCEPTION.

SENSATION SEEKING **High-risk sports** such as hang gliding, rock climbing and skydiving are activities in which the high risk of injury or death plays a prominent role. In skydiving, there was an average of 36 fatalities in each of the years from 1996 to 2001. It is estimated that there is one fatality per 65,000 jumps worldwide per annum. Risk factors include equipment failure and losing track of altitude.

Zuckerman et al. (1964) proposed a construct of sensation seeking by which humans seek to decrease tension via "optimal stimulation." Zuckerman's (1984) Sensation Seeking Scale measures four dimensions of sensation seeking: Thrill and Adventure Seeking (the desire to engage in thrill seeking, risk, adventurous activities such as hang gliding); Experience Seeking (seeking arousal through mind, sense and nonconforming lifestyle); Disinhibition (release through traditional sensation-seeking outlets, such as drinking and gambling) and Boredom Susceptibility (aversion to repetition, routine and boring people, and restlessness when escape from tedium is not possible). Skydivers have been found to score highly on the Sensation Seeking Scale. There is some evidence that firstborns are underrepresented in high-risk sports. This may be explained by the fact that firstborns have their needs met in more conventional ways, whereas those born later may be forced to pursue nontraditional activities in order to gain parental or peer approval.

Bibliography

Skydiving Fatalaties – Unofficial Records. Http://www.skydivingfatalaties.com

Zuckerman, M. (1979). *Sensation seeking: Beyond the optimal level of arousal*. Hillsdale, NJ: Erlbaum

Zuckerman, M. (1991). *Psychobiology of personality*. New York: Cambridge University Press.

SENSORIMOTOR INTEGRATION Sensory integration. It concerns the ongoing relationship between behavior and brain functioning. Intrasensory and intersensory integration are outcomes of both sensorimotor and perceptual-motor training. **Intrasensory integration** refers to improved function within one sensory system. **Intersensory integration** refers to improved function between several sensory systems. Modalities providing sensory input that must be organized and processed are touch and pressure, kinesthesis, the vestibular system, temperature, pain, smell, taste, vision, audition and the common chemical sense. The **common chemical sense** controls complex reactions to such activities as peeling an onion.

SENSORY INTEGRATION DISORDER A neurological disorder that results from the brain's inability to integrate certain sensory information. Signs of sensory integration disorder include: oversensitivity to touch, movement, sights or sounds; underreactivity to touch, movement, sights or sounds; tendency to be easily distracted; social and/or emotional problems; activity level that is unusually high or unusually low; physical clumsiness or apparent carelessness; impulsiveness, lacking in control; difficulty in making transitions from one situation to another; inability to unwind or calm self; poor self concept; and delays in speech, language or motor skills; delays in academic achievement. Sensory integrative problems are found in up to 70% of children with learning disabilities. It is also common in autism and attention-deficit hyperactivity disorder. It is typically detected in young children.

Tacitile defensiveness is a type of sensory integration disorder in which there are behavioral and emotional responses, which are aversive, negative and out of proportion to certain types of tactile stimuli that most people would find to be non-painful. Behavioral indicators include avoidance responses to touch stimulation (e.g. avoidance of going barefoot), aversive responses to non-painful touch (e.g. aversion or struggle when hugged), and emotional responses to touch stimulation (e.g. responding with physical aggression to light touch to arms, face or legs). About 60% to 90% of boys with fragile X syndrome and some girls with the full mutations are described as having tactile defensiveness, such as being very sensitive to textures and tags on clothing. Strategies to help a child with tactile defensiveness include: use of firm pressure when touching the child; straight, downward firm pushes on top of the head or on both shoulders in order to calm the child; avoidance of touching or approaching the child from behind; and having the child go first or last in a line.

Another class of tactile disintegration disorder is body image and object awareness problems related to body boundaries, feeling the difference between self and not self, and processing information that comes from touch. It includes: **stereoagnosia** (the inability to identify shapes, textures, and other characteristics of three-dimensional objects by touch alone); **body part agnosia** (inability, when eyes are closed, to recognize which body part has been touched; and **tag agnosia** (when individuals do not realize they have been tagged as part of a game).

Bibliography

Dyspraxia Foundation. Http://www.dyspraxia.org.uk
The National Fragile X Organization. Http://www.fragilex.org
Sensory Integration International. Http://www.sensoryint.com
Sensory Integration Network. Http://www.sinetwork.org

SEPTUM   A dividing wall or membrane between body spaces or masses of soft tissue.

SEPTUM PELLUCIDI   *See under* HEAD INJURIES.

SERINE   A three-carbon, nonessential, glycogenic (glucogenic) amino acid.

SERIOUS EMOTIONAL DISTURBANCE   *See* EMOTIONAL DISTURBANCE.

SEROTONIN   5-hydroxytryptamine. It is the primary inhibitory neurotransmitter modulating the excitatory catecholamine systems in the central nervous system. It is also found in the neural pathways of the peripheral ganglia. **5-hydroxytryptophan (5-HT)** is an intermediate in the serotonin pathway.

Serotonin is involved in many behaviors, such as depression and obsessive-compulsive disorder. Depression is effectively treated with drugs such as fluoxetine (Prozac) that specifically block the reuptake of serotonin into the pre-synaptic axon terminal. Obsessive-compulsive disorder is effectively treated by serotonin reuptake inhibitors, suggesting that this condition may be due to dysregulation in serotonin synapses. Sleep-onset latency is decreased with tryptophan, which is the amino acid needed by the brain for the synthesis of serotonin. Thus, serotonin may play a role in sleep induction. Milk is a good source of tryptophan, thus the folk practice of a glass of milk before bedtime may have some validity.

It has been suggested that carbohydrate craving and occasional binge eating symptoms may occur as a result of tryptophan and serotonin deficiency. Both tryptophan and serotonin may be involved in regulating mood, sensitivity to pain and sleep. Tryptophan may also be involved in appetite regulation. As a consequence of overtraining, the amount of tryptophan in the diet may be insufficient. Carbohydrates stimulate the release of tryptophan and serotonin in the brain. If the levels of tryptophan and serotonin in the brain become too low, depression may result and the need for carbohydrate ingestion is signaled so that more tryptophan can enter the brain.

See also under OBESITY.

Bibliography

Insel, P., Turner, R.E. and Ross, D. (2004). *Nutrition.* 2nd ed. Sudbury, MA: Jones and Bartlett.

Scharf, M.B. and Barr, S. (1988). Craving carbohydrates: A possible sign of overtraining. *Annals of Sports Medicine* 4(1), 19-20.

SEROTYPE   It is a taxonomic subdivision of a species or subspecies distinguishable from other strains therein based on its characteristic antigens or proteins.

SERUM   The fluid that separates from blood, lymph and other fluids of the body when clotting takes place in them. **Blood serum** is plasma without its fibrinogen.

SESAMOID BONES   *See under* OSSICLES.

SEVER'S DISEASE   Traction apophysitis of the calcaneus that occurs as a result of chronic traction from the Achilles tendon. It is common in the 9 to 11 year-old age group, and is self-limiting within 12 to 18 months. It is the pre-adolescent analogue of Osgood-Schlatter's disease. It is commonly observed in skeletally immature soccer players. Risk factors include inappropriate footwear.

Bibliography

American Academy of Pediatrics (2001). Injuries in youth soccer. A subject review. *Pediatrics* 105(3), 659-661.

SEX   i) *See under* GENDER; GENDER DIFFERENCES. ii) *See* SEX BEHAVIOR.

SEX BEHAVIOR   The effects of sexual activity the night before sport depend on the intensity of it. If the sexual activity is light and leads to rest and relaxation, then it may enhance athletic performance the following day.

Regular moderate exercise can have a positive effect on sex behavior. Exercise may improve libido (sexual desire) and overall sexual satisfaction. Possible explanations include decreased fatigue and heightened sexual pleasure due to increased muscle tone. In older men, increased levels of testosterone improve libido and increased cardiovascular function may result in greater blood supply to the penis during coitus (sexual intercourse). Overtraining may have a detrimental effect on libido. There is evidence that sexual activity is associated with quality of life and longevity.

Testosterone seems to promote sexual desire in both sexes. Testosterone contributes to sexual arousal, but sexual activity also produces higher levels of testosterone. For most women, however, psychological factors influence sexual desire far more than hormone levels.

Viagra (sildenafil citrate), an oral drug taken one hour prior to sexual activity, improves erectile function in the majority of men with erectile dysfunction who receive it. Vasodilation of the arteries in the penis allows more blood to flow into the penis. The veins that normally carry blood away from the penis get compressed, restricting the flow of blood out of the penis. More blood flows in and less flows out, making the penis larger. It is not an aphrodisiac and therefore will not work without sexual stimulation. Side effects include headache and facial flushing.

In a laboratory setting, healthy males with their usual female partners achieved an average peak heart rate of 110 bpm with woman-on-top coitus and an average peak heart rate of 127 bpm with man-on-top coitus, with an average of 2.5 METS and 3.3 METS, respectively. There are wide interindividual differences in heart rate response to coitus, however. Coitus will, in most men, represent only a moderate 'stress' on the heart in terms of the responses that impact on myocardial oxygen requirement (heart rate and systolic blood pressure). Sexual activity is usually regarded as being safe if a person can cope comfortably with walking about 300 yards on level ground, or can climb two flights of stairs briskly without getting chest pain or breathlessness. If angina occurs during sex, prior administration of nitrates may help. ACE inhibitors may relieve breathlessness during sex, because they can improve exercise tolerance.

In patients with coronary artery atherosclerosis,

coitus, compared with vigorous physical activity and intense emotional responses, represents a small risk of triggering an acute myocardial infarction. Sexual activity has been found to double the relative risk of acute myocardial infarction in healthy individuals and patients with a prior history of angina or myocardial infarction. The absolute risk of sexually triggered myocardial infarction is low, because the baseline risk of myocardial infarction is low for most individuals and the increased risk due to sexual activity is transient. Regular exercise decreases the risk of myocardial infarction by sexual activity.

Girls who play sports are more likely to be virgins than those who do not play sports. They wait longer before having sex for the first time, have sex less often, and have sex with fewer partners, than female nonathletes. Female teenage athletes are far less l ikely to get pregnant than their peers who are not athletes.

A total of 2,298 college athletes (from seven major geographically represented collegiate institutions in the USA) and 683 randomized nonathlete controls completed a confidential survey questionnaire between the summer of 1993 and winter of 1994, assessing lifestyle and health-risk behaviors over the previous 12 months. Athletes were found to exhibit significantly higher risk-taking behaviors than their nonathlete peers in a number of areas, especially those involving alcohol and sex. Athletes were found to: ride more often as a passenger with a driver under the influence of alcohol or drugs; to have a greater quantity and frequency of alcoholic beverage consumption; and to have less-safe sex, a greater number of sexual partners and less use of contraceptives. Athlete subgroups at highest risk include male athletes and athletes participating in contact sports. Athletes at risk for one high-risk behavior demonstrated an increased risk for multiple risk-taking behaviors. *See also under* HEADACHES.

Bibliography

Butt, D.S. (1990). The sexual response as exercise: A brief review and theoretical proposal. *Sports Medicine* 9(6), 330-343.

Cheitlin, et al. (1999). American College of Cardiology (ACC)/American Heart Association (AHA). Use of sildenafil (Viagra) in patients with cardiovascular disease. Expert consensus document. *Journal of the American College of Cardiology*

(1), 273-282.

Drory, Y. et al. (1995). Myocardial ischemia during sexual activity in patients with coronary artery disease. *American Journal of Cardiology* 75, 835-837.

Erkut, S. and Tracy, A. (2000). *Protective effects of sports participation on girls' sexual behavior.* Wellesley, MA: Center for Research on Women.

Kloner, R.A. (1998). Viagra: What every physician should know. *Ear, Nose and Throat Journal* 77(9), 783-786.

Levin, S. (1993). Does exercise enhance sexuality? *The Physician and Sports Medicine* 21(3), 199-203.

Muller, J.E. (2000). Triggering of cardiac events by sexual activity: Findings from a case-crossover analysis. *American Journal of Cardiology* 86(2A), 14F-18F.

Nattiv, A., Puffer, J.C. and Green, G.A. (1997). Lifestyles and health risks of collegiate athletes: A multi-center study. *Clinical Journal of Sport Medicine* 7(4), 262-272.

Sabo, D. et al. (1998). *The Women's Sports Foundation report: Sport and teen pregnancy.* East Meadow, NY: Women's Sports Foundation.

Stein, R.A. (2000). Cardiovascular response to sexual activity. *American Journal of Cardiology* 86(2A), 27F-29F.

SEX CHROMATIN TEST See under HEREDITY.

SEX GLANDS The gonads (testes in males; ovaries in females).

SEXUALLY TRANSMITTED DISEASES STDs. Many STDs cause no symptoms, but even when symptoms occur it can be difficult to distinguish between two different infections. With 4 million annual cases, **chlamydia** (chlamydial infection) is the most common STD in the USA. Infection from *Chlamydia trachomatis* is usually asymptomatic, especially in female patients. If symptoms develop, they usually occur 7 to 14 days after infection. Symptoms in women usually include vaginal discharge, dysuria, lower abdominal pain and, occasionally, menstrual abnormalities. Complications of chlamydia include pelvic inflammatory disease, perihepatitis (Fitz-Hugh-Curtis syndrome) or conjunctivitis from exposure to genital secretions. Symptomatic male patients usually have dysuria and mild urethral discharge only, but can have abrupt symptoms including swelling of the epididymis with fever and chills. In young men, epididymitis is usually caused by *Chlamydia trachomatis*. It is important to rule out other causes of scrotal tenderness, such as testicular torsion, acute orchitis, tumor and hydrocele.

Gonorrhea (gonococcal infection) is the second

most common STD in the USA, affecting approximately 1 million people. Most patients are asymptomatic, especially women. If symptoms do occur, they are difficult to distinguish from a chlamydial infection. Complications of gonorrhea include epididymitis, pharyngitis and pelvic inflammatory disease, which can lead to infertility and ectopic pregnancy. *Neisseria gonorrhoeae* is easier to transmit than *Chlamydia trachomatis*, but, like chlamydia, gonorrhea transmits more readily from a male than from a female.

Candidiasis is infection with candida, which is a yeast-like fungus. It is the most common cause of vaginal discharge. Other causes of vaginal discharge include bacterial vaginosis and trichomoniasis. **Bacterial vaginosis** is caused by *Gardnella vaginalis* and a malodorous vaginal discharge is the only symptom. If a patient is not treated, complications may include pelvic inflammatory disease, premature labor, chorioamnionitis and endometritis. Bacterial vaginosis may not be a true STD, because the causative organism has been recovered in many women who have never been sexually active. **Trichomoniasis** is caused by the protozoan *Trichomonas vaginalis*. Many patients are asymptomatic. If symptoms develop, patients usually have a profuse yellow discharge and vulvovaginal irritation on pelvic examination.

In the USA, genital herpes, syphilis and chancroid are the most common causes of sexually transmitted genital ulcers. **Herpes simplex virus**, the single leading cause, affects approximately 20% of young adults. Genital ulcers increase the likelihood of acquiring and transmitting HIV. Asymptomatic people can also transmit herpes simplex virus, the incubation time for which is 2 to 20 days. Once ulcers resolve (usually after 14 days), the virus resides in the sensory ganglia and establishes latency. About 80% of patients with primary genital herpes simplex virus will develop recurrences, which are usually less severe than the primary infections. Besides recurrent infections, other complications include herpetic whitlow (herpes simplex virus of the finger), autonomic dysfunction and neonatal transmission. Acyclovir is a medication that shortens the duration of lesions, viral shedding and clinical

symptoms, as well as decreasing new lesion formation. **Syphilis**, caused by *Treponema pallidum*, is the second most common cause of sexually transmitted ulcers in the USA. Primary syphilis usually develops within 3 to 5 weeks after exposure. An untreated primary lesion usually resolves within 6 weeks, but lymphadenopathy can last for months. Secondary syphilis usually begins 3 to 8 weeks after the appearance of the primary chancre (a small hard painless nodule at the site of entry of a pathogen). Without treatment, syphilis resolves spontaneously within 3 to 12 weeks. The patient then remains in an asymptomatic stage called latency. About 25% of these patients have relapses of secondary syphilis, while 33% develop tertiary syphilis, which may appear as neurologic, cardiovascular, soft tissue or cutaneous symptoms. The third most common type of sexually transmitted genital ulcer is **chancroid**, which is caused by a species of bacteria called *Hemophilus ducreyi*.

Genital warts (condylomata acuminata) are benign proliferations of the epidermis caused by one or more than 70 serotypes of the human papillomavirus. Many people infected with human papillomavirus have no symptoms. Genital warts appear as single or multiple bumps in the genital areas of men and women, and are transmitted by skin-to-skin contact during vaginal, anal, or (rarely) oral sex with someone who is infected. About two thirds of people who have sexual contact with a partner with genital warts will develop warts, usually within 3 months of contact. In women, warts occur on the outside and inside of the vagina, on the opening of the uterus (cervix), or around the anus. In men, genital warts are less common. If present, they are usually seen on the tip of the penis. They also may be found on the shaft of the penis, on the scrotum, or around the anus. More than 100 different types of human papillomavirus exist, most of which are harmless. About 30 types are spread through sexual contact. Some serotypes of the human papillomavirus can cause malignant disease (types 16 and 18 cause 80% of cervical cancers found in the USA). A distinction is made between high-risk and low-risk human papillomavirus. High-risk human papillomavirus may cause abnormal Pap smear results, and could lead to cancers of the cervix, vulva, vagina, anus, or penis. Low-risk human papillomavirus may cause abnormal Pap results or genital warts.

Bibliography

Clark, J.R. (1997). Sexually transmitted diseases: Detection, differentiation and treatment. *The Physician and Sportsmedicine* 25(1).

National Institute of Allergy and Infectious Diseases. Http://www.niaid.nih.gov

SEXUAL REFLEX The reflex of erection and ejaculation produced by stimulation of the genitals.

SHARPEY'S FIBERS *See under* PERIOSTEUM.

SHEAR FORCE A force that causes deformation in an angular direction. It tends to cause a portion of the object to slide, displace or shear with respect to another portion of the object. If two external forces are equal, parallel and applied in the opposite direction, but are not in line with each other, they constitute shear loading. This causes shear stress and strain. Shear stress is equal to the shear force divided by the cross sectional area (parallel to the direction of the applied force). Maximum shear stress acts on the surface parallel to the plane of the applied force.

See under BONE; KINETIC CHAIN EXERCISE; MENISCI; STRUCTURE.

SHEPHERD'S FRACTURE *See under* ANKLE JOINT, INJURIES.

SHIN SPLINTS *See under* LOWER LEG PAIN.

SHIVERING *See under* COLD STRESS.

SHOCK (MECHANICS) A transitory state in which the equilibrium of a system is disrupted due to non-uniform distribution of application of stress to the system. A **shock wave** is a spatial propagation of mechanical discontinuity in a system as a result of shock. In heel-strike running, the leg is extended at impact and effectively stiff, resulting in a high level of shock. **Shock absorption** refers to the damping of vibrations in a system. The muscle-tendon unit has the highest energy-absorbing capacity of all muscle

and connective tissue, but this capacity decreases as fatigue increases. As a consequence of fatigue to muscle-tendon units, there is increased strain on associated structures such as bones and joints. A shock absorbent material acts to change the momentum of an impact over a longer period of time than a material that is not shock absorbent. *See also* RESILIENCE.

Chronology

•1936 • Jesse Owens ran the 100 meters in 10.2 seconds. He ran on a clay track that absorbed more energy than modern tracks.

•1977 • The 'tuned' track at Harvard designed by Tom McMahon, Gordon McKay and Peter Greene incorporated the notion that an indoor track mounted on a sprung wooden beam might increase running speed. It enabled an increase in speed of about 3% and decreased injuries by half.

•1996 • The track at the Olympic Games in Atlanta was the fastest in Olympic history. Comprising sheets of vulcanized rubber, the manufacturer Mondo claimed it had a shock absorption rating of 35.6% against the allowable minimum of 35%.

Bibliography

McMahon, T.A. and Greene, P.R. (1978). Fast running tracks. *Scientific American* 239(6), 148-163.

McMahon, T.A. and Greene, P.R. (1978). The influence of track compliance on running. *Journal of Biomechanics* 12, 893-904.

SHOCK (PHYSIOLOGY) Severe disturbance of the circulatory system characterized by decreased blood pressure, weak rapid pulse, generalized tissue hypoxia, thirst and pallor. **Circulatory shock** occurs when blood vessels are inadequately filled with blood and cannot circulate normally. As a consequence, tissue demands for blood flow are not met. If circulatory shock persists, necrosis and organ damage may occur. The most common type of circulatory shock is hypovolemic. **Vascular shock** occurs when extreme vasodilation causes an abnormal expansion of the vascular bed. Blood pressure falls rapidly as a result of a large decrease in peripheral resistance. The most common types of vascular shock result from losses of vasomotor tone due to anaphylaxis (**anaphylactic shock**), failure of autonomic nervous system regulation (**neurogenic shock**) and septicemia (**septic shock**). Septicemia may especially result from severe systemic bacterial infection or bacterial toxins. A transient type of vascular shock may occur as a result of prolonged sunbathing. The heat of the sun on the skin causes cutaneous blood vessels to dilate. Standing up abruptly causes blood to pool briefly (because of gravity) in the dilated vessels of the lower limbs rather than promptly returning to the heart. Blood pressure falls and dizziness occurs as a result of the brain not receiving an adequate supply of oxygen. **Cardiogenic shock** occurs when the heart is unable to sustain adequate circulation. It is usually caused by myocardial damage (e.g. following myocardial infarction). *See also* SPINAL SHOCK.

SHOULDER GIRDLE   Two gliding joints: the sternoclavicular joint and the acromioclavicular joint. The sternoclavicular joint is the only connection between the axial skeleton and the upper appendage. Every movement of the shoulder girdle involves the sternoclavicular joint and the acromioclavicular joint.

The **sternoclavicular joint** involves articulation of the clavicle (collar bone) with the sternum (chest bone). The **acromioclavicular joint** involves articulation of the clavicle with the acromion process of the scapula (shoulder blade). **Elevation** involves upward movement of the shoulder girdle. Muscles that produce elevation are: *trapezius* (upper fibers), *levator scapulae*, *rhomboid major* and *rhomboid minor*. **Depression** involves downward movement of the shoulder girdle. Muscles that produce depression are: *trapezius* (lower fibers), *pectoralis minor*, *latissimus dorsi* and *subclavius*. **Protraction** involves movement of the shoulder girdle forward on a plane parallel to the ground. Muscles that produce protraction are: *serratus anterior, pectoralis minor* and *subclavius*. **Retraction** involves movement of the shoulder girdle backward on a plane parallel to the ground. Muscles that produce retraction are: *trapezius* (middle fibres), *rhomboid major, rhomboid minor* and *latissimus dorsi*. Muscles that produce **lateral displacement of the inferior angle of the scapula** are *serratus anterior* and *trapezius* (upper and lower fibers). Muscles that produce **medial displacement of the inferior angle of the scapula** are: *rhomboid major, rhomboid minor, latissimus dorsi, levator scapulae* and *trapezius*.

Acromioclavicular joint stability is provided by the superior and inferior acromioclavicular ligaments, and the coracoclavicular ligaments (conoid and trapezoid ligaments). The **acromioclavicular ligaments** protect against posterior translation and axial distraction of the clavicle. The **trapezoid ligament** resists axial compression and secondarily, superior translation. The **conoid ligament** primarily resists superior and anterior translation. Both the *trapezius* and *deltoid* muscles are dynamic stabilizers of the acromioclavicular joint. An **acromioclavicular separation** is a sprain of the ligaments supporting the acromioclavicular joint, and is second only to glenohumeral instability as the most common type of shoulder instability. The acromioclavicular joint is typically injured from falling with an adducted arm, striking the shoulder against the ground, and forcing the joint inwards and upwards. As a consequence, the ligaments and the joint capsule may tear, and a partial separation or dislocation (subluxation) occurs. If the strong coracoclavicular ligaments also tear, a complete separation occurs. Osteoarthritis of the acromioclavicular joint is common and increases with age. Fractures of the distal clavicle and acromioclavicular dislocations may predispose this joint to osteoarthritis. Atraumatic osteolysis of the distal clavicle occurs in various disease states such as rheumatoid arthritis.

Sternoclavicular joint stability is provided by a fibrous capsule reinforced by the sternoclavicular and costoclavicular ligaments. Sternoclavicular joint dislocations may be direct or, more commonly, indirect. When the injury mechanism is direct, a force is applied to the anteromedial aspect of the clavicle, pushing the clavicle posteriorly behind the sternum. This may happen to an athlete who is lying supine on the ground and is jumped on, or to an athlete who is kicked directly in the sternoclavicular region. When the injury mechanism is indirect, it typically results from a violent compression of the shoulder toward the midline combined with an anterior or posterior force. This may occur in an athlete who is lying on one side with the upper shoulder compressed. If the upper shoulder is rolled posteriorly, an ipsilateral anterior dislocation results. If the upper shoulder is rolled posteriorly, an ipsilateral posterior dislocation occurs. This may occur during a pile-up in American football or rugby, for example. The incidence of sternoclavicular joint dislocations is less than 1% of all joint dislocations, and the sternoclavicular joint is the least commonly injured joint of the shoulder girdle.

See also CLAVICLE; SCAPULA; SCAPULO-HUMERAL RHYTHM.

Bibliography

Johnson, R.J. (2001). Acromioclavicular joint injuries. Identifying and treating 'separated shoulder' and other conditions. *The Physician and Sportsmedicine* 29(11), 31-35.

SHOULDER JOINT Glenohumeral joint. A ball and socket joint, where the head of the humerus fits into a shallow cavity (**glenoid fossa**) in the scapula. The shoulder joint is unstable, because of a relative surface-area mismatch of the larger humeral head in the smaller glenoid fossa. Stability is largely provided, statically, by soft tissue structures including the glenoid labrum; and dynamically, by the rotator cuff and large muscles of the shoulder. The **glenohumeral ligaments** are discrete thickenings in the joint capsule. The cavity of the shallow glenoid is deepened by the **glenoid labrum**, a fibrocartilaginous thickening surrounding the articular surface of the glenoid cavity. It contributes to stability of the shoulder joint by functionally deepening the glenoid fossa, and acting as an anchoring point for the glenohumeral ligaments and joint capsule. The **superior glenohumeral ligament** originates from the glenoid rim (of the glenoid cavity) just anterior to the insertion of the long head of the biceps tendon and inserts into the lesser tuberosity of the humerus. It prevents inferior subluxation of the glenohumeral joint when the arm is by the side. The **middle glenohumeral ligament** originates from the anteriosuperior labrum and the adjacent supraglenoid tubercle, and inserts onto the lesser tuberosity, contributing to anterior stability. The **inferior glenohumeral ligament** consists of the capsule attached to the middle and lower part of the glenoid, and inserts onto the humeral neck just inferior to the head. This is the ligament that becomes detached in the presence of a Bankart lesion (*see under*

SHOULDER JOINT, DISLOCATIONS). It is probably the most important anterior and inferior stabilizer of the glenohumeral joint with the arm in abduction and external rotation. The humeral head is centered in the glenoid by a compressive force that is created by the contraction of the rotator cuff muscles. The *supraspinatus* muscle is particularly important in depressing the head of the humerus against the superior pull of the *deltoid* muscle. The long head of the *biceps brachii* muscle inserts into the superior rim of the glenoid and also acts as a humeral head depressor.

The movements of flexion, extension, abduction, adduction, lateral and medial rotation, horizontal flexion and extension are permitted at the shoulder joint. **Circumduction** involves combinations of the latter movements. **Flexion** involves movement of the humerus forwards. Muscles that produce flexion are: *deltoid* (anterior fibers), *pectoralis major* (clavicular fibers; from full extension), *biceps brachii* and *supraspinatus*. **Extension** involves movement of the humerus backwards. Muscles that produce extension are: *deltoid* (posterior fibers), *teres major*, *latissimus dorsi* and *pectoralis major* (sternocostal fibers; when arm is flexed). **Abduction** involves sideways movement of the humerus away from the midline of the body. Muscles that produce abduction are: *deltoid* (middle fibers), *supraspinatus* and *infraspinatus*. **Adduction** involves sideways movement of the humerus towards the midline of the body. Muscles that produce adduction are: *pectoralis major, latissimus dorsi, teres major, teres minor, triceps brachii* (long head; assists if arm is adducted) and *coracobrachialis*. **Lateral rotation** involves outward rotation of the humerus. Muscles that produce lateral rotation are: *deltoid* (posterior fibers), *infraspinatus* and *teres minor*. **Medial rotation** involves inward rotation of the humerus. Muscles that produce medial rotation are: *pectoralis major, teres major, latissimus dorsi, deltoid* (anterior fibers) and *subscapularis*. See also SCAPU-LOHUMERAL RHYTHM.

SHOULDER JOINT, DISLOCATIONS
Shoulder joint laxity involves excessive range of movement, but is not pathological as long as the person remains asymptomatic and is able to keep the

humeral head centered in the glenoid fossa. **Instability** occurs when joint laxity becomes symptomatic. It may take the form of dislocation or subluxation. A **dislocation** is a glenohumeral injury in which the articular surface of the humeral head and articular surface of the glenoid cease to be in contact with each other; i.e. there is total loss of congruity of the joint surfaces. A **subluxation** is a partial dislocation and involves an abnormal movement of the humeral head on the glenoid; i.e. there is a loss of congruity that is incomplete. **Voluntary subluxation** results from a person's ability to sublux at will. **Habitual subluxation** occurs with a particular movement(s). **Anterior glenohumeral dislocation** may be caused by direct force applied to the posterior aspect of the shoulder, or indirect force applied through the arm in an extended, abducted and externally rotated position. **Subcoracoid dislocation** is the most common form of anterior dislocation. **Posterior glenohumeral dislocation** may be caused by direct force applied to the anterior aspect of the shoulder, or indirect force applied to the posterior aspect of the shoulder.

Orthopedically, glenohumeral instability is viewed in terms of a spectrum with 'AMBRI' at one end and 'TUBS' at the other end. **AMBRI instability** is **A**traumatic, **M**ulti-directional, **B**ilateral, treated by **R**ehabilitation with **I**nferior capsular shift surgically. **TUBS instability** is **T**raumatic, **U**nidirectional, with **B**ankart lesion, treated with **S**urgery. A **Bankart lesion** is a detachment (tear) of the anterior labrum from the glenoid due to subluxation or dislocation. 90% of acute dislocations have a tearing of the glenoid labrum from the glenoid. In some cases, the glenoid rim is fractured during the dislocation. This is called a **bony Bankart lesion**. It has been implicated as the primary injury resulting from traumatic dislocation. 95% of all instability is anterior in direction and is the result of a single trauma. A greater percentage of posterior instability is attributable to atraumatic causes. A **Hills-Sachs lesion** is a fracture in the shoulder on the posterolateral aspect of the articular surface of the humeral head. It is caused by compression of the humeral head against the anterior rim of

the glenoid fossa. It occurs in about 30% of acute shoulder dislocations and in 75% of recurrent dislocations. In anterior dislocation, the lesion is in the rear of the humeral head; in the posterior dislocation, the lesion is in the front of the head (a **reverse Hills-Sachs lesion**). A **SLAP lesion** (**S**uperior **L**abrum, **A**nterior and **P**osterior) is a tear of the glenoid labrum anterior and posterior to the biceps insertion. **Multidirectional instability** encompasses a spectrum of atraumatic, microtraumatic and macrotraumatic types of injuries, but the majority of injuries are atraumatic and microtraumatic.

SHOULDER JOINT, FRACTURE Fractures of the upper part of the humerus occur most frequently as a result of falling onto an outstretched arm, but may also result from a direct fall onto the shoulder during sports such as rugby, skiing and horseback riding.

SHOULDER POINTER *See under* CLAVICLE.

SHY-DRAGER SYNDROME Idiopathic orthostatic hypotension. Multiple system atrophy. It is a progressive disorder of the central and autonomic nervous systems. There are 3 types of Shy-Drager syndrome: **Parkinsonian** type, which may include symptoms of Parkinson's disease; **cerebellar** type, which may include problems such as loss of balance and tendency to fall; and **combination** type, which may include symptoms of both types 1 and 2. Orthostatic hypotension, which can occur in all three types of the syndrome, and symptoms of autonomic failure such as constipation, impotence in men, and urinary incontinence usually predominate early in the course of the disease. Treatment is aimed at controlling symptoms, using anti-hypotensive, anti-parkinsonian and alpha-adrenergic drugs. Shy-Drager syndrome usually ends in death 7 to 10 years after the onset of symptoms. Pneumonia is the most common cause of death.

Bibliography

National Institute of Neurological Disorders and Stroke. Http://ninds.nih.gov

SIBUTRAMINE   *See under* OBESITY.

SICKLE CELL ANEMIA   *See under* ANEMIA.

SICKLE CELL TRAIT   *See under* ANEMIA.

SIGNS   Readily apparent manifestations of changes in body functions. Vital signs are objective measurements that are made to determine general health and cardiorespiratory function. Vital signs include pulse, respiration, blood pressure and body temperature.

SINDING-LARSEN-JOHANSSON SYNDROME   It is a traction apophysitis in which the lower pole of the patella is injured by the pull of the patellar tendon. The lesion is considered a calcification in an avulsed portion of the patellar tendon, and is self limiting. It is a juvenile form of jumper's knee. The causes and pathology are the same as for Osgood-Schlatter's disease. Both Sinding-Larsen-Johansson syndrome and Osgood-Schlatter's disease occur during the ages of 8 to 13 years in girls and 10 to 15 years in boys.

SINE   In a right-angled triangle, it is the ratio of the side opposite to the angle in question to the side that is the hypotenuse.

SINOATRIAL NODE   *See* SINUS NODE.

SINUSITIS   Inflammation of the paranasal sinuses due to bacterial infection. The paranasal sinuses are: the **frontal** sinuses, over the eyes in the brow area; the **maxillary** sinuses, inside each cheekbone; **ethmoid** sinuses, behind the bridge of the nose and between the eyes; and **sphenoid** sinuses, behind the ethmoids in the upper region of the nose and behind the eyes.

Air trapped within a blocked sinus, along with pus or other secretions, may cause pressure on the sinus wall. This results in painful sinus attacks. Similarly, when air is prevented from entering a paranasal sinus by a swollen membrane at the opening, a vacuum can be created that also causes pain. When the sinus openings become narrow, mucus cannot drain properly and ideal conditions are created for bacteria to multiply. Most healthy people harbor bacteria, such as *Streptococcus pneumoniae* and *Hemophilus influenzae*, in their upper respiratory tracts with no problems until the body's defenses are weakened or drainage from the sinuses is blocked by a common cold or some other viral infection. Bacteria that live harmlessly in the nose or throat can multiply and invade the sinuses, causing an acute sinus infection. Vasomotor rhinitis, caused by humidity, cold air, alcohol, perfumes and other environmental conditions, may be complicated by sinus infections.

Oral steroids such as prednisone are used to treat chronic sinusitis. In children, problems are often eliminated by removal of adenoids obstructing nasal-sinus passages.

Swimmers who are susceptible to sinusitis may be advised to wear nose-clips during training and competition. Scuba diving should be restricted until sinus symptoms have resolved because of the risk of barotrauma.

Bibliography
O'Kane, J.W. (2002). Upper respiratory infection. Helpful steps for physicians. *The Physician and Sportsmedicine* 30(9).

SINUS NODE   The cells that produce the electrical impulses which cause the heart to contract. *See* CARDIAC CYCLE; CARDIAC ARRHYTHMIAS.

SINUS TARSI   *See under* SUBTALAR JOINT.

SITTING HEIGHT   *See under* STATURE

SKELETAL MUSCLE   *See* MUSCLE.

SKELETON   The framework made of bones upon which the rest of the body is built. The **axial skeleton** is that part of the skeleton consisting of the spine, skull, hyoid bone, ribs and sternum. It includes the atlanto-axial joint, the occipito-axial joint, the occipito-atlantal joint, the costovertebral joints and the sternocostal joints. The **appendicular skeleton** is that part of the skeleton consisting of the upper and lower limbs. The shoulder girdle and pelvic girdle link the appendicular skeleton (the arms and legs) to the axial skeleton. Only 177 of the 206 bones in the adult human skeleton are engaged in voluntary movement.

The structural functions of bone are: to provide support for the body against gravity, to act as a lever system to transfer muscular forces; and to protect vital internal organs. Bone also has metabolic functions (e.g. as a repository for calcium).

Each bone in the body is uniquely designed to perform its particular function. Bones can be divided into four categories: long, short, flat and irregular. **Long bones**, such as the femur of the leg, consist of a shaft, which is usually thicker at the end where tendons and other connective tissue attach, and is thinner towards the middle. Long bones are designed to withstand stress and serve as levers. **Short bones,** such as the carpals of the wrist, are also important in movement, but their role is not as great as long bones. **Flat bones**, such as the sternum, have hard smooth surfaces and their main function is to protect vital organs. **Irregular bones** are those that are not classified as long, short or flat, such as the vertebrae of the spine.

The **arm** (**upper limb**) is comprised of the shoulder joint, elbow joint, radio-ulnar joint, wrist joint, intercarpal joints, carpometacarpal joints, metacarpophalangeal joints and interphalangeal joints.

The **lower limb** (**leg**) is comprised of the following joints: hip joint, knee joint, tibiofibular joint, ankle joint, subtalar joint, intertarsal joints, midtarsal joints, tarsometatarsal joints metatarsophalangeal joints and interphalangeal (toe) joints.

SKIER'S HIP   Traumatic intertrochanteric and subtrochanteric fractures.

Bibliography
Frost, A. and Bauer, M. (1991). Skier's hip: A new clinical entity? Proximal femur fractures sustained in cross-country skiing. *Journal of Orthopedic Trauma* 5(1), 47-50.

SKI INJURIES   The knee is the most common site for Alpine skiing injuries, accounting for 20 to 32% of all injuries. The inadequate release of ski bindings has been implicated in lower limb injuries. The ski-release binding is the mechanism that attaches the boot to the ski so that the heel is held down in a fixed position until the bindings are released. The mechanism consists of spring-actuated toe and heel-pieces that respond to torsional and upward forces, respectively. The forces are transmitted through the lower limb and ski boot to the binding mechanism, and vice versa. Release is determined by the spring tensions in the adjustable toe and heelpieces. Ski bindings should release in response to certain transmitted forces in time to prevent injury to the skier, but not 'prematurely.' The forces transmitted through the boot-binding-ski system to the lower limb during skiing can be large, and there is unlikely to be a binding that will respond correctly in all potential release situations. *See also* KNEE LIGAMENTS; STRUCTURE.

Bibliography
Finch, C.F. and Kelsall, H.L. (1998). The effectiveness of ski bindings and their professional adjustment for preventing Alpine skiing injuries. *Sports Medicine* 25(6), 407-416.

SKILL   *See* LEARNING; MOTOR SKILL.

SKIN   The integumentary or covering body system. The skin is protective. It has two principal layers: the epidermis (outer layer) and dermis (inner layer). The epidermis and dermis are supported by a subcutaneous layer, which connects the skin to the underlying muscles.

Wrestling fosters skin infection such as herpes simplex virus (HSV-1), tinea corporis and impetigo. **Herpes gladiatorum** is a cutaneous infection caused by HSV-1, which is spread through direct skin-to-skin contact in sports such as wrestling and rugby. It is characterized by grouped vesicles on an erythematous base, is capable of latency and has a tendency to recur at the site of the primary lesion. The incubation period for primary infection is 2 to 14 days. ***Tinea corporis gladiatorum*** is caused by dermatophytes, usually of the genus *Trichophyton*. It is characterized by often circular, pruritic patches that are typically well demarcated and scaly with raised borders and central healing, producing rings.

With respect to their implications for wrestlers, bacterial infections falls into three classes: those that are contagious like impetigo; those in which the wrestler risks further morbidity with continued competition, like cellulites, furuncles, and carbuncles; and those in which continued competition is permitted, like a local (nonvirulent) bacterial overgrowth associated with folliculitis, abrasions or dermatitis.

Water, perspiration and abraded skin can weaken the *stratum corneum* (the protective outer layer of the epidermis), providing an excellent medium for bacteria to proliferate. **Impetigo contagiosa** is a superficial skin infection caused by either staphylococci or streptococci bacteria. It is particularly common in sports with close skin-to-skin contact, such as wrestling. **Folliculitis** is a superficial infection of the upper portion of the hair follicle and surrounding areas characterized by mildly tender papules or pustules surrounded by erythema. **Furunculosis** is an infection of the deeper hair follicle cavity, and the lesions usually contain pus. **Furuncles** (abscesses, boils) are large, well-defined, erythematous and fluctuant nodules that commonly occur in areas of increased sweating and friction, such the buttock, belt line, anterior thigh and axilla. Both folliculitis and furunculosis are caused by *Staphylococcus aureus*. Hot tubs, whirlpools and swimming pools may be colonized with *Pseudomonas aeruginosa*, leading to 'hot tub folliculitis.' **Carbuncles** are due to infection of the subcutaneous tissues involving the hair follicles, usually caused by staphylococci bacteria.

Pitted keratolysis is a foot malady that typically occurs in active people who wear socks that retain moisture. Numerous bacteria have been implicated. Callus formation is another factor contributing to pitted keratolysis in athletes. *Corynebacterium* organisms produce enzymes that degrade calluses and thrive in environments with high amounts of keratin. Socks that are made of either cotton or a synthetic material designed for absorption are essential.

See also ABRASION; ACNE; BLISTER, CALLUS; CHAFING; TALON NOIR.

Bibliography

Dienst, W.L. et al. (1997). Pinning down skin infections: Diagnosis, treatment, and prevention in wrestlers. *The Physician and Sportsmedicine* 25(12), 45-56.

Levy, J.A. (2004). Common bacterial dermatoses. *The Physician and Sportsmedicine* 32(6).

SKINFOLD FAT Subcutaneous fat. Adipose tissue found under the skin. Measurements of skinfold thickness with calipers are probably the most well established and widely used field method of assessing body composition. More than 100 regression equations have appeared in the literature to predict body fat from skinfolds. A number of problems of estimating body fat content by skinfolds have been revealed by cadaver dissection studies reported by Clarys et al. (1984). In particular, it seems that the best predictors of adipose tissue are different from those generally used. Furthermore, two identical thicknesses of adipose tissue may contain significantly different concentrations of fat. Skinfolds are significantly related to external (subcutaneous) adipose tissue, but the relation to internal adipose tissue is less evident and the relation with intramuscular adiposity is unknown.

Standard skinfolds include the following: abdominal (vertical fold 2 cm to the right of the umbilicus); biceps (vertical fold on the anterior aspect of the arm over the belly of the biceps muscle 1 cm above the level used to mark the triceps site); pectoral (diagonal fold half the distance between the anterior axillary line and the nipple in men or one-third of the distance between the anterior axillary line and the nipple in women); medial calf (vertical fold at the maximum girth of the calf on the midlines of the medial border); midaxillary (vertical fold on the midaxillary line at the level of the xiphoid process of the sternum); subscapular (diagonal fold at 45-degree angle, 1 to 2 cm below the inferior angle of the scapula); and suprailiac (diagonal fold in line with the natural angle of the iliac crest taken in the anterior axillary line immediately superior to the iliac crest); thigh (vertical fold on the anterior midline of the thigh midway between the proximal border of the patella and the inguinal fold); and triceps (vertical fold on the posterior midline of the upper arm halfway between the acromion and olecranon processes, with the arm held freely to the side).

The equations to convert from body density to

body fat (Siri, 1961; Brozek et al, 1963) are based on assumptions derived primarily from body density measurements in a group of young men ('reference man') and later 'confirmed' on the basis of 3 White, male cadavers ('reference body'). Water, protein and mineral were 73.8%, 19.4% and 6.8% respectively, of fat-free mass in the 'reference man,' supporting the initially recommended overall mean fat-free mass density of 1.100 g/cm³, but slight differences between the two equations are magnified with increasing fatness, thus affecting women more than men. These fixed value assumptions do not take into account the greater variability in the density of the fat-free mass of women compared to men, because of decreased fractional bone mineral content and episodic increases in body water. With pregnancy, the most significant deviation from density assumptions is increased water content of the fat-free mass. Menopause is associated with a substantial decrease in bone mineral content. This is primarily due to the estrogen withdrawal, but chronological age is also a factor. Thus, there is a tendency to overestimate fatness from density in women. Although the dissectible bone was comparable at 20% of fat-free mass in women and men in the study by Clarys et al. (1984), bone mineral content as a fraction of fat-free mass is estimated to be 6% in women compared to 6.6% in men, and individual variations in this component can have very large effects on estimates of body fat from body density.

The 10 to 20% greater bone mineral density in lack men and women introduces a significant underestimate in the interpretation of body density results with the standard two-compartment models. Existing equations used to calculate body composition come from body density in Caucasians and would tend to overestimate fat-free mass (underestimate body fat) when applied to African Americans.

In highly trained and select groups of athletes such as American football players, the densities of the fat-free mass could theoretically exceed 1.10 g/cm³. See also BODY COMPOSITION.

Bibliography

Behnke, A.R. and Wilmore, J.H. (1974). Evaluation and regulation of body build and composition. Englewood Cliffs, NJ: Prentice Hall.

Brozek, J. et al. (1963). Densitometric analysis of body composition: Revision of some quantitative assumptions. Annals of the New York Academy of Science 110, 113-140.

Clarys, J.P., Martin, A.D. and Drinkwater, D.T. (1984). Gross tissue masses in adult humans: Data from 25 dissections. Human Biology 56, 459-473.

Clarys, J.P. et al (1987). The skinfold: Myth and reality. Journal of Sports Sciences 5, 3-33.

Siri, A.W. (1961). Body composition from fluid spaces and density: Analysis of methods. In J. Brozek and A. Hanschels (eds). Techniques for measuring body composition. pp223-244. Washington, DC: National Academy of Science, National Research Council.

Vogel, J.A. and Friedl, K.E. (1992). Body fat assessment in women. Special considerations. Sports Medicine 13(4), 245-269.

SKIN INJURIES   See ABRASION; BLISTER; CONTUSION; LACERATION; PUNCTURE WOUNDS.

SKIPPING   A form of locomotion that involves a combination of stepping and hopping, both of which involve transfer of body weight from one leg to the other as the leading leg alternates. Motor milestones are as follows: skipping one-footed (4 years), skipping skillfully about 20% of the time (5 years) and skipping skillfully most of the time (6 years).

SLATER-HARRIS FRACTURES   Classification is based on the specific location of the fracture line(s) across the epiphyseal region of the bone. Type I is complete separation of the epiphysis from the metaphysis. Type II is separation of the epiphysis from the metaphysis as a fracture through a small part of the metaphysis. Type III is fracture of the epiphysis. Type IV is fracture of both the epiphysis and metaphysis. Type V is crushing injury of the epiphysis without displacement.

SLEEP-WAKE CYCLE   A biological rhythm which, more specifically, has a circadian rhythm. It is not known whether the sleep-wake cycle is driven by neurotransmitters or by core temperature. **Sleep** is a state of unconsciousness in which the brain is relatively more responsive to internal than to external stimuli. Sleep involves non-rapid eye movement (non-REM) sleep (about 80% of total sleep) and rapid eye movement (REM) sleep (about 20%). Waking usually transitions into non-REM sleep. Non-REM and REM sleep alternate through the night with approximately 90-minute intervals between REM periods, of which there are 3 to 5. Stages 3 and 4 tend to become shorter, or even disappear, and REM periods tend to get longer and closer together as the hours pass. There are four stages of non-REM with stages 3 and 4 (the deepest) involving delta sleep, which is characterized by high frequency, low amplitude brain waves. When restrictions are made on total sleep, delta sleep is maintained at the expense of other stages. Delta sleep comprises about 15 to 20% of total sleep time. Growth hormone secretion and cell division are at their peak during delta sleep. During REM, the brain is extremely active while the body is entirely inactive (hence why REM sleep has also been called 'paradoxical sleep') and metabolic rate, respiration and core temperature are at their lowest. Non-REM sleep may be important for memory consolidation.

Horne (1988) proposed that high-intensity exercise is needed to affect non-REM sleep. This may explain why physically fit people are more likely to have enhanced non-REM sleep following exercise: unfit people may simply be unable to reach and maintain the rate of energy expenditure to bring about non-REM increases. Research on sleep and performance has generally involved people submitting to sleep deprivation, which in the real world occurs as a result of sleep disorders, work-shift patterns, and social activities Cognitive performance deteriorates approximately in proportion to the duration of sleep deprivation. On the other hand, tasks that are well learned, simple and/or involve large muscle groups show little degradation. Although sleep deprivation of 30 to 72 hours does not affect aerobic and anaerobic capacity, it does decrease time to exhaustion. One theory of decreasing performance in sleep deprivation is the occurrence of micro-sleep, in which theta or delta brain waves briefly interrupt the beta or alpha waves of a wakeful state.

There is some evidence that 'napping' can enhance arousal, mood and cognitive performance. A nap should be taken about 8 hours after awakening and should last a maximum of 15 to 20 minutes, or more than 90 minutes, in order to minimize '**sleep inertia,**' which is a grogginess upon awakening from deep sleep that can last around 30 minutes. It is natural to awaken from REM sleep; this is associated with a fresher feeling. Long naps can also affect the body clock, leading to disruption of the sleep-wake cycle. Resting by lying quietly can be beneficial to performance. It is possible that the primary beneficial effect of both napping and lying quietly is the process of relaxation. Excessive amounts of REM sleep have been associated with depression.

When alcohol is a large proportion of daily energy intake, the network of signals for energy homeostasis appears to adapt, with abnormal patterns of sleep and growth hormone release, along with gradual acquisition of an addictive physical dependency on alcohol. During both drinking periods and withdrawal, alcoholics commonly experience problems falling asleep and decreased total sleep time. Alcoholics are more likely to suffer from certain sleep disorders, such as sleep apnea. Conversely, sleep problems may predispose some people to developing alcohol problems.

In **obstructive sleep apnea**, the muscles of the pharynx, tongue and neck lose their tone during sleep, causing soft tissues of the posterior pharynx to collapse and obstruct airflow while the diaphragm and abdominal muscles continue to contract against the occluded airway. About 2.5 million people in the USA suffer from sleep apnea, with the highest incidence being in obese middle-aged men. Many such patients have small nasal and oral passages, hypertrophied tonsils, or anatomical abnormalities of the jaw that predispose to upper airway obstruction. Partial obstruction of the pharynx gives rise to snoring. Complete obstruction may lead to arterial hypoxemia and bradycardia. Eventually there is momentary arousal, muscular tone returns, the obstruction is abolished, and gas exchange and hemodynamics normalize. Pulmonary and systemic arterial hypertension, secondary polycythemia, and a variety of cardiac arrhythmias may develop. Treatment includes administration of continuous positive airway pressure via a tight facemask to prevent upper away closure during sleep along with weight reduction. **Obesity hypoventilation syndrome (Pickwickian syndrome)** is a condition related to obstructive sleep apnea in which a very obese person does not breathe a sufficient amount of oxygen during sleep or while awake.

Bibliography
Brower, K.J. (2001). Alcohol's effects on sleep in alcoholics. *Alcohol Research and Health* 25(2), 110-125.

Chambers, M.J. (1991). Exercise: A prescription for a good night's sleep. *The Physician and Sportsmedicine* 19(8), 106-114.

Horne, J.A. (1988). *Why we sleep: The function of sleep in human and other mammals.* Oxford: Oxford University Press.

Lands, W.E. (1999). Alcohol, slow-wave sleep, and the somatotropic axis. *Alcohol* 18(2-3), 109-122.

Reilly, T. et al. (1997). *Biological rhythms and exercise.* Oxford: Oxford University Press.

Russo, M.B. (2004). Normal sleep, sleep physiology, and sleep deprivation: General principles. Http://www.emedicine.

Sarvis, J.C. (1994). Sleep and athletic performance: Overview and implications for sport psychology. *The Sport Psychologist* 8, 111-125.

Shephard R.J.(1984). Sleep, biorhythms and human performance. *Sports Medicine* 1, 11-37.

Van Helder, T. and Radomski, M.W. (1989). Sleep deprivation and the effect on exercise performance. *Sports Medicine* 7, 235-247.

SLIDING   *See under* GALLOPING.

SLIPPED CAPITAL FEMORAL EPIPHYSIS   *See under* FEMORAL NECK.

SLUMP   *See under* BURNOUT.

SMITH'S FRACTURE   *See under* ELBOW FRACTURES.

SMOKELESS TOBACCO   Spit tobacco. In the USA, over 12 million people use some form of smokeless tobacco (National Cancer Society). This includes 15 to 20% of all adolescent men. Chewing tobacco and snuff – tobacco leaves that are shredded and twisted into strands – are two types of smokeless tobacco products. Snuff dipping involves placing a pinch of tobacco between the gums and cheek. Tobacco chewing involves absorption of nicotine through the mucus lining of the mouth. Snuff may also be 'snorted' through the nose. Use of smokeless tobacco is increasing among male adolescents and young male adults, due at least in part to effective advertising campaign depicting famous people using snuff tobacco. Consumption of smokeless tobacco was stimulated in the USA by media promotion using professional athletes. This followed decreased cigarette smoking in the mid-1960s after the publication of the *Surgeon General's First Report on Smoking and Health*. The nicotine content of smokeless tobacco is equivalent to that of cigarettes and will therefore produce habituation and addiction. The use of smokeless tobacco may expose the long-term user to a number of adverse physiologic effects on the cardiovascular system that are similar to those attributed to smoking. Smokeless tobacco also contains N-nitrosamines, which have a potential carcinogenic effect on the tissues with which they come into contact in the oral cavity. One can of chew tobacco has three times more cancer-causing chemicals than one pack of cigarettes. The risk of cancer of the cheek and gum may reach nearly 50% among long-term snuff users.

Smokeless tobacco use among major and minor league baseball players in the USA is in the range of 34 to 39%. Smokeless tobacco use by baseball players has been found to have neither a negative nor a positive effect on athletic performance as measured by batting average and run average.

Chronology
•1886 • Baseball cards, packed with tobacco products, were introduced by the Allen & Ginter Company in Virginia.

•1964 • The Advisory Committee to the US Surgeon General reported that "cigarette smoking is causally related to lung cancer in men; the magnitude of the effects of cigarette smoking far outweighs all other factors."

•1965 • In the USA, Congress passed legislation setting up the National Clearinghouse for Smoking and Health.

•1965 • In the UK, the government banned cigarette adverts on television.

•1971 • Congress passed laws that prohibited advertising of tobacco.

•1994 • Oral Health America's National Spit Tobacco Education Program (NSTEP) was founded as "an effort to educate the baseball family and the American public about the dangers of smokeless or spit tobacco, and break the long-standing link between this potentially deadly drug and America's pastime. Each year, anywhere from 10 to 16 million Americans put their health at risk by using spit tobacco products. The National Spit Tobacco Education Program (NSTEP)'s mission is to prevent people, especially young people, from starting to use spit tobacco, and to help all users quit." NSTEP has worked with Major and Minor League Baseball to provide spit tobacco education, prevention and awareness to players at Spring Training camps throughout Florida and Arizona. •2000 • A study conducted by Herb Severson of the Oregon Research Institute reported that spit tobacco use among Major League ballplayers had declined significantly, from 38.55% in 1998 to 33.7% in 2000. Use among Minor League players declined from 35.2% in 1998 to 26.6% in 2001. 67% of current users had tried to quit.

Bibliography

National Spit Tobacco Education Program. Http://www.nstep.org

Sinusas, K. and Coroso, J.G. (1995). Smokeless tobacco use and athletic performance in professional baseball players. *Medicine, Exercise, Nutrition and Health* 4(1), 48-50.

Wichmann, S. and Martin, D.R. (1994). Snuffing out smokeless tobacco use. *The Physician and Sportsmedicine* 22(4), 97-110.

SMOKING *See* CIGARETTE SMOKING.

SMOOTH MUSCLE Muscle that is found in hollow structures of the body such as the urinary and digestive tracts, and other places such as the eye.

SNAPPING-HIP SYNDROME A symptom complex characterized by an audible snapping sensation and usually, but not necessarily, associated with hip pain during certain movements of the hip joint. There are many causes of snapping hip and they are classified as intra-articular (e.g. subluxation of the hip) or extra-articular (e.g. iliopsoas bursitis).

See also ILIOTIBIAL BAND FRICTION SYNDROME.

SNEEZE *See under* COUGH.

SOCCER TOE *See* REVERSE TURF TOE.

SOCIAL FACILITATION The positive effect on performance of an audience or co-actors. A co-actor is a person performing the same task at the same time, in view of the other co-actors. Zajonc (1965) hypothesized that social facilitation could be explained by the mere presence of other people. On the other hand, Cottrell et al. (1968) hypothesized

that social facilitation depends on the other people having the potential to evaluate a person's performance. The research evidence has tended to support the latter hypothesis. **Evaluation apprehension** is a facet of social anxiety that may be the product of a larger and more general motivational state based on a need for inclusion in a social collective and a corresponding fear of social exclusion. Social facilitation is the 'flip-side' of social loafing.

Chronology

•1897 • Norman Triplett's experiments at the University of Indiana on audience effects and motor performance were published in the *American Journal of Psychology*. The performance of cyclists was investigated under three conditions: a) paced efforts against a clock; b) paced efforts against a standard; and c) paced efforts in actual competition against other cyclists. Triplett concluded that the presence of another competitor in a race served "to liberate latent energy in the cyclists not ordinarily available." Other than Triplett's experiments, the majority of the studies conducted up until the early 1920s focused on the relationship between psychology and motor learning. Triplett was a keen sports fan, and even at one stage became temporary head track coach at Kansas State while a search for a new coach was taking place.

Bibliography

Cottrell, N.B. (1968). Performance in the presence of other human beings: Mere presence, audience and affiliation effects. In: Samuels, R.A. et al. (eds). *Social facilitation and imitative behavior*. Boston: Allyn and Bacon.

Wankel, L. (1984). Audience effects in sport. In: Silva, J.M. and Weinberg, R.S. (1984). *Psychological foundations of sport*. pp293-314. Champaign, IL: Human Kinetics.

Zajonc, R.B. (1965). Social facilitation. *Science* 149, 269-274.

SOCIAL LOAFING A process that is manifested in the '**Ringelmann effect**' (the tendency of people to exert less effort in collective performance). Sport teams may be particularly vulnerable to social loafing. Possible explanations include the '**free rider effect**,' i.e. if players feel that their team mates are working less hard or effectively than themselves, then they may believe that their team mates are less motivated or less able than themselves. Since playing the role of a 'sucker' is thought to be aversive, players may choose to decrease their efforts rather than work hard to aid any free riders and/or those who are perceived as less competent. The importance of individual effort decreases as the size of a team or group increases, because there is a greater probability that someone else will solve the problem. Lack of identifiability can also decrease an individual's motivation and the individual may work only as hard as he needs to in order to gain credit or avoid blame. Karau and Williams' (1993) **Collective Effort theory** proposes that individuals will exert effort on a collective task only to the degree that they expect their efforts to help them obtain personally-valued outcomes. It is suggested that social loafing is decreased in the following situations: when individuals believe that others can evaluate their collective performance (e.g. via competition); when individuals work in smaller groups; when individuals perceive their contributions to the collective product as unique; when individuals have a standard with which to compare their group's performance; when individuals work on tasks that are intrinsically interesting to them; when individuals work with others they respect or in a situation that activates a salient group identity; when individuals expect their co-actors to perform poorly; and when individuals have a dispositional tendency to view favorable collective outcomes as valuable (i.e. being a 'team player').

Bibliography

Hardy, C.J. (1990). Social loafing: Motivational losses in collective performance. *International Journal of Sport Psychology* 21(4), 305-327.

Karau, S.J. and Williams, K.D. (1993). Social loafing: A meta-analytic review and theoretical integration. *Journal of Personality and Social Psychology* 65, 681-706.

Karau, S.J. and Williams, K.D. (1995). Social loafing: Research findings, implications and future directions. *Psychological Science* 4(5), 134-139.

SOCIAL SUPPORT   An exchange of resources between at least two individuals, perceived by the provider or recipient to be intended to enhance the well being of the recipient. Sarason et al. (1990) argue that perceived social support is more important for well-being than actual social support. Seven types of social support are listening (non-judgmentally), emotional (providing comfort and care), emotional challenge (encouraging reflection on attitudes, values and feelings), reality confirmation (helping to support the recipient's perspective), task

appreciation (acknowledging the recipient's effort and expressing so), task challenge (promoting motivation and skill) and personal assistance (providing services or help in relation to non-sport needs). Social support is particularly important in the context of sport injury and rehabilitation processes.

Bibliography

Hardy, C.J. and Crace, R.K. (1993). The dimensions of social support when dealing with sport injuries. In Pargman, D. (ed). *Psychological bases of sport injuries.* pp121-144. Morgantown, WV: Fitness Information Technology.

Rosenfeld, L.B. and Richman, J.R. (1997). Developing effective social support: Team building and the social support process. *Journal of Applied Social Psychology* 9, 133-153.

Sarason, I.G., Sarason, B.R. and Pierce, G.R. (1990). Social support, personality and performance. *Journal of Applied Sport Psychology* 2, 117-127.

SOCIOLOGY OF SPORT   An area of study concerned with the social structure, social patterns and social organization of groups and subcultures in sport. Theoretical approaches in sociology include functionalism, conflict and hegemony.

Functionalist theory is based on the premise that social order is underpinned by consensus, common values and inter-related subsystems. Sport is a source of inspiration to both society and the individual. The weakness of this approach is the assumption that the existence and popularity of sport proves that it is serving positive functions. By ignoring the possibility of internal conflicts within social systems, it assumes that sport serves the needs of all subsystems and individuals in an equal manner.

Conflict theory is based on the premise that social order is underpinned by coercion, exploitation and subtle manipulation of individuals. Sport is a distorted form of physical activity shaped by the needs of autocratic or production-conscious societies. Sport is an 'opiate,' rather than an inspiration, and lacks the creative and expressive elements of play. The weakness of this approach is that it ignores factors other than political and economic structures. It focuses too much attention on elite-level spectator sport and overemphasizes the extent to which all sport involvement is controlled by power elites.

In contrast to conflict theory, **Hegemony**

theory rejects the idea that people are manipulated by a system. As conceived by Gramsci (1971), hegemony is based on a form of control that is persuasive rather than coercive. It proposes that cultural experiences can be both exploitative and worthwhile. It thus rejects the original Marxist position that the state is a mere instrument through which the power elites conspire to attain their own interests. Smith (2002) provides an insight into the relationship between sport, religion and political action, showing that the appropriation of a cultural activity can begin to dismantle the hegemonic control by the dominant group. The Nation of Islam focused on Muhammad Ali as representative of both Black oppression and progress, and used his success, reputation and charisma to confirm their position in the USA and to enhance their civil rights struggle. As a Black Muslim, Ali was the victim of White Christian persecution; while as world champion, he became a hero for those promoting Black pride and for those protesting the Vietnam War. Ali was embraced, as long as he was not a threat to the Nation of Islam and its leadership, and his sporting success did not openly conflict with his religious teachings. When Ali became bigger than the Nation of Islam, however, he was marginalized and sport returned to being what it had once been in the Nation of Islam's thinking – a Christian activity, responsible for all kinds of wickedness in the USA.

The work of investigative journalists (e.g. Simson and Jennings, 1992) has strongly influenced the sociology of sport. Sugden and Tomlinson (2002) describe a "critical sociology of sport," which is similar in method to that of investigative journalism.

See also CULTURE; GENDER; IDEOLOGY; SUBCULTURE.

Chronology

•1964 • The International Committee for Sociology of Sport was founded.

•1968 • The American Sociological Association included a discussion on the sociology of sport and the American Association for the Advancement of Science sponsored a session on the psychology and sociology of sport at its annual conference.

•1978 • The International Society on Comparative Physical Education and Sport was founded.

Bibliography

Coakley, J. (2004). *Sports in society. Issues and controversies.* 8th ed. Boston, MA: McGraw-Hill.

Coakley, J. and Dunning, E. (2000, eds). *Handbook of sports studies.* London: Sage.

Edwards, H. (1973). *Sociology of sport.* Homewood, IL: Dorsey Press.

Eitzen, D.S. and Sage, G.H. (2003). *Sociology of North American sport.* 7th ed. Boston, MA: McGraw-Hill.

Frey, J.H. and Eitzen, D.S. (1991). Sport and society. *Annual Review of Sociology* 17, 503-522.

Gramsci, A. (1971). *Selections from the Prison Notebooks.* Trans. Q.Hoare and G. Nowell-Smith. London: Lawrence and Wishart.

Gruneau, R. (1999). *Class, sports, and social development.* Champaign, IL: Human Kinetics.

Hargreaves, J. (1985). *Theatre of the great: Sport and hegemony in Britain.* Oxford: Blackwell/Polity Press.

Jennings, A. (1996). *The new lords of the rings: Olympic corruption and how to buy gold medals.* London: Pocket.

Jennings, A. (2000). *The great Olympic swindle:When the world wanted its games back.* London: Simon and Schuster.

Leonard, W. (1998). *Sociological perspectives of sport.* 5th ed. San Francisco, CA: Benjamin Cummings.

Simson, V. and Jennings, A. (1992). *The lords of the rings: Power, money and drugs in the modern Olympics.* London: Simon and Schuster.

Smith, M. (2002). Muhammad Speaks and Muhammad Ali. Intersections of the Nation of Islam and sport in the 1960s. In Magdalinski, T. and Chandler, T.J.L. (eds). *With God on their side: Sport in the service of religion.* London: Routledge.

Sugden, J. and Tomlinson, A. (2002). Critical sociology of sport: Theory and methods. In Sugden, J. and Tomlinson, A. (eds). *Power games. A critical sociology of sport.* pp3-21. London: Routledge.

Tomlinson, A. (1999). *The game's up: Essays in the cultural analysis of sport, leisure and popular culture.* Aldershot, England: Ashgate Publishing Ltd.

Williams, R. (1977). *Marxism and literature.* Oxford: Oxford University Press.

Yiannakis, A. and Melnick, M.J. (2001, eds). *Contemporary issues in sociology of sport.* Champaign, IL: Human Kinetics.

SODIUM An element, which is a 'macromineral' in the human body and is involved with acid-base balance, body water balance and in the functioning of nerves. Sodium, potassium and chlorine are electrolytes, in that they are dissolved in the body as ions. Sodium and chlorine are the main minerals in blood plasma and extracellular fluid. Sodium is almost completely located in extracellular fluid with very little in intracellular fluid. The sodium ions draw fluid from inside the cells to the extracellular fluid and help to maintain balance between intracellular fluid and extracellular fluid volumes. If the concentration of sodium in extracellular fluid is decreased, more fluid will move into intracellular fluid causing the cell to swell and the extracellular fluid to decrease. If sweat loss exceeds five liters a day, then sodium intake needs to be in excess of the recommended dietary allowance. If so, then the addition of sodium to fluid replacement beverages may enhance recovery from exercise. Large quantities of dilute solutions low in sodium can cause hyponatremia.

For adults, the adequate intake (AI) for sodium and chloride are 500 and 750 mg/day, respectively. In the USA, about 75% of the salt intake is derived from salt added during food processing or manufacturing rather than salt added during cooking or eating. In order to decrease the risk of hypertension and its complications, the National High Blood Pressure Education Program and the National Heart, Lung and Blood Institute of the National Institute of Health recommend consuming no more than 6 g/day of salt (2.4 g/day of sodium). Potato chips (8 oz, salted) contain 1,348 mg of sodium.

Bibliography
Luetkemeier, M.J., Coles, M.G. and Askew, E.W. (1997). Dietary sodium and plasma volume levels with exercise. *Sports Medicine* 23(5), 279-286.

Oregon State University. The Linus Pauling Institute. Micronutrient Information Center. Http://lpi.oregonstate.edu/infocenter

SODIUM BICARBONATE A substance that has been used by athletes as an ergogenic aid for anaerobic exercise. It is also known as baking soda, as it is used in food preparation. It can be ingested orally to augment the body's buffering capacity in order to counteract the build-up of lactic acid. The research evidence on the effectiveness of sodium bicarbonate is equivocal. It seems reasonable to suggest that bicarbonate administration before high-intensity exercise will only enhance performance when the intensity and duration of the exercise are sufficient to result in significant muscle acidosis and adenine nucleotide loss. Any ergogenic effect of sodium bicarbonate would likely be due to increased transport of lactate and hydrogen ions from the intracel-lular compartment of working muscle into the extracellular fluid. This increased transport delays the onset of the critical intramuscular pH that impairs the metabolic and contractile function of muscle.

Chronic administration of sodium bicarbonate can cause hypercalcemia and alkalosis that can cause changes in electrolyte balance and respiration, potentially with serious consequences.

Bibliography
Gledhill, N. (1984). Bicarbonate ingestion and anaerobic performance. *Sports Medicine* 1, 177-180.

Linderman, J.K. and Fahey, T.D. (1991). Sodium bicarbonate ingestion and exercise performance: An update. *Sports Medicine* 11(2), 71-77.

Linderman, J.K. and Gosselink, K.C. (1994). The effects of sodium bicarbonate ingestion on exercise performance. *Sports Medicine* 18(2), 75-80.

Maughan, R.J., King, D.S. and Lea, T. (2004). Dietary supplements. *Journal of Sports Sciences* 22, 95-113.

SODIUM CHROMOGLYCATE Cromolyn sodium (Intal). A drug that is a mast cell stabilizer, thus it selectively suppresses the release of chemical mediators (such as histamine) arising from antigen/antibody reaction or degranulating agents. It is very effective dealing with allergic rhinitis and also decreases symptoms of asthma during exercise or from cold dry air. *See also* EXERCISE-INDUCED BRONCHOCONSTRICTION.

SODIUM-POTASSIUM PUMP One of the active transport mechanisms for moving substances through semi-permeable membranes. Energy from ATP 'pumps' ions 'uphill' against the electrochemical gradient through the membrane by a specialized protein carrier enzyme (sodium-potassium ATPase) that serves as the pumping mechanism. It maintains the resting potential of neurons by conveying three sodium ions out of the cell for every two potassium ions transported to the interior. The sodium-potassium pump is an example of futile cycling. During muscular activity, the potassium ions that are pumped out of the cell due to depolarization should be transported back in via sodium/potassium ATPase. Instead, many of the potassium ions are lost to the interstitial space where it equilibrates with plasma.

SOLAR PLEXUS CONTUSION 'Winding.' It occurs when a blow to the epigastric area affects the neural solar plexus, leading to temporary reflex spasm of the diaphragm and paralysis of breathing. Occasionally, it is due to a forceful expiration of the residual volume of air normally present in the lungs. This leads dyspnea - an inhibition of inspiration for the next few seconds. It is believed that solar plexus contusion is caused by diaphragmatic spasm and transient contusion to the sympathetic celiac plexus. The **celiac plexus** is a network of nerve fibers in the abdomen that is controlled by the autonomic nervous system.

SOLUBLE MEDIATORS *See under* IMMUNITY.

SOLUTION A liquid containing dissolved particles or other liquids in a homogenous single liquid phase.

SOLVENT The liquid into which solids (solutes) dissolve. Water is the universal solvent for biochemical reactions. Substances that are readily soluble in water are said to be hydrophilic. They usually contain ionic bonds, such as sodium chloride, or have one or more polar covalent bonds.

SOMATOMEDINS *See* INSULIN-LIKE GROWTH FACTORS.

SOMATOSTATIN *See under* NEUROTRANSMITTER.

SOMATOTROPIN *See* GROWTH HORMONE.

SOMATOTYPING A method used to measure somatotype (body shape). The somatotype is expressed as three components. The first component, **endomorphy**, refers to relative fatness and 'roundness.' The second component, **mesomorphy**, refers to the relative robustness of the musculoskeletal system. The third component, **ectomorphy**, refers to relative linearity (thinness). Sheldon et al. (1940) used photographs taken at the front, rear and side of the subject, in order to rate the somatotype by inspection. This method was used to measure athletes of the 1960 Olympic Games

(Tanner, 1964). The most common method used today is the Heath-Carter (1967) method, which is a modification of Parnell's (1958) method. Endomorphy is rated by taking skinfold fat measurements. Mesomorphy is rated by taking bone widths and limb girths. Ectomorphy is rated by the **ponderal index**, which is the ratio of body height to the cubed root of body weight. A standardized somatotype rating form is used to yield a three-digit expression for somatotype.

Bibliography

Bale, P. (1995). *Bibliography of research papers on physique, somatotyping and body composition*. 3rd ed. Eastbourne, UK: Chelsea School Research Centre.

Bloomfield, J., Ackland, T.R., and Elliott, B.C. (1994). *Applied anatomy and biomechanics in sport*. Melbourne: Blackwell Scientific Publications.

Heath, B.H. and Carter, J.E.L. (1961). A modified somatotype method. *American Journal of Physical Anthropology* 27, 57-74.

Parnell, R.W. (1958). *Behaviour and physique*. London: Edward Arnold.

Sheldon, W.H., Stevens, S.S. and Tucker, W.B. (1940). *The varieties of human physique*. New York: Harper Brothers.

Tanner, J.M. (1964). *The physique of Olympic athletes*. London: Allen and Unwin.

SPASM *See* MUSCLE SPASM.

SPASTICITY The most common type of motor disorder. It is abnormal muscle tightness and stiffness characterized by hypertonic muscle tone during voluntary movement. The resulting hypertonic state causes muscles to feel and look stiff. Hypertonicity results in co-contraction of agonists and antagonists. This makes the release of objects difficult or impossible.

Abnormal postures are caused by retention of primitive reflexes and immaturity of postural reflexes. Inability to move the head without associated muscle tension in the arms results in many abnormal postures. Among the abnormal postures associated with spasticity are the scissors gait and the hemiplegic gait.

Spasticity is mainly caused by damage to the motor cortex and the cortical tracts that carry motor commands downward through the brain. Damage to the basal ganglia and cerebellum further exacerbates spasticity. Damage to the cerebellum results in exaggerated stretch (myotatic) reflexes that in some persons may be so disruptive that their limbs need to be strapped down. When reflex disturbances are severe, persons with spasticity remain nonambulatory.

About 65% of people with cerebral palsy have spasticity as their predominant type.

SPATIAL AWARENESS   An individual's understanding of the external space. **Subjective (egocentric) localization** involves an immature and limited spatial awareness in which all or most aspects of a child's understanding of the surroundings are noted in reference to herself. **Objective awareness** is a more advanced level of awareness based on establishing objective frames of reference in space. In the course of development, involvement in movement activity may facilitate spatial awareness. *See also* AWARENESS.

SPEAR TACKLER'S SPINE   Originally described in 1993, after data was reviewed from the National Football Head and Neck Injury Registry, it is characterized by: developmental narrowing of the cervical spinal canal; straightening or reversal of the normal cervical lordotic curve; pre-existing minor post-traumatic radiographic evidence of bony or ligament injury; and a past history of using spear tackling techniques.

In general, there is consensus that basic necessities for return to collision sports include: normal strength, painless range of motion, a stable vertebral column, and adequate space for the neurological elements. Some neurosurgeons believe that if normal cervical lordosis is restored and spear tackling is avoided, then there is not a high degree of risk of reinjury. Most neurosurgeons, however, argue that spear tackler's spine remains a contraindication for further participation in contact sports.

Chronology
•1976 • Spearing, a tackling technique in which the helmet is used, in effect, as a weapon, was outlawed in American football. The number of fatalities in high-school football decreased from 20 in 1965 to 4 in 1985. The National Collegiate Athletic Association (NCAA) and the National Federation of State High School

Association prohibited use of the head as the initial point when blocking and tackling.

Bibliography
Morganti, C. (2003). Recommendation for return to sports following cervical spine injuries. *Sports Medicine* 33(8), 563-573.
Torg, J.S. et al. (1993). Spear tackler's spine. An entity precluding participation in tackle football and collision activities that expose the cervical spine to axial energy inputs. *American Journal of Sports Medicine* 21(5), 640-649.

SPECIFIC GRAVITY   The density of a substance relative to the density of water. It is the ratio of the density of a solid or liquid to the density of water at 4 degrees Celsius. It can also refer to the ratio of the density of a gas to the density of dry air at standard temperature and pressure, but this specification is less often used. Specific gravity is a dimensionless quantity; i.e. it is not expressed in units. Water has a specific gravity equal to 1. Materials with a specific gravity less than 1 are less dense than water, and will float on the pure liquid; substances with a specific gravity more than 1 are denser than water, and will sink.

SPECIFIC HEAT   *See under* HEAT.

SPECIFIC WEIGHT   Weight per unit of volume. The SI units are Newtons per cubic meter (N/m^3).

SPEECH OR LANGUAGE IMPAIRMENT Under federal legislation in the USA, it is a communication disorder, such as stuttering, impaired articulation, language impairment or voice impairment, which adversely affects a child's educational performance.

SPEED   Time rate of motion. It is the magnitude of velocity. *See under* ACCELERATION; GENDER; GROWTH; POWER.

SPEED, TRAINING   In human movement, speed is a function of quickness, reactive ability, strength, endurance and skill to effectively coordinate one's movements in response to the external conditions under which the motor task is to be executed. **Quickness** is a general quality of the central nervous system, being displayed most powerfully during reflexive motor reactions and production of the simplest unloaded movements. There is far greater potential to enhance speed of movement than quickness.

Specific sprint exercises can be categorized as either overspeed (facilitated) running or overload (hindered) running. In **overspeed training**, the athlete is made to run faster than he normally can by artificial means. Techniques include downhill running, high-speed treadmill running and towing using either a motorized device or another runner. It is possible to achieve a higher stride rate in overspeed or supramaximal running as compared with normal maximal running. **Overload training** techniques are aimed at increasing stride length. Techniques include uphill running and 'speed chute' running. In the latter, the athlete pulls a parachute while sprinting, which results in a resistance to the order of 4 to 10 kg, depending on the size of the chute. High resistance is used to improve the acceleration phase, medium resistance to increase speed-endurance, and low resistance is used in the phase of maximum running speed. Except at rapid speeds, running speed is mainly increased by lengthening the stride.

Nerve conduction velocity along the motor axon has been shown to increase in response to a period of sprint training. However, it is difficult to determine if nerve conduction velocity is likely to contribute to improved sprint performance. Maximizing motor neuron excitability would be expected to benefit sprint performance, because an increase in motor neuron excitability, as measured by the Hoffman reflex (H-reflex), has been reported to produce a more powerful muscular contraction. At rest, however, the H-reflex has been reported to be lower in athletes trained for explosive events compared with endurance-trained athletes. This may be explained by the relatively high percentage of fast-twitch muscle fibers and the consequent high activation thresholds of motor units in power-trained populations. Stretch reflexes appear to be enhanced in sprint athletes, possibly due to increased muscle spindle sensitivity as a result of sprint training.

Bibliography

Brown, L., Ferrigno, V.A. and Santana, J.C. (2000, eds). *Training for speed, agility and quickness.* Champaign, IL: Human Kinetics.

Delecluse, C. (1997). Influence of strength training on sprint running performance. *Sports Medicine*, 24(3), 147-156.

Dintiman, G. and Ward, R. (2003). *Sports speed.* 3rd ed. Champaign, IL: Human Kinetics.

Ross, A., Leveritt, M. and Riek, S. (2001). Neural influences on sprint running: Training adaptations and acute responses. *Sports Medicine* 31(6), 409-425.

Siff, M.C. (2000). Biomechanical foundations of strength and power training. In Zatsiorsky, V. (ed). *Biomechanics in sport. Performance enhancement and injury prevention. Vol. IX of the Encyclopedia of Sports Medicine.* pp103-139. Oxford: Blackwell Science.

SPHINCTER A ring-like band of muscle fibers that closes off a duct, tube or orifice.

SPHINGOMYELIN *See under* CHOLINE.

SPHYGMOMANOMETER Apparatus used to measure blood pressure consisting of a stethoscope, inflatable unit, rubber bag, valve, hand pump and pressure gauge. The cuff is placed at heart level and wrapped around the left arm above the elbow such that the brachial artery is depressed. Turbulence in the artery creates sounds called **Korotkoff sounds.** The basic rhythm of the heart sounds is 'lub-dup,' pause, 'lub-dup,' pause, etc. The pause is the quiescent period – the period of time when there is total heart relaxation. The length of the cardiac cycle is about 0.8 sec (atrial systole 0.1 sec, ventricular systole 0.3 sec and quiescent period 0.4 sec). The stethoscope is placed on the axis of the elbow. The cuff is inflated to about 180 mm Hg. The pulse will disappear. The valve is opened to slowly release the pressure. When the pulse is first heard again in the stethoscope, the pressure is recorded as systolic blood pressure. As pressure is further released, the pulse gets louder, but suddenly it becomes muted or disappears. At this point, diastolic blood pressure is recorded. There are now electronic sphygmomanometers available; these do not depend on a stethoscope.

SPHYRION FIBULARE Malleolare laterale. It is an anatomical landmark that is the most distal tip of the lateral malleolus. It is more distal than the sphyrion tibiale.

SPHYRION TIBIALE An anatomical landmark

that is the most distal border of the medial malleolus of the tibia.

SPINA BIFIDA   *See under* NEURAL TUBE DEFECTS.

SPINAL ACCESSORY NERVE   Cranial nerve XI. A pure motor nerve that may have components from nerve roots of the 3rd and 4th cervical vertebrae (C3 and C4). It innervates the upper, middle and lower *trapezius* muscle in addition to the *sternocleidomastoid* muscles. It becomes superficial just posterior to the *scaleneus* muscles, where it is susceptible to injury by a direct blow to the neck. Injuries to the spinal accessory nerve have been reported in sports requiring the use of a stick, such as ice hockey.

SPINAL COLUMN   Vertebral column. *See* SPINE.

SPINAL CORD   The part of the central nervous system within the spinal column that is composed of numerous tracts (pathways), containing nerve fibers that carry impulses to and from the brain. It is a hollow tube containing numerous nerve cells and bundles of nerve fibers. It extends from the brainstem to the 1st and 2nd lumbar vertebrae (LI and L2). There are 31 pairs of spinal nerves that travel from the spinal cord to various parts of the body. The spinal cord is composed of central gray matter, containing cell bodies of neurons, and surrounding white matter carrying ascending and descending motor and sensory tracts. The white matter can be divided into three major motor and sensory tracts: the dorsal (posterior) tract, the lateral corticospinal (pyramidal) tract and the anterior spinothalamic tract. **Ascending tracts** carry nerve impulses to the brain; **descending tracts** carry nerve impulses to muscles and glands.

The inferior portion of the spinal cord lies below the lumbosacral enlargement and is known as the **conus medullaris,** below which there is a continuation of nerve roots known as the cauda equina. *See also* NERVOUS SYSTEM; REFLEXES; SPINAL PARALYSIS.

SPINAL DEVIATIONS   *See* KYPHOSIS; LOR-DOSIS; SCOLIOSIS.

SPINAL GALANT REFLEX   A primitive reflex that is present from birth until 3 to 9 months. It is elicited by stroking an infant's lower back at one or other side of the spine with the response that the lower back flexes toward the part that has been stroked. It is involved in the earliest 'wriggling' type movements that an infant makes. If it is not integrated, it can affect posture, gait and other forms of locomotion.

SPINAL NERVES   *See under* SPINAL CORD.

SPINAL PARALYSIS   A broad term for conditions caused by injury or disease to the spinal cord and/or spinal nerves. Causes of spinal paralysis may be traumatic (e.g. motor accident), congenital (e.g. spina bifida) or degenerative (e.g. multiple sclerosis). Forces responsible for producing spinal cord injury include compression, shear, laceration and distraction. 5 to 10% of patients with head injury have an associated spinal cord injury. 25 to 50% of patients with spinal cord injury have an associated head injury. Alcohol use is often associated with spinal cord injury. Sport and recreation account for 5 to 15% of all spinal cord injuries. 66% of spinal cord injuries that occurred in sport occurred as a result of diving accidents, the majority in the lower cervical spine leading to complete spinal paralysis. Diving causes 10 times more spinal cord injuries than any other sports. Of the estimated 200,000 to 500,000 Americans with spinal cord injury, the division between complete and incomplete lesions is about equal. Approximately 11,000 new injuries occur each year of which 82% occur in males.

Spinal paralysis involves both the central nervous system and the autonomic nervous system. Severity of spinal paralysis depends on the level of the lesion and whether it is complete (total) or incomplete (partial). The higher the lesion, the greater is the loss of function. **Complete spinal paralysis** occurs when there is a complete loss of motor and sensory function below the level of the lesion. **Incomplete spinal paralysis** occurs when there is some residual function at the lowest level of the spinal cord. It can be classified into one of three clinical syndromes: anterior cord syndrome, central cord syndrome or the Brown-Séquard syndrome. **Anterior cord syndrome** often occurs as a result of forced hyperflexion. It typically presents as loss of motor function and loss of pain and temperature sensation below the injury; dorsal column functions (joint position, touch and vibration) are preserved. The prognosis is poor. **Central cord syndrome** usually occurs as a result of forced hyperextension and may be associated with buckling of the ligamentum flavum or underlying degenerative arthritis. It typically presents as loss of distal upper extremity pain, temperature and strength, with relative preservation of lower extremity strength and sensation. **Brown-Séquard syndrome** is often secondary to penetrating trauma and typically presents as loss of ipsilateral strength, vibratory and joint position sense, and loss of contralateral pain and temperature sensation below the level of the injury. Some bowel and bladder function is retained.

Tetraplegia (quadriplegia) means involvement of all four limbs and the trunk. Persons with complete tetraplegia have no trunk or sitting balance. They use high-backed chairs and are strapped in for safety. About 50% of persons with tetraplegia have incomplete lesions, meaning that they are able to walk. High-level tetraplegia refers to complete lesions of the 1st to 4th cervical vertebrae (C1 to C4). These persons are dependent upon motorized chairs for ambulation. Persons with complete lesions at C3 and above cannot breathe independently and must carry portable oxygen tanks.

Paraplegia means involvement of the legs, but often includes trunk balance as well. It involves damage to any of the 12 thoracic nerves, 5 lumbar nerves, or sacral nerves 1 and 2. Persons with lesions of the 1st to 6th thoracic vertebrae (T1 to T6) have no useful sitting balance and must be strapped in their chairs. A complete lesion of the 7th thoracic to 1st lumbar vertebrae (T7 to L1) allows some useful sitting balance, whereas from L2 and beyond there is normal trunk control. Persons with low-level lesions can walk without assistance (except for braces), but are still classified as paraplegics.

Symptoms and complications of spinal cord injury include: loss of bladder and bowel function; spasticity; autonomic hyper-reflexia; absence of vasodilation and vasoconstriction below the level of the lesion; postural hypotension; pressure sores; diminished pulmonary function; contractures; and diminished exercise capacity. All persons with spinal paralysis above the 2nd sacral vertebra (S2) (except those with poliomyelitis) have some kind of bladder dysfunction, requiring that they void (urinate) in a different way. Most commonly, voiding is accomplished using intermittent catheterization, which involves inserting a tube into the urethra for a few seconds and draining urine into a small disposable bag. Frequent emptying of the bladder is important, because retention of urine leads to urinary and kidney infections, a major cause of illness and death among persons with spinal paralysis. If defecation is difficult, surgical procedures (ileostomy or colostomy) can create an opening (stoma) in the abdomen. A tube is inserted into the stoma and connects the intestine with a bag that fills up with fecal matter. The bag must be emptied and cleaned periodically. These bags are not worn during swimming; the stoma is covered with a watertight bandage.

Loss of vasocontriction function below the lesion results in diminished venous return. Impairment of vasomotor function due to venous pooling (caused mainly by sympathetic nervous system dysfunction) means that the vessels cannot constrict and force the blood through the venous valves and back to the heart. This results in lowered stroke volume. Venous pooling increases the cross-sectional area of veins, creating stress on the vascular walls that is relieved by some of the fluid in the blood leaking into the surrounding tissue. This results in edema. Decreased sympathetic outflow results in a decreased blood flow to the working muscles. Lesions above T1 result in diminished sympathetic outflow to the heart. This results in decreased cardiac output and oxygen uptake. The higher the lesion, the lower is maximal oxygen uptake. Tetraplegics and high-level paraplegics have abnormally low resting heart rates. This condition is called **chronotropic incompetence (sick sinus syndrome)**. Likewise, their cardiac response to aerobic exercise is blunted, because of sympathetic nervous system impairment. Lesions at or above T5 affect heart rate response to arm exercise, whereas lesions at or below T10 affect cardiac responses to leg exercises. Tetraplegics and high-level paraplegics (lesions above T6) may only reach a maximum heart rate of 120 bpm during arm ergometry. Persons with lesions below T6 exhibit maximum heart rates similar to able-bodied persons. Maximum heart rates and target zones used in aerobic exercise programs for able-bodied persons are not appropriate in high-level spinal paralysis.

Sexual function is innervated by the same nerves as urinary function (S2 to S4). Lesions above the sacral region (except in poliomyelitis) may make it necessary for sexual activity to be modified. Loss of sexual function, however, does not mean a corresponding loss of sexuality. With spinal paralysis, the spinal center for sexual function is generally intact; it is the communication from the brain to the spinal center that is usually disrupted. Unless some sensation in the area of the sexual organs, the usual sensation of orgasm is lost, but a 'phantom orgasm' may be experienced elsewhere in the body. Women with spinal paralysis can bear children. Menstruation is not affected.

Exercise is important in order to prevent secondary conditions such as diabetes and pressure sores, to prevent deconditioning and obesity, and to provide psychological and recreational benefits. Obesity and osteoporosis are consequences of a sedentary lifestyle, and there is a greater risk of cardiovascular disease than in sedentary people without spinal paralysis. In tetraplegia, training intensity should be between 50 and 70% of maximal heart rate. Arm ergometry is a preferred type of exercise. In paraplegia, training intensity should not exceed 70%. Suitable exercise includes wheelchair ergometry, swimming and sports such as basketball.

Sunburn is a special problem, because persons with spinal paralysis cannot feel discomfort caused by sun on skin when there is no sensation. Spinal paralysis above T8 renders the body incapable of adapting to temperature changes. **Poikilothermy** is the name for the condition in which the body assumes the same temperature as the environment.

Patients at the age of 20 years at the time of sustaining spinal cord injury have life expectancies of approximately 33 years as tetraplegics, 39 years as low tetraplegics, and 44 years as paraplegics. At the age of 60 years at the time of sustaining spinal cord injury, life expectancy is approximately 7 years as tetraplegics, 9 years as low tetraplegics, and 13 years as paraplegics.

Among patients with incomplete paraplegia, the leading causes of death among incomplete paraplegics are cancer and suicide. Among complete paraplegics, the leading causes are suicide and heart disease.

See also AUTONOMIC HYPER-REFLEXIA; CONTRACTURES; WHEELCHAIR.

Chronology

•1995 • Christopher Reeve, the actor who played "Superman," was riding in an equestrian contest. When his horse stopped suddenly at a rail jump, Reeve was thrown forward, head first over the horse, and landed on the ground in a near-perpendicular position. The weight of Reeve's 6 ft, 4 inch, 230 lb body shattered his 1st and 2nd cervical vertebrae and severely damaged his spinal cord. Reeve's condition was classified initially as Grade A on the American Spinal Injury Association scale, which means that the patient has no sensory or motor function below the shoulders. Experts predicted that Reeve would never be able to breathe on his own without the assistance of a ventilator or to regain the movement and feeling he had lost.

•1999 • Christopher Reeve's foundation merged with the American Paralysis Association to form the Christopher Reeve Paralysis Foundation, which awards grants to top international neuroscientists.

•2000 • Christopher Reeve began participation in Washington University School of Medicine's Activity-Based Recovery Program, which is based on the theory that patterned neural activity might stimulate the central nervous system to become functional as it does during development. Reeve's program consisted largely of functional electrical stimulation, which involves a specially designed recumbent bicycle system that uses computer-controlled electrodes placed on a patient's legs to stimulate the leg muscles in specific patterns. Reeve used the bicycle for one hour per day three times a week, building muscle mass and bone density, decreasing spasticity, and improving cardiovascular fitness. The incidence of infections and use of antibiotic medications was decreased by over 90%. Once muscle recovery had been stimulated, aqua therapy was added to Reeve's exercise program. This form of physical therapy performed in water focused on those muscle groups for which voluntary control had been recovered (e.g. the right hemidiaphragm, *extensor carpi radialis* and *vastus medialis*).

•2002 • Christopher Reeve's condition was improved to the

extent that he was reclassified as Grade C, with improved neck function and intact sacral motor and sensory function. He was able to move some of his joints without assistance (his right hand, the fingers of his left hand, and his feet). It is not clear what led to Reeve's improvement, but it is possible that a small number of nerves around the site of his injury were left alive, but atrophied. The exercise may have reactivated these nerves or induced new nerve connections to grow around the site of injury.

•2004 • Christopher Reeve, 52 years-old, died of cardiac arrest, having recently been treated for a pressure sore wound that became severely infected. A month before he died, Reeve revealed that he had fought off three dangerous infections during this year: "The most recent was a blood infection caused by an abrasion on my left hip that I probably picked up one day when I was on the exercise bike. It seemed benign, but developed into strep[tococcus]. Then a lot of major organs shut down. We're trying to figure out what's going on."

Bibliography

Dawodu, S.T. (2001). Spinal cord injury: Definition, epidemiology, pathophysiology. Http://www.emedicine.com

Hoiland, E. (2002). Promising progress for Christopher Reeve's spinal injury.

Http://faculty.washington.edu/chudler/reeve.html

McDonald, J.W. et al. (2002). Late recovery following spinal cord injury. Case report and review of the literature. *Journal of Neurosurgery (Spine 2)* 97, 252-265.

National Center on Physical Activity and Disability. Http://www.ncpad.org

National Spinal Cord Injury Association. Http://www.spinal-cord.org

Spinal Cord Injury Information Network. Http://www.spinal-cord.uab.edu

SPINAL MUSCLE ATROPHY

A hereditary disease characterized by progressive hypotonia and muscular weakness. It is the second most common disease, after cystic fibrosis, inherited as an autosomal recessive trait. The characteristic muscle weakness occurs due to a progressive degeneration of the alpha motor neurons from anterior horn cells in the spinal cord. The weakness is more severe in the proximal musculature than in the distal segments. In certain patients, the motor neurons of cranial nerves (especially the 5th to 12th) can also be involved. Sensation, which originates from the posterior horn cells of the spinal cord, is spared, along with intelligence.

In the USA, spinal muscle atrophy occurs in about 1 in 15,000 to 20,000 persons. Males are more commonly affected than females. Several spinal muscle atrophies have been identified including Hoffman disease, Kugelberg-Welander disease and Oppenheim's disease. In school settings, however, these are usually called the floppy baby syndromes or congenital hypotonia since the major indicator is flaccid muscle tone. Most of these atrophies are present at birth or occur shortly thereafter. The conditions vary in severity, with some leveling off, arresting themselves, and leaving the child with chronic, nonprogressive muscle weakness. Others are fatal within 2 or 3 years of onset. Typically, in severe cases, there is a loss of muscle strength, followed by a tightness of muscles, then contractures, and finally nonuse. Stretching exercises are particularly important to combat contractures. It is sometimes difficult to distinguish spinal muscle atrophy from muscular dystrophy. It can be distinguished from cerebral palsy, however, because there is no spasticity, no ataxia, no seizures and no associated dysfunctions.

The younger the patient is at onset, the worse the prognosis is. Death usually occurs due to respiratory compromise.

Bibliography

Herrera, J.A. (2003). Spinal muscle atrophy. Http://www.emedicine.com

SPINAL SHOCK

A state of transient physiological reflex depression of spinal cord function below the level of injury with associated loss of all sensorimotor functions. It usually occurs in conjunction with a severe spinal cord injury. There is an initial increase in blood pressure, due to the release of catecholamines, followed by hypotension. Flaccid paralysis, including of the bowel and bladder, is observed, and sometimes a sustained priapism develops. These symptoms tend to last several hours to days until the reflex arcs below the level of the injury begin to function again.

Bibliography

Dawodu, S.T. (2001). Spinal cord injury: Definition, epidemiology, pathophysiology. Http://www.emedicine.com

SPINAL STABILIZATION

See under INTRA-

ABDOMINAL PRESSURE.

SPINAL STENOSIS   Narrowing of the vertebral canal, as a result of prolapsed intervertebral disk, wear of the facet joints and osteophyte formation. *See also* CERVICAL STENOSIS.

SPINE   Spinal Column. Vertebral column. Backbone. The spine is part of the axial skeleton. It is a jointed hollow rod made up of vertebrae and the spinal cord. The different parts of the vertebral column are connected together by ligaments. Joints (articulations) are formed between the vertebral bodies, the laminae, the articular processes, the spinous processes and the transverse processes. All the above are gliding joints, with the exception of the articulations of the vertebral bodies that are amphiarthrodial (limited movement).

The spine can be divided into five regions: cervical (neck), thoracic (dorsal; chest), lumbar (low), sacral and coccygeal. Of the 33 vertebrae, 7 are cervical, 12 are thoracic, 5 are lumbar, 5 are sacral and 4 are coccygeal. The sacrum and coccyx, along with the two pelvic bones (the ilium and ischium) make up the pelvic girdle. The two pelvic bones are joined together anteriorly by the pubic symphysis, which is an amphiarthrodial joint. At the posterior, there is the sacro-iliac joint, which is also amphiarthrodial. In adults, the sacral and coccygeal vertebrae are fused.

From birth to two months, the spine has a single C-curve, with the convexity to the back, and the legs are flexed. During the early months of life, when the baby starts to raise its head and kick its legs, the spine becomes relatively straight. The cervical curvature develops at about 4 to 5 months of age when the infant sits upright. Development of cervical curvature is facilitated by the prone-on-elbow crawling position, combined with labyrinthine and optical righting reflexes. Creeping, occurring at about 8 months, further strengthens abdominal and lumbar spine muscles. During early standing with support, there is flat-back posture. The lumbar curve develops as the child starts to support the weight of the body on the feet and begins to walk. This occurs at about 14 months. This is accompanied by the development

of the other curves until the spine adopts the normal curves of an adult. The lumbar curve does not reach full development until about the age of 17 years.

The range of movement of the joints varies in each region of the spine. For each type of movement, the greatest range of movement is allowed in the cervical region. In the thoracic region, flexion, extension and circumduction are very limited, but rotation is very free in the upper part and non-existent in the lower part. In the lumbar region, flexion, extension and lateral movement are free, but there is little rotation. Flexion and extension occur predominantly at the lower two lumbar segments. Rotation at each lumbar segment is limited to only a few degrees, because of the vertical orientation of the lumbar facets.

The muscles of the back can be classified according to their length. The long back muscles (*erector spinae*; also known as *sacrospinalis*) lie superficial and pass at least seven vertebrae. These are: *iliocostalis* (pelvis to ribs), *longissimus* (spinous outgrowths to transverse outgrowths and ribs) and *spinalis* (between spinous outgrowths). The back muscles of average length are: *semi-spinalis* (pass 4 to 7 vertebrae) and *multifidi* (pass 2 to 3 vertebrae). The back muscles of short length (vertebra to vertebra) are: *intertransversarii* (between transverse outgrowths), *interspinales* (between spinous outgrowths) and *rotatores* (between spinous and transverse outgrowths). The *semispinalis*, *multifidi* and *rotatores* form a group that is known as the *transversospinalis*.

Flexion is movement of the spine forward. Muscles that flex the spine are: *sternocleidomastoid, longus colli, scaleni, rectus abdominis* and *psoas major*. Muscles that flex the head are: *longus capitis* and *rectus capitis anterior*. **Extension** is upward movement of the spine. Muscles that extend the spine are: *splenius capitis, splenius cervicis, iliocostalis lumborum, iliocostalis thoracis, iliocostalis cervicis, longissimus thoracis, longissimus cervicis, spinalis thoracis, spinalis cervicis, spinalis capitis, multifidi, rotatores* and *interspinalis*. Muscles that extend the head are: *rectus capitis posterior major/minor, obliquus capitis superior* and *splenius capitis/cervicis*. **Lateral movement** is sidewards bending. Muscles that laterally flex the spine are *scaleni* (acting on one side), *splenius capitis,* *splenius cervicis, iliocostalis lumborum, iliocostalis thoracis, iliocostalis cervicis, intertransversarii, obliquus externus abdominis, obliquus internus abdominis* and *quadratus lumborum.* Muscles that laterally flex the head are: *rectus capitis lateralis, obliquus capitis superior, splenius capitis* and *splenius cervicis.* **Rotation** is movement of the spine in a transverse plane. Muscles that produce rotation of the spine are: *sternocleidomastoid, scaleni* (acting on one side), *splenius capitis* (acting on one side), *semispinalis thoracis, semispinalis cervicis, multifidi, rotatores, obliquus externus abdominis* and *obliquus internus abdominis.* Muscles that produce rotation of the head are: *sternocleidomastoid, scaleni* (acting on one side), *rectus capitis posterior major, obliquus capitis inferior* (rotates atlas) and *splenius capitis.* Muscles that **compress the abdominal contents** are: *obliquus externus abdominis, obliquus internus abdominis, transversus abdominis* and *rectus abdominis.* In males, the *cremaster* muscle pulls the testes toward the body.

The joints between the vertebral arches are called **intervertebral facet joints.** These facet joints are oriented in such a way as to limit rotation of the vertebrae and thus decrease the wearing away of the intervertebral disks. The **facet joint** is a synovial joint consisting of two articular surfaces: the inferior facet, which is dorsal and medial, and the superior facet, which is volar and lateral. With normal lumbar concavity, the facet joint bears about 20% of the compressive load. Due to the 90-degree orientation of the lumbar facet joints, motion in the sagittal plane (i.e. flexion and extension) is greater than the motion in either the transverse plane (i.e. rotation) or frontal plane (i.e. lateral flexion and extension). Rotation in the lumbar spine is limited to a few degrees. Rotation greater than 3 degrees may result in tensile failure of the annular fibers. The facet joint capsule, in conjunction with other mid-line ligamentous structures, prevents excessive lumbar flexion. The **pars interarticularis** is a thin (1 to 2 mm) bony bridge between the pedicle and lamina. Isolated extension, and extension combined with rotation, are the motions most commonly associated with injuries to the pars interarticularis and facet joint. These injuries (e.g. spondylolysis) are typically due to chronic, repetitive loading. **Facet joint syndrome** affects older adults and involves wear in the intervertebral facet joints.

An **intervertebral disk** is a viscoelastic structure consisting of the annulus fibrosus and nucleus pulposus, and is separated from the vertebra by a thin layer of hyaline cartilage. The **nucleus pulposus** consists of fine fibers embedded in a mucoprotein gel. Its water and proteoglycan content is highest during youth and decreases with age. Mechanical consequences of this age loss include decreases in disk height, elasticity and load-bearing capacity. Due to less gravity pushing down on the vertebrae, astronauts are up to 2 inches taller while they are in space; but once they come back to Earth, they return to their normal height. The **annulus fibrosis** consists of concentric bands of annular fibrocartilage that surround the nucleus pulposus to form the perimeter of the disk. Due to the relative incompressibility of the nucleus pulposus, compressive load is transmitted as a tensile load to the annulus fibrosus. This is an example of Poisson's effect. Mechanically, the annulus fibrosus behaves as a coiled spring, holding the vertebral bodies together, while the nucleolus pulposus acts like a ball bearing that the vertebrae roll over during flexion/extension and lateral bending. In addition to exhibiting viscoelastic properties (creep and stress relaxation), intervertebral disks exhibit hysteresis. Disks are able to withstand greater than normal loads when compressive force is rapidly applied, which protects the disk from catastrophic failure until extremely high loads are applied.

Prolapse of an intervertebral disk is an acute injury and typically results from hyperflexion of the spine, often in conjunction with lateral bending. Intervertebral disks have no blood or lymph supply and only a limited nerve supply. Structures in the spine that are pain sensitive include: the outer fibers of the annulus fibrosus; the capsule and synovium of the facet joints; ligaments; nerve fibers; fascia; and muscle. Disk degeneration transfers weight bearing and rotational loads to the facet joints and may produce facet joint inflammation, arthropathy and a degenerative cascade in the lumbar spine.

See also LOW BACK PAIN; LUMBAR SPINE; NECK INJURIES; PELVIC GIRDLE; POSTURE; SPINAL DEVIATIONS; SPONDYLOLISTHESIS; THORACIC SPINE.

Bibliography

National Aeronautics and Space Administration. Http://www.nasa.gov

SPLANCHNIC Relating to viscera.

SPLEEN An organ located in the upper quadrant of the abdominal cavity that maintains a reserve of ready-to-use blood cells for the body. Injury to the spleen is not common, but occurs most often because of a fall or a direct blow to the left upper quadrant of the abdomen when some existing systemic disorder has caused enlargement of the spleen. Acute cases of infectious mononucleosis result in enlargement of the spleen (**splenomegaly**) in 40 to 60% of all cases. Splenomegaly predisposes the spleen to rupture during episode of blunt trauma as is common in many contact sports. Splenomegaly is the most common cause of death from blunt trauma of the abdomen in sport. This is because the spleen can splint itself and stop hemorrhaging, only to produce delayed hemorrhage days, weeks or months later after a minor jarring motion such as a cough. Mononucleosis is thus an automatic disqualification from contact and vigorous noncontact sports for at least three weeks.

SPONDYLITIS Inflammation of the synovial joints of the vertebrae.

SPONDYLOLISTHESIS Forward slippage of a superior vertebra on the inferior vertebra. Spondylolysis and spondylolisthesis have a higher incidence in athletes than non-athletes.

See also under HAMSTRINGS.

SPONDYLOLYSIS A defect in the pars interarticularis, most commonly at the site of maximal shear stress (5th lumbar vertebra). In sport, it is typically a stress fracture through the pars interarticularis. It is caused by repeated, high compressive loading to the spine, especially in combination with flexion-extension and rotation. It is most common in adolescent athletes, especially gymnasts due to the hyperexten-sion movements in routines such as the back walkover. It is also common in young adults, especially offensive linesmen in American football. A high incidence of spondylolysis in weightlifters (36% versus 5% in the general population) was one reason why the press was removed as an Olympic lift after the 1972 Olympic Games. Spondylolysis creates the necessary conditions for spondylolisthesis to occur.

SPORT A subset of leisure and work activities that involve both physical activity and competition. A key difference between play and sport is that sport involves institutionalization of games with formalized sets of rules, national regulations and a governing administrative superstructure of adults. The organizational structure provides for the maintenance and control of the activity through interpretation of rules by adults who act as officials. Sport is also characterized by formally recorded histories and traditions.

Guttmann (1988) differentiates between play, games, contests and sports. Play may be either spontaneous or organized. Organized play involves either non-competitive games or competitive games (contests). **Contests** may be intellectual contests or physical contests (sports). Chess could be regarded as an intellectual contest. What activities should be classified as sport is often debated. Britain is one of the few countries not to recognize chess as a sport, because according to the Sports Council the game is not sufficiently "physical."

Characteristics of modern sports (Guttmann, 1978) are: secularism (primitive sports were related to some transcendent realm of the sacred); equality (rules are the same for all contestants); bureaucratization (at all levels from local to international level); specialization (many sports have evolved from earlier less differentiated games); rationalization (e.g. technologically-advanced equipment); and quantification (including records).

Coakley (2004) describes sports as institutionalized competitive activities that involve vigorous physical exertion or the use of relatively complex physical skills by individuals whose participation is motivated by a combination of personal enjoyment and external rewards. **Institutionalization** refers to the process through which behaviors and organization become patterned or standardized over time and from one situation to another.

Political processes in sport are concerned with questions about: what qualifies as a sport; the rules of a sport; the organization and control of sporting events; sporting venues; participant eligibility; and the distribution of extrinsic rewards, such as prizes. Many sport organizations are described as 'governing bodies,' because they are the context for political decision-making that affects everyone connected with the particular sports.

Chronology

•700 BC • The *Iliad* and the *Odyssey*, epic poems by Homer, contain the first descriptions of sport and organized athletics. According to a later myth, Homer was a blind traveling poet. The *Iliad* and the *Odyssey*, however, were more likely a combination of various folktales evolving over centuries into their final form. The *Iliad* ("a poem about Troy") describes a few weeks in the tenth year of the Trojan War, while the *Odyssey* recounts the return journey of Odysseus after the war. In the *Iliad*, Patroclus, the closest friend of Achilles, is killed by the god Apollo. The Greek gods served not to illuminate the supernatural, but to symbolize recognizable aspects of human behavior. Homer describes the games in celebration of the funeral of Patroclus, who was killed in battle. The first athletic event was boxing. Leather helmets, and leather gloves impregnated with metal studs, were worn; but the victor was not allowed to kill his opponent. When competitors were called for, Epeius announced, "This is what I say, and this is what will happen. I will tear my opponent's flesh and smash his bone. Let all his friends stand by to carry him away when I have finished with him." Euryalus took up the challenge made by Epeius, and knocked him out. The prize was a mule. In Greek, 'athlon' means prize and is the origin of the word 'athletics.'

•1845 • Alexander J. Cartwright, a banker, organized a group of men into a social and fraternal club called the Knickerbocker Base Ball Club. Cartwright developed the first formal rules of baseball. The first recorded game of baseball was played at the Elysian Fields in Hoboken, New Jersey, between the Knickerbockers and the New York Base Ball Club. Cartwright left New York and headed for the Californian gold rush in 1849, taking his bat, ball and rulebook with him. By 1860, the New York game spread to Maine and had become established all the way to Oregon and California. Baseball evolved from the games of rounders and town ball and was played in various forms as early as 1734 in Harvard. Baseball was described in a book in England published in 1744. The story that Abner Doubleday invented baseball in Cooperstown, New York, is a myth, created by Albert G. Spalding, a major league pitcher who formed the first major sporting goods company. In 1901 Henry Chadwick, one of the earliest sportswriters, wrote an article claiming that baseball was of British rather than American origin. Two years later, however, Spalding established a commission to pursue the origin of baseball. His motivation was to promote baseball by showing that it was an American invention. The committee was chaired by Abraham Mills, who was a past president of the National League. After three years of research, it was concluded that Doubleday invented baseball at Coopertown in 1839, but at that time Doubleday was apparently in the midst of officer training at West Point.

•1853 • The Caledonian Games were first held in America, including many running and throwing events. These games provided competition among the various Caledonian social clubs that had developed to perpetuate the traditions and athletic games of Scotland. Events included throwing the 56 lb for height and tossing the caber. Donald Dinnie (born in 1837), Scotland's greatest athlete, toured the US Caledonian circuit in 1870. He was 6 foot 11 inches and a body weight of 218 lb. He earned a great amount of money. The spread of the Caledonian Games to the whole country over the next two decades was an important influence on the development track and field athletics in the USA.

•1869 • In rowing, Oxford beat Harvard on the River Thames. This was the first international intercollegiate sporting contest. It was managed from the USA by Harvard graduate William Blaikie, who developed the training plan for the Harvard crews.

•1869 • The first intercollegiate football game was played: Rutgers versus Princeton. The game was played with two teams of 25 men each under rugby-like rules. Princeton used yelling (an imitation of the Confederate rebel yell from the Civil War) to frighten the Rutgers players. In the second game, they asked fellow students to yell for them. This was the start of organized yelling from the sidelines. In 1873, Princeton, Yale, Columbia and Rutgers formed the Intercollegiate Association for Football.

•1873 • The first collegiate track contest was held in the USA at Princeton. It was organized by George Goldie, a Scotsman who was director of the gymnasium at Princeton from 1869 to 1911, and called the Caledonian Games. The Games survived until 1947, before the modern intercollegiate schedule of sports took over.

•1878 • Yale undergraduate, Walter Camp, recommended to a football convention at Springfield that the number of players be reduced from 15 to 11. This resolution was defeated. A convention two years later brought forth the start of modern football with the invention of the scrimmage: "It was [Camp's] contention that the old-fashioned scrum was nothing but a scramble. The ball was set down on the field and both teams clustered around it, with all the rushers kicking at the ball and trying to drive it from the forest of legs all around it. This seemed to Camp an absurd and disorderly way to start play. Neither side could practice strategy, because neither knew when, or at what point, the ball would come out of the scrum. ... Camp declared that the game needed sharp revision; that it should be a game of brains, not chance. He maintained that neither the players, nor the public would be interested in the game unless it became orderly. ... It needed finesse, generalship, consistent and continued strategy." (Powel, 1926, p52-3) Camp's rule was that, "A scrimmage takes place when the holder of the ball puts it on the ground before him and puts it into play either by kicking the ball, or by snapping it back with his foot." As part of the same rule establishing the scrimmage, Camp invented the position of quarterback: "the man who first receives the ball from the snap back shall be called the quarterback, and shall not rush forward with the ball under penalty of foul." At a football convention in 1881, Camp presented the following rule: "If on three consecutive fairs and downs a team shall not have advanced the ball five yards, nor lost 10, they must give up the ball to the opponents at the spot of the 4th down." This rule requires the 5-yard line marks from which the name 'grid iron' comes from. Later, Camp was also the first coach who made successful use of the forward pass. After graduating from Yale in 1880, Camp spent two years in Yale Medical School before becoming a businessman and a volunteer adviser to the Yale team. He eventually became Yale's football coach and is known as 'the Father of American Football.'

•1885 • Albert G. Spalding established the *Spalding Library of American Sports* to provide up-to-date information on training methods, techniques, and 'records.' It was also a medium for advertising his growing equipment business. By the end of the century, Spalding had issued about 300 separate publications, written by journalists, physical educators, athletes, and coaches.

•1912 • At the Olympic Games in Stockholm, electric timing and a public address system were introduced.

•1920 • The Golden Age of Sports, in which America developed an obsession with sports, was marked by the creation of spectator sport and stars, such as Babe Ruth (baseball), Red Grange (football), Bobby Jones (golf) and Joe Louis (boxing).

•1932 • Official automatic timing was introduced to the Olympic Games, when Omega unveiled its Olympic chronograph with a fly-back hand. It was the first time in the history of the Games, that a single manufacturer supplied identical stopwatches with observatory precision-rating certificates for timekeeping, and it increased the accuracy and reliability of results dramatically. The photo-finish camera was also introduced to the Olympics.

•1936 • The Olympic Games was the first televised sporting event. Thousands of local residents watched the Games free on 25 large screens housed in newly constructed television halls around Berlin. Due to a weak signal from the main stadium, viewers were typically only able to see dark-colored horses at the polo events (hence the term 'dark horse').

•1948 • The Olympic Games were first shown on home television. The British Broadcasting System (BBC) bought the rights to transmit the Games at a cost of US$3,000 to an official audience of 500,000 people in the UK.

•1952 • At the Olympic Games in Helsinki, an electric scoreboard was first used.

•1960 • At the Olympic Games in Rome, computers, made by IBM, were used for the first time to relay results information and electronic results boards were introduced for field events.

•1963 • The first skateboard contest was held at the Pier Avenue Junior School in Hermosa, California. A boom in skateboarding occurred with more than 50 million boards being sold within a three-year period, before skateboarding was banned by many cities in response to health and safety concerns.

•1964 • Seiko was the official timer of the Olympic Games in Tokyo, unveiling its new, fully electronic automated timing system. The system linked a starting pistol with a quartz timer and a

photo-finish apparatus to record finish times, making it possible to record results to the nearest 0.01 second. The Games were transmitted worldwide by live satellite broadcasting.

•1970 • The International Swimming Federation ruled that automatic timing (and judging) equipment should take preference over human times (and judges).

•1973 • The International Swimming Federation agreed that times and placings would be determined only to hundredths of a second and that competitors whose times were equal to hundredths would be adjudged to have finished in a dead heat.

•1974 • The International Amateur Athletics Federation (IAAF) decided that in track events up to 400 meters, where the best fully automatic electric times were slower than the human timed records, the electric times should also be accepted as world records.

•1977 • Imperial distance events, except for the mile, were dropped from international athletics. All records at sprint distances up to 400 m were accepted only if timed fully automatically.

•1984 • At the Olympic Games in Los Angeles, 200 IBM personal computers linked up to three mainframe computers for the management, results and information systems.

•1986 • The National Football League (NFL) introduced instant video replay to assist decision-making for disputed plays. In the 1991 season, 570 plays were reviewed and 90 calls were reversed. NFL officials later admitted that at least nine of these were reversed incorrectly. The NFL discontinued playbacks, but in 1998 the owners voted to reinstate playbacks. Computer technology made it much easier and quicker to use.

•1995 • The first Extreme Games, created by ESPN as a made-for-TV festival of alternative sports for teenagers, were held in Newport, Rhode Island (USA). It featured sports such as bungee jumping, freestyle biking, mountain biking, skateboarding, snowboarding and windsurfing.

•1996 • MSG Network in New York City used SuperVision, developed by QuesTec, in Major League baseball. Two cameras, one located on the first-base line, the other on the third-base line, follow the pitch. A computer program isolates the ball and uses triangulation to locate its position at each point.

•1999 • The International Olympic Committee (IOC) pronounced the World Chess Federation to be a "recognized federation" under Rule 29 of the Olympic Charter. British Minister for Sport, Tony Banks, expressed his wish to have the definition of sport changed in order to embrace chess, but this would require amendments to the Physical Training and Recreation Act (1937) and the National Lottery Act (1993).

•2000 • At the Olympic Games in Sydney, Orad Hi-Tec Systems Ltd introduced the first use of virtual imaging in Olympic history. Its Virtual World Record Line on TV and the Internet connected directly to the electronic timing in the swimming pool and featured a superimposed line on the water's surface and graphics depicting the existing world records. These graphics enabled viewers to watch athletes approach and exceed the current world record as the events unfolded.

•2000 • Philadelphia City Council passed bill 147, municipal law

10-610, "prohibiting skateboarding on all public property unless otherwise authorized." Skateboarding is legal on sidewalks, public streets and bike paths, but it is banned in LOVE Park and the Municipal Services Plaza. Philadelphia is regarded the American capital for street skating. It was one of the reasons why Philadelphia staged ESPN's Extreme Games in 2001 and 2002. According to American Sports Data, Inc., there were 12.46 million skateboarders in 2001, which was a 73% increase over three years. Baseball had 11.41 million participants in 2001, which was a 7% increase over three years and a 25% decrease over 14 years. •2004 • DC Shoes of Vista, California, announced a $1 million gift to the City of Philadelphia if it reopens LOVE Park to skateboarding. DC Shoes would give $100,000 each year for 10 years to pay for "maintenance, security and upkeep" of LOVE Park.

Bibliography

Caspersen, C.J., Powell, K.E. and Christenson, G.M. (1985). Physical activity, exercise and physical fitness. *Public Health Reports* 100, 125-131.

Coakley, J.J. (2004). *Sport in society. Issues and controversies*. 8th ed. Boston, MA; Irvin McGraw-Hill.

Cordes, K.A. and Ibrahim, H.M. (2003). *Applications in recreation and leisure. For today and the future*. 3rd ed. Boston, MA: McGraw-Hill.

Dyson, J. (1993). *Leisure. How to find out in sport and recreation*. London; Sport and Recreation Information Group.

Guttmann, A. (1978). *From ritual to record*. New York: Columbia University Press.

Guttmann, A. (1988). *A whole new ball game. An interpretation of American sports*. Chapel Hill: The University of North Carolina Press.

IEEE-USA. Http://www.todaysengineer.org/July04/history.asp

Powel, H. (1926). *Walter Camp, the father of American football. An authorized biography*. Boston, MA: Little, Brown & Co.

Roberts, G. (1993). Motivation in sport: Understanding and enhancing the motivation and achievement of children. In: Singer, R. Murphy, M. and Tennant, L.K. (eds). *Handbook of research on sport psychology*. pp405-420. New York: MacMillan.

Wade, M.G. and Baker, J.A.W. (1995). *Introduction to kinesiology: The science and practice of physical activity*. Madison, Wisconsin: W.C.B. Brown and Benchmark.

Zarnowski, F. (1998). The amazing Donald Dinnie: The nineteenth century's greatest athlete. *Iron Game History* 5(1), 3-11.

SPORT COMMITMENT

A psychological construct representing the desire and resolve to continue sport participation. Five factors that influence sport commitment are: positive emotions associated with participating in the activity; the attractiveness of alternative activities; resources invested in the activity that cannot be recovered if participation is discontinued; social expectations or norms that create perceived obligation to continue the activity;

and valued opportunities that are present only with continued involvement with the activity.

Bibliography

Scanlan, et al. (1993). An introduction to the Sport Commitment Model. *Journal of Sport & Exercise Psychology* 15, 1-15.

Scanlan, T.K. et al. (1993). The Sports Commitment Model: Measurement development for the youth-sport domain. *Journal of Sport & Exercise Psychology* 15, 16-38.

SPORTS BIOMECHANICS   *See under* BIOMECHANICS.

SPORTS HISTORY   The study of change and continuity over time in sport and physical education.

Bibliography

Greenberg, S. (1991). *The Guinness Olympics fact book*. London: Guinness Publishing.

Grover, K. (1989, ed). *Fitness in American culture. Images of health, sport and the body*. Amhert, MA: University of Massachusetts Press.

Guttmann, A. (1976). *The Olympics: A history of the Modern Games*. Chicago: University of Illinois Press.

Guttmann, A. (1988). *A whole new ball game. An interpretation of American sports*. Chapel Hill: University of North Carolina Press.

Hackensmith, C.W. (1966). *History of Physical Education*. New York: Harper and Row.

Levinson, D. and Christensen, K. (1996, Eds). *Encyclopaedia of world sport*. Santa Barbara, CA: AB-CLIO Ltd.

Lovesey, J. (1996, ed). 1000 makers of sport. *The Sunday Times* Supplements, June and July.

McIntosh, P.C. (1968). *Physical Education in England since 1800*. London: Bell and Hyman.

McIntosh, P.C. et al. (1981). *Landmarks in the history of physical education*. London: Routledge and Kegan Paul.

Mechikoff, R.A. and Estes, S.G. (2002). *A history and philosophy of sport and physical education. From ancient civilization to the modern world*. 3rd ed Boston, MA: McGraw-Hill.

Park, R.J. (1992). Athletes and their training in Britain and America, 1800-1914. In Berryman, J.W. and Park, R.J. (eds). *Sport and exercise science: Essays in the history of sports medicine*. pp57-107. Urbana, IL: University of Illinois Press.

Polidoro, J.R. (2000). *Sport and physical activity in the modern world*. San Francisco, CA: Benjamin Cummings.

Rice, E.A., Hutchinson, J.L. and Lee, M. (1958). *A brief history of physical education*. 4th ed. New York: The Ronald Press Company.

Siedentop, D. (2004). *Introduction to physical education, fitness and sport*. 5th ed. Boston, MA: McGraw-Hill.

Struna, N.L. (1997). Sport history. In: Massengale, J.D. and Swanson, R.A. (eds.). *The history of exercise and sport science*.

pp143-179. Champaign, IL: Human Kinetics.

Swanson, R.A. and Spears, B. (1995). *History of sport and physical education in the United States*. 4th ed. Boston, MA: WCB/McGraw-Hill.

Van Dalen, D.B. and Bennett, B.L. (1973). *A world history of physical education*. 2nd ed. Englewood Cliffs, NJ: Prentice Hall.

Wiggins, D.K. (1995, ed). *Sport in America. From wicked amusement to national obsession*. Champaign, IL: Human Kinetics.

Wuest, D.A. and Butcher, C.A. (2003). *Foundations of physical education and sport*. 14th ed. Boston, MA: WCB/McGraw-Hill.

Zeigler, E.F. (1979). *History of physical education and sport*. Englewood Cliffs, NJ: Prentice Hall.

SPORTS INJURIES   *See under* INJURY.

SPORTS MEDICINE   The term 'sports medicine' has been used in two ways. Firstly, to refer to a branch of medicine concerned with the diagnosis, treatment, rehabilitation and prevention of traumatic and non-traumatic conditions (injuries and disease) affecting the athlete. Secondly, it has been used as an 'umbrella term' that covers both medical and scientific aspects of sport and exercise. In fact, the term 'sports medicine' was first used to describe an area of clinical practice and research concerned with athletic performance at the 2nd Winter Olympic Games in 1928.

See KINESIOLOGY; SPORTS INJURIES.

Chronology

•1910 • Siegried Weissbein of Berlin published *Hygiene des Sports*, probably the first book to deal comprehensively with sports medicine.

•1912 • The German Imperial Committee for the Scientific Study of Sport and Physical Exercise was founded.

•1924 • The USA sent its first medical delegation to the Olympic Games.

•1928 • 33 physicians representing 11 countries met in St. Moritz, Switzerland, the site of the Winter Olympic Games to organize an international sports medicine association. Later in the same year at the Summer Olympic Games in Amsterdam, the Association Internationale Medico-Sportive (AIMS) was founded and the 1st International Congress on Sports Medicine was held.

•1931 • The first books on sports medicine in English were published, in England G.B. Heald's *Injuries and Sport*; and in the USA, W.E. Meanwell and Knute Rockne's *Training, Conditioning and the Care of Injuries*. Meanwell was team physician at the University of Wisconsin and Rockne was the Notre Dame football coach.

•1933 • At the 2nd International Congress of Sports Medicine, the name Association International Medico-Sportive (AIMS) was changed to Fèdèration Internationale Medico-Sportive et Scientifique (FIMS).

•1934 • At the 3rd International Congress on Sports Medicine, the word "Scientifique" was dropped from the name of FIMS.

•1936 • The 4th International Congress on Sports Medicine included approximately 1500 physicians from 40 nations, including the USA.

•1946 • The Federation of Sports Medicine of the USSR was founded.

•1950 • A department of sports medicine was opened in the German College of Physical Culture in Leipzig in the German Democratic Republic (East Germany), which became a sovereign state in 1949.

•1952 • The Federation of Sports Medicine of the USSR became a member of the International Federation of Sports Medicine (FIMS).

•1953 • In the German Democratic Republic (GDR), the Ministry of Health established its own Sport-Medical Committee that developed into the German Society for Sports Medicine in 1958.

•1953 • The British Association of Sport and Medicine (BASM) was founded when a group of doctors, led by Sir Adolphe Abrahams and Sir Arthur Porritt, met at the Westminster Hospital in London. Non-medical practitioners were permitted to join in the early 1960s.

•1954 • The American College of Sports Medicine (ACSM) was founded. Of the eleven founding members, eight had a background in physical education or were employed by departments of physical education. Eight were members of the American Association for Health, Physical Education & Recreation (AAHPER), and seven were members of the American Academy of Physical Education (AAPE). Four of the founders made contributions to cardiology and four made contributions to physiology. One of the common interests of the founders was the production and measurement of physical fitness. In 1962, there were 514 members and it is now the leading organization for sports medicine in the USA with around 16,000 members.

•1954 • A delegation of physicians from the USSR attended the 10th International Congress of Sports Medicine for the first time.

•1956 • In the German Democratic Republic (GDR), the Ministry of Health agreed to recognize the principle of sports-medical doctors on condition that they completed their five-year general medical course, passed all their exams and worked for a year in sports medicine. It later became six years general and three years clinical sports medicine.

•1962 • The American Academy of Orthopedic Surgeons established a Committee on Sports Medicine.

•1962 • John G.P. Williams' *Sports Medicine* was the first book published in English to use the term 'sports medicine.'

•1963 • The first European Congress of Sports Medicine in Prague included delegates from 23 countries.

•1963 • The Institute of Sports Medicine was founded by the British Association of Sport and Medicine, the Physical Education Association and the British Olympic Association.

•1963 • The Australian Sports Medicine Federation was formed.

•1963 • In the German Democratic Republic (GDR), the Government set up a sports-medical service as part of the State Secretariat for Physical Culture and Sport. All 15 regions had their own sports medicine centers. The 240 districts each had a small sports medicine service.

•1964 • The Fédération Internationale de Médecine du Sport (FIMS) established a Scientific Commission. One of the objectives was to stimulate research in both basic and practical aspects of sports medicine.

•1970 • The American Academy of Pediatric Sports Medicine was founded. It is affiliated with the American Pediatric Medical Association.

•1972 • The American Orthopedic Society for Sports Medicine was founded.

•1977 • In the USSR, sports medicine was officially approved of as an independent discipline, following a special resolution of the State Committee on Science and Technology. Since 1918, the whole area of "sports medicine" had been described as "medical supervision" of sport and physical education.

•1977 • The American Osteopathic Academy of Sports Medicine was founded.

•1979 • The American Academy of Sports Physicians was founded.

•1984 • The first International Congress of Sports Traumatology was held.

•1985 • The North American Society for Pediatric Exercise Medicine was founded.

•1987 • The British Olympic Medical Centre was set up to provide facilities for treatment of sports injuries, physiological testing and nutritional advice for accredited competitors in all sports.

Bibliography

Berryman, J.W. (1995). *Out of many, one: A history of the American College of Sports Medicine*. Champaign, IL: Human Kinetics.

Bloomfield, J. and Fitch, P.A. (1996). *Science and medicine in sport*. Oxford: Blackwell Scientific Publications.

Dirix, A., Knuttgen, H.G. and Tittel, K. (eds, 1988). *The Olympic book of sports medicine*. Oxford: Blackwell Scientific Publishers.

Hackney, R.G. and Wallace, W.A. (1999). *Sports medicine handbook*. London: BMJ Publishing Group.

Harries, M. et al. (1998). *Oxford textbook of sports medicine*. 2nd ed. Oxford: Oxford University Press.

International Federation of Sports Medicine. Http://www.fims.org

Irvin, R., Iversen, D. and Roy, S. (1998). *Sports medicine. Prevention, assessment, management and rehabilitation of athletic injuries*. 2nd ed. Boston, MA: Allyn & Bacon.

Kent, M. (1994). *Oxford dictionary of sport science and medicine*. Oxford: Oxford University Press.

Kjaer, M. et al. (2003). *Textbook of sports medicine. Basic science and clinical aspects of sports injury and physical activity*. Malden, MA: Blackwell Science.

Maughan, R.J. (1999, ed). *Basic and applied sciences for sports medicine*. Oxford: Butterworth-Heinemann.

Mellion, M.B. (1999). *Sports medicine secrets*. 2nd ed. Philadelphia, PA: Hanley and Belfus.

Payne, S.D.W. (1990, ed). *Medicine, sport and the law*. Oxford: Blackwell.

Safran, M.R., McKeag, D.B. and Van Camp, S.P. (1998). *Manual of sports medicine*. Philadelphia, PA: Lippincot-Raven.

Sallis, R.E. and Massimino, F. (1997, eds). *ACSM's Essentials of sports medicine*. St Louis, MO: Mosby.

Sherry, E. and Wilson, S. (1998). *Oxford handbook of sports medicine*. 2nd ed. New York: Oxford University Press.

SPORTS NUTRITION   See DIET; NUTRIENTS; NUTRITION.

SPORTS PEDAGOGY   The study of teaching and coaching in sport and physical education.

Bibliography

Bain, L.L. (1997). Sport pedagogy. In: Massengale, J.D. and Swanson, R.A. (eds.). *The history of exercise and sport science*. Pp15-37. Champaign, IL: Human Kinetics.

Pieron, M. and Graham, G. (1986, eds). *Sport pedagogy*. Champaign, IL: Human Kinetics.

SPORTS PHILOSOPHY   The search for deeper meanings of various issues, such as the importance of sport and physical education to the educational process; mind versus body arguments; how games and play fit within the framework of physical education; the role of society in sport; and ethical aspects of sport. Estes and Mechikoff (1999) provide an introduction to the following areas of philosophy: metaphysics (study of the nature of reality); ontology (study of the nature of being); cosmology (study of the nature of the material universe); theology (study of the nature of God); epistemology (study of the nature of knowledge); axiology (study of the nature of values); aesthetics (study of the nature of beauty); politics (study of the nature of the common good); and ethics (study of the nature of right and wrong). With respect to epistemology, six ways of knowing used in kinesiology are: authority (being told what is true); rationalism (knowing through the use of reason); empiricism (knowing through observation); pragmatism (knowing through testing observations and inferences in action); somatics (knowing through awareness or subjective experience); and narrativism (knowing through story telling).

See AMATEURISM; CHARACTER-BUILDING; COMMERCIALISM;   DRUGS;   GENDER; HEALTH;   HUMAN MOVEMENT;   KINESIO-LOGY; MIND-BODY RELATIONSHIP; PHYSICAL EDUCATION; RELIGION; SPORT; VALUES.

Bibliography

Estes, S.G. and Mechikoff, R.A. (1999). *Knowing human movement*. Boston, MA: Allyn and Bacon.

Holowchak, M.A. (2002, ed). *Philosophy of sport: Critical reading, crucial issues*. Upper Saddle River, NJ: Prentice Hall.

Kretchmar, R.S. (1994). *Practical philosophy of sport*. Champaign, IL: Human Kinetics.

Kretchmar, R.S. (1997). Philosophy of sport. In: Massengale, J.D. and Swanson, R.A. (eds.). *The history of exercise and sport science*. pp181-201. Champaign, IL: Human Kinetics.

Mechikoff, R. and Estes, S. (2002). *A history and philosophy of sport and physical education: From ancient civilization to the modern world*. 3rd ed. Boston, MA: McGraw-Hill.

Morgan, W., Meier, K. and Schneider, A. (2001). *Ethics in sport*. Champaign, IL: Human Kinetics.

National Association for Sport and Physical Education (2004). *Minimum competencies for teaching undergraduate sport philosophy courses*. Approved by the Sport Philosophy Academy of the National Association for Sport and Physical Education. Reston, VA.

SPORTS PHYSIOTHERAPY

SPORTS PHYSIOTHERAPY   It is a branch of physiotherapy emphasizing active rehabilitation and therapeutic exercise. Athletes often seek medical advice directly from a physiotherapist rather than a doctor, thus sports physiotherapists require knowledge of the etiology of athletic injury. At athletic contests, sports physiotherapists play an important role in first aid. *See also* ATHLETIC TRAINING.

Chronology

•1972 • In Britain, the Association of Chartered Physiotherapists in Sports Medicine was founded. It runs training courses for physiotherapists in sports medicine.

•1984 • The first International Congress of Sport Physiotherapy was held.

Bibliography

Association of Chartered Physiotherapists in Sports Medicine. Http://www.acpsm.org

Zuluaga, M. et al. (1995). *Sports physiotherapy: Applied science and practice*. Melbourne: Churchill Livingstone.

SPORTS PSYCHOLOGY

SPORTS PSYCHOLOGY   The study of human behavior and mind in sport. It can be traced back to the 1920s, but up until 1960 it was mainly concerned with motor learning and sport skill acquisition. It then became recognized as a subdiscipline of physical education. By the 1980s, it had become part of sports science.

Educational sport psychologists are primarily concerned with psychological skills training. **Clinical sport psychologists** deal with problems such as eating disorders, substance abuse and severe depression. In the USA and Canada, licensure is required in order to sell sport-related psychological services to the public.

In a survey of 96 NCAA Division I universities, it was determined that 53% of the athletic departments in the sample used some form of sport psychology consulting. The most often used consultant positions were part-time consultants hired by either individual sport programs (n=19, 37%) or the athletic departments (n=10, 20%), and full-time consultants hired by the athletic departments (n=7, 14%).

Miller and Kerr (2002) proposed an athlete-centered sport system in which performance and personal excellence co-exist. Many college athletes have strong athletic identities that preclude their exploration of other, available roles; and may lead to problems such as: restricted exploration of external interests, emotional and psychological distress upon withdrawal from sport roles; a willingness to engage in risk behaviors; and immature career and lifestyle planning.

Some sport psychologists and coaches argue that the psychological skills and abilities that are necessary for elite athletes to perform consistently at high levels are transferable to the business world. Jones (2002) describes his transition from sport psychologist to business consultant. A one-to-one session involving an athlete and a sport psychologist is commonly referred to as consulting; the same process in business is more commonly known as coaching.

See also PSYCHOLOGY; PSYCHOLOGICAL SKILLS TRAINING.

Chronology

•1918 • Knute Rockne became head coach at Notre Dame and served until his death in a plane crash in 1931. Rockne was one of the most successful coaches in the history of football. During his 13 years as head coach, he had a record of 105 won, 5 tied and 12 lost. At half time in the 1928 Army game, Rockne motivated his dispirited team by telling them that George Gipp, on his deathbed, had asked the team to "win one for the Gipper." A movie, *Knute Rockne: All American*, was made in 1940 with Ronald Reagan playing George Gipp and Pat O'Brien playing Rockne.

•1918 • Coleman R. Griffith, as a doctoral student at the University of Illinois, became the first person to conduct systematic sport psychology research. He investigated psychological factors in basketball and football. During his years at Illinois, Griffith did collaborative research on Red Grange, Knute Rockne and Dizzy Dean. In 1924, Rockne received a letter from Griffith asking him about his pre-game pep talks: "Dear Coach Rockne: I have been interested for some years in many of the problems of psychology and athletics.... I have heard it said that you do not key your men up to their games: that you select such men as play the game joyously for its own sake and that you try to develop in them as much of this spirit as you can." In reply to this, Rockne stated, "I do not make any effort to key [my players] up, except on rare, exceptional occasions. I keyed them up for the Nebraska game this year, which was a mistake, as we had a reaction the following Saturday against Northwestern." (Quoted in LeUnes, 1986)
•1920 • A sport psychology laboratory was established by Carl Diem at the Deutsche Hochschule fuer Leibesuebungen in Berlin.
•1925 • Coleman Griffith, the 'father of American sports psychology,' officially became director of the Athletic Research Laboratory at the University of Illinois. The laboratory was closed in 1932. In 1938, Griffith was appointed as psychologist for the Chicago Cubs Baseball Club.
•1925 • A sport psychology laboratory was established by A. Z. Puni at the Institute of Physical Culture in Leningrad.
•1962 • Thomas Tutko and Bruce Ogilvie, clinical psychologists, began using personality scales to study personality traits of various athletic teams in the San Francisco area and founded the Institute for the Study of Athletic Motivation (later to become the Institute of Athletic Motivation). In 1966, they published a book called *Problem Athletes and How to Deal With Them.*
•1965 • The first International Conference of Sports Psychology was held in Rome and the International Society of Sports Psychology was formed.
•1966 • The North American Society for the Psychology of Sport and Physical Activity (NASPSA) was founded. A year later, the first annual meeting was held before the American Alliance for Health, Physical Education and Recreation (AAHPER) conference.
•1967 • The National Society of Sport Psychology was founded in Russia.
•1968 • The Fédération Europeène de Psychologie des Sports et Des Activities Corporèlles (FEPSAC) was founded. It is a collective member of the International Society of Sports Psychology.
•1969 • In *Athletics for Athletes*, Jack Scott criticized how athletes were treated and advocated reforms that would focus on personal development of the athletes.
•1976 • A sport psychologist was assigned to be with the US teams at the Olympic Games. A year later, the US Olympic Committee appointed its first part-time director of sport psychology.
•1980 • The US Olympic Committee established a Sport Psychology Advisory Board.
•1982 • The Elite Athlete Project was developed by the Sports Medicine Council of the US Olympic Committee. It led to the first systematic services in sport psychology for US Olympic teams.

•1985 • Following the recommendation in 1984 of the North American Society for the Psychology of Sport and Physical Activity (NASPSA) not to incorporate professional issues at its conferences, the Association for the Advancement of Applied Sport Psychology (AAASP) was founded to promote the development of psychological theory, research and intervention strategies in sport psychology. It was composed of three interrelated sections: intervention/performance enhancement, social psychology and health psychology.
•1986 • The American Psychological Association founded Division 47: Exercise and Sport Psychology. It furthers the scientific, educational and clinical foundations of exercise and sport psychology.
•1988 • In order to satisfy objections from the Canadian Psychological Association, the Canadian Association of Sport Sciences removed the word "psychology" from its sport psychology registry and renamed it The Canadian Registry for Sport Behavioral Professionals.
•1988 • The US Olympic Team was accompanied by an officially recognized sport psychologist for the first time.
•1989 • The American Association for the Advancement of Sport Psychology (AAASP) approved certification criteria for the title Certified Consultant, AAASP. In 1998, there were 133 Certified Consultants.
•1994 • The CHAMPS/Life Skills Program of the National Amateur Athletic Association (NCAA) was launched, addressing five core components: academics, athletics, personal development, community service, and career development. CHAMPS is an acronym for Challenging Athlete's Minds for Personal Success. Originally it was implemented in 49 institutions. By the end of 2003, there were CHAMPS/Life Skills programs in place at 472 NCAA institutions and conference offices, with more being added each year.

Bibliography

Anshel, M.H. (2003). *Sport psychology: From theory to practice.* 4th ed. San Francisco: Benjamin Cummings.

Biddle, S.J.H. (1995, ed). *European perspectives on exercise and sport psychology.* Champaign, IL: Human Kinetics.

Butler, R.J. (1996). *Sports psychology in action.* Oxford: Butterworth-Heinemann.

Butler, R.J. (1997). *Sports psychology in performance.* Oxford: Butterworth-Heinemann.

Carron, A.V. and Hausenblas, H.A. (1998). *Group dynamics in sport.* 2nd ed. Morgantown, WV: Fitness Information Technology.

Cashmore, E. (2002). *Sport psychology. The key concepts.* London: Routledge.

Cockerill, I. (2002). *Solutions in sport psychology.* London: Thomson.

Cox, R.H. (2002). *Sport psychology: Concepts and applications.* 5th ed. Boston, MA: McGraw-Hill.

Duda, J.L. (1998). *Advances in sport and exercise psychology measurement.* Morgantown, WV: Fitness Information Technology.

Gill, D.L. (1997). Sport and exercise psychology. In: Massengale, J.D. and Swanson, R.A. (eds.). *The history of exercise and sport science*. pp293-320. Champaign, IL: Human Kinetics.

Gill, D.L. (2000). *Psychological dynamics of sport and exercise*. 2nd ed. Champaign, IL: Human Kinetics.

Halden-Brown, S. (2003). *Mistakes worth making. How to turn sports errors into athletic excellence*. Champaign, IL: Human Kinetics.

Hardy, L., Jones, G. and Gould, D.D. (1996). *Understanding psychological preparation for sport. Theory and practice of elite performers*. Chichester, UK: Wiley.

Hill, K.L. (2001). *Frameworks for sport psychologists. Enhancing sport performance*. Champaign, IL: Human Kinetics.

Horn, T. (2002, ed). *Advances in sport psychology*. 2nd ed. Champaign, IL: Human Kinetics.

Jones, G. (2002). Performance excellence: A personal perspective on the link between sport and business. *Journal of Applied Sport Psychology* 14, 268-281.

Lavallee, D. et al. (2004). *Sport psychology. Contemporary themes*. New York: Palgrave MacMillan.

LeUnes, A. and Nation, J.R. (2002). *Sport psychology: An introduction*. 3rd ed. Pacific Grove, CA: Wadsworth.

Lidor, R., Morris, T., Bardaxoglu, N. and Becker, B. (2001). *The world sport psychology sourcebook*. 3rd ed. Morgantown, WV: Fitness Information Technology, Inc.

Miller, P.S. and Kerr, G.A. (2002). Conceptualizing excellence: Past, present, and future. *Journal of Applied Sport Psychology* 14, 140-153.

Moran, A.P. (2004). *Sport and exercise psychology: A critical introduction*. London: Psychology Press / Routledge.

Morgan, W.P. (1996, ed). *Physical activity and mental health*. Washington, DC: Taylor & Francis.

Murphy, S. (1996). *The achievement zone*. New York: Putnam.

Ostrow, A.C. (1996, ed). *Directory of psychological tests in sport and exercise sciences*. Morgantown, WV: Fitness Information Technology.

Pitino, R. (1997). *Success is a choice: Ten steps to overachieving in business and life*. New York: Broadway Books.

Porter, K. (2003). *The mental athlete*. Champaign, IL: Human Kinetics.

Rosenberg, B. (2003). Life Skills scores perfect 10. Program to help acclimate student-athletes celebrates decade of excellence. *NCAA News*, November 24.

Silva, J.M. and Stevens, D.E. (2002, eds). *Psychological foundations of sport*. Boston, MA: Allyn & Bacon.

Singer, R. Murphy, M. and Tennant, L.K. (1993, eds). *Handbook of research on sport psychology*. New York: MacMillan.

Van Raalte, J.L. and Brewer, B.W. (1996). *Exploring sport and exercise psychology*. Washington, DC: American Psychology Association.

Voight, M. and Callaghan, J. (2001). The use of sport psychology services at NCAA Division I Universities from 1998-1999. *The Sport Psychologist* 15(1), 91-102.

Wann, D.L. (1997). *Sports psychology*. Upper Saddle River, NJ: Prentice Hall.

Weinberg, R.S. and Gould, D. (2003). *Foundations of sport and exercise psychology*. 3rd ed. Champaign, IL: Human Kinetics.

Weinberg, R. and McDermott, M. (2002). A comparative analysis

of sport and business organizations: Factors perceived critical for organizational success. *Journal of Applied Sport Psychology* 14, 282-298.

Williams, J.M. (2001, ed). *Applied sport psychology: Personal growth to peak performance*. 4th ed. Boston, MA: McGraw-Hill.

SPORTS SCIENCE A broad discipline that is mainly concerned with the processes that explain behavior in sport and how athletic performance can be improved. Sports science involves a number of disciplines, including kinanthropometry, biomechanics, exercise physiology, sport psychology and sociology of sport. Sports science contributes to sports medicine primarily with regard to the etiology and prevention of injury and disease. Australia has a high reputation in sports science, due to the way in which sports science has been infused into Australian coaching techniques and the way in which Australia has been able to identify talent and monitor training (Bloomfield, 2001). *See also* KINESIOLOGY.

Chronology

•1958 • In India, the Ad Hoc Enquiry Committee on Games and Sports was appointed to investigate the low standards of sports and the performance of Indian teams in international competition. Three years later, the National Institute of Sports was established to produce coaches of high caliber in as many sports as possible.

•1958 • The International Council of Sport and Physical Education was founded. In 1983, it became known as the International Council of Sports Science and Physical Education.

•1977 • In Britain, the Society of Sports Sciences was founded. In 1984, it merged with the newly formed British Association of Sports Sciences.

•1981 • The Australian Institute of Sport was opened and a Sports Science Unit was established.

•1982 • In the UK, the Sports Council (founded in 1965) established a working party to investigate closer links between the many organizations representing sports science and sports medicine.

•1983 • The Australian Government formally recognized the link between science, research and sporting performance with the establishment of the National Sports Research Program, which was to become the National Sports Research Centre in 1992.

•1984 • The British Association of Sports Science (BASS) was founded, following the dissolution of the Biomechanics Study Group, the British Society of Sports Psychology and the Society of Sports Sciences.

•1987 • The Talent Search Program was begun in Australia. It would scour the high schools of Australia for 14- to 16-year olds who had the potential to be elite athletes. In the same year, an editorial of the *Australian Journal of Science and Medicine in Sport* stated, "Sports science and medicine has certainly made progress in

Australia in the last few years. It has become an established area of study in three universities and several institutes of technology and advanced education throughout the country. It forms the theory base for both the national coaching accreditation and sports trainers' schemes. It is now an accepted ingredient in the preparation of the high performance athlete."

•1988 • In the Department of Human Movement Studies at the University of Queensland, a majority of members voted to: (a) move from the Faculty of Education to the Faculty of Science; (b) emphasize applied sport science and exercise management; and (c) marginalize sociology in the curriculum (McKay et al., 1990).

•1988 • In the UK, the Sports Council (UK) stated in *Sport and the Community: A Strategy for Sport 1988-1993*, "The need has never been greater for British sports people, especially, but not only, top level performers, to have access to adequate medical and scientific support when and where they need it. Yet medicine remains an area of contention, beset by a traditionally muddled British approach."

•1993 • The British Association of Sports Sciences (BASS) changed its name to the British Association of Sports and Exercise Sciences (BASES).

Bibliography

Bloomfield, J. (2001). The contribution of sports science and sports medicine to the development of the Australian sports system. Http://www.ausport.gov.au/fulltext/2001/acsms/papers/BLOO.pdf

McKay, J., Gore, J.M. and Kirk, D. (1990). Beyond the limits of technocratic physical education. *Quest* 42(1), 52-76.

SPORTS SOCIOLOGY   *See* SOCIOLOGY OF SPORT.

SPORTS VISION   An area of practice and study that combines vision science, motor learning, biomechanics, sport psychology and neuroanatomy as they relate to visual/perceptual motor performance. It is concerned with the assessment, correction and enhancement of vision, as well as the protection of eyes during sporting activity.

Bibliography

All About Vision. Http://www.allaboutvision.com

Bahill, A.T. and LaRitz, T. (1984). Why can't batter keep their eyes on the ball? *American Scientist* 72, 249-253.

Bard, C., Fleury, M. and Goulet, C. (1994). Relationship between perceptual strategies and response adequacy in sport situation. *International Journal of Sport Psychology* 25, 266-281.

Blundell, N.L. (1985). The contribution of vision to the learning and performance of sports skills: Part I. The role of selected visual parameters. *Australian Journal of Science and Medicine in Sport* 17, 3-11.

D & J Brower Opticians. Http://www.brower.co.uk

Knudson, D. and Kluka, D. (1997). The impact of vision and vision training on sport performance. *Journal of Physical Education, Recreation, and Dance* 68(4), 17-24.

Loran, D.F.C. and MacEwen, C.J. (1995, eds). *Sports vision*. Oxford: Butterworth Heinemann.

Starkes, J., Helsen, W. and Elliot, D. (2002). A ménage a trios: The eye, the hand and on-line processing. *Journal of Sports Sciences* 20, 217-224.

Visual Fitness Institute. Http://visualfitness.com

Watts, R.G. and Bahill, A.T. (1990). *Keep your eye on the ball. The science and folklore of baseball*. New York: W.H. Freeman and Co.

Wilson, T.A. and Falkel, J. (2004). *SportsVision: Training for better performance*. Champaign, IL: Human Kinetics.

SPOT REDUCTION   The belief that fat can be lost from a specific body site by exercising a local muscle group. It is probably a myth, because research has shown that fat is lost from all over the body during an aerobic exercise program and not just from the sites involved in producing muscular work. In elite tennis players, it has been found that the girth of the dominant arm is significantly larger than that of the non-dominant arm, but there are no significant differences in subcutaneous fat. There is no evidence that fatty acids are preferentially released to a greater degree from the subcutaneous fat directly over the active muscle.

See also ABDOMINAL OBESITY; BODY WEIGHT REDUCTION.

SPRAIN   An acute injury to a ligament. A **first-degree sprain** is the acute minor trauma of tearing a few ligamentous fibers, resulting in mild pain, swelling and disability, but no joint instability. A **second-degree sprain** is the acute, moderate trauma of tearing a moderate number of ligamentous fibers, resulting in moderate pain, swelling and disability, but slight or no joint instability. A **third-degree sprain** is the acute and complete tear of a ligament, resulting in pain and swelling that may be minimal to severe, disability that is severe and joint instability.

SPRINTING   *See under* ACCELERATION.

SPUTUM   Phlegm. It is a mass of saliva ejected from the mouth mixed with mucus or pus exuded from the respiratory passages, as in bronchitis or bronchiectasis.

STABILIZER   *See under* MUSCLE ACTION.

STABILITY   *See* BALANCE; CENTER OF GRAVITY; EQUILIBRIUM.

STABILITY BALL   *See* SWISS BALL.

STACKING   A term coined by Harry Edwards in 1967 to refer to the assignment of a player to a position, an achieved status, on the basis of ascribed status. African Americans are disproportionately found in those positions requiring physical rather than cognitive or leadership abilities. In American football, for example, African Americans tend to be precluded from leadership positions such as quarterback. Furthermore, there is a lack of African Americans in administrative, managerial and officiating roles. It has been hypothesized that stacking can be explained in terms of stereotypes in the sporting world of African American cognitive and leadership abilities that, in turn, can be traced to the Caucasian European colonials of the 1700s, who believed they were intellectually superior to African American individuals. Another hypothesis is that African American youths may segregate themselves into specific sport roles, because they wish to emulate African American stars (McPherson, 1975). Empirical evidence to reject the latter hypothesis has been provided by Eitzen and Sanford (1975) who found that African American athletes changed from central to non-central positions more frequently than Caucasians as they moved from high school to college to professional competition.

Coakley (1998) argues that remnants of stacking still exist in professional basketball and American football, but have shifted to reflect changes in coaching strategies and associated changes in responsibilities for players in different positions, e.g. college quarterbacks run the ball now and they seldom call their own plays in the huddle. The cognitive processes involved in coaching have affected the extent to which racial ideology is expressed in player position patterns.

During the 1998 NFL season, stacking was evidenced in the following positions: quarterback (91% African American), center (83% Caucasian), wide receiver (92% African American), running back (87% African American), cornerback (99% African American) and safety (91% African American). *See also* RACE.

Bibliography
Coakley, J.J. (2004). *Sport in society. Issues and controversies*. 8th ed. Boston, MA: Irwin McGraw-Hill.

Eitzen, D.S. and Sage, G.H. (2003). *Sociology of North American sport*. 7th ed. Boston, MA: McGraw-Hill.

Eitzen, D.E. and Sanford, D.C. (1975). The segregation of Blacks by playing position in football: Accident or design? *Social Science Quarterly* 55, 948-959.

McPherson, B.D. (1975). The segregation by playing position hypothesis in sport. *Social Science Quarterly* 55, 960-966.

STALENESS   *See under* OVERTRAINING.

STARCH   *See under* CARBOHYDRATE.

STARGARDT DISEASE   *See under* MACULAR DISEASE.

STARTLE REFLEX   A primitive reflex that may not appear until 2 to 3 months after the Moro reflex disappears. It can be elicited by a rapid change of head position or striking the surface that supports the infant, with the response that the arms and legs flex immediately.

STASIS   (i) An abnormal state in which the normal flow of a liquid, such as blood, is slowed or stopped. (ii) Inactivity resulting from a static balance between two forces.

STATURE   Height. It is a measure of the distance from the bottom of the feet (with the heels together) to the highest point (**vertex**) of the head. There are four general techniques for measuring stature: free standing stature, stature against the wall, recumbent length and stretch stature. Each technique gives a slightly different value. From birth to 2 years, or until a child can stand without assistance, total body length (recumbent length) is measured while the child is supine.

Middle-distance runners, jumpers, throwers and sprint swimmers tend to be of above-average height. Gymnasts and divers tend to be of below-average height.

Sitting height-to-stature ratio, expressed as a percentage, is the contribution of the legs and trunk to total height. It is measured by having the subject sit on a high bench such that the feet do not touch the floor and the spine is kept erect. Boys have longer trunks than girls until they are about 12 years old. During adolescence and adulthood, women have shorter legs than men of equal stature. See also under GROWTH.

STEADY STATE   The state of a physiological system in which its output per unit time becomes constant. The time to achieve a steady state is usually different for each physiological system. A system is not in a steady state when it reaches the limit of its output. Exercise can be defined as being of high intensity when it exceeds an individual's capability to maintain a steady state condition.

STEM CELL   A 'generic' cell that can make exact copies of itself indefinitely. A distinction can be made between embryonic and adult stem cells. **Embryonic stem cells** are obtained from either aborted fetuses or fertilized eggs that are left over from *in vitro* fertilization. In the 3- to 5-day-old embryo (blastocyst), stem cells in developing tissues give rise to the multiple specialized cell types that make up the heart, lung, skin and other tissues. Embryonic stem cells can produce cells for almost every tissue in the body. The use of embryonic stem cells, however, is controversial for ethical reasons. An **adult stem cell** (**somatic stem cell**) is an undifferentiated cell found among differentiated cells in a tissue or organ. An adult stem cell is specific to a certain cell type. It can renew itself and can differentiate to yield the major specialized cell types of the tissue or organ. Adult stem cells are found in both children and adults, thus the term 'adult' stem cell is somewhat of a misnomer. The primary roles of adult stem cells in a living organism are to maintain and repair the tissue in which they are found. In some adult tissues, such as bone marrow, muscle and

brain, discrete populations of adult stem cells generate replacements for cells that are lost through normal wear and tear, injury or disease. A single adult stem cell should be able to generate a line of genetically identical cells, known as a **clone**, which then gives rise to all the appropriate differentiated cell types of the tissue. Stem cells may be useful for *in vitro* research and testing in the treatment of disease and development of drugs. It is thought that Parkinson's disease may be one of the first diseases to be amenable to treatment using stem cells transplantation, partly because of the knowledge of the specific cell type (dopaminergic neurons) needed to relieve the symptoms of the disease.

Bibliography
National Institutes of Health. Http://stemcells.nih.gov

STENOSIS   A stricture or narrowing of any canal or vessel. In the heart, it occurs when a valve does not open completely.

STEPPING REFLEX   *See* WALKING REFLEX.

STEREOTYPE   An overgeneralization about the behavior or other characteristics of members of particular groups.

STEREOTYPY   Self-stimulatory behavior. Stimming. It involves repetitive body movements or repetitive movement of objects. These purposeless, rhythmical and patterned movements are normal in infants, but are pathological in children and adults when they persist as rocking, waving, wriggling or banging mannerisms. Kicking stereotypies are among the first to appear, usually at about 4 weeks of age. Visual stereotypies include staring at lights, repetitive blinking, moving fingers in front of the eyes and hand-flapping. Auditory stereotypies include tapping ears, snapping fingers and making vocal sounds. Tactile stereotypies include rubbing the skin with one's hands or with another object; and scratching. Vestibular stereotypies include rocking front to back, or side to side. Taste stereotypies include placing body parts or objects in one's mouth and licking objects. Smell stereotypies include smelling objects and sniffing people.

Stereotypies tend to appear just before infants display voluntary control of body parts and seem to provide needed input for maturation of the central nervous system. Throughout the first year, many stereotypies cease and new ones emerge. Most sterotypies are integrated by about 12 months. In children and adults, stereotypies can become independent movement disorders that significantly interfere with normal activities or result in self-inflicted bodily injury, but typically they coexist with such conditions as attention-deficit hyperactivity disorder, severe mental retardation, autism, deaf-blindness, or blindness. It has been suggested that people with stereotypies may be hyposensitive and crave stimulation. Alternatively, people with stereotypies may be hypersensitive and these behaviors have a calming effect. Stereotypies interfere with attention and learning, but may often be effective positive reinforcers if a person is allowed to engage in these behaviors after completing a task. *See* AUTISM; OBSESSIVE COMPULSIVE DISORDER; PERVASIVE DEVELOPMENTAL DISORDERS; TICS.

STERNOCLAVICULAR JOINT *See under* SHOULDER GIRDLE.

STERNO-COSTAL JOINTS Gliding joints where the cartilages of the true ribs articulate with the sternum, except for the first rib, which is synarthrodial (immovable). Elevation and depression (slight) of the ribs are permitted.

STERNUM Breastbone. The sternum is rarely fractured in sports, but it may occur as a result of rapid deceleration and high impact into an object. Stress fractures may be caused by indirect force, such as vigorous muscle contraction in a baseball pitch.

STEROIDS A class of lipids, containing no fatty acids, which includes sterols, sterol glycosides, saponins, bile acids, vitamin D, and hormones of the adrenal cortex and gonads. The most abundant steroids are the **sterols**. Cholesterol is the major sterol in animal tissues and it is an important com-ponent of plasma lipoproteins and of the outer cell membrane. **Phytosterols**, which are sterols found in plants, are poorly absorbed by humans and decrease intestinal absorption of cholesterol. *See also* ANABOLIC STEROIDS.

STIEDA'S PROCESS *See under* OSSICLES.

STIFFNESS *See under* ELASTIC MODULUS.

STIMULANTS A group of drugs that increase arousal and activity. They produce effects on both the central nervous system and the peripheral nervous system. Amphetamines, ephedrine, cocaine and caffeine are sympathomimetics, thus mimic the effects of the stress hormones epinephrine and norepineph-rine. Amphetamines are the most potent and cause the release of excitatory neurotransmitters such as dopamine to stimulate the central nervous system.

See also CLENBUTEROL; COCAINE; EPHEDRINE; GINSENG; NICOTINE; YOHIMBINE.

Chronology
•1988 • A United States Olympic Committee (USOC) spokesper-son explained that between 6 and 10 track-and-field athletes who failed drug tests at the Olympic Trials would be allowed to com-pete in the Olympic Games, because the drug use was either "pre-declared" or "inadvertent." All the positive tests were for over-the-counter stimulants from herbal teas or cold medications.

STIMULI Events, occurrences or changes that evoke behavioral responses from organisms.

STITCH Side stitch. It is a sharp pain in the upper abdominal area that may occur during exercise. A stitch may be located on the right or left side of the body. It is more frequent when exercise takes place immediately after a meal.

One theory to explain stitch is change in blood flow, such that blood is shunted away from the diaphragm and other respiratory muscles to the stomach, intestines and limb muscles. This leads to ischemic pain. Another theory, which seems more plausible, is related to foot impact with the ground. The bouncing of the body causes pain through pull of the peritoneal ligaments of the viscera on the diaphragm. This would explain why running, but not swimming or cycling is associated with stitches.

The pain is exacerbated by deep expiration and relieved by deep inspiration. Improvements in breathing from training may help prevent the stitch. Avoiding exercise immediately after eating a large meal or ingesting a liter or more of fluid may also help.

Bibliography
Plunkett, B.T. and Hopkins, W.G. (1999). Investigation of the side pain 'stitch' induced by running after fluid ingestion. *Medicine and Science in Sports and Exercise* 31 (8), 1169-1175.
Stamford, B. (1985). A 'stitch' in the side. *The Physician and Sportsmedicine* 13(5), 187.

STOMA *See under* SPINAL PARALYSIS.

STOMACH *See under* GASTRO-INTESTINAL SYSTEM.

STPD **S**tandard **T**emperature and **P**ressure **D**ry. It refers to gas volume at standard conditions of temperature (zero degrees Celsius) and pressure (760 mm Hg) and dry (free of water vapor).

STRABISMUS A muscle imbalance resulting in the inability of both eyes to look directly at an object at the same time. Types of strabismus include: esotropia (an inward turn), exotropia (an outward turn), hypertropia (an upward turn) and hypotropia (a downward turn).

STRAIN i) *See* ELASTIC MODULI. ii) *See* MUSCLE STRAIN.

STREAMLINING *See under* DRAG.

STRENGTH The maximum force or torque that can be developed during maximal voluntary contraction of muscle(s). **Static strength** involves virtually no movement of joints. The force is applied against a resistance that is virtually immovable. The muscle contraction is mainly isometric, because force is generated by a muscle without shortening of the muscle fibers, thus no movement of joint(s) occurs. Static strength can be measured using a

dynamometer, which is an instrument in which a spring is compressed and moves a pointer when an external static isometric force is applied to it. An example is the handgrip dynamometer. **Dynamic strength** involves movement of joints. The muscle contractions are mainly isotonic. Dynamic strength can be measured in various ways, such as the 'one-repetition maximum' (1-RM), i.e. the maximum weight that can be lifted for only one repetition on a particular movement involving one or more joints. The heaviest weight that can be lifted through a full range of joint motion cannot be greater than the strength at the weakest point (the 'sticking point').

Absolute strength refers to the total force that can be exerted. There is a positive correlation between muscle cross-sectional area and absolute strength. There is also a positive correlation between body mass and absolute strength. **Relative strength** is strength in relation to body weight (or lean-body weight). In some sports, such as gymnastics, relative strength is more important than absolute strength.

Strength is governed primarily by the ability of each muscle fiber to generate force and the ability of motor nerves to stimulate a large number of muscle fibers. It is possible to increase strength without any change in muscle size. The use of resistance training to improve strength must ultimately involve the use of low repetitions with heavy weights. The first adaptations from resistance training, exhibited after 2 weeks of four training sessions per week, are always mainly due to improvement in intermuscular coordination. Substantial gains in strength are evident, but without a concomitant increase in muscle mass. Neuronal adaptations occur after 6 to 8 weeks of four training sessions per week. In order to enable significant improvements in strength and power over a period of several years, it is necessary to make gains in muscle mass. After approximately 9 to 12 weeks of training, related to the type of training and sex of subjects, the rate of increase drops off dramatically.

See also BODYBUILDING; ISOKINETIC MOVEMENT; MOTOR UNITS; POWER; RESISTANCE TRAINING.

Bibliography
Schmitbleicher, D. (1992). Training for power events. In: Komi,

P.V. (ed). *Strength and power in sport*. pp381-395. Oxford: Blackwell Scientific Publishers.

Siff, M.C. (2000). Biomechanical foundations of strength and power training. In Zatsiorsky, V. (ed). *Biomechanics in sport. Performance enhancement and injury prevention. Vol. IX of the Encyclopedia of Sports Medicine*. pp103-139. Oxford: Blackwell Science.

STRENGTH, MATERIAL   *See under* ELASTIC MODULUS.

STRESS CONCENTRATION   A phenomenon that occurs when high localized stresses result from sudden changes in the shape of a structure that is under stress. **Stress risers** (points of focused stress) tend to occur at locations of discontinuity within tissue. Examples of stress risers are abrupt tissue interfaces (e.g. bone-tendon junctions) and fracture sites.

STRESS FRACTURES   Fatigue fractures of bone secondary to repetitive stress that may occur at all ages beyond 7 years. Stress fractures may occur when there is an imbalance between bone injury and bone remodeling. Stress fractures are most commonly oblique, but might be compression-type, transverse or longitudinal (least common).

In terms of loading, a distinction can be made between two types of stress fracture: fatigue and insufficiency. **Fatigue-type stress fractures** result from abnormally increased load on normal bone. Stress fractures occur after the application of a normal load at high frequency (e.g. long distance running), a heavy load at normal frequency (e.g. increasing the gradient for hill running) or a heavy load at high frequency (e.g. intensive weight training). **Insufficiency-type stress fractures** result from normal loads on deficient bone (e.g. in osteoporosis).

Theories about the cause of stress fractures include the Fatigue theory and the Overload theory. The **Fatigue theory** postulates that excessive forces are transmitted to bone when the surrounding muscle becomes fatigued. The **Overload theory** is concerned with the effects of repeated muscle contraction on the deformation of bones, e.g. contraction of the calf muscles causes the tibia to bend forward like a drawn bow; after repeated contrac-

tions the tibia is unable to tolerate the stress and fracture occurs.

The most commonly afflicted bones are the tibia, fibula, metatarsal shaft, calcaneus, femur, pars interarticularis of the lumbar vertebrae, ribs and humerus. Stress fractures are less common in the upper extremity, but may occur in the proximal humerus, coracoid process and acromial process. Stress fractures are common in distance running and jumping sports, but are also found in weightlifting (acromion), aerobics (fibula), hurdling (patella), sprinting (tarsal bones), gymnastics (pars interarticularis), fast bowling in cricket (pars interarticularis), rowing (ribs) and racquet sports (ulna and humerus). Stress fractures occur more frequently in female athletes than in male athletes. Obesity has been proposed as a risk factor for stress fractures by increasing weight-bearing forces on the bones. *See also* ELBOW JOINT, THROWING INJURIES; FEMORAL NECK STRESS FRACTURE; MARCH FRACTURE; METATARSAL FRACTURES; STRESS REACTION.

Bibliography
Brukner, P. Bennell, K. and Matheson, G. (1999). *Stress fractures*. Champaign, IL: Human Kinetics.

STRESSORS   Stimuli that disrupt homeostasis and cause physiological responses or adaptations. **External stimuli** include heat, cold, odor, food, water, hypoxia, noise, light, darkness, injury, electric shock, physical threat, bacteria and viruses. **Internal stimuli** include heat, cold, sleep, hunger, thirst, infection, ion imbalance, fear, muscle tension, internal clock, emotions, autonomic change and abstract thoughts. **Adaptive responses (adaptations)** are physiological changes that minimize bodily strain, and represent the body's attempts to counteract stressors and re-establish homeostasis. Adaptations may be either short-term (accommodation), intermediate in duration (acclimation/acclimatization) or long term (genetic adaptation). **Accommodation** refers to an immediate physiological change in the sensitivity of a cell or tissue to change(s) in the external environment. **Acclimatization** is induced by exposure to natural environments, whereas **acclimation** is induced experimentally in artificial environments. **Genetic adaptation** refers to semi-permanent morphological, physiological or other changes that occur over many generations within one species that favor survival in a particular environment. *See* HEREDITY.

Bibliography

Armstrong, L.E. (2000). *Performing in extreme environments.* Champaign, IL: Human Kinetics.

STRESS, PSYCHOLOGICAL In scientific psychology, there are three categories of theory on stress: i) stimulus-based theories that regard stress as a noxious or aversive characteristic of a person's environment; ii) response-based theories that regard stress as a response to noxious or aversive stimuli; and iii) theories that regard stress as a process.

McGrath (1970) proposed that four elements must be considered when studying stress as a social psychological process: the physical and social environment that places some demand on the person; the person's perception of the demand and the decision about how to respond to it; the person's response to the perceived demand; and the consequences resulting from the response. Stress is regarded as a substantial imbalance between perceived demand and perceived response capability under conditions where failure to meet demand has important consequences. If the imbalance is such that perceived demand is greater than perceived response capability, and if it is perceived as unpleasant and there is high arousal, then it can be said to be anxiety. If such an imbalance is pleasant and it is coupled with high arousal, then it is excitement or what some authors have called 'eustress.' Successful athletes often speak of reactions to heightened arousal and 'being nervous' or 'psyched up' in a positive manner. When perceived demand is lower than perceived capability to cope, and it perceived as pleasant, then relaxation may be experienced; or when unpleasant, then boredom may be experienced.

Kobasa's (1979) construct of **psychological hardiness** describes the personalities of people who

have the tendency to interpret stressful situations in a positive manner. People with hardy personalities are characterized by: an ability to feel deeply involved in or committed to what they do; the belief that they can control or influence events in their life; and a tendency to appraise potentially stressful situations as challenging rather than threatening.

Pressure occurs when one or more factors (such as parental demands) increase the importance of performing well on a particular occasion. On the assumption that pressure increases self consciousness (the tendency to focus attention on oneself), possibly via heightened arousal, which in turn disrupts performance, Baumeister (1984) predicted the following: individuals who are habitually self-conscious will find it easier to cope with situations that promote self-consciousness (i.e. high-pressure situations), because they are accustomed to performing while self-conscious. Low self-conscious individuals, on the other hand, will choke more easily in pressure situations, because they are not accustomed to performing while self-conscious. There is some empirical support for these predictions. '**Choking**' is the inability to perform up to previously exhibited standards in pressure situations.

The '**yips**' is a motor phenomenon of involuntary movements affecting golfers that is manifested by symptoms of jerks, tremors or freezing in the hands and forearms. Smith et al. (2003) regard the yips on a continuum from the neurologic disorder of dystonia to the psychologic disorder of choking. In many golfers, the pathophysiology of the 'yips' may be an acquired deterioration in the function of motor pathways, such as those involving the basal ganglia that are exacerbated when a threshold of high stress and physiologic arousal is exceeded. In other golfers, the 'yips' may result from severe performance anxiety.

Coronary-prone behavior pattern ('**Type A personality**') comprises high levels of ambition, aggressiveness, hostility, competitiveness and time urgency. It is an especially powerful independent risk factor for coronary heart disease.

Coping consists of all the things people do to control, tolerate or decrease the effects of life's stressors. A typical **stress management** strategy used by a sports psychologist to help an athlete cope with stress includes the following: appraisal of the problem, stress education (investigating the nature of the athlete's stress), relaxation training and cognitive interventions.

See also SYSTEMATIC DESENSITIZATION.

Bibliography

Baumeister, R.F. (1984). Choking under pressure: Self conscious-ness and paradoxical effects of incentives on skilful perfor-mance. *Journal of Personality and Social Psychology* 46, 610-620.

Cox, T. (1978). *Stress*. London: MacMillan.

Kobasa, S.C. (1979). Stressful life events, personality and health: An inquiry into hardiness. *Journal of Personality and Social Psychology* 37, 1-11.

McGrath, J.E. (1970). Major methodological issues. In: McGrath, J.E. (ed). *Social and psychological factors in stress*. pp19-49. New York: Holt, Rinehart and Winston.

Rotella, R.J. and Lerner, J.D. (1993). Responding to competitive pressure. In: Singer, R. Murphy, M. and Tennant, L.K. (eds). *Handbook of research on sport psychology*. pp528-541. New York: MacMillan.

Smith, A.M. et al. (2003). The 'yips' in golf: A continuum between a focal dystonia and choking. *Sports Medicine* 33(1), 13-31.

STRESS REACTION   A condition in which there are microfractures in bone. If force on the bone is increased, an actual stress fracture may result. *See under* LOWER LEG PAIN.

STRESS RELAXATION   A phenomenon that occurs when a material is strained (deformed) to a given dimension and maintained at that strain. In this situation, the stress within the material gradually decreases with time. If the load is removed, the material gradually returns to its original size and shape. Viscoelastic materials such as connective tissue may exhibit stress relaxation and also creep. Creep occurs with constant stress while strain increases, whereas stress relaxation has a constant strain while stress decreases. *See* CARTILAGE; CREEP.

STRESS, ULTIMATE   *See under* ELASTIC MODULUS.

STRESS URINARY INCONTINENCE   *See under* INCONTINENCE.

STRETCHING   It is the method used to improve or maintain flexibility. A **stretch** is defined as a linear deformation of tissue that increases its length. Muscle and connective tissue are viscoelastic. The **elastic elements** enable recoverable deformation, while the **viscous elements** enable permanent deformation. The latter is what is required for the development of flexibility. The conditions for this to take place optimally include a higher-than-normal tissue temperature (hence the need for a 'warm-up') and a low force applied over an extended period of time. It is not clear what length of time is optimal, but 10 to 30 seconds is the normal guide. It has been found that greater range-of-movement increases occur after warm-up followed by stretching than after stretching alone. Recent evidence suggests that stretching immediately before exercise does not prevent overuse or acute injuries, but that warm up is important.

Sapega et al. (1981) argued that when a relaxed muscle is stretched, most (if not all) of the resistance to stretch comes from the connective tissue within and around the muscle, rather than the muscle fibers themselves. More recently, however, it has been argued that the role of connective tissue, as the major resistance to stretch, has been overestimated and that intrinsic myogenic structures and mechanisms, such as the passive properties of titin and adaptive responses in sarcomere number, have been under-estimated.

There are three types of stretching: static stretch-ing, dynamic stretching and 'proprioceptive neuro-muscular facilitation.' **Static stretching** involves passive stretch of muscles to the point of 'slight discomfort' or 'slight stretch.' By holding the stretch for about 10 to 30 seconds, there is a decrease in tension of the muscle being stretched. Although one 30-second stretch per muscle group is sufficient to increase the range of motion in most healthy people, it is likely that longer periods or more repetitions are required in some people, injuries and muscle groups. It seems that the changes in the viscoelasticity of muscle-tendon units depends on the duration rather than the number of stretches.

The increase in resistance during stretching is explained by the stretch reflex. There are at least three explanations for the decreased tension associ-ated with a holding stretch. First, muscle spindles may become desensitized and subsequently become adapted to stretch, hence decreasing the stretch reflex. Second, if passive tension from the stretch is great enough, Golgi tendon organs and joint receptors will be activated, thus initiating **autogenic inhibition (inverse stretch reflex)**. In turn, the autogenic inhibition will inhibit the motor neuron of the muscle under stretch. Muscle tension will decrease, thereby facilitating relaxation. The third explanation implicates creep and stress relaxation, which are time-dependent mechanical properties of muscle and connective tissue.

Dynamic (ballistic) stretching involves repetitive contractions of agonist muscle(s) in order to stretch the antagonist muscles. This method may be effective, but is dangerous because injury may result if the forces generated by the agonists are greater than the extensibility limits of the antagonists and the connective tissues of the joint.

Proprioceptive neuromuscular facilitation (PNF) is actually a technique that was originally developed for treating patients with neuromuscular disorders. The original concepts have been modified for stretching techniques in sports. All involve some combination of contraction and relaxation of agonist and/or antagonist muscles.

For an athlete stretching her hip extensors (hamstrings) with the assistance of her coach, the stages of **passive PNF** are: i) the coach flexes the athlete's hip until slight discomfort is felt by the athlete; ii) the athlete contracts her hamstrings for ten seconds to push against resistance provided by the coach (to decrease the risk of injury, the coach should tell the athlete to "meet my resistance" and not permit maximal muscular contraction); iii) the athlete relaxes for 10 seconds; and iv) The coach flexes the athlete's hip further. **Active PNF** starts with i) to iii) of passive PNF. The athlete then actively contracts her *quadriceps femoris* muscles to further flex her hip. The athlete relaxes for 10 seconds and then continues with iv) and ii) of passive PNF.

There is evidence that PNF techniques can lead to a greater improvement in flexibility over a period of time, when compared to the other techniques. Active PNF appears to be superior to passive PNF.

Nevertheless, both the theory and practice of PNF are controversial. For example, while it has been claimed that prior contraction of the muscle to be stretched will evoke more inhibitory activity from Golgi tendon organs, Hutton (1992) argues that there is no research evidence to support such a claim. In fact, it has been found that PNF procedures produce greater muscle activity (as measured by electromyography) in stretched muscle. It has been proposed that effectiveness of PNF procedures may be due to an analgesic effect of 'stretch tolerance,' i.e. subjects feel less pain for the same force applied to the muscle. The result is increased range of motion, even though true stiffness does not change.

In 1998, the American College of Sports Medicine added flexibility training to its exercise recommendations: stretching the major muscle groups using static or PNF techniques with a minimum frequency of 2 or 3 days per week and 3 to 4 repetitions per stretch. The intensity is holding at a position of 'mild discomfort' for 10 to 30 seconds (static) or a 6-second contraction followed by 10 to 30 seconds of assisted stretch for PNF.

In terms of the effect of stretching on performance and injury prevention, Witvrouw (2004) distinguishes sporting activities on the basis of whether or not they involve high-intensity stretch-shortening cycles. When the type of sports activity contains low-intensity, or limited stretch-shortening cycles (e.g. swimming, cycling, jogging), there is no need for a very compliant muscle-tendon unit since most of its power generation is a consequence of active (contractile) muscle work that needs to be directly transferred (by the tendon) to the articular system to generate motion. Therefore, stretching (in order to make the tendon more compliant) may not be advantageous. There is strong evidence that stretching has no beneficial effect on injury prevention in these sports. The stiffer the muscle-tendon unit, the faster the force is transferred to the bones, and the resulting movement of the joint is quicker. Church et al. (2001) found that performing active PNF before a vertical jump test may be detrimental to performance. Kokkonen, Nelson and Cornwell (1998) found that acute, static stretching of the hip, thigh and calf muscles before the performance of a one-repetition maximum lift resulted in a decreased one-repetition maximum for both knee flexion and knee extension. If it is assumed that the musculo-tendinous unit becomes less stiff as a result of acute stretching, it is conceivable that stretching could compromise the generation of maximal muscular force. Stretching could also induce autogenic inhibi-tion of a muscle that could also compromise force production. Therefore, vigorous static or PNF stretching that is designed to enhance flexibility should be performed after practice or competition.

Sports involving bouncing and jumping activities, with a high intensity of stretch-shortening cycles, (e.g. basketball) require a muscle-tendon unit that is compliant enough to store and release the high amount of elastic energy that benefits performance in such sports. If athletes in these sports have muscle-tendon units with insufficient compliance, the demands in energy absorption and release may rapid-ly exceed the capacity of the muscle-tendon unit. This may lead to an increased risk for injury of this structure. Therefore, athletes in these sports should increase the compliance of the muscle-tendon unit. Stretching programs can significantly influence the viscosity of the tendon and make it significantly more compliant. Musculotendinous stiffness is significant-ly related to isometric and concentric performance, but not to eccentric performance. Wilson et al. (1992) showed that the enhancement in rebound bench press performance observed consequent to flexibility training was caused by a decrease in stiff-ness of muscle-tendon units, increasing the utiliza-tion of elastic strain energy during the rebound bench press lift. Using ultrasonography to quantify the viscoelastic properties of human tendon struc-tures *in vivo*, Kubo et al. (2001) found that stretching decreased the viscosity of the tendon structures but increased the elasticity. The tendon structures became more compliant by decreasing stiffness. The mechanism by which the increase in compliance occurs immediately after stretching and in the long term cannot be determined from the available research. A possible mechanism involves the move-ment of the mobile elements within the tissues, i.e. liquid and polysaccharides may be redistributed within the collagen matrices. After a periodic stretching program, the changes are more likely to involve structural changes to collagen.

Bibliography

Alter, M.J. (1996). *Science of stretching*. 2nd ed. Champaign, IL: Human Kinetics.

Alter, M.J. (1998). *Sport stretch*. 2nd ed. Champaign, IL: Human Kinetics.

Church, J.B. et al. (2001). Effect of warm-up and flexibility treat-ments on vertical jump performance. *Journal of Strength and Conditioning Research* 15(3), 332-336.

Etnyre, B.R. and Abraham, L.D. (1988). Antagonist muscle activ-ity during stretching: A paradox reassessed. *Medicine and Science in Sports and Exercise* (2), 184-188.

Hutton, R.S. (1992). Neuromuscular basis of stretching exercises. In: Komi, P.V. (ed). *Strength and power in sport*. pp29-38. Oxford: Blackwell Scientific Publications.

Kokkonen, J., Nelson, A.G. and Cornwell, A. (1998). Acute mus-cle stretching inhibits maximal strength performance. *Research Quarterly for Exercise and Sport* 69(4), 411-415.

Kubo, K. et al. (2001). Influence of static stretching on viscoelas-tic properties of human tendon structures in vivo. *Journal of Applied Physiology* 90, 520-527.

Magid, A. and Law, D.J. (1985). Myofibrils bear most of the rest-ing tension in frog skeletal muscle. *Science* 230, 1280-1282.

McAtee, R.E. (1999). *Facilitated stretching*. 2nd ed. Champaign, IL: Human Kinetics.

Moore, M.A. and Hutton, R.S. (1980). Electromyographic inves-tigation of muscle stretching techniques. *Medicine and Science in Sports and Exercise* 12(5), 322-329.

Nelson, A.G. and Kokkonen, J. (2001). Acute ballistic muscle stretching inhibits maximal strength performance. *Research Quarterly for Exercise and Sport* 72(4), 415-419.

Pollock, M.L. et al. (1998). The recommended quantity and qual-ity of exercise for developing and maintaining cardiorespira-tory and muscular fitness, and flexibility in healthy adults. *Medicine and Science in Sports and Exercise* 30(6), 975-991.

Sapega, A.A. et al. (1981). Biophysical factors in range-of-motion exercise. *The Physician and Sportsmedicine* 9(12), 57-65.

Shellock, F.G. and Prentice, W.E. (1985). Warming-up and stretching for improved physical performance and prevention of sports-related injuries. *Sports Medicine* 2, 267-278.

Shrier, I. and Gossal, K. (2000). Myths and truths about stretch-ing. Individualized recommendations for healthy muscles. *The Physician and Sportsmedicine* 28(8), 57-63.

Wilson, G.J., Elliot, B.C. and Wood, G.A. (1992). Stretch short-en cycle performance enhancement through flexibility train-ing. *Medicine and Science in Sports and Exercise* 24, 116-123.

Witvrouw, E. et al. (2004). Stretching and injury prevention: An obscure relationship. *Sports Medicine* 34(7), 443-449.

STRETCH MARKS   Striae distensae. Stretch marks are the result of an increased level of circulat-ing glucocorticoids throughout the bloodstream.

This hormone becomes elevated during adolescence, obesity, pregnancy, weight lifting, Cushing's disease and medications (e.g. oral steroids, such as prednisone, used for asthma attacks). Glucocorticoids affect the dermis by preventing the fibroblasts from forming collagen and elastin fibers, which are necessary to keep rapidly growing skin taut. Dermal tearing occurs as the skin is stretched, due to lack of supportive material. The collagen bundles mix with some abnormally thin elastin fiber, but are unable to fully realign themselves correctly. The thinned out skin initially appears red from inflammation, and then dusky purple, but eventually turns white, leaving a mature stretch scar.

Common sites of striae distensae include the abdomen and breasts of pregnant women, and on the shoulders of bodybuilders. In the USA, it occurs in about 90% of pregnant women, 70% of adolescent females and 40% of adolescent males (many of whom participate in sport). It is also a side effect of anabolic steroids.

Tretinoin (Retin-A), a vitamin-A derivative that is applied topically, has been shown to be beneficial in the treatment of early red or pink striae distensae. It is postulated that Retin-A decreases fibroblast proliferation and collagen synthesis. It has been used effectively in the treatment of acne. There has been concern, however, that Retin-A could be a teratogen.

New approaches to improve stretch marks include treatment with a type of infrared laser, which stimulates production of new collagen in depressed stretch marks where a loss of elastic tissue and collagen play an important role. Ultraviolet light technology is used to treat white stretch marks associated with pregnancy or rapid weight fluctuation.

Bibliography

Alaiti, S. and Obagi, Z.E. (2003). Striae distensae. Http://www.emedicine.com
American Society of Dermatologic Surgery. Http://www.asds-net.org

STRETCH REFLEX Myotatic reflex. When a muscle is stretched the muscle spindles are also stretched, which causes nerve impulses to be sent from the spindles to the spinal cord, indicating the stretch. Impulses are then sent from the spinal cord to the muscle, causing a reflex contraction that resists the stretch. An example of the stretch reflex is the **patellar ('knee-jerk') reflex** that that is elicited when the quadriceps tendon is tapped just below the patella with a reflex hammer. This stretches the *quadriceps femoris* (and the muscle spindles within it) and produces a reflex contraction of the *quadriceps femoris* via their alpha motor neurons with the result that the lower leg is extended. Other stretches reflexes include: the Achilles tendon reflex, biceps tendon reflex, posterior tibial reflex and triceps brachii reflex.

The stretch reflex also operates when a person anticipates receiving a weight; the threshold level of the muscle spindle is adjusted so that as soon as any change occurs, a reflex contraction results. (Consider what happens when a person lifts an empty box after thinking that it would be heavy.) The stretch reflex has also been termed **autogenic facilitation**, because it involves the facilitation of the alpha motor neurons of the same muscle.

The information entering the spinal cord via Type I afferent neurons is also sent to the cerebellum and the sensory areas of the cerebral cortex to be used for feedback on muscle length and velocity. In the spinal cord, there are excitatory inter-neuron connections made with the alpha motor neurons of synergist muscles to facilitate their muscle activity along with the agonist. There may also be inhibitory inter-neuron connections that create reciprocal inhibition (relaxation of antagonist muscles).

There is evidence that the stretch reflex has two components, one of which is the result of phasic (ballistic) stretching and the other the result of tonic (static) stretching. The phasic component is well developed in both the flexor and extensor muscles, but the static component is well developed only in the extensor muscles, which are involved in maintenance of posture.

Stretch reflexes appear to be enhanced in sprint athletes, possibly because of increased muscle spindle sensitivity as a result of sprint training.

Bibliography

Ross, A., Leveritt, M. and Riek, S. (2001). Neural influences on sprint training: Training adaptations and acute responses. *Sports Medicine* 31(6), 409-425.

STRETCH-SHORTENING CYCLE   It is an eccentric contraction followed by a concentric contraction of the same muscle group, with a very brief isometric phase in between. If the shortening contraction of the muscle occurs within 0 to 0.9 seconds after the stretch, the stored energy is recovered and used. Holding the stretch for too long before shortening occurs leads to the loss of stored elastic energy through conversion to heat. Research on weightlifting has found that the stretch-shortening cycle can be exploited to enable about 20% greater weight to be lifted than would be possible if a 4-second pause occurred between the eccentric and concentric phases of the bench press. The greater a muscle is pre-stretched from its resting length before shortening occurs, the greater the force the muscle will be able to exert. Pre-stretching involves the stretch reflex as the muscle resists overstretching.

Four mechanisms have been proposed to explain the greater positive work that a muscle can do with a stretch-shorten cycle: time to develop force, elastic energy, force potentiation and reflexes. **Force potentiation** refers to the force from individual cross-bridges being enhanced as a consequence of the preceding stretch, but this effect appears only at relatively long muscle lengths. The relative contribution of each mechanism varies across movements. The rapid stretch-shortening cycle seems to be influenced by the elastic energy mechanism. A countermovement jump can be completely explained by the extra time that muscles have to generate force prior to the beginning of the shortening contraction. Thus, force potentiation seems an unlikely contributor. The role of reflexes is controversial. A stretch-shortening cycle faster than 130 ms does not experience a contribution from the stretch reflex.

Sports skills such as golf and baseball exploit the stretch-shortening cycle. If a strong application of force is desired in a sporting action such as a golf swing, the preparatory movement or backswing should be rapid (to increase the phasic response) and

long (to increase the tonic response). When accuracy is required the backswing should be short and slow, with a pause before the force application. This allows the phasic frequencies of the primary endings of the muscle spindle to slow down to tonic level. *See* PLYOMETRIC TRAINING.

Bibliography
Schmitbleicher, D. (1992). Training for power events. In: Komi, P.V. (ed). *Strength and power in sport.* pp381-395. Oxford: Blackwell Scientific Publishers.

Siff, M.C. (2000). Biomechanical foundations of strength and power training. In Zatsiorsky, V. (ed). *Biomechanics in sport. Performance enhancement and injury prevention. Vol. IX of the Encyclopedia of Sports Medicine.* pp103-139. Oxford: Blackwell Science.

STRIKING   Imparting force to objects in an overarm, sidearm, or underarm pattern. Motor milestones are as follows: faces the object and swings in a vertical plane (2 to 3 years), swings in a horizontal plane and stands to the side of the object (4 to 5 years), and mature striking pattern with body rotation and weight transfer (6 to 7 years).

STROKE   Apoplexy. A type of cardiovascular disease caused by an embolus or thrombus that occludes one or more arteries leading to the brain. A stroke occurs when the blood supply to part of the brain is suddenly interrupted (**ischemic stroke**) or when a blood vessel in the brain bursts, spilling blood into the spaces surrounding the brain cells (**hemorrhagic stroke**). Ischemic strokes are associated with coronary heart disease. 70 to 80% of strokes are ischemic. Hemorrhagic strokes are linked with high blood pressure, weak or malformed arteries and veins within the brain, and leukemia.

Symptoms of stroke include: numbness or weakness in the face, arm or leg, especially to one side of the body; dizziness; visual difficulty; and speech difficulty. **Cerebrovascular accident** is a general term used to describe cerebrovascular symptoms and neurological impairment caused by an ischemic or hemorrhagic lesion. If the stroke occurs in the right-hemisphere of the brain, the left side of the body (and the right side of the face) will be affected, producing some or all of the following: paralysis on the left side of the body; vision problems; memory loss; and a behavioral style that is quick and inquisitive. If the stroke occurs in the left-hemisphere of the brain, the right side of the body (and the left side of the face) will be affected, producing some or all of the following: paralysis on the right side of the body; speech and language problems; memory loss; and a behavioral style that is slow and cautious.

Stroke is the third leading killer of Americans and more than 2 million individuals in the USA are coping with the residual effects of stroke. Recovery of muscle function, including speech, can progress for several months or stop abruptly, leaving the individual permanently disabled. Typically, muscle function gradually progresses from hypotonus to spasticity to synergies, before voluntary movement is restored. During the spasticity stage, contractures must be prevented by daily range of motion exercises. The synergies are similar in function to primitive reflexes. Most people with complete stroke have difficulty with both sitting and standing balance, and postural reflexes must be relearned.

After the age of 55 years, the risk of having a stroke more than doubles for each decade of life. The incidence and prevalence of stroke are about equal in men and women. However, at all ages, more women than men die of stroke. The chance of stroke is greater in people who have a family history of stroke. African Americans have a much higher risk of disability and death from a stroke than Caucasians, in part due to greater incidence of high blood pressure, a major risk factor for stroke in African Americans. The risk of stroke is greater for a person who has already had one. High blood pressure and cigarette smoking are important risk factors for stroke. Diabetes mellitus is an independent risk factor for stroke and is strongly correlated with high blood pressure. Individuals with diabetes often also have high cholesterol and are overweight, increasing their risk even more. High hematocrit is a risk factor for stroke, because more red blood cells thicken the blood and make clots more likely. Other risk factors include carotid artery disease, atrial fibrillation and transient ischemic attack.

Stroke in sport is rare, but most cases involve external trauma or excessive head rotation, flexion or extension with resulting dissection of a major extracranial vessel. Ischemic symptoms usually occur within the next few days, but may be delayed by up to a month. Arterial dissections, often spontaneous, may be related to a history of trauma to the neck. The largest report of carotid arterial dissection with stroke in sport was of 10 cases that occurred while skiing.

Transient ischemic attack is an incomplete stroke that involves a temporary disruption of blood flow to the brain. Symptoms of a transient ischemic attack usually occur suddenly and are similar to those of stroke, but do not last as long. Most symptoms disappear within an hour, but they may persist for up to 24 hours. Often, transient ischemic attacks are warnings of severe cerebral pathology and impending major strokes.

Childhood stroke must not be confused with cerebral palsy. The major difference is that stroke is followed by gradual improvement, whereas cerebral palsy is nonprogressive.

Bibliography

American Stroke Association. Http://strokeassociation.org
MacGowan, D. and Caronna, J.J. (1998). Stroke in sport. In Jordan, B., Tsairis, P. and Warren, R.F. (eds). *Sports neurology*. 2nd ed. pp289-299. Philadelphia, PA: Lippincott-Raven.
Noelle, B. et al. (1994). Cervicocephalic arterial dissections related to skiing. *Stroke* 24, 526-527.

STROKE VOLUME The volume of blood ejected into the main artery by each ventricular beat. Stroke volume increases with exercise intensity, reaching a plateau at about 50% of maximal oxygen uptake. During maximal exercise, it may increase 1.5 times from its resting value. *See* CARDIAC OUTPUT.

STROMA *See under* BREAST; CONNECTIVE TISSUE.

STRUCTURE A physical entity of a definite size and shape that usually carries a load, transmits motion or secures other structures in a position. It may comprise a single material or composites of different materials. A **homogenous material** has a uniform distribution of the material constituents. An **isotropic material** has uniform mechanical properties in all directions. *See also* BENDING.

Bibliography

Gordon, J.E. (1978). *Structures or why things don't fall down.* London: Penguin.

STRYCHNINE   A poisonous alkaloid that was discovered in St. Ignatius' beans (*Strychnos Ignatii*); it also occurs in other species of *Sir ychnos* (e.g. *Nux vomica*). It is used primarily as a pesticide, especially to kill rats. It acts on the nervous system by antagonizing the action of glycine, an amino acid responsible for transmitting inhibitory nerve impulses that control muscle contraction. It may also increase brain levels of glutamic acid, an amino acid that acts as a transmitter for excitatory nerve impulses that excite muscle control. Skeletal muscles become hyperexcitable and prone to convulsions. High doses of strychnine may lead to respiratory failure and death. In human medicine, it is used as a heart stimulant. Most of the drugs used in the early modern Olympics were a mixture of strychnine and alcohol.

Chronology

•1903 • Harry Andrews, trainer to Alfred Shrubb (the greatest distance runner in the world at that time), published his training manual. Andrews discussed ergogenic aids: "Strychnine in lozenge form is ... used. I tried this once on a man during a bad time, and it had no effect at all. So I reverted to hot beef tea, and got my man home all right." The training manual was endorsed by Oxo, the food company that made the beverage.

•1904 • At the Olympic Games in St. Louis, the winner of the marathon, Thomas Hicks of the USA, collapsed after finishing. He had been given repeated doses of strychnine and brandy during the race.

•1917 • An advert designed to look like a regular newspaper article showed baseball batter great Ty Cobb attributing a successful comeback to Nuxated iron, a combination of *Nux vomica* and iron. It promised health, strength and even greatness: "Greatest baseball batter of all time says Nuxated iron filled him with renewed life after he was weakened and all run down…"

•1989 • In testifying before the Dublin Commission, Robert Kerr confessed his knowledge that athletes in strength events from Eastern-block countries were using small amounts of strychnine as a stimulant 30 to 60 minutes before competition.

Bibliography

Green, J. (1986). *Fit for America. Health, fitness, sport and American society.* New York: Pantheon Books.

Todd, J. and Todd, T. (2001). Significant events in the history of drug testing and the Olympic movement 1960-1999. In: Wilson, W. and Derse, E. (eds). *Doping in elite sport. The politics of drugs in the Olympic movement.* pp65-128. Champaign, IL: Human Kinetics.

STUDENT'S ELBOW   *See* OLECRANON BURSITIS.

STURGE-WEBER DISEASE   Sturge-Weber-Dimitric syndrome. It is a rare disease characterized by multiple vascular lesions (angiomas) involving the skin of the face, mucus membranes, and meninges. It is characterized by port-wine stains on the face. **Port-wine stains** are the most common kind of abnormality of blood vessel development and involve dilated capillaries in the skin. 1 in 200 persons are born with a port-wine stain in the USA. Sturge-Weber syndrome occurs in 8% to 15% of live births with an associated port-wine stain. Infants with Sturge-Weber syndrome are at increased risk of developing epilepsy, developmental delays, mental retardation, hemiparesis and vision loss. The cause is unknown and neither a hereditary component nor specific risk factors have been recognized.

Bibliography

Sturge-Weber Foundation. Http://www.sturge-weber.com

STY   An infection of the sebaceous gland of an eyelash or eyelash follicle.

STYLION   An anatomical landmark that is the most distal point of the styloid process of the radius. *See under* ANATOMICAL SNUFF BOX.

SUBCLAVIAN VEIN   Axillary vein. *See under* EFFORT THROMBOSIS.

SUBCLINICAL DISEASE   A disease or disorder that is present, but not severe enough to produce symptoms that can be detected or diagnosed.

SUBCORTICAL   *See under* BRAIN.

SUBCULTURE   A subsystem of a larger culture, characterized by a distinguishing pattern of values.

The term subculture has been applied to particular sport or leisure activities. It has also been applied to activities on the basis of age, gender, social class, occupation, geographical region and ethnicity. To understand sport in social and cultural terms, it is necessary to consider the effects of individuals belonging to several subcultures at the same time. The relationship of a subculture to its 'parent' culture(s) must also be understood.

A distinction can be made between group culture and subculture. A **group culture** has a set of values that is confined to a small group, linked by informal means of communication, whereas a subculture has a set of values that spreads to other groups by more formal means of communication.

Rugby, triathlon and windsurfing are among the sporting subcultures that have been investigated by sociologists. With regard to the behavior of rugby players in both the UK and North America, what may appear to be spontaneous deviance is actually highly ritualized and internally policed behavior. The attractiveness of triathlon to the educated middle class in the 1980s was related to the centrality of personal challenge and personal control in the sport. It provided a contrast to the lack of perceived challenge and personal control in their occupational life.

In contemporary Western society, consumption, lifestyles and identity are profoundly linked. People manipulate or manage appearances, and thereby create and sustain an identity. The adoption of subcultural identity is a way of asserting cultural identity and a sense of community in a society, fragmented by divisions of class, race and gender; i.e. it gives people a sense of belonging. In the emergence of new, individualized forms of extreme sports, such as windsurfing, in-line skating, mountain biking and snowboarding, consumers seek a particular and desirable lifestyle. These activities are perceived as being 'cool' and go hand-in-hand with fashion and music. Wheaton and Tomlinson (1998) identify the core principles of windsurfing's culture, the gender identities most prevalent within it, and the tension between the dominant masculinity and the potentially empowering dimensions of the activity for women. Commitment, not the conspicuous display

of equipment or subcultural style, is central to the meanings the windsurfers in the UK give to their participation and subcultural identity.

Boyd (2003) discusses the intertwining of hip-hop culture and basketball in the USA, with respect to race, class and identity.

Bibliography

Boyd, T. (2003). *Young, Black, rich and famous. The rise of the NBA, the Hip Hop invasion and the transformation of American culture*. New York: Doubleday.

Cashmore, E. (2000). *Sports culture: An A-Z guide*. London: Routledge.

Coakley, J. and Donnelly, P. (1999). *Inside sports*. London: Routledge.

Crosset, T. and Beal, B. (1997). The use of 'subculture' and 'sub-world' in ethnographic works on sport: A discussion of definitional distinctions. *Sociology of Sport Journal* 14(1), 73-85.

Hilliard, D.C. (1988). Finishers, competitors and pros: A description and speculative interpretation of the triathlon scene. *Play and Culture* 1(4), 300-313.

Wheaton, B. (2000). 'Just do it:' Consumption, commitment, and identity in the windsurfing subculture. *Sociology of Sport Journal* 17(3), 254-274.

Wheaton, B. and Tomlinson, A. (1998). The changing gender order in sport? The case of windsurfing subcultures. *Journal of Sport and Social Issues* 22(3), 252-274.

Young, K. (1988). Performance, control, and public image of behavior in a deviant subculture: The case of rugby. *Deviant Behavior* 9(3), 275-293.

SUBDURAL HEMATOMA *See under* HEAD INJURIES.

SUBHYALOID Situated under the hyaloid membrane. It is a transparent membrane that envelopes the vitreous humor of the eye and separates it from the retina.

SUBSTANCE ABUSE A maladaptive pattern of substance use, leading to clinically significant impairment or distress, as manifested by one or more of the following, within a 12-month period: recurrent substance use resulting in a failure to fulfill major role obligations at work, school, or home; recurrent substance use in situations in which it is physically hazardous; recurrent substance-related legal problems; continued substance use despite having persistent or recurrent social or interpersonal problems caused by or exacerbated by the effects of the substance; and the symptoms have never met the criteria for substance dependence for this class of substance.

Bibliography

American Psychiatric Association (1994). *Diagnostic and statistical manual of mental disorders.* 4th ed. Washington, DC: American Psychiatric Association.

SUBSTANCE P   A neurotransmitter distributed widely in the central nervous system.

SUBSTANCE-RELATED DISORDERS   A maladaptive pattern of substance use, leading to clinically significant impairment or distress, as manifested by three or more of the following within the same 12-month period: tolerance; withdrawal; substance taken in larger amounts or over a longer period of time than intended; persistent desire or unsuccessful efforts to cut down or control use; great amount of time is spent in activities necessary to obtain the substance or recover from its effects; important social, occupational, or recreational activities are given up or decreased, because of use; and the substance use is continued despite knowledge of having a persistent or recurrent physical or psychological problem that is likely to have been caused or exacerbated by the substance.

There does not appear to be a superior treatment method, but social support is very important.

Bibliography

American Psychiatric Association (1994). *Diagnostic and statistical manual of mental disorders.* 4th ed. Washington, DC: American Psychiatric Association.

SUBSTRATE   A specific chemical compound acted upon by an enzyme in a metabolic reaction. Carbohydrates, fats, proteins and alcohol are substrates in energy metabolism.

See ENERGY SUBSTRATE UTILIZATION; PHOSPHORYLATION.

SUBSTRATE-LEVEL   PHOSPHORYLATION *See under* PHOSPHORYLATION.

SUBTALAR JOINT   A joint formed by three artic-

ulations between the inferior surface of the talus with the superior surface of the calcaneus. These articulations are referred to as posterior, middle and anterior facets. The upper surface of the calcaneus has three smooth facets (posterior, middle and anterior), which articulate with corresponding facets on the lower surface of the talus to form the subtalar joint. The anterior and middle facets are located on the medial side and are usually continuous with each other. The middle and posterior facets are separated from each other by a deep groove that, together with a corresponding groove on the talus, forms a channel between the two bones (i.e. the **sinus tarsi**). The **posterior facet** is the largest and is formed by a concave facet on the undersurface of the talus and a convex facet on the body of the calcaneus. The **anterior facet** and **middle facet** are smaller and are formed by two convex facets on the inferior body of the talus and two concave facets on the calcaneus.

The supporting connective tissues can be categorized as superficial, intermediate and deep layers. The **superficial layer** includes the lateral, posterior and medial talo-calcaneal ligaments, as well as the lateral root of the inferior extensor retinaculum and the calcaneo-fibular ligament, which is immediately posterior to the lateral talocalcaneal ligament. The **intermediate layer** consists of the intermediate root of the inferior extensor retinaculum and the cervical ligament, which limits inversion. The **deep layer** consists of the medial root of the inferior extensor retinaculum and the interosseus talo-calcaneal ligament inside the tarsal canal. This ligament prevents eversion, valgus of the heel and depression of the longitudinal arch of the foot. The subtalar joint is covered by a thin capsule and does not communicate with other joints. The subtalar joint is very stable and rarely dislocates.

Functionally, the subtalar joint includes the talocalcaneal part of the talocalcaneonavicular joint. In conjunction with the midtarsal joint, the subtalar joint is responsible for transforming tibial rotation into forefoot supination and pronation. Rotation about the subtalar joint axis includes inversion/eversion (transverse plane), but also dorsal/plantar flexion (sagittal plane) and abduction/adduction (frontal plane). The normal axis is positioned 42 degrees from the transverse plane, 16 degrees from the sagittal plane and 45 degrees from the frontal plane. Triplanar motions of supination and pronation are clinically referred to as subtalar inversion and eversion. Average subtalar motion is 20 to 30 degrees of inversion and 5 to 10 degrees of eversion. Ankle dorsal flexion and tibial internal rotation are associated with subtalar eversion (pronation). Ankle plantar flexion and tibial external rotation are associated with subtalar inversion (supination). *In vivo*, it is difficult to distinguish between rotations about the ankle and subtalar joints.

The subtalar joint is the key to the biomechanics of the foot and ankle. It must evert at heel strike to unlock the foot/ankle complex, making it sufficiently flexible to absorb energy. It must invert at toe-off to lock the joints for rigidity and efficient transfer of energy from the Achilles tendon through the ankle and forefoot.

Four types of subtalar injuries can be distinguished according to the injury mechanism and the ligamentous damage. In type 1 injuries, a forceful supination of the hindfoot is associated with either a plantar flexion or dorsal flexion of the ankle. With the plantar-flexed ankle, the anterior talofibular ligament, and possibly the cervical ligament, is torn first, followed by disruption of the calcaneofibular ligament and the lateral capsule. In type 2 injuries, rupture of the interosseus talocalcaneal ligament also occurs. With the ankle in dorsal flexion, type 3 injuries can be sustained with severe soft tissue lesions in combination with rupture of the calcaneofibular ligament, cervical ligament and the interosseus talocalcaneal ligament. The anterior talofibular ligament remains intact and is not injured as it is without tension in that position. Type 4 injuries are a combination of severe talotibial and subtalar ligament injuries. This injury is produced by forceful supination of the hindfoot while the ankle is primarily in dorsal flexion, but subsequently rotates into plantar flexion. In triple jump and basketball, the abrupt impact and deceleration of the calcaneus with the inertial progression of movement of the talus may cause injury to the interosseus talo-calcaneal ligament. *See also* FOOT; MIDTARSAL JOINT.

Bibliography
Karlsson, J., Eriksson, B.I. and Renström, P.A. (1997). Subtalar ankle instability. A review. *Sports Medicine* 24(5), 337-346.

SUBUNGUAL HEMATOMA   *See under* TOE NAILS.

SUCCINATE   An intermediate in the Krebs cycle synthesized from succinyl CoA.

SUCCINYL COA   An intermediate in the Krebs cycle synthesized from alpha ketoglutarate.

SUCROSE   A disaccharide composed of glucose and fructose. The common name is table sugar.

SUDDEN DEATH   Sudden cardiac death. Non-traumatic, non-violent, unexpected death due to cardiac causes within one hour of the onset of symptoms (witnessed event) or within 6 hours of witnessed normal state of health (unwitnessed event). Sport-related deaths are defined as those with symptoms occurring within one hour of sports participation.

Sudden death can be classified as certain, probable or presumptive. **Certain sudden death** is marked by obvious anatomical evidence at autopsy, such as myocardial infarction or ruptured aorta. **Probable sudden death** occurs when there is left ventricular hypertrophy without definite criteria for hypertrophic cardiomyopathy. **Presumptive sudden death** is due to mitral valve prolapse.

The major mechanisms involved in exercise-related sudden death are related to hemodynamic and electrophysiological changes brought about by exercise in the susceptible individual. Fatal arrhythmia seems to be the most common mechanism of death. Between 1 and 5 cases of sudden death per million athletes occur annually.

In young athletes (under 35 years old), the majority of these cases are caused by defined and hereditary cardiovascular disorders. **Hypertrophic cardiomyopathy** is the single most common cardiovascular cause of sudden death in young athletes in the USA.

Maron et al. (1996) analyzed a total of 158

sudden deaths that occurred in trained athletes throughout the USA from 1985 to 1995. Of the 158 sudden deaths among athletes, 24 (15%) were explained by noncardiovascular causes. Among the 134 athletes who had cardiovascular causes of sudden death, the median age was 17 years (range, 12 to 40 years); 120 (90%) were male; 70 (52%) were White and 59 (44%) were Black. The most common sports involved were basketball (47 cases) and football (45 cases), together accounting for 68% of sudden deaths. A total of 121 athletes collapsed during or immediately after a training session (78 cases) or a formal athletic contest (43 cases). The most common structural cardiovascular diseases identified at autopsy as the primary cause of death were hypertrophic cardiomyopathy (48 athletes, 36%), which was disproportionately prevalent in Black athletes compared with White athletes (48% vs. 26% of deaths).

Hypertrophic cardiomyopathy has a prevalence of 1 per 500 in the general population of the USA and is higher in African Americans. It is inherited as an autosomal dominant trait. Research has revealed more than 100 mutations in genes encoding proteins for the cardiac sarcomere that result in hypertrophic cardiomyopathy. It is characterized by asymmetric left ventricular hypertrophy (usually involving the ventricular septum), left ventricular wall thickness of 16 mm or more, a ratio between the septum and free wall of more than 1.3, and a nondilated left ventricle. Symptoms, which may or may not be present, include: dyspnea, angina, light-headedness and syncope during exertion. Most athletes with hypertrophic cardiomyopathy remain asymptomatic until the time of death.

It is difficult to differentiate hypertrophic cardiomyopathy from athlete's heart. Keys to the differential diagnosis include: evidence of heterogeneous left ventricle hypertrophy; left atrial enlargement; unusual ECG patterns; and family history of gene mutations. The most definitive evidence for the presence of hypertrophic cardiomyopathy in an athlete with increased wall thickness comes from the demonstration of the disease in a relative. Children with genetic forms of hypertrophic cardiomyopathy usually show little or no left ventricular wall thickening before the age of 14 years. However, abrupt and marked increases in wall thickness may occur before the age of 18 years, coinciding with growth and maturation.

Maron (2002) documents the case of a male 17 year-old player who stumbled off the court during a high-school basketball game and collapsed. He was found to be pulseless and apneic. Cardiopulmonary resuscitation (CPR) was initiated immediately by the boy's father (a cardiovascular surgeon) for about 5 minutes. Ventricular fibrillation was documented, and external defibrillation, performed three times, ultimately restored his sinus rhythm. An echocardiogram performed the following day showed a markedly increased left ventricular wall thickness compared with normal values 27 months earlier, anterior ventricular septum of 25 mm, posterior septum of 21 mm and posterobasal left ventricular free wall of 23 mm. The patient recovered completely without neurologic impairment. An implantable cardioverter-defibrillator was placed for prevention of sudden death.

Patients with hypertrophic cardiomyopathy judged to be at high risk should be considered for an **implantable cardioverter-defibrillator**, which shocks the heart to normalize an irregular heart beat, such as ventricular tachycardia or fibrillation, if the heart's own electrical signals become disordered. These devices are now the size of a matchbox and sited just below the collarbone so that they can easily be accessed and adjusted. An implanted defibrillator is only appropriate for hypertrophic cardiomyopathy patients at high risk of death.

Athletes with unequivocal hypertrophic cardiomyopathy should not participate in competitive sports, except perhaps some low-intensity ones. This recommendation includes those athletes with or without symptoms, and with or without left ventricular outflow obstruction.

Idiopathic left ventricular hypertrophy is another cause of sudden death in young athletes and accounts for about 10% of cases. It is marked by an unexplained increase in cardiac mass that exceeds that limits of physiologic hypertrophy in athlete's heart. The increase in cardiac mass does not meet criteria for hypertrophic cardiomyopathy, because the hypertrophy is symmetric (concentric) and histologic examination does not show the cellular disarray characteristic of hypertrophic cardiomyopathy. It is not known whether idiopathic left ventricular hypertrophy is a separate disease or whether it may be a variant of hypertrophic cardiomyopathy.

Bibliography

Futterman, L.G. and Myerburg, R. (1998). Sudden death in athletes. An update. *Sports Medicine* 26(5), 335-350.

Maron, B.J. (2002). Hypertrophic cardiomyopathy. Practical steps for preventing sudden death. *The Physician and Sports Medicine* 30(1), 19-24.

Maron, B.J. (1993). Sudden death in young athletes: Lesson from the Hank Gathers affair. *New England Journal of Medicine* 329, 55-57.

Maron, B.J., Isner, J.M. and McKenna, W.J. (1994). 26th Bethesda Conference: Recommendations for determining eligibility for competition in athletes with cardiovascular abnormalities: Task Force 3: Hypertrophic cardiomyopathy, myocarditis and other myopericardial diseases and mitral valve prolapse. *Journal of the American College of Cardiology* 24(4), 880-885.

Maron, B.J. et al. (1996). Sudden death in young competitive athletes: Clinical, demographic, and pathological profiles. *Journal of the American Medical Association* 276(3), 199-204.

Maron, BJ. et al. (2000). Efficacy of implantable cardioverter-defibrillators for the prevention of sudden death in patients with hypertrophic cardiomyopathy. *New England Journal of Medicine* 342(6), 365-373.

Perrault, H. and Turcotte, R.A. (1994). Exercise-induced cardiac hypertrophy. Fact or fallacy? *Sports Medicine* 17(5), 288-308.

Van Camp, S.P. (1993). What we can learn from Reggie Lewis' death? *The Physician and Sportsmedicine* 21(10), 73-80.

SUICIDE The act of killing oneself intentionally. In the USA, there are approximately 30,000 suicides each year. 12 out of every 100,000 Americans kill themselves. Suicide is the eighth leading cause of death in the USA, and the third leading cause of death in 15 to 24 year-olds. Rates of suicide are highest, however, among the elderly (age 65 and over). White men who are 85 years of age and older have a suicide rate that is six times that of the overall national rate. It has been estimated that there may be 8 to 25 attempted suicides per one suicide death. About 2 million Americans have made one or more attempts at suicide. More than four times as many men as women die by suicide, but women attempt suicide more often during their lives than men. Firearms are the most commonly used method of suicide for men and women, accounting for 60% of suicides. 80% of all suicides involving firearms are committed by Caucasian males.

Between 40 and 60% of those who die by suicide are intoxicated with alcohol at the time of death. An estimated 1 to 6% of individuals with alcohol dependency will die by suicide. At the time of death, 50 to 75% of alcohol dependent individuals, who commit suicide, are suffering from depression.

Psychological autopsy studies show that more than 90% of completed suicides had one or more mental disorders. It is estimated that 60% of people who commit suicide have had a mood disorder. An estimated 2 to 15% of individuals who have been diagnosed with major depression die by suicide. Depression and suicidal behavior have both been linked to decreased serotonin in the brain. Suicide risk is greatest in depressed individuals who feel hopeless about the future, those who have just been discharged from the hospital, those who have a family history of suicide, and those who have made a suicide attempt in the past. It is estimated that 3 to 20% of persons who have been diagnosed with bipolar disorder die by suicide.

Impulsiveness – the tendency to act without thinking through a plan or its consequences – has been linked to suicidal behavior, usually through its association with mental disorders and/or substance abuse. The mental disorders with impulsiveness most linked to suicide include: borderline personality disorder among young females; conduct disorder among young males and anti-social behavior in adult males; and alcohol and substance abuse among young and middle-aged males.

As of July 2000, 6 out of 339 (1.77%) England cricketers had taken their own lives. Among Australian, New Zealand and South African cricketers, the rates are 5 out of 182 (2.75%), 2 out of 52 (3.92%) and 7 out of 170 (4.12%), respectively. These rates are above national average in each country. Frith (2001) documents the suicides of 152 former first-class cricketers and explains their suicides in terms of stress, especially the uncertainty on a day-to-day basis. According to Frith, loss of cricket contributed substantially to the death of former professional cricketers: "facing life without the familiar routine and the benefits and, most of all, the camaraderie, the fellowship."

Seven times as many major league baseball players committed suicide during the first 75 years of the National League as American males from the general population.

Glick and Horsfall (2001) document the case of a basketball player who spent 13 years playing in the National Basketball Association (NBA). The player had a history of lowered mood or depression since his teens for which he had never sought treatment. Throughout his career he used alcohol, but never to excess, as a way of coping with lowered mood. On being released by his team, he felt that his life had no future. He drank steadily for several months and refused therapy or help from former players. He died of a self-inflicted gunshot wound within a year of his release.

Bibliography

American Association of Suicidology. Http://www.suicidology.org

American Foundation for Suicide Prevention. Http://www.afsp.org

Aronson, S.C. (2004). Major Depressive Disorder. Http://www.emedicine.com

Frith, D. (2001). Silence of the heart: Cricket suicides. Edinburgh, UK: Mainstream Publishing.

Glick, J.I.D. and Horsfall, J.L. (2001). Psychiatric conditions in sports. Diagnosis, treatment and quality of life. The Physician and Sportsmedicine 29(8).

National Institute of Mental Health. Http://nimh.nih.gov

National Strategy for Suicide Prevention. Http://www.mental-health.org/suicideprevention

Suicide Prevention Action Network USA. Http://www.spanusa.org

Zoss, J. (1996). Diamonds in the rough: The untold history of baseball. Chicago: Contemporary Books.

SULCUS   A shallow impression or groove.

SULFUR   Sulphur. A non-metallic element that as a mineral in the human body is present in all cells, especially in cartilage and keratin of skin and hair.

SULFUR DIOXIDE   Sulphur dioxide. *See under* AIR POLLUTION.

SUMMATION OF VELOCITY PRINCIPLE   The velocity of the distal end of a linked system is built up by summing the individual velocities of all the segments involved in the sequence. This coordination occurs so that the movement of one segment begins as the velocity of the previous (larger) segment has reached its maximum.

Bibliography

Bunn, J.W. (1972). The scientific principles of coaching. 2nd ed. Englewood Cliffs, NJ: Prentice Hall.

SUPEROXIDE DISMUTASE   *See under* FREE RADICALS.

SUPERSTITION   *See under* OPERANT CONDITIONING; RITUALS.

SUPRASCAPULAR NERVE   The suprascapular nerve innervates the supraspinatus, infraspinatus and glenohumeral joint capsule. During overhead motions such as spiking in volleyball, the suprascapular nerve and its adjoining arteries are subjected to rapid stretching.

SUPRASTERNALE   An anatomical landmark that is located as the superior border of the sternal notch (or incisura jugularis) in the midsagittal plane.

SURAL NERVE   A nerve that lies within the superficial posterior compartment and increased pressures may cause numbness over the lateral aspect of the leg and foot. Uncommonly, sural nerve entrapment is found in patients who have exercise-induced leg pain.

SURFACE TENSION   It relates to a resisting force created at the surface of a liquid in contact with a gas, structure or another liquid. The greater the surface tension surrounding a spherical object, such as an alveolus, the greater the force required to overcome the pressure within the sphere and cause it to enlarge.

SURFACTANT   A lipoprotein mixture of phospholipids, proteins and calcium ions produced by alveolar epithelial cells. It mixes with the fluid that encircles the alveolar chamber. Its action interrupts the surrounding water layer to decrease the alveolar membrane's surface tension. This effect greatly decreases the energy required for alveolar inflation and deflation.

SURVIVAL BEHAVIOR   *See under* MOTIVATION.

SWAYBACK See LORDOSIS.

SWEAT *See under* THERMOREGULATION.

SWEET SPOT With a tennis racket, the sweet spot can be defined as a combination of the node of the first harmonic, center of percussion and maximum coefficient of restitution. The **center of percussion** is where the initial shock to the player's hand is at a minimum. In the original wooden rackets, center of percussion was near the throat. In a modern racket, it is much closer to the center of the head. The **node of the first harmonic** is the minimum amount of uncomfortable vibration that the player feels in her hand and arm. The **maximum coefficient of restitution** is where the ball rebounds from the strings with maximum speed (or power). In general, these three points are found at separate locations on the face of the racket.

Bibliography
Brody, H. (1987). *Tennis science for tennis players*. Philadelphia: University of Pennsylvania Press.

SWIMMER'S EAR Otitis externa. It is a bacterial or fungal infection involving the lining of the external auditory canal. It is most often caused by either *Pseunomas aeroginosa* or *Staphylococcus aureus*. The external auditory canal contains cerumen (wax), which is hydrophobic to repel water from the walls of the canal and acidic to create an inhospitable environment for bacterial growth. If the cerumen is washed out of the external auditory canal, the skin lining can become macerated (softened) by moisture, and the pH level can increase. Other factors that contribute to infection include excessive

cleaning of the external auditory canal, narrow ear channels and, possibly, eustachian tube dysfunction. Swimming caps, drying drops before and after swimming, water-impermeable earplugs, and blow-drying the external auditory canal after swimming may be helpful in preventing swimmer's ear.

Bibliography
Levy, J.A. (2004). Common bacterial dermatoses. *The Physician and Sportsmedicine* 32(6). Http://www.physsportsmed.com

SWIMMER'S SHOULDER It is a partial rotator cuff tear associated with repetitive swimming or throwing activities. In swimming, especially the butterfly, the blood supply to the tendon of the *supraspinatus* muscle may be disturbed due to excessive rotation of the arm about the shoulder joint. This can result in a localized area of necrosis in the supraspinatus tendon that, in turn, can lead to edema and an inflammatory reaction. Most cases of swimmer's shoulder are due to impingement of the rotator cuff, the biceps tendon, bursae and other soft tissue structures of the subacromial space. The mechanism of injury is excessive translation of the humeral head, secondary to loss of dynamic stability of the glenohumeral joint. Anterior subluxation of the glenohumeral joint may result from repeated use of the backstroke.

Technique modifications to prevent swimmer's shoulder on the front crawl include a high-elbow position on the recovery that is achieved by rotating the body about its long axis by at least 45 degrees in each direction, with the head kept in a neutral position on the spine. During the entry- and catch-phases of the stroke, the hand should be kept in front and at a position just outside the line of the shoulder. Asymmetric body roll or unilateral breathing may increase impingement by causing a compensatory crossover pull-through on the side with less roll on the non-breathing side. Swimmers with painful shoulders tend to have weakness in the *serratus anterior* and increased activity of the *rhomboids* during the pull. This gives rise to a mechanical imbalance that increases anterior impingement of the biceps and supraspinatus tendons. Lack of shoulder flexibility for internal rotation and horizontal adduction are further risk factors for anterior impingement. *See also* BREAST-STROKER'S KNEE.

Bibliography

Johnson, J.N., Gauvin, J. and Fredericson, M. (2003). Swimming biomechanics and injury prevention. New stroke techniques and medical considerations. *The Physician and Sportsmedicine* 31(1), 41-48.

Kammer, C.S.K., Young, C.C., and Niedfeldt, M.W. (1999). Swimming injuries and illnesses. *The Physician and Sportsmedicine* 27(4), 51-60.

SWIMMING REFLEX   A primitive reflex in which swimming-like movements can be elicited. The reflex is elicited by holding the infant over a solid surface or the surface of water (or even in water), causing coordinated, rhythmical, swimming-type movements of the arms and legs. A breath-holding reflex is elicited when the infant's face is placed in the water; swimming movements are more pronounced from this position. The swimming reflex operates from the 2 weeks after birth through the 5th month. *See* INFANT SWIM PROGRAMS.

SWISS BALL   Pezzi ball. Stability ball. A training tool, used widely in physical therapy, to promote neuromuscular and proprioceptive development and to develop muscular control, especially of lumbopelvic rhythm.

SYMMETRICAL TONIC NECK REFLEX   A reflex that is not present at birth, but which develops between 4 to 6 months of age and persists until 10 to 12 months. It may be elicited by extension or flexion of the head and neck from a supported sitting position. If the head and neck are extended, the arms extend and the legs flex. If the head and neck are flexed, the arms flex and the legs extend. Like the asymmetrical tonic neck reflex, the symmetrical tonic neck reflex does not occur each time the infant's head is extended or flexed. The symmetrical tonic neck reflex contributes to motor milestones, such as lifting and supporting the upper body on the arms and rising to a four-point creeping position.

Failure of this reflex to become integrated causes a number of problems, including difficulty in maintaining a 'tuck position' as the head changes position from flexion to extension in exercises that require the head to be held down in a tucked position at the same time as the knees are tucked in to the chest. There is difficulty in creeping on the hands and knees. The symmetrical tonic neck reflex also interferes with using the hands when the head position changes.

In 75% of children with learning disabilities there is retention of the symmetrical tonic neck reflex.

SYMPATHETIC-ADRENAL-MEDULLARY AXIS   *See under* HORMONES.

SYMPATHETIC NERVOUS SYSTEM   *See under* AUTONOMIC NERVOUS SYSTEM.

SYMPATHETIC TONE   A state of partial vasoconstriction of blood vessels maintained by impulses from nerve fibers of the sympathetic branch of the autonomic nervous system.

SYMPHYSION   An anatomical landmark that forms the superior border of the pubic symphysis at the mid-sagittal plane.

SYNAPSES   *See under* AUTONOMIC NERVOUS SYSTEM.

SYNCOPE   The sudden loss of postural tone and consciousness with subsequent spontaneous recovery. It frequently occurs because of a transient decrease in blood flow to the brain, usually for more than 8 to 10 seconds. It is usually benign, but in some cases it can be life threatening.

Cardiac syncope includes mechanical (e.g. valvular obstruction), electrical (e.g. arrhythmias), neurally mediated (vasovagal) and orthostatic causes. **Noncardiac syncope** is much less common and includes decreased intravascular volume (e.g. from heat exhaustion), metabolic conditions (e.g. hypoglycemia), Valsalva's maneuver, drugs (e.g. stimulants) and intracranial conditions (e.g. head injuries).

The least-serious cause of syncope, **vasovagal reaction**, results from venous dilation and increased vagal tone with ensuing bradycardia. The enhanced tone of the vagus nerve in endurance athletes probably explains why they are more susceptible to exercise-induced vasovagal syncope than non-athletes. Vasovagal or unknown etiologies account for 75% of all syncopal episodes. Such episodes typically occur while the victim sits or stands, following an unpleasant or anxiety-provoking event. Light-headedness, dizziness, profuse sweating and nausea may be experienced. Consciousness is regained rapidly after the victim lies down.

See under POSTURE.

Bibliography
Hargarten, K.M. (1992). Syncope. Finding the cause in active people. *The Physician and Sportsmedicine* 20(5), 179-186.
Wang, D., Sakaguchi, S. and Babcock, M. (1997). Exercise-induced vasovagal syncope: Limiting the risks. *The Physician and Sportsmedicine* 25(5), 64-74.

SYNDACTYLISM It is webbing or fusion of two or more digits on the foot due to failure of early interdigital tissue to degenerate. It is often inherited as an autosomal dominant trait. Webbing of toes is usually corrected surgically, and extra toes may be removed to facilitate purchase of shoes. The most debilitating defect is absence of the big toe, which plays a major role in static balance and in the push-off phase of locomotor activities. However, a child with good coordination can overcome syndactylism and achieve athletic success.

SYNDESMOSIS A form of articulation in which the bony surfaces are united by an interosseous ligament. *See* ANKLE JOINT.

SYNDROME A combination of signs and symptoms that characterize an abnormal condition, and that appear together with sufficient regularity to warrant designation by a special name.

SYNERGIST *See under* MUSCLE ACTION.

SYNOSTOSIS The joining of two or more bones to form one bone. It is an important indicator of age. A synostosis can form where ligaments closely approximate two bones, and the ligament calcifies to form a bony joint. Examples of synostoses are: radioulnar synostosis and craniosynostosis.

SYNOVIAL FLUID *See under* JOINT.

SYNOVIAL INJURY Synovitis, peritenonitis or bursitis. The pathophysiology of the synovial membrane is inflammatory dominant.

SYNOVIAL LIPOMASTOSIS *See* HOFFA'S DISEASE.

SYNOVITIS Non-specific inflammation of the lining of a joint. **Transient synovitis of the hip** is the most common cause of non-traumatic hip pain in children. The cause is unknown, but it has been suggested that it may be secondary to viral infection, trauma or an auto-immune process.

SYNTHETASE Synthase. A class of enzymes that synthesize a specific compound, e.g. glycogen synthetase is involved in the synthesis of glycogen.

SYSTEMATIC DESENSITIZATION A behavioral therapy used to treat anxiety, which is based on the classical conditioning procedure of counter-conditioning. Wolpe (1958) argued that anxiety is learned through classical conditioning, whereby the presence of certain stimuli causes an excessively high response by the sympathetic nervous system.

Systematic desensitization involves replacing sympathetic innervation with behaviors associated with parasympathetic innervation (a process called '**reciprocal inhibition**'). Having learned a modification of progressive relaxation, a hierarchy of anxiety-provoking situations is drawn up. Systematic desensitization involves the subject getting deeply relaxed, then imagining or thinking about anxiety provoking situations (starting with the least anxiety-provoking and proceeding to the next one when the previous one has been counter-conditioned). It is assumed that the decrease in anxiety that occurs to imagined stimuli transfers to corresponding real events.

Visual-motor behavior rehearsal (VMBR) is a procedure developed by Suinn as a modification of Wolpe's systematic desensitization procedure. VMBR involves a combination of relaxation and imagery. A shortened version of Jacobsen's progressive relaxation technique is followed by the use of imagery for mental practice of specific skills. There is some evidence for the effectiveness of VMBR; more so for decreasing anxiety than enhancing athletic performance.

Bibliography

Suinn, R.M. (ed) (1976). *Psychology in sports. Methods and applications*. Minneapolis, Minnesota: Burgess Publishing.

Wolpe, J. (1958). *Psychotherapy by reciprocal inhibition*. Stanford, California: Stanford University Press.

SYRINGOMYELIA   A disorder in which there is an obstruction in the normal flow of cerebrospinal fluid, redirecting it to the spinal cord. This results in the formation of a **syrinx**, which is a cyst that fills with cerebrospinal fluid. The syrinx expands and elongates over time, destroying the center of the spinal cord. The condition may lie dormant and undetected for months or years, but symptoms usually begin in young adulthood. Symptoms include pain, weakness and stiffness in the back, shoulders, arms or legs. Other symptoms may include headaches and loss of the ability to feel extremes of hot or cold. Syringomyelia may also adversely affect sweating, sexual function, and bladder and bowel control.

There are two forms of syringomyelia: communicating and noncommunicating. **Communicating syringomyelia** may be related to a congenital abnormality of the brain called Arnold Chiari I malformation, in which the lower part of the cerebellum protrudes from its normal location in the back of the head into the cervical portion of the spinal canal. A syrinx may develop in the cervical region of the spinal cord. It is called 'communicating' syringomyelia, because of the relationship that was once believed to exist between the brain and spinal cord in this type of syringomyelia. **Noncommunicating syringomyelia** occurs as a complication of trauma, meningitis, hemorrhage or tumor. The syrinx develops in a segment of the spinal cord damaged by one or more of these conditions.

In the USA, approximately 21,000 people have syringomyelia. Some cases of syringomyelia are familial, but this is rare. Surgery is usually recommended for syringomyelia patients, with the main aim being to provide more space for the cerebellum at the base of the skull and upper neck, without entering the brain or spinal cord. If a tumor is causing syringomyelia, the tumor can be surgically removed, almost always eliminating the syrinx. However, syringomyelia may recur after surgery. In some patients it may be necessary to drain the syrinx, using a shunt to drain cerebral fluid into a cavity of the body (usually the abdomen).

Chronology

•1948 • In the year of his last appearance in the US Masters golf tournament, Robert Tyre ("Bobby") Jones was diagnosed with syringomyelia. In 1930, Jones had completed the 'Grand Slam' by winning the British Amateur, British Open, US Open and US Amateur championships. He died from complications of the disease in 1971, at the age of 69 years.

Bibliography

American Syringomyelia Alliance Project. Http://www.asap.org.

National Institute of Neurological Disorders and Stroke. Http://www.ninds.nih.gov.

SYSTEMIC   Pertaining to the human body as a whole.

T

TACHYCARDIA A heart rate of over 100 beats per minute.

TACKLER'S EXOSTOSIS *See under* HUMERUS.

TACTILE DISINTEGRATION DISORDERS *See under* SENSORY INTEGRATION.

TAILOR'S BUNION Inflammation of the bursa over the lateral aspect of the 5th metatarsophalangeal joint.

TALIPES Clubfoot. A number of foot deformities in which the foot is severely twisted out of shape. The Achilles and tibial tendons are always shortened (usually from contractures) causing a tendency to walk on the toes or forefoot. Bony changes occur mainly in the talus, calcaneus, navicular and cuboid. Tibial torsion is usually present. It is usually congenital or acquired as a result of a neuromuscular condition. It occurs in about 1 in 700 babies born in the USA each year and is one of the most common birth defects.

Any two types of talipes can coexist. **Talipes calcaneus** involves contracture of the foot in the dorsal-flexed position. **Talipes valgus** involves contracture of the foot with toes and sole of foot turned outward, causing the individual to walk on the inside edge of the feet. It is associated with athetoid cerebral palsy, arthritis and flat feet. **Talipes equines** involves contracture of the foot in plantar-flexed position and results in toe walking. It is the most severe form of talipes. **Talipes varus** involves contracture of the foot with toes and the sole of foot turned inward, causing the individual to walk on the outside edge of the feet. It is associated with spastic hemiplegic cerebral palsy and/or scissors gait.

Mild forms of the conditions are treated with braces and orthopedic shoes. More severe forms require a combination of corrective surgery and braces.

Bibliography
National Organization of Rare Disorders. Http://www.rarediseases.org

TALOCALCANEAL JOINT *See* SUBTALAR JOINT.

TALOCALCANEONAVICULAR JOINT The talonavicular joint and the subtalar joint.
See under MID-TARSAL JOINT; SUBTALAR JOINT.

TALONAVICULAR JOINT *See under* MID-TARSAL JOINT.

TALON NOIR Black heel. It is associated with sports involving frequent, sudden starts and stops (e.g. basketball). The repeated lateral shearing force of the epidermis sliding over the *rete arteriosum subpapillare* (a network of vessels between the papillary and reticular strata of the dermis) causes intra-epidermal and, ultimately, intracorneal hemorrhage. Talon noir appears as a blue-black plaque composed of multiple pigmented puncta, usually on the posterior or posterolateral heel. The condition is self limiting and will resolve spontaneously over time.

Bibliography
Basler, R.S., Hunzeker, C.M. and Garcia, M.A. (2004). Athletic skin injuries. Combating pressure and friction. *The Physician and Sportsmedicine* 32(5), 33-40.

TALUS The bone connecting the leg to the foot. It does not have any muscle attachments.

TANGENT i) In a right-angled triangle, it is the ratio of the side opposite the angle in question to the side adjacent to that angle. ii) A line that just touches the circumference of a circle.

TANGENTIAL ACCELERATION The change in linear velocity per unit time of a body moving along a curved path; the component of acceleration of a body in angular motion directed along a tangent to the path of motion. It is one of two perpendicular components of linear acceleration, the other being radial acceleration. It is calculated as the product of the radius of rotation and angular acceleration. At the instant that a thrown ball is released, its tangential and radial acceleration become equal to zero, because a thrower is no longer applying force.

TAPER   A progressive, nonlinear decrease of the training load during a variable period of time, in an attempt to decrease the physiological and psychological stress of daily training and optimize sports performance. The aim of the taper should be to minimize accumulated fatigue without compromising adaptations. This is best achieved by maintaining training intensity, decreasing training volume (by up to 60 to 90%), and slightly decreasing training frequency (by no more than 20%). The optimal duration of the taper ranges from between 4 and more than 28 days. Strength and power should be maintained by performing two training sessions per week. For peak performance, training should not cease more than 5 to 6 days before competition. Progressive, nonlinear tapers are more beneficial to performance than step tapers. Performance usually improves by about 3% (usual range 0.5 to 6%).

The use of taper is justified, because it has been associated with favorable physiological changes. Resting, maximal and submaximal heart rates do not change, unless athletes show clear signs of overreaching before the taper. Submaximal ventilation may decrease and the respiratory exchange ratio may be slightly decreased or stable. There may be hematological changes, such as increased blood volume. Daily energy expenditure is decreased, promoting a positive energy balance, and muscle glycogen concentration increases progressively. Peak blood lactate concentration is increased, with blood lactate at submaximal intensities being unchanged or decreased. Oxidative enzyme activities can increase and the contractile properties of muscle fibers may be enhanced. Decreased blood creatine kinase concentrations suggest recovery from training stress and muscle damage. Psychological changes in the athlete include: a decrease in total mood disturbance and somatic complaints; decreased perception of effort; physical relaxation; and improved quality of sleep.

Bibliography

Houmard, J.A. and Johns, A.R. (1994). Effects of taper on swim performance. Practical implications. *Sports Medicine* 17(4), 224-232.

Mujika, I. And Padilla, S. (2003). Scientific bases for precompetition tapering strategies. *Medicine and Science in Sports and Exercise* 35(7), 1182-1187.

Mujika, I. et al. (2004). Physiological changes associated with the pre-event taper in athletes. *Sports Medicine* 34(13), 891-927.

Schmitbleicher, D. (1992). Training for power events. In: Komi, P.V. (ed). *Strength and power in sport*. pp381-395. Oxford: Blackwell Scientific Publishers.

TARSAL BONES   *See under* INTERTARSAL JOINTS.

TARSAL CANAL   *See under* TARSAL TUNNEL SYNDROME.

TARSAL COALITION   A condition that occurs when one or more joints in the foot fail to form properly during development. The most common sites are the calcaneonavicular joint and the talocalcaneal joint. Instead of forming the usual synovial joint, the joint is replaced by fibrous tissue, cartilage or bone. As a result, dynamic flexibility of the foot is compromised and the foot is subjected to undue stress.

TARSAL TUNNEL SYNDROME   A neuritis of the posterior tibial nerve. The **tarsal tunnel** is a fibroosseous canal formed by the flexor retinaculum and the bones of the foot posterior to the medial malleolus. It contains the posterior tibial nerve, artery and vein, and the *tibialis posterior, flexor digitorum longus* and *flexor hallucis longus* muscles. Entrapment of the main trunk of the tibial nerve, or of one of its branches, in the tarsal tunnel has been found in mountain climbers, runners and other athletes. The most common cause of tarsal tunnel syndrome is a space-occupying lesion, such as a synovial or ganglion cyst. In runners, the os trigonum may compress the tibial nerve at the tarsal tunnel.

TARSOMETATARSAL JOINTS   Lisfranc's joint.

These are gliding joints between the tarsal bones and metatarsals. Movement is limited to slight gliding of the bones upon each other.

TAU *See under* TIMING ACCURACY.

TAURINE An amino acid synthesized in humans from dietary cysteine or methionine with vitamin B_6 also required. It is so named because it was first discovered in bulls. Dietary essentialness of taurine has not been demonstrated in humans, but it is needed for the formation of bile salts. In the central nervous system, taurine works along with GABA, glycine and glutamine as a neuromodulator or membrane-active amino acid helping the cell to hold on to potassium.

TAY-SACHS DISEASE A fatal, genetic disorder in which harmful quantities of a fatty substance, called ganglioside GM2, accumulates in nerve cells of the brain. It is typical of descendants of Central and Eastern European Jews, known as Ashkenazim. About 1 in every 30 American Jews carries the Tay-Sachs gene. The disorder is caused by insufficient activity of the enzyme hexosaminidase A, which catalyses the degradation of gangliosides. It is inherited as an autosomal recessive trait. When both parents are found to carry a genetic mutation in hexosaminidase A, there is a 25% chance with each pregnancy that the child will be affected with Tay-Sachs disease. Infants with Tay-Sachs disease appear to develop normally for the first few months of life before a relentless mental and physical deterioration sets in, as nerve cells become distended with fatty material. The child becomes blind, deaf and unable to swallow. Muscle atrophy and paralysis sets in. Children with Tay-Sachs disease usually die before the age of 5 years.

Bibliography
National Tay Sachs and Allied Diseases Association. Http://www.ntsad.org

TEAM A type of group having a relatively high degree of structure, organization and task definition. A **group** is one or more persons who are interacting with one another in such a manner that each person influences, and is influenced by, each other person. Tuckman (1965) proposed a four-stage model to explain how a group moves from being a collection of individuals to being a team. In the 'forming stage,' team members familiarize themselves with each other, assess each other's strengths and weaknesses, decide individually whether or not they belong in the group and, if so, in what role. In the 'storming stage,' there is resistance to the leader, resistance to control by the group and interpersonal conflict. **Conflict** occurs when two or people perceive their individual goals as being mutually exclusive (i.e. they perceive that accomplishing one person's goal keeps another person's goal from being achieved). During the 'norming stage,' conflict is resolved and there is development of cooperation, group cohesiveness, role definition and mutual respect for others. In the 'performing stage,' the focus is on effective problem solving and team members helping each other to succeed.

Team performance can be analyzed in terms of communication processes. The observational system used by Hanin (1992) contains five categories of behavior: orienting, stimulating, evaluating, task-irrelevant and performance-related. Orienting behavior is the planning and coordinating of interaction. Stimulating behavior is urging teammates to maintain or increase activity level. Evaluative behavior is positive or negative evaluations of players' actions. Task-irrelevant behavior is positive or negative messages having no direct bearing on the task at hand. Performance-related behavior is task-oriented, individual and collective actions and interactions. Within a particular sport, the typical communication profile is very stable, especially in successful teams. For example, in volleyball the category of stimulating tends to rank first.

Hanin's research with top teams shows that there are usually three practical problems to be confronted: i) coping with major conflicts and aggressive behavior of leaders toward lower-status players; ii) inexperienced and emotionally-unstable players receiving no support from their team-mates or coach; and iii) insufficient communication between low- and high-status players, or inappropriate behavior that provokes interpersonal conflicts.

Further barriers to effective team performance include 'group think,' subgroups, 'psychological homogeneity,' value incompatibility and social loafing. '**Group think**' is a term coined by Irving Janis to describe a set of behaviors consistently exhibited by high-power groups that have made disastrous decisions. Information that had been available to prevent tragedy never reached the top levels of the hierarchy. Group think is characterized by: illusion of invulnerability; belief in the inherent morality of the group; stereotyping members of out-groups; closed-mindedness; single mindedness or mindlessness; collective rationalizations; self-censorship; pressure on dissenters; and illusion of unanimity. By way of underestimating a previously defeated opponent, 'group think' may be involved in team sport 'upsets' (i.e. when an 'underdog' defeats a 'hot favorite').

A **subgroup (clique)** may have a negative effect on team performance if it has certain values that are at odds with the goal structure of the remaining team members. **Psychological homogeneity** occurs when a team is composed of members with very similar needs for individual prominence and achievement motivation. A high degree of psychological homogeneity may make it difficult for a group of individuals to function as a team. Every member who acquires a functional role on a team can be regarded as a 'leader' in the sense that fulfillment of responsibilities assigned to that role contributes to the overall effectiveness of the team. Troubles occur when the jockeying for positions on a team does not result in clear role differentiation and group consensus with respect to which group members are best qualified to fill those roles.

In order to be a team rather than a collection of individuals, a group requires rules, procedures, customs, traditions, rituals and values. Team values are reflected and objectified in the goals that team members seek through their collective action. **Norms** are the rules or standards of behavior regarded as socially acceptable, and they help ensure the attainment of a team's values or goals. Most norms are informal and develop over time. The norms should logically flow from the goals to which the group is committed. **Sanctions** are the rewards and punishments imposed on individual members in order to encourage or discourage certain types of behavior. The problems caused by incompatibility of values, norms and sanctions can be effectively eliminated when team members are given an opportunity to participate in goal, norm and sanction setting.

Conformity involves behaving in ways that are consistent with the group's norms and standards. **Deindividuation** is a psychological state that occurs when a person, who is a member of a group, loses his or her sense of individuality and increasingly conforms to the dictates of the group.

Collective efficacy is a belief or perception shared by members of a team regarding their aggregate capabilities, i.e. it is 'belief in the team.' There is evidence that collective efficacy may be more related to team performance than the sum of each team member's self efficacy.

See also COHESION; HOME ADVANTAGE; SOCIAL LOAFING; TEAM BUILDING.

Bibliography

Carron, A. V. and Dennis, P. W. (1998). The sport team as an effective group. In Williams, J.M. (ed). *Applied sport psychology: Personal growth to peak performance.* 3rd ed. pp128-141. Mountain View, CA: Mayfield.

Hanin, Y.L. (1992). Social psychology and sport: Communication processes in top performance teams. *Sport Science Review* 1(2), 13-28.

Lirgg, C.D. and Feltz, D.L. (1994). Relationship of individual and collective efficacy to team performance. *Journal of Sport and Exercise Psychology* 16, S17.

Lumsden, D.L. and Lumsden, G. (1999). *Communicating in groups and teams: Sharing leadership.* 3rd ed. Belmont, CA: Wadsworth.

Melnick, M.J. (1982). Six obstacles to effective team performance: Some small group considerations. *Journal of Sport Behavior* 5(3), 114-123.

Tuckman, B.W. (1965). Developmental sequence in small groups. *Psychological Bulletin* 63, 384-399.

Yukelson, D.P. (1984). Group motivation in sport teams. In: Silva J.M. and Weinberg, R.S. (eds). *Psychological foundations of sport.* pp229-239. Champaign, IL: Human Kinetics.

TEAM BUILDING Interventions that aim to increase group effectiveness by enhancing group cohesiveness. In sport, most team-building interventions are filtered through a coach, manager or leader. Carron et al. (1997) provided a model of team building has four stages. The first three stages typically take place in a workshop with coaches. The introductory stage and conceptual stage give coaches an overview of the benefits of cohesion and a frame of reference. In the practical stage, coaches brainstorm with their group in order to identify specific strategies to use for team building with their group. In the intervention stage, coaches implement the team-building protocols.

Crace and Hardy (1997) emphasize awareness of individual and team values, identification of interfering factors, and development of interventions to improve mutual respect and cohesion.

Yukelson (1997) offers the following guidelines to coaches: get to know your athletes as unique individuals; develop pride in group membership and a sense of team identity; develop team goals and team commitment; provide for goal evaluations; make roles clear; have periodic team meetings to discuss progress; and use team leaders or representatives to keep coaches informed of attitudes; and feelings in the group.

Bibliography

Carron, A.V., Spink, K.S. and Prapavessis, H. (1997). Team building and cohesiveness in the sport and exercise setting: Use of indirect interventions. *Journal of Applied Sport Psychology* 9, 61-72.

Crace, R.K. and Hardy, C.J. (1997). Individual values and the team building process. *Journal of Applied Sport Psychology* 9, 41-60.

Rosenfeld, L.B. and Richman, J.M. (1997). Developing effective social support: Team building and the social support process. *Journal of Applied Sport Psychology* 9(1), 133-153.

Yukelson, D. (1997). Principles of effective team building intervention in sport: A direct services approach at Penn State University. *Journal of Applied Sport Psychology* 9, 73-96.

TEAM SPIRIT *See under* COHESION.

TEETH A tooth consists of the root and the crown. The **root** is attached to the socket by periodontal ligaments. The **pulp**, housed in the pulp chamber and root canals, contains nerves and blood vessels. The **crown** is the visible part of the tooth and is formed by the yellowish, softer dentin that is covered by enamel.

Loss of baby teeth starts at age 5 or 6 years, and by the age of 12 years, the larger, permanent teeth are developed.

Injuries to teeth can be divided into three categories: fracture, luxation and avulsion, but they often occur in combination. A **fracture** typically splits a tooth into two fragments, one attached to the socket and the other free. A fracture can be classified as a root fracture, broken tooth (crown fracture) or chipped tooth. A broken tooth can involve the pulp. A **luxation** shifts the tooth's position at the level of the root, but does not remove it from the socket. Luxations may be extruded, laterally displaced or intruded. The **extruded tooth** appears longer than the surrounding teeth. A **laterally displaced tooth** is positioned ahead of or behind the normal tooth row. An **intruded tooth** is pushed into the gum, thus appearing shorter than the surrounding teeth. An **avulsion** removes the entire tooth from its socket. Teeth that have been knocked out should be taken to a dentist as soon as possible (ideally after being placed in a 0.9% saline solution). The longer the delay, the less chance there is for successful replantation. After two hours, there is little chance of saving the tooth.

The most commonly injured tooth is the **maxillary central incisor** that is positioned front and center; it receives 80% of all dental injuries. Nearly all such injuries are preventable through regular use of mouth protection. Dental injuries are most common in soccer and basketball.

See also FLUORINE; MOUTHGUARDS.

Bibliography

American Academy of Pediatrics (2001). Injuries in youth soccer. A subject review. *Pediatrics* 105(3), 659-661.

Roberts, W.O. (2000). Field care of the injured tooth. *The Physician and Sportsmedicine* 28(1), 101-102.

TEMPERATURE (i) The degree of sensible heat or cold; a measure of the average kinetic energy due to thermal agitation of the particles in a system. The Standard International units derived from the Kelvin are Celsius (degrees C) and Fahrenheit (degrees F). 0 degrees Celsius is equal to 273.15 Kelvin. 32 degrees Fahrenheit is equal to 0 degrees Celsius. (ii) The level of heat natural to a living being. In **cold-blooded animals**, body temperature varies with environmental temperature. **Normal temperature** refers to the temperature of core areas of the body. **Rectal temperature** is most representative of core temperature (37.1 degrees Celsius). **Oral (sublingual) temperature** is minus 0.6 degrees C below rectal temperature. **Axillary (under arm) temperature** is minus 0.7 degrees Celsius below rectal temperature. During exercise, body temperature rises to around 40 degrees Celsius. (iii) *See* FEVER.

TEMPERATURE REGULATION *See* THERMOREGULATION.

TEMPOROMANDIBULAR JOINT A hinge joint that connects the lower jaw (**mandible**) to the temporal bone. It is stabilized by ligaments and separated into upper and lower compartments by the **temporomandibular disc**, which is a fibrocartilagenous meniscus located between the mandibular condyle and mandibular fossa. The condyles of the mandible glide over the joint socket of the temporal bone. The condyles slide back to their original position when the mouth is closed. This temporomandibular disc absorbs shock to the temporomandibular joint from chewing and other movements.

When the temporomandibular disc does not move with the condyle, it can result in partial or total dislocation. With subluxation (partial dislocation), the condyle moves into the fossa, but there is a delayed movement of the disc. This delay causes crepitation. With total dislocation, the condyle moves and the disc does not move at all. The dislocated disc acts as a wedge, keeping the jaw locked open or closed.

The most common form of temporomandibular disorder is myofascial pain, which is discomfort or pain in the muscles that control jaw function and the neck and shoulder muscles. **Jaw clicking** is fairly common in the general population, but does not require treatment unless there is pain or other symptoms. Other injuries may involve intracapsular bleeding (hemarthrosis), inflammation of the capsular ligaments (capsulitis), meniscal displacement, or fracture. **Bruxism** is habitual grinding of the teeth when sleeping. Mostly women suffer from it. It causes muscle soreness and puts stress on the

temporomandibular joint, producing pain.

In diving, tempomandibular joint pain may occur as a result of clenching too hard onto the mouthpiece.

Bibliography
Academy of General Dentistry. Http://www.agd.org/consumer/topics/sports
The National Institute of Dental Research. Http://www.nidcr.nih.gov

TEMPORAL AWARENESS An understanding of time relationships, such as coincidence-anticipation timing, which is intricately related to eye-hand coordination and eye-foot coordination. Temporal awareness develops simultaneously with spatial awareness.

TENDON The smallest unit in the tendon is **tropocollagen**, a protein composed of type I collagen and created by fibroblasts. Fibrils of tropocollagen lie parallel to one another within the extracellular matrix, and they are capable of resisting loads. Groups of parallel fibrils form **fibers**. Groups of fibers constitute **fascicles** and these are the smallest functional unit in the tendon. The fascicles are enveloped by a sheath of connective tissue called the **endotenon**. This sheath contains the tendon's nervous, vascular and lymphatic structures. The endotenon is surrounded by the epitenon and paratenon. The **epitenon** (tendon sheath) is found only in tendons exposed to high friction forces against surrounding structures. The **paratenon (peritenon)** is designed to decrease friction forces between the tendon and other surrounding structures.

Tendons have the ability to deform under high tensile stresses and to return to their original length once they are unloaded. Through intramolecular and intermolecular cross-links, collagen contributes greatly to the tensile strength of tendons. It is the type, quantity, cross-sectional area and structural organization of collagen that determines the tensile stress that a tendon can accommodate without failure. In the case of the Achilles tendon, the largest tendon in the body, it can receive up to eight-times the body's weight during running when a force of 7000 N is applied. By being able to elongate up to

70% of its original length before rupture, elastin is largely responsible for tendon flexibility. If strain does not exceed 4%, the tendon will return to its original length when unloaded. Tendons resist shearing forces less effectively than tensile forces, and provide little resistance to compressive force. Overuse injuries occurs in tendon after repetitive strain, such that it is no longer able to withstand further loading. Injuries to tendon are often located in areas of poor circulation, e.g. in the Achilles tendon, injuries may be located 2 to 5 cm proximal to its attachment to the calcaneus where there is decreased vascularity. **Tendon rupture (tear)** is loss of continuity of some or all fibers of a tendon. Tendons begin to degenerate and lose their elasticity by the age of 30 years, but this can be delayed by regular exercise.

Following a lack of consensus in the literature about the classification and terminology of tendon injuries, the following classification has received wide support. **Paratenonitis (peritenonitis)** is inflammation of only the paratenon (peritenon), either lined by synovium or not. It includes what was formerly termed tenosynovitis (e.g. de Quervain's syndrome), tenovaginitis and peritendinitis. **Tendinosis** is intratendinous degeneration as a result of atrophy due to factors such as aging, micro-trauma or vascular compromise. It was formerly termed tendinitis. Paratenonitis and tendinosis may be combined in what was also formerly termed tendinitis. Conditions that have traditionally been labeled as Achilles tendinitis, patellar tendinitis, lateral epicondylitis and rotator cuff tendinitis are in fact tendinosis. An increasing body of evidence supports the notion that these overuse tendon conditions do not involve inflammation. Tendinitis is a rather rare condition, but may occur occasionally in the Achilles tendon in conjunction with a primary tendinosis. **Tendinitis** is now regarded as symptomatic degeneration of the tendon with vascular disruption and inflammatory-repair response. It was formerly called tendon strain or tear. **Enthesopathy (tenoperiostitis)** is an injury in which tendon fibers are either microtorn or inflamed at their bony attachment. It occurs most frequently in the elbow area (lateral or medial epicondylitis), in the groin at the attachment of the *adductor longus* muscle, in the knee at the proximal and distal attachments of the patellar tendon, in the Achilles tendon insertion to the calcaneus and in the attachment of the plantar fascia into the calcaneus (plantar fasciitis). Bone-tendon (i.e. osteotendinous) junctions are poorly supplied with blood, because the fibrocartilage creates a 'barrier.' Growing individuals rarely suffer enthesopathy, because their tendons and muscles are relatively stronger than bone. Instead, they sustain inflammation and fragmentation of bone, e.g. Osgood-Schlatter's disease.

Common sites of overuse tendon injuries include: the Achilles tendon; patella ('jumper's knee'); common wrist extensor origin, usually involving the origin of the *extensor carpi radialis brevis* (lateral epicondylitis, i.e. 'tennis elbow'); common wrist flexor origin and *pronator teres* (medial epicondylitis, i.e. 'golfer's elbow'); *supraspinatus* ('swimmer's shoulder,' impingement syndrome); other rotator cuff tendons (i.e. *infraspinatus*, *teres minor* and *subscapularis*); long head of *biceps brachii*; *extensor pollicis brevis* and *abductor pollicis longus* (de Quervain's syndrome); posterior tibia ('shin splints'); leg adductors ('groin strain'); and hamstrings.

See also OVERUSE INJURIES.

Bibliography

Hawary, R.E., Stanish, W.D. and Curwin, S.L. (1997). Rehabilitation of tendon injuries in sport. *Sports Medicine* 24(5), 347-358.

Hess, G.P. et al (1989). Prevention and treatment of overuse tendon injuries. *Sports Medicine* 8(6), 371-384.

Józsa, L. and Kannus, P. (1997). *Human tendons. Anatomy, physiology and pathology*. Champaign, IL: Human Kinetics.

Khan, K.M et al. (1992). Histopathology of common tendinopathies: Update and implications for clinical management. *Sports Medicine* 27(6), 393-408.

Kahn, K.M. et al. (2000). Overuse tendinosis, not tendinitis. *The Physician and Sportsmedicine* 28(5), 38-48.

TENNIS ELBOW   *See* LATERAL EPICONDYLITIS.

TENNIS LEG   *See under* GASTROCNEMIUS.

TENSILE FORCE   *See* TENSION.

TENSION   Traction. A loading mode in which equal and opposite loads are applied outward from the surface of the structure, tending to pull an object apart. In general, a tensile force will cause the length of the body to be increased and the width to be narrowed. Tensile stress and strain result inside the structure. Maximal tensile stress occurs on a plane that is perpendicular to the applied load. Under tensile loading, the structure lengthens and narrows.
   See BENDING; ELASTIC MODULI.

TERATOGEN   Any substance that may cause the unborn child (embryo or fetus) to develop in an abnormal manner. The most dangerous period of time is generally between the 3rd and 8th weeks of gestation. This is the time during which the placenta develops and so the mother's blood supply becomes shared with the fetus. **Thalidomide**, a tranquilizing drug, is one of the most powerful teratogens. 95% of all live births in the USA are healthy and well formed.
   See COCAINE; FETAL ALCOHOL SYN-DROME.

TERMINAL VELOCITY   The maximum, free-falling velocity of an object. It is determined by the amount of air resistance the object encounters. The most important factor influencing the resistance of fluids such as air is the relative velocity of the object. Having jumped from an airplane, the velocity of a skydiver will increase up to some terminal velocity. The magnitude of air resistance increases as the square of relative velocity. The velocity of the skydiver and associated equipment, such as the parachute, increases until the force due to air resistance is equal to the weight of the skydiver and associated equipment (i.e. acceleration due to gravity). After these forces become equal, velocity will remain constant and the skydiver and associated equipment will have reached a terminal velocity.
   The greater terminal velocity of a skier, compared to a skydiver, is a function of cross-sectional area. A skydiver's 'spread-eagle' position presents about twice the frontal area to air resistance as that of a speed skier in a 'tucked' position. If the skydiver adopted an aerodynamic position like that of a speed skier, his terminal velocity would be at least twice that of the speed skier.
   A badminton shuttlecock has a small mass, but a large effective cross-sectional area (measured at the top of the feathers). The initial velocity of the shuttle can exceed 200 miles per hour (mph), but its terminal velocity is about 15 mph.

Bibliography
Zumerchik, J. (1997, ed). *Encyclopedia of sports science*. New York: Macmillan Library Reference.

TESTOSTERONE   A steroid hormone that is androgenic, because it promotes male sex characteristics, and anabolic in that it controls the growth of muscle. It also decreases body fat and increases the number of red blood cells. Its secretion is controlled by luteinizing hormone. In males, 95% of testosterone is produced by the testes, from cholesterol or acetyl CoA; and 5% by the adrenal cortex. Adrenocortical and ovarian testosterone is important in women as it is responsible for some secondary sexual characteristics, such as pubic and axillary hair growth, and also for its influence on sexuality.
   Circulating testosterone is mainly bound to protein, primarily sex hormone binding globulin, but also to albumin and cortisol-binding globulin. **Sex hormone binding globulin** (**SHBG**) is a glycoprotein, synthesized in the liver, which binds testosterone and 5 alpha-dihydrotestosterone strongly; and binds estradiol somewhat less strongly. The '**free androgen index**' is the ratio of total testosterone to SHBG. It is a useful indicator of abnormal status in conditions such as hirsutism. Testosterone is converted to **dihydrotestosterone** in the target tissue.
   High-intensity exercise is associated with increased secretion of testosterone. There is evidence that a subset of endurance-trained men (particularly runners) suffer a decrease in total and free testosterone, in addition to alterations in the release of luteinizing hormone and other pituitary hormones. There is no evidence that endurance training causes **male factor infertility**, which

encompasses all potential causes of infertility in men and contributes to approximately 50% of reproductive failure in reproductive couples. Infertility is said to be present when a couple, attempting to conceive, have not achieved a pregnancy after one year of regular unprotected sexual intercourse. 15 to 20% of couples have such difficulty. Although exhaustive endurance training can decrease plasma testosterone levels, for men of normal fertility status, changes in reproductive status do not always occur. For men who already have difficulty with spermatogenesis, exercise could exacerbate the problem by raising testicular temperatures.

While a relationship between endogenous testosterone levels and aggressive behavior has been observed in various animal species, it is less consistent in humans.

As a natural hormone, **epitestosterone** can contribute to the regulation of androgen-dependent events, such as the control of growth. Testosterone administration can be detected by measuring the **ratio of concentrations of testosterone to epitestosterone**. Until 2005, this ratio could not exceed 6:1, but it was then changed to 4:1. The World Anti-Doping Agency (WADA) Code states that if a laboratory has reported the presence of a T/E ratio greater than 4:1, further investigation is obligatory in order to determine whether the ratio is due to a physiological or pathological condition. In normal men, thirty times more testosterone compared with epitestosterone is produced endogenously, but only 1% of the testosterone is excreted unchanged compared with 30% of epitestosterone. This results in a urinary ratio of testosterone to epitestosterone that is equal to unity. It follows that athletes could take mega-doses of testosterone with epitestosterone in a ratio of about 30:1 and still maintain a normal urinary ratio, but the ratio of testosterone to luteinizing hormone would be abnormally high. Some athletes who have tested positive with ratios in the range of 6:1 to 9:1 have denied doping. It is possible that some of these individuals excrete smaller quantities of epitestosterone, perhaps due to an enzymatic deficiency in their biosynthesis of epitestosterone. These athletes would be expected to have normal urinary testos-

terone-to-luteinizing hormone ratios, because the homeostatic mechanism tends to keep the concentration of testosterone in the blood constant.

The use of an isotope ratio mass spectrometer can detect differences in the ratio of carbon isotopes in different compounds. This technology can be used to determine whether competitors have taken synthetic testosterone. Drug companies use plant sterols from soybeans to produce synthetic testosterone. Compared with carbon atoms in natural testosterone, the carbon atoms in a sample of synthetic testosterone have a slightly lower ratio of carbon-13 isotope to carbon-12. By measuring this ratio, researchers can determine if some of the carbon in a testosterone sample originated from outside the body.

Administration of dihydrotestosterone also inhibits secretion of luteinizing hormone, but due to the decreased excretion of testosterone as well as of luteinizing hormone and epitestosterone, it is unlikely to alter these ratios significantly. Dihydrotestosterone is a more potent anabolic agent than testosterone, since it is known to bind more strongly than testosterone to the androgen receptors.

See ALCOHOL; ANABOLIC STEROIDS; ANDROGEN SUPPLEMENTS; HUMAN CHORIONIC GONADOTROPIN; SEX BEHAVIOR.

Chronology

•1771 • John Hunter induced male characteristics in the hen by transplanting testes from the cock. This was one of the first recorded uses of hormones.

•1889 • Charles Brown-Séquard, a 72-year old French physiologist believed that old age and dwindling sexual powers could be reversed. He claimed rejuvenation upon injection of an extract derived from the testes of dogs and guinea pigs. He reported to the Société Biologie in Paris that these injections had proved effective, but his personal observations were greeted with hostility and skepticism.

•1931 • German scientist Adolf Butenandt extracted a bioactive male hormone from human urine. Eight years later, Butenandt and Leopold Ruzicka were chosen to receive the Nobel Prize in chemistry for their discovery of testosterone.

•1945 • Inspired by Paul de Kruif's *The Male Hormone*, which recorded research into the effects of testosterone, bodybuilders in America began using testosterone preparations.

•1980 • At the Olympic Games, International Olympic Committee (IOC) drug testing expert Manfred Donike unofficially screened urine samples for exogenous testosterone. Using his new test, which measured the ratio of testosterone to epitestosterone, 20% of all athletes tested – males and females – would have failed the test. The 20% included 16 gold medallists. Donike used these unofficial test results to convince the IOC to add his testosterone screen to their testing protocols.

•1983 • Testosterone was added to the International Olympic Committee (IOC)'s list of banned substances. When testosterone is injected, it both raises the testosterone level and lowers the epitestosterone level. If an athlete's ratio exceeded the 6:1 maximum, then there would be evidence of doping.

•1991 • The American javelin thrower Brian Couser was cleared of a doping offence after it was discovered that he had cancer of the testicle. To fight the disease, his body had been generating extra testosterone.

•1993 • Having tested positive for an anabolic steroid at the 1988 Olympic Games, Ben Johnson failed another drugs test at an athletics meeting in Montreal, for an unacceptably high testosterone-to-epitestosterone ratio (T/E ratio), and received a life ban from the International Amateur Athletics Federation (IAAF).

•1994 • British middle-distance runner, Diane Modahl, failed a drugs test when a testosterone-to-epitestosterone ratio of 42-to-1 was found. Later, she successfully claimed that her urine had become degraded, because it had been stored at too high a temperature. In 1999, the House of Lords rejected a case Diane Modahl made against the British Athletic Federation (BAF) in connection with her failed drug test. She argued that the laboratory in Lisbon, which analyzed her urine sample, was not properly accredited, because it had moved to temporary premises without notifying the International Olympic Committee (IOC) and that two members of the original BAF panel who found her guilty of committing a doping offence were biased.

•1996 • Mary Slaney, of the USA, the greatest female middle-distance runner of her generation, allegedly failed a drug test during the American trials for the Olympics, but was still selected. She was found to have a testosterone-to- epitestosterone ratio of 10-to-1. Slaney's lawyer claimed that the testing was flawed, while her sponsors Nike said that she was menstruating during the trials and also taking oral contraceptives. International Olympic Committee (IOC) testing criteria cannot distinguish between androgens from banned anabolic steroids and those caused by oral contraceptives. The US Supreme Court refused Decker's right to appeal the International Amateur Athletic Federation (IAAF) ban. In 2003, Slaney was formally inducted into the USA Track & Field Hall of Fame.

•1999 • Lance Armstrong, a 27-year old Texan, won the Tour de France. Three years earlier, while suffering from testicular cancer, doctors gave him little more than a 20 per cent chance of survival. The cancer had spread to his lungs and brain. *Le Monde* newspaper alleged that Armstrong was tested positive for a banned anti-inflammatory drug at the start of the Tour. Armstrong argued that the only drug he took was an authorized skin cream to relieve saddle sores. Armstrong also won the Tour in 2000, 2001, 2002, 2003 and 2004 to become only the fifth rider to win five Tours and the only rider to win six.

Bibliography

Arce, J.C. and De Souza, M.J. (1993). Exercise and male factor infertility. *Sports Medicine* 15(3), 146-169.

Bahrke, M.S., Yesalis, C.E. and Wright, J.E. (1990). Psychological and behavioural effects of endogenous testosterone levels and anabolic-androgenic steroids among males. *Sports Medicine* 10(5), 303-337.

Höberman, J. (1992). *Mortal engines: The science of performance and the dehumanization of sport.* New York: Basic Books.

Levin, S. (1993). Does exercise enhance sexuality? *The Physician and Sportsmedicine* 21(3), 199-203.

World Anti-Doping Agency. Http://www.wada-ama.org

TETRAHYDROGESTRINONE   *See under* ANABOLIC STEROIDS.

TETRALOGY   A group or series of four. **Tetralogy of Fallot** is a congenital heart defect that combines four structural anomalies: obstruction to pulmonary flow; ventricular septal defect (abnormal opening between the right and left ventricles); dextroposition of the aorta (aortic opening overriding the septum and receiving blood from both ventricles); and right ventricular hypertrophy (increase of volume of the myocardium of the right ventricle).

THALAMUS   *See under* BRAIN.

THALIDOMIDE   *See under* LIMB DEFICIENCIES; TERATOGEN.

THELION   An anatomical landmark that is located at the nipple.

THENAR EMINENCE   *See under* HAND MUSCLES.

THEOBROMINE   *See under* CAFFEINE.

THEOPHYLLINE   *See under* ADENOSINE; CAFFEINE.

THERMAL INJURIES   *See under* SCAR TISSUE.

THERMIC EFFECT OF FOOD   *See under* ENERGY EXPENDITURE.

THERMODYNAMICS   The branch of science and

engineering concerned with energy transformations. At the theoretical level, a thermodynamic system is a system that is separated from the surroundings by real (or imaginary) boundaries across which energy is transferred (in various forms).

Energy transfer may be work transfer, heat transfer or energy transfer by mass flow. **Work transfer** is a form of energy that crosses the boundary of a thermodynamic system because of displacement of all or part of the system boundary in the presence of a force or torque. Regarding the thermodynamics of skeletal muscles, which are the only body structures able to generate force and do work, the surroundings are the body segments on which they act. Work is done by the system on its surroundings (positive), or the surroundings do work on the system (negative). **Heat transfer** is a form of energy that crosses the system boundary because of a temperature difference between the system and the surroundings (conduction, convection and radiation) or because of a partial vapor pressure difference (evaporation). By convention, heat transfer from the system to the surroundings is defined as negative. Conversely, heat transfer to the system from the surroundings is defined as positive. Unlike mechanical engines, biological engines cannot convert heat energy into other forms. Energy may be transferred by **mass flow** in various forms, including chemical, kinetic, pressure and thermal. When thermal energy is transferred across a system by mass flow it is called enthalpy flow. **Enthalpy flow** is the product of the mass (m) of substance entering (positive) or leaving (negative) the system, the specific heat at constant pressure (Cp) of the substance and its absolute temperature, i.e. $H = mCpT$. The main source of enthalpy in the human thermodynamic system is respiratory gases.

In a **closed system**, no mass is transferred across the system boundary and a non-flow process takes place. In an **open system**, mass transfer occurs across the boundary. The flow process may be steady or non-steady. In general, an athlete is an open system and the mass flows (mainly caused by breathing) are non-steady.

The universe is a closed system, i.e. neither matter nor energy enters or leaves the system. The

matter and energy present in the universe at the time of the primordial explosion are all the matter and energy it will ever have. After each and every energy exchange and transformation, the universe as a whole has less potential energy than it did before. Life can exist, however, because the universe is running down. The universe as a whole is a closed system, but the earth is not a closed system, because it receives energy input from the sun. Less than one percent of the solar energy reaching the earth becomes the energy that drives all the processes of life. This occurs through a series of operations performed by the cells of plants and other photosynthetic organisms. Living systems change energy from one form to another, transforming the radiant energy from the sun into the chemical and mechanical energy used by all living things.

The **first law of thermodynamics** is that energy can be changed from one form to another, but it cannot be created or destroyed. A system's internal energy can change only by the exchange of heat or work with the surroundings. The total energy of any system plus its surroundings thus remains constant, despite any changes in form. In the case of chemical reactions, this means that the energy of the products of the reaction plus the energy released in the reaction is equal to the initial energy of the reactants.

The **second law of thermodynamics** states that processes always go in the direction of randomness or disorder. It means that efficiency of energy exchange is always imperfect in that some energy will escape from a system as entropy (usually in the form of heat). **Entropy (ΔS)** is the measure of the amount of disorder (loss of higher-level energy) in a system. The amount of energy does not change, but the ability of that energy to do work is decreased. There is more disorder associated with more numerous and smaller objects than with fewer, larger ones. Ice at 0 degree Celsius has low entropy, but water at 0 degrees Celsius has high entropy. There will always be many more ways of putting a large number of molecules into a disorderly arrangement than into an orderly one. Therefore, the entropy of an ordered state is lower than that of a disordered state of the same system. When ΔS is positive, the reaction becomes more disordered and something is catabolized. When ΔS is negative, the reaction becomes less disordered and something is anabolized. Life involves a temporary decrease in entropy, paid for by the expenditure of energy. Energy must be expended to pay the price of organization. In other words, living organisms spend energy to overcome entropy.

Enthalpy change (ΔH) is the total heat exchange in a reaction or process. Enthalpy is an expression of heat change in a constant-pressure reaction. *In vivo* chemical reactions occur under nearly constant-pressure conditions. The oxidation of a fatty substance, such as palmitic acid, occurs very differently in the human body than it does in a calorimeter. Nevertheless, the values of ΔS and ΔH for the process are exactly the same in both pathways, because a quantity like ΔS or ΔH depends only on the final and initial states. For most biochemical reactions, the distinction between ΔS and ΔH is of little consequence. Most of these reactions occur in solution and do not involve the consumption or formation of gases. ΔH can be thought of as a measure of the energy change in a process.

The **free energy change** (ΔG) is equal to enthalpy change (ΔH) minus ΔS multiplied by the absolute temperature (T), i.e. $\Delta G = \Delta H - T\Delta S$. ΔG is the part of the total energy change in a reaction or process that is capable of doing work at constant temperature and pressure. ΔG for a biochemical reaction can be defined as the difference in free energy content between the reactants and the products under standard conditions. If ΔG is zero, the reaction will be in a state of equilibrium. Every reaction has a characteristic ΔG that can be calculated by assuming standard conditions of temperature (298 degrees Kelvin), pressure (101 kPa) and pH (7).

An **exergonic reaction** or process, e.g. ATP hydrolysis, is one in which free energy is released and ΔG is negative. An **endergonic reaction** or process, e.g. protein synthesis, is one in which free energy must be added and ΔG is positive. Exergonic reactions provide the free energy to perform all the endergonic reactions that maintain the functioning of cells and tissues. Coupling of endergonic to exergonic reactions is one of the most important

principles in biochemistry. Exergonic reactions can drive endergonic reactions, provided the sum of the two is exergonic. Muscle contraction must be driven by simultaneous hydrolysis of ATP. Amino acids cannot be joined together to make a peptide unless GTP is simultaneously hydrolyzed. Glucose molecules cannot be joined together to make glycogen unless UTP is simultaneously hydrolyzed.

Exergonic reactions usually occur spontaneously since they do not require energy. They occur because the products possess less energy in the covalent bonds than the reactants had possessed. No matter how 'spontaneous' a chemical reaction is, however, some energy is required to start the reaction. The input of energy is called **activation energy**. If a large amount of activation energy is required, then the reaction will tend not to go forward (all else held constant). If a small amount of activation energy is required, then the reaction will tend to go forward very readily.

Exergonic and endergonic refer to ΔG and spontaneity, not heat released or absorbed. In exergonic reactions, ΔH may be zero or may even be positive, but ΔG is always negative. The greater the increase in ΔS, the more negative ΔG will be, i.e. the more exergonic the reaction will be. Heat released or absorbed is referred to as **exothermic** or **endothermic**, respectively. In general, an exergonic chemical reaction is also an exothermic reaction, i.e. it gives off heat and thus has a negative ΔH.

Bibliography

Bartlett, R. (1997). *Introduction to sports biomechanics*. London: E & FN Spon.

Houston, M.E. (2001). *Biochemistry primer for exercise science*. 2nd ed. Champaign, IL: Human Kinetics.

Mathews, C.K. (2000). *Biochemistry*. San Francisco, CA: Benjamin/Cummings.

THERMOGENESIS   The generation of heat. Thermogenic mechanisms are classified as either obligatory or facultative (adaptive). **Obligatory thermogenesis** is the energy released as heat during cellular and organ functions in the body, and the bulk of this heat is produced by the basal metabolism. **Facultative (adaptive) thermogenesis** is heat production that does not result in mechanical work or net synthesis. It is not known precisely how thermogenesis occurs, but it is likely that some mechanism for uncoupling of oxidative phosphory lation is involved; i.e. energy substrates are oxidized, but heat is produced instead of ATP. Increased activity of brown fat, sodium-potassium pump activity and futile cycling have been implicated in thermogenesis. The thermic effect of food (diet-induced thermogenesis) includes facultative and obligatory thermogenesis.

A **futile cycle** is a substrate cycle in which the two opposing reactions occur at comparable rate in the same cell. Such a cycle accomplishes nothing except the waste of the free energy difference between the two reactions or, possibly, the generation of heat. An example is the reversible reaction in which glucose and ATP form glucose 6-phosphate and ADP, or the reverse; together with the reversible reaction in which glucose 6-phosphate and water form glucose and inorganic phosphate, or the reverse. The net reaction is the reversible reaction in which ATP forms ADP and inorganic phosphate, or the reverse. Flight-or-fight hormones, such as epinephrine, stimulate and promote futile cycling in cells. Sympathomimetic agents can increase substrate availability in muscle and white adipose tissue, and thyroid hormone action. Intense exercise increases epinephrine levels and triggers futile cycling, thereby causing the body to burn extra calories after exercise. Exercise also increases metabolism by increasing muscle temperature and disturbing cell function. The contribution of the futile cycles to facultative thermogenesis is presently unknown, but it could be significant.

THERMORECEPTORS   *See under* MECHANO-RECEPTORS.

THERMOREGULATION   It is the balance between heat gain and heat loss. Thermoregulation is important because body core temperature must be kept between 36 and 38 degrees Celsius for normal functioning of the body. Thermoregulatory mechanisms are activated by thermal receptors in the skin that send information to the hypothalamus and the cerebral cortex, and by the temperature of the blood perfusion in the anterior region of the hypothalamus, which then activates other regions of the hypothalamus.

Heat gain from the metabolism and the environment occurs by radiation and conduction. **Heat loss** occurs by radiation, conduction, convection and evaporation. **Conduction** is the transfer of heat from the warmer to the cooler of two objects or bodies that are in direct contact. Ice packs and cold-water baths are examples of heat transfer by conduction. The rate of heat lost by conduction depends on the temperature gradient between the skin and the surrounding matter, as well as the thermal properties of the matter (e.g. water conducts heat about 25-times more than air).

Radiation involves the transfer of heat by electromagnetic waves. When the body is warmer than the environment, heat is transferred from the body to the environment. When the temperature of the environment is greater than that of the body, the body absorbs heat from the environment and the only mechanism for heat loss is from evaporation.

Convection is heat transfer with the movement of air or water currents next to the surface of the skin. When convection is slow, the air next to the skin is warmed and provides insulation from heat loss by conduction. When convection is high, the warm air next to the skin is replaced by cooler air and heat is lost. Convection increases with speed of movement of the body through air or water. Moving air from a fan or a windy day are examples of heat transfer by convection.

Evaporation involves heat loss due to the vaporization of water from the surface of the skin and respiratory passages to the environment. A distinction can be made between eccrine and apocrine glands. Eccrine glands are more widely distributed than apocrine glands. The **eccrine glands**, dispersed at variable densities all over the surface of the body, are controlled by the sympathetic nervous system. Eccrine glands secrete a fluid (perspiration) that is mainly water and salt (sodium chloride) with trace amounts of electrolytes. The evaporation of perspiration cools the skin and the blood that has been directed from the core to the periphery. Perspiration is basically odorless, but it can take on an unpleasant smell when it comes into contact with bacteria on the skin. **Apocrine glands** are mainly found in areas abundant in hair follicles, such as the armpits, pubic region and areolae of the breasts. The secretion of apocrine glands is more viscous than eccrine glands. Apocrine glands secrete a fatty sweat directly onto the tubule of the gland. During emotional stress, the wall of the tubule contracts and the sweat is pushed to the surface of the skin where bacteria begin breaking it down. This may cause a strong odor. **Antiperspirants** block the sweat ducts with aluminum salts, thereby decreasing the amount of perspiration that reaches the skin. **Deodorants** eliminate the odor, but not the perspiration, and turn the skin acidic, which makes it less attractive to bacteria.

Exercise increases body-core temperature. Heat production can increase 15 to 20 times during heavy exercise. The relationship between exercise intensity and body core temperature is linear up to 75% of maximal oxygen uptake and curvilinear thereafter. Training has been shown to enhance sweat production by eliciting changes in the sensitivity of eccrine glands, total sweat output and distribution of gland activity. *See also* COLD STRESS; HEAT STRESS.

THIAMIN *See* VITAMIN B$_1$.

THIOLASE   The enzyme that catalyzes the thio-lytic cleavage reaction in beta oxidation. This is the last step in beta oxidation: a fatty acyl CoA derivative, in the presence of coenzyme A (CoA) is cleaved to produce acetyl CoA and a fatty acyl CoA of a fatty acid that contains two carbon atoms less than the fatty acid that entered the cycle.

THORACIC OUTLET   It is comprised of three anatomic spaces (scalene triangle, costoclavicular space and pectoralis minor space) through which neurovascular structures pass from the neck and thorax into the arm. The boundaries of the **scalene triangle** are the *scalenus anterior*, *scalenus posterior* and first rib (inferior). The subclavian vein lies anteromedial to the *scalenus anterior* and the sub-clavian artery and brachial plexus run posterolateral to this muscle. The boundaries of the **costoclavicular**

space are the clavicle (superior), first rib (inferior), costoclavicular ligament (anteromedial) and *scalenus medius*/long thoracic nerve (posterolateral). The **pectoralis minor space** is a remote area located outside the thoracic outlet. It involves the ligamentous insertion of the *pectoralis minor* muscle.

THORACIC OUTLET SYNDROME   A group of distinct disorders that affect the nerves in the brachial plexus and various nerves and blood vessels of the thoracic outlet.

True neurologic thoracic outlet syndrome is a rare, typically painless disorder that is caused by congenital anomalies. It generally occurs in middle-aged women and almost always on one side of the body. Symptoms include weakness and wasting of hand muscles, and numbness in the hand.

Disputed (non-specific) thoracic outlet syndrome is believed by many scientists to be a brachial plexus injury, while other scientists dispute that it exists. The most prominent symptom of the disorder is pain. Other symptoms include weakness and fatigue.

Arterial thoracic outlet syndrome is a rare disorder that occurs on one side of the body. It is caused by a congenital anomaly. Symptoms can include sensitivity to cold in the hands and fingers, numbness or pain in the fingers, and finger ulcers or severe limb ischemia.

Venous thoracic outlet syndrome is a rare disorder that often develops suddenly, frequently following unusual, prolonged limb exertion. The exact cause is unknown.

Traumatic thoracic outlet syndrome may be caused by trauma, such as a motor vehicle accident or a hyperextension injury (overextending an arm overhead while reaching for an object). Pain is the most common symptom, and it often occurs with tenderness.

The etiology of thoracic outlet syndrome is usually related to congenital bands, an anomaly of one of the three anatomic spaces, or a history of repetitive trauma. **Congenital bands** are fibrous thickenings of the *scalene* muscle. These may be located in the muscle fibers or in discrete locations connecting the muscles. Congenital bands are the most common causes of venous thoracic outlet syndrome and neurogenic thoracic outlet syndrome. Anatomic anomalies include cervical ribs that arise from the lower neck and articulate with the upper aspect of the first thoracic rib, causing compression. The cervical ribs are usually found in the middle *scalene* muscle. Bilateral cervical ribs are seen in 63% to 80% of individuals with symptoms. Agenesis of the anterior part of the first thoracic rib may result in abnormal congenital fusion with the second rib, resulting in arterial problems. Neck trauma is the most common predisposing factor for neurogenic thoracic outlet syndrome. A history of trauma and repetitive stress injuries is present in 80% of individuals with symptoms.

In sport, thoracic outlet syndrome is most often seen in athletes who engage in repetitive motions that place the shoulder at the extreme of abduction and external rotation, e.g. freestyle, butterfly and backstroke in swimming. Venous thoracic outlet syndrome most commonly develops in young male athletes in whom upper extremity musculature is overdeveloped as a result of work of physical conditioning. In weightlifters, hypertrophy of the *scalene* muscles can impinge the subclavian vessels and the brachial plexus in the *scalene* or costoclavicular triangles. Hypertrophy of the *pectoralis minor* muscle may impinge the same nerves and vessels in the pectoralis minor space during hyperabduction and external rotation of the shoulder.

Thoracic outlet syndrome is three times more common in females than males. Differential diagnoses include effort thrombosis.

Bibliography

Kalra, A., Thornburg, M. and Spadone, D. (2002). Thoracic outlet syndrome. Http://www.emedicine.com
National Institute of Neurological Disorders and Stroke. Http://ninds.nih.gov
Reeves, R.K., Laskowski, E.R. and Smith, J. (1998). Weight training injuries: Part 2: Diagnosing and managing chronic conditions. *The Physician and Sportsmedicine* 26(3), 54-73.

THORACIC SPINE   A structure that has limited flexibility in humans because it is splinted by the ribs. Many problems are postural in origin and are usually due to excessive kyphosis. Disk displace-

ments in the thoracic spine are rare. Facet and costovertebral articulations in the thoracic region are commonly injured, usually from compression of the chest, e.g. when a football player falls onto a ball with another player on top of him. The **thoracolumbar junction** is a region of potentially high stress during flexion-extension movements of the trunk. See also SPINE.

THREONINE   An essential, four-carbon amino acid that is considered glucogenic (glycogenic), because two of its carbons form pyruvate that could lead to their incorporation in glucose.

THROMBIN   An enzyme in blood that facilitates blood clotting.

THROMBOCYTES   *See under* LEUKOCYTES.

THROMBOEMBOLISM   *See under* THROMBOSIS.

THROMBOPHLEBITIS   Inflammation of a vein associated with thrombosis.

THROMBOSIS   It is the formation or presence of a thrombus. A **thrombus** (blood clot) is a mechanical mass that forms within the cardiovascular system on denuded endovascular or prosthetic (artificial) flow surfaces. Thrombi are composed of insoluble fibrin, deposited platelets, accumulating leukocytes and entrapped red blood cells in variable flow-dependent patterns. **Thrombotic disorders** are diseases characterized by formation of a thrombus that obstructs vascular blood flow locally or detaches and embolizes to occlude blood flow downstream (**thromboembolism**). Deep vein thrombosis and pulmonary embolism are different manifestations of venous thromboembolism. The incidence of venous thromboembolism is 1 to 2 per 1,000 people. It is estimated that more than 250,000 cases of venous thromboembolism are diagnosed each year in the USA. At least 50,000 of these cases are fatal.

Deep vein thrombosis occurs when venous thrombi develop within a deep vein at a site of vascular trauma and in areas of sluggish blood flow (e.g. in the venous sinuses of the calf and within a valve cusp). A proximal deep vein thrombosis in the leg is one that is located within the popliteal, femoral or iliac veins. The typical symptoms of deep vein thrombosis include leg pain, edema, erythema and warmth in the affected area.

Pulmonary embolism occurs if the clot breaks away and travels to the lung. Most patients with deep vein thrombosis develop pulmonary embolism and the majority of cases are unrecognized clinically. The most common symptoms of pulmonary embolism in individuals without preexisting cardiopulmonary disease are dyspnea, pleuritic chest pain, cough, leg edema, leg pain, hemoptysis and palpitations. Nearly 50% of patients with deep vein thrombosis have an asymptomatic pulmonary embolism at the time of their diagnosis. Untreated, about one third of patients who survive an initial pulmonary embolism die of a future pulmonary embolism. Thrombus in the popliteal segment of the femoral vein is the cause of pulmonary embolism in more than 60% of cases. Fatal pulmonary embolism is also common from a thrombus that originates in the axillary/subclavian veins or in the veins of the pelvis. Pulmonary embolism is the third most common cause of death in the USA, with at least 650,000 cases occurring each year. The highest incidence of recognized pulmonary embolism occurs in hospitalized patients, with recent surgery and pregnancy being risk factors.

Fibrinolysis is widely regarded as the primary treatment of choice for all patients with pulmonary embolism and even for all patients who have deep vein thrombosis without evidence of pulmonary embolism. Heparin is the single most important treatment. Through activation of antithrombin III, it slows or prevents clot progression and decreases the risk of further embolism. Heparin does not dissolve an existing clot.

Research evidence suggests that spontaneous deep vein thrombosis and pulmonary embolism are nearly always related to some underlying hypercoagulable state that may be congenital or acquired. Risk factors include: previous episode of thrombosis; hormonal therapy; recent surgery; malignancy;

pregnancy; thrombophilic disorders, such as factor V Leiden mutation; and primary or acquired deficiencies of natural anticoagulants, such as antithrombin III, protein C and protein S. Angiography is the diagnostic reference standard. This involves radiography of blood vessels after the injection of a contrast medium. Of patients with venographically proven spontaneous deep vein thrombosis, 25 to 50% have a genetic predisposing factor. The most common congenital risk factor for deep vein thrombosis is inborn resistance to activated protein C. Most patients with this syndrome have a genetic mutation in factor V (Arg506Gln mutation) known as 'factor V Leiden,' but there are other mechanisms that can produce a resistance to activated protein C.

Warfarin is an oral drug that inhibits gamma-carboxylation of the vitamin K-dependent coagulation factor II (prothrombin), factor VII (proconvertin), factor IX (Christmas factor; plasma thromboplastin component) and factor X (Stuart-Prower factor). Warfarin also inhibits carboxylation of the natural anticoagulants, protein C and protein S, resulting in a rapid decline of their levels. Patients on warfarin should avoid consumption of foods that contain a significant amount of vitamin K (e.g. leafy green vegetables, soybean).

There is a link between long-haul air travel and venous thromboembolism. Risks are associated with any flight of more than 2 hours in length where passengers are seated and immobile for long periods of time. The risk appears to be small and largely confined to those with recognized risk factors, such as a previous episode of thrombosis, hormonal therapy, recent surgery, malignancy and pregnancy. Travel-related factors include stasis associated with prolonged periods of immobility, physiological stresses resulting from exposure to the cabin environment (low humidity and hypoxia) in long-haul flight and other in-flight factors. The term **'traveller's thrombosis'** is more accurate than **'economy class syndrome,'** because it can occur when using other forms of transport such as long car journeys. Presenting the case of a 32-year-old male for whom sitting for long periods at a computer represented the major risk factor for his life-threatening venous thromboembolism, the term 'eThrombosis' has been proposed to describe venous thromboembolism associated with immobility from prolonged sitting.

Movement, avoidance of dehydration and alcohol, and appropriate pharmacological prophylaxis for high-risk travelers can decrease the likelihood of venous thromboembolism. Physical prophylaxis, such as use of compression stockings or in-flight exercise devices, may also be of general benefit to passengers. Compression stockings should provide a compression gradient of 30 to 40 mm Hg or higher. This will decrease the capacitive venous volume by about 70% and increase the measured velocity of blood flow in the deep veins by at least fivefold.

Post-thrombotic syndrome is characterized by leg pain, edema, other signs of venous insufficiency, and eventually leg ulceration as a result of prolonged venous hypertension. At least 30% of patients with venous thromboembolism develop this chronic debilitating disease. Sized-to-fit compression stockings may decrease the risk of post-thrombotic syndrome.

Effort thrombosis (primary upper-extremity deep vein thrombosis; Paget-Schroetter syndrome) is known as 'effort' thrombosis, because 70% of cases have been associated with unaccustomed or vigorous activity. Athletic activity has been cited as a cause in about 20% of all cases. It is primarily a condition of the young, healthy and active. Effort thrombosis generally has a traumatic pathogenesis. Sometimes it results from a blow to the shoulder. More commonly, it develops as a result of chronic repetitive minor trauma to the axillosubclavian vein during vigorous activity. Impingement by structures in the thoracic outlet (e.g. hypertrophied *scalenus anterior* muscle) may often predispose a person to primary upper-extremity deep vein thrombosis from trauma. Nonfatal pulmonary embolism occurs in about 12% of patients who have primary upper-extremity deep vein thrombosis.

Bibliography

Beasley, R. et al. (2003). eThrombosis: The 21st century variant of venous thromboembolism associated with immobility. *European Journal of Respiratory Physiology* 21(2), 374-376.

deWeber, K. (1999). Effort thrombosis with sepsis. *The Physician and Sportsmedicine* 27(5), 74-86.

Giangrande, P.L. (2001). Air travel and thrombosis. *International Journal of Clinical Practice* 55(10), 690-693.

Giangrande, P.L. (2002). Air travel and thrombosis. *British Journal of Haematology* 117, 509-512.

Iqbal, O. et al. (2003). Air travel-associated venous thromboembolism. *Medical Principles and Practice* 12(2), 73-80.

Koenig, W. and Ernst, E. (2000). Exercise and thrombosis. *Coronary Artery Disease* 11(2), 123-127.

THROMBOXANES *See under* FATTY ACIDS.

THROMBUS *See under* THROMBOSIS.

THROWING Imparting force to an object in the general direction of intent. Motor milestones are: body faces target, feet remain stationary with the ball thrown with forearm extension only (2 to 3 years); body rotation added (3.5 to 5 years); stepping forward with the leg on the same side as the throwing arm (5 to 6 years); and mature throwing pattern (6 years).

See under ELBOW JOINT, INJURIES.

THUMB *See* CARPOMETACARPAL JOINTS; METACARPOPHALANGEAL JOINTS.

THYMINE A nitrogenous, pyrimidine base found in DNA.

THYROID GLAND An endocrine gland located in the neck just below the larynx. It secretes iodine-containing hormones. A minute amount of iodine is required from the diet for the thyroid gland. Deficiency of iodine causes enlargement of the thyroid. The thyroid gland secretes thyroxine and triidothyronine. **Thyroglobulin** is a glycoprotein that is synthesized by the thyroid follicular cell and iodinated once it has been synthesized.

Thyroid hormones include **triidothyronine** (T3) and **thyroxine** (T4). These iodine-containing amino acid hormones increase metabolic rate, mobilize fuels and are involved in growth. They are controlled by thyroid-stimulating hormone and metabolic rate. Exercise is associated with an increase in free triidothyronine and thyroxine. The trained individual will have a lower concentration of free triidothyronine at rest and a higher turnover during exercise. The trained individual will have a higher concentration of free thyroxine at rest and a higher turnover during exercise.

Thyroid-stimulating hormone (thyrotropin) is secreted by the anterior pituitary gland. The secretion of thyroid-stimulating hormone (TSH) is controlled by hypothalamic TSH-releasing factor and thyroxine. Thyroid-stimulating hormone stimulates production and release of thyroxine from the thyroid gland. It is secreted more during exercise, but there is no evidence for a training effect.

The only use for pharmacological thyroid hormones is replacement therapy in thyroid disease. The problem for athletes wishing to use thyroid hormones as an ergogenic aid is that these hormones tend to break down muscle. *See also* ENERGY EXPENDITURE; HYPERTHYROID MYOPATHY; HYPOTHYROID MYOPATHY.

THYROXINE   *See under* THYROID GLAND.

TIBIAL BOWING   Bowing of the diaphysis of the tibia with the apex of the deformity directed anterolaterally, anteromedially, or posteromedially. Each type of bowing tends to have a classic etiology. Anterolateral bowing is associated with pseudoarthrosis of the tibia and neurofibromatosis. Anteromedial bowing is associated with fibular hemimelia. Posteriomedial bowing is a congenital bowing of the tibia (with the apex directed posteriorly and medially) and a calcaneovalgus foot deformity. Both of these deformities tend to resolve so that there is little clinical disability, but a leg length inequality commonly develops and often requires treatment. Most children with posteromedial tibial bowing have a limb-length inequality averaging 3 cm, but this can vary from about 2 to 6 cm. Typically, a limb-length inequality of 2 cm or less is not a functional problem.

Bibliography
McCarthy, J. (2003). Tibial bowing. Http://emedicine.com

TIBIALE LATERALE   An anatomical landmark that is the most superior aspect of the lateral border of the head of the tibia (lateral tibial condyle). It is found within the depression or dimple of the knee bounded by a triad of prominences: the epicondylar femur, anterolateral portion of the head of the tibia and head of the fibula. The tibiale laterale is approximately in the same transverse plane as the tibiale mediale.

TIBIALE MEDIALE   An anatomical landmark that is the superior extremity of the tibia and the most proximal point of the glenoid margin on the medial border of the head of the tibia.

TIBIAL NERVE   Like the common peroneal nerve, the **posterior tibial nerve** is a continuation of the sciatic nerve. It is derived from the 4th lumbar to 3rd sacral (L4-S3) nerve roots. The tibial nerve travels from the popliteal fossa into the deep posterior compartment of the leg, where it is well protected by overlying muscle until it reaches the tarsal tunnel posterior to the medial malleolus. At that level, the posterior tibial nerve divides into three main branches: the lateral plantar nerve, medial plantar nerve and calcaneal nerve. The posterior tibial nerve innervates the *soleus*, *gastrocnemius*, *flexor digitorum longus*, *flexor hallucis longus*, *tibialis posterior* and intrinsic foot muscles. It also provides sensation to the posterior calf and the sole of the foot. Because it is so well protected by overlying muscles, the tibial nerve is much less prone than the peroneal nerve to acute injury. Tibial nerve injuries tend to occur with severe trauma such as a tibia fracture sustained during baseball while sliding into base.

See also TARSAL TUNNEL SYNDROME.

TIBIAL STRESS REACTION   *See under* LOWER LEG PAIN.

TIBIAL TORSION   Malleolar torsion. Twisting of the tibia around its longitudinal axis from the knee to the ankle. Normal range of external (lateral) rotation is 45 to 70 degrees; and for internal (medial) rotation it is 10 to 45 degrees. Internal tibial torsion is a condition in early childhood in which the tibia is twisted inwards axially, causing the child to toe-in as he walks ('pigeon toe gait'). It is considered normal, unless it does not resolve beyond 18 to 24 months of age. It frequently occurs in young children who are in a non-weight bearing position for a prolonged period of time as a result of injury or illness. About 30% of 2 year olds have in-toe gait because of tibial torsion and this decreases to around 8 or 9% between the ages of 12 and 14 years. The condition is bilateral in about two thirds of affected infants (left side affected more than right). Severe in-toeing can cause a child to trip or run awkwardly, and it can interfere with participation in sport. Internal tibial torsion improves with time. External tibial torsion often worsens, because the natural progression is toward increasing external torsion.

The ability to compensate for tibial torsion depends on the amount of inversion and eversion present in the foot and on the amount of rotation possible at the hip. Internal torsion causes the foot to adduct and the patient tries to compensate by everting the foot and/or by externally rotating the hip. Similarly, persons with external tibial torsion invert at the foot and internally rotate at the hip.

Bibliography
Ask Dr. Chris. Http://guardian.curtin.edu.au: 16080/cga/faq/torsion.html
Patel, M. (2004). Tibial torsion. Http://www.emedicine.com

TIBIAL TUBEROSITY   A protuberance on the upper anterior surface of the tibia.

TIBIAL VALGUS   Curvature of the tibia outwards from its proximal to distal end. It results in extra tensile stress being placed on the medial side of the knee and the lateral side of the ankle. It is usually combined with femoral varus and results in a knock-kneed appearance.

See also under FEMORAL VARUS.

TIBIAL VARUS   Blount's disease. An uncommon growth disorder characterized by disordered ossification of the medial aspect of the proximal tibial physis, epiphysis and metaphysis. This progressive deformity is manifested by varus angulation and internal rotation of the tibia in the proximal metaphyseal region immediately below the knee.

The term 'osteochondrosis deformans tibiae' is not accurate, because it describes a disorder in which the primary or secondary centers of ossification undergo avascular necrosis. Avascular necrosis has never been found in Blount's disease.

Blount's disease can occur in growing children of any age and is classified into three forms: infantile (in children less than 3 years), juvenile (in children 4 to 10 years) and adolescent (in those aged 11 years and older). Adolescent Blount's disease does not appear to be as progressive or common as the infantile form. The infantile form is generally more prevalent in females and Blacks and those with marked obesity.

The varus angulation results in extra tensile stress being placed on the lateral aspect of the knee joint and the medial side of the ankle as the foot rotates to interface with the horizontal ground. It is often combined with rearfoot valgus. If it is not compensated, the feet or ankles may impact one another during the swing phase of gait. Tibial varus may also be found with femoral valgus, and may cause iliotibial band friction syndrome.

Bibliography
DeOrio, M.J. (2003). Blount's disease. Http://www.emedicine.com

TIBIO-FEMORAL JOINT   *See under* KNEE JOINT.

TIBIO-FIBULAR JOINT   A joint comprising three articulations between the tibia and fibula. For each, the movement is limited to very slight gliding of the articular surfaces upon each other.

TICS   Involuntary, sudden, rapid, recurrent, non-rhythmic, stereotyped motor movements or vocalizations that may occur in an infrequent or almost continuous manner. Tics include eye blinking, neck jerking, throat clearing, sniffing, and repeating words or phrases. **Coprolalia** is a complex vocal tic involving the uttering of obscenities. Complex motor tics include touching, squatting, retracing steps, and twirling when walking. Tics occur frequently during daytime hours, but are diminished or absent during sleep. 10% of boys experience tics at some time during childhood. Tics are slightly less common in girls. Most tics resolve spontaneously.

Tic disorders frequently occur in association with compulsions and attention-deficit hyperactivity disorder. The best known of the tic disorders is **Tourette's syndrome**. It occurs in 4 to 5 children per 10,000 and affects three to four times as many males as females. It is estimated that 100,000 Americans have full-blown Tourette's syndrome. Age of onset is between 2 and 18 years, but over 60% of affected children exhibit their first tics between the ages of 5 to 8 years. Diagnostic criteria for Tourette's syndrome (DSM-IV-TR) are: both multiple motor tics and one or more vocal tics must be present at some time, although not necessarily concurrently; the tics must occur many times a day (usually in bouts) nearly every day or intermittently over more than one year, during which time there must not have been a tic-free period of more than 3 consecutive months; the age of onset must be less than 18 years; and the disturbance must not be due to the direct physiological effects of a substance (e.g. stimulants) or a general medical condition (e.g. Huntington's disease). Mental disorders, especially obsessions, compulsions and attention-deficit hyperactivity disorder, are often associated with Tourette's syndrome. The cause of Tourette's syndrome is unknown, but it is thought to be due to an abnormality in dopamine or other brain neurotransmitters. Tourette's syndrome is inherited as an autosomal dominant trait. Penetrance in female and male gene carriers is approximately 70% and 99%, respectively. There is no cure for Tourette's syndrome, but the condition does improve in many individuals as they mature. Anti-psychotic drugs, such as haloperidol, may help suppress the tics even thought psychosis is not the problem. Haloperidol can cause side effects, such as stiffness, weight gain, blurred vision, sleepiness, and dulled, slowed thinking. People with Tourette's syndrome often have a difficult time in social situations. Individuals with Tourette's syndrome are often drawn to athletics, partly because they have good speed, accuracy and reaction time. A number of accomplished professional sportsmen are known to have Tourette's syndrome, including Jim Eisenreich, the Philadelphia Phillies baseball outfielder.

Transient tic disorder is characterized by single or multiple motor tics, which are brief, repetitive, difficult-to-control movement and/or vocalizations that often resemble nervous mannerisms. Tics must have occurred almost every day for at least 4 weeks, but not have been present for more than a year. The onset is before the age of 18 years. The cause of transient tic disorder can be physical or psychological. It may be a mild variant of Tourette's syndrome.

Chronic motor or vocal tic disorders begin before the age of 18 years and are recurrent, involuntary movements or vocalizations over which the individual appears to have no control. Chronic motor tics may be unilateral or bilateral, and the movement is usually preceded by an urge to make the movements. Chronic motor tics may involve any part of the body including the face, arms, legs, or trunk.

Bibliography

American Psychiatric Association. (2000). *Diagnostic and statistical manual of mental disorders*. 4th ed. Text Revision. Washington, DC: American Psychiatric Association.

Lees, A.J. (1998). Abnormal movement disorder. In Jordan, B., Tsairis, P. and Warren, R.F. (eds). *Sports neurology*. 2nd ed. pp301-308. Philadelphia, PA: Lippincott-Raven.

Tourette Syndrome Association, Inc. Http://tsa.mgh.harvard.edu

TIDAL VOLUME   The volume of gas inspired or expired during each inspiratory cycle. The ratio of **tidal volume to inspiratory capacity** is the ratio of the tidal volume to the air potentially available for that breath. It is measured from the end-expiratory lung volume to the maximum inspiratory volume. *See also under* GROWTH.

TILTING REFLEXES   *See* EQUILIBRIUM REFLEXES.

TIME   The second is a base unit of the Standard International (SI) system. One second (s) is defined in terms of one characteristic frequency of a cesium clock (9,192,631,770 cycles of radiation associated with a specified transition of the cesium-133 atom). The Standard International (SI) units derived from time concern acceleration, frequency, momentum, speed and velocity.

TIMING ACCURACY

Visual-based timing involves making an action coincide with the arrival of an approaching object. **Visual reaction time** is the time between the onset of a visual stimulus and the initiation of an appropriate action.

It has been found that elite cricket batsmen are unable to react to unpredictable movement of the ball in less than about 200 milliseconds. This is similar to the reaction times of normal persons responding to the sudden onset of uncertain visual information. Normal persons can time an action to coincide with the arrival of an approaching object with an accuracy of at least +/-10 milliseconds. This is similar to the accuracy shown by elite sportsmen in some sporting situations.

When the visual scene is moving continuously before the eyes, such as when faced with a flying ball, the eyes fix on one highlight after another in the visual field, jumping from one to the next at a rate of two to three jumps (saccades) per second. The brain suppresses the visual image during the saccades so that one is not conscious of the movements from point to point. The eyes can also remain fixed on a moving object (pursuit movement). With a fast bowler in cricket, the ball takes about 600 ms to reach the batsman. The batsman must therefore select an appropriate trajectory for his bat based on information from the first two thirds of the ball's flight. Batsmen's eye movements monitor the moment when the ball is released, make a predictive saccade to the place where they expect it to hit the ground, wait for it to bounce and then (using smooth pursuit tracking) follow its trajectory for 100 to 200 ms after the bounce (Land and McLeod, 2000). It does not seem necessary to track the ball thereafter. Information provided by these fixations may allow precise prediction of the ball's timing and placement. A short latency for the first saccade appears to distinguish good from poor batsmen. It is also possible that subtle combination of pursuit tracking and saccadic movement as the batsman locates the bounce point is a key factor in distinguishing the expert from the good batsmen.

An important optical variable for timing accuracy is '*tau*,' which would seem to be computed by the central nervous system on the basis of optical flow produced by an approaching object, such as a ball. It indicates the time remaining until the object reaches the plane of the observer's eye. **Optical flow** refers to the movement of the patterns of light rays from the environment over a person's retina. *Tau* is figured as the size of the retinal image divided by the rate of change of the image. The retinal image of an approaching object expands as the object approaches.

The finding that cricket batsmen are not looking at the ball for most of the pre-bounce period, which is when one would expect they would try to obtain early *tau* information, is evidence that *tau* is not used as the main method of determining time of contact between bat and ball.

During the final six strides of a long jump, the elite athlete makes stride-length adjustments so that she can hit the board accurately. Almost 50% of these adjustments are made on the last stride. The visual system picks up time-to-contact information from the board, and directs the locomotor control system to make appropriate stride-length modifications for the strides remaining until contact with the take-off board. *See also* ANTICIPATION.

Bibliography

Land, M.F. and McLeod, P. (2000). From eye movements to actions. *Nature Neuroscience* 3(12), 1340-1345.

Lee, D.N., Lishman, J.R. and Thomson, J.A. (1982). Regulation of gait in long jumping. *Journal of Experimental Psychology: Human Perception and Performance* 8, 448-459.

Magill, R.A. (2004). *Motor learning and control. Concepts and applications*. 7th ed. Boston: MA: McGraw-Hill.

McLeod, P. and Jenkins, S. (1991). Timing accuracy and decision time in high-speed ball games. *International Journal of Sport Psychology* 22(3/4), 279-295.

TINNITUS A persistent ringing or buzzing noise in the ears.

TISSUE A unit of two or more cells. Five categories of tissue are: epithelial tissues; connective tissues; muscle; tissues in the nervous system; and wandering corpuscles of the blood and lymph.

TITIN A giant intramuscular protein, which is

composed of a single chain of more than 27,000 amino acids. It has a molecular weight that is ten times greater than the average protein. It helps to keep the thick filament centered between two Z lines during muscle contraction. Titin is very elastic. *See under* MUSCLE; STRETCHING.

TOBACCO *See under* CARBON MONOXIDE; CIGARETTE SMOKING; NICOTINE; SMOKE-LESS TOBACCO.

TOCOPHEROLS *See* VITAMIN E.

TOCOTRIENOLS *See* VITAMIN E.

TOE NAILS Body structures that protect the toes from pressure on the forefoot and from trauma. The great toe (hallux) is most commonly injured. A chronic force across the soft tissues on either side of the toenail promotes the formation of an in-grown toenail. **In-grown toe nail** is usually caused by ill-fitting shoes pressing against the edge of the nail. **Subungual hematoma** ('black toe') results from hemorrhage between the nail plate and the nail bed secondary to separation of these two structures after repeated contact of the shoe against the nail. It is common among tennis players and skiers, but is becoming less frequent in runners due to increased room in the toe box of the latest-designed shoes. Shoes that permit forward sliding of the foot also predispose an athlete to subungual hematoma.

TOLERABLE UPPER INTAKE LEVELS *See under* DIETARY REFERENCE INTAKE.

TONE *See* MUSCLE TONE.

TONIC Continuous, sustained.

TONIC LABYRINTHINE REFLEX-PRONE A primitive reflex that is normal from birth to 4 months. It is elicited by any change in the position of the head with the result that flexor tone is increased. Failure of this reflex to become integrated leads to abnormal distribution of muscle tone and inability of body segments to move independently of one

another. It compromises any activity done against gravity from a prone position.

TONIC LABYRINTHINE REFLEX-SUPINE A primitive reflex that is normal from birth to 4 months. It is elicited by any change in the position of the head with the result that extensor tone is increased. Failure of this reflex to become integrated leads to domination by extensor tone, which holds the shoulders retracted and prevents or compromises head raising, bringing the limbs to the midline and rotation of the body.

TONIC NECK REFLEX *See* ASYMMETRIC TONIC NECK REFLEX; SYMMETRIC TONIC NECK REFLEX.

TONIC VIBRATION REFLEX An artificial reflex that has both clinical and experimental uses. It is elicited by small-amplitude, high-frequency (50 to 150 Hz) vibration of muscle. It has the same neural circuit as the tendon-tap reflex. It involves the muscle spindle and the homonymous motor units activated by excitation of the muscle spindles. It appears that vibration activates both mono- and polysynaptic pathways. Although vibration produces a reflex response, both tendon-tap (stretch) and H reflexes are depressed during vibration, and prolonged vibration can decrease maximum voluntary contraction force. Vibration of an antagonist muscle can be used to decrease the spasticity in an agonist muscle.

Vibration disrupts the information conveyed by the muscle spindle about muscle length, thus can produce illusions about joint position. For example when the elbow flexor muscles are vibrated at 100 Hz, the elbow joint angle is perceived to be about 10 degrees more extended than it actually is. These illusions are not present when vibration is superimposed on a voluntary contraction.

Bibliography
Enoka, R.M. (2002). *Neuromechanics of human movement*. 3rd ed. Champaign, IL: Human Kinetics.

TONSILS Glands located at the back and sides of

the mouth, comprising lymphatic tissue, but generally have little purpose beyond childhood.

TONUS *See* MUSCLE TONE.

TOOTH *See under* DENTAL INJURIES.

TORQUE Moment of force. Moment. It is the effectiveness of a force to produce rotation about an axis. The force may be centric (acting through the center of gravity), eccentric (not acting through the center of gravity) or it may be a couple. The distance from the pivot point to the point where the force acts is called the **moment arm**. It is the product of moment of inertia and angular acceleration. The Standard International unit is the Newton.meter (N.m).

Torque is produced by muscles when they pull on bones, and the result is rotary (angular) motion of the body segments.

The **magnitude of the torque** depends on the force of muscle contraction and the perpendicular distance between the angle of pull and the axis of the joint. The muscle's **angle of pull** is defined as the angle between the line of action and that portion of the mechanical axis of a bone (or segment) that lies between the point of application of the muscle force and the joint, which acts as the axis. The **mechanical axis of a bone (or segment)** is a straight line that connects the midpoint of the joint at one end with the midpoint of the joint at the other end or, in the case of a terminal segment, with the midpoint of its distal end.

The greater the perpendicular distance between the angle of pull and the axis of the joint, the greater the torque produced for a given force of contraction. The perpendicular distance between the line of action and the axis of the joint depends on the angle of the joint. The size of a muscle's angle of pull changes with every degree of joint motion. As the muscle's angle of pull changes, so do the sizes of the horizontal and vertical components. The **vertical component** is always perpendicular to the lever and is the rotary component. It is the part of the force that moves the lever. The **horizontal component** is parallel to the lever and is the non-rotational component. It does not contribute to the lever's movement. The angle of pull of most muscles in the resting position is less than 90 degrees, and it usually remains so during the movement. This means that the non-rotary component of force is directed toward the axis, which gives it a stabilizing effect. It pulls the bone lengthways toward the joint. When the angle of pull is 90 degrees, the force is completely rotary. When it is 45 degrees, the rotary and stabilizing (non-rotary) components are equal. The muscle's angle of pull usually remains less than 45 degrees, thus more of the muscle's force serves to stabilize the joint than to move the lever. There are some muscles (e.g. *coracobrachialis*) whose angles of pull are always so small that their rotary component would seem to be negligible. Using trigonometry to determine the components of muscular force, the hypotenuse coincides with a portion of the muscle's line of pull, and the adjacent side coincides with the mechanical axis of the bone into which the muscle is inserted.

The sum of two or more torques may result in no motion, linear motion or rotational motion. The **principle of torques (summation of moments)** states that the resultant torques of a force system must be equal to the sum of the torques of the individual forces of the system about the same point. **Clockwise moments** are negative; **counterclockwise moments** are positive. When the sum of counterclockwise torques equals the sum of clockwise torques, no rotation will occur. When the sum of clockwise torques does not equal the sum of the counterclockwise torques, the torque will be the difference between the two sets of opposing forces and will be in the direction of the larger.

The further a tendon is inserted from the center of a joint, the greater the torque that can be generated around the joint, because the muscle force acts through a longer moment arm. This entails a greater mechanical advantage, but with a loss of maximum speed.

See also COUPLE; ISOKINETIC MOVEMENT; LEVER.

Bibliography

Hamilton, N. and Luttgens, K. (2002). *Kinesiology. Scientific basis of human motion*. 10th ed. Madison, WI: Brown & Benchmark.

TORSION It is deformation of a structure, such as a bar, which occurs because of a torque about the longitudinal axis of the structure. If torque is applied about the longitudinal axis at opposite ends of a bar, then twisting will occur. Shearing stresses act throughout the entire structure on planes that are perpendicular to the longitudinal axis. As in bending, the magnitude of these stresses is proportional to their distance from the neutral axis. The farther the stresses are from the neutral axis, the higher their magnitude.

Torsional rigidity is the ratio of the torque about the centroidal axis of a bar (e.g. shaft) at one end of the bar to the resulting torsional angle. The **torsional angle** is the total relative rotation of the ends of a bar when subjected to a torque. **Torsional modulus** is the ratio of the torsional rigidity of a bar to its length. *See under* FRACTURE.

TORSIONAL MISALIGNMENTS Misalignments that occur when one segment is rotated about its longitudinal axis relative to the next adjacent segment.

See FEMORAL TORSION; TIBIAL TORSION.

TORTICOLLIS Wry neck. It is presentation of the neck in a twisted or bent position. The Latin word 'torti' means twisted and 'collies' means neck. It is characterized by involuntary contractions of the neck, leading to abnormal postures and movements of the head. Torticollis is a symptom as well as a disease, and there are many underlying pathologies.

Acute torticollis develops overnight in young and middle-aged adults and manifests itself as painful neck spasms. Cervical muscle spasm is visible and palpable. Symptoms usually resolve spontaneously within two weeks.

Spasmodic torticollis (cervical dystonia) is the most common of the focal dystonias. It is characterized by involuntary contraction of the neck muscles, causing abnormal movements and posture of the head and neck. It is thought to be due to abnormal functioning of the basal ganglia. It affects 3 in every 10,000 people in the USA, where approximately 90,000 people are known to be sufferers. It is more common in women than men. Cases of inherited spasmodic torticollis have been reported, usually in conjunction with early-onset generalized dystonia, which is associated with the DYT1 gene. Spasmodic torticollis generally appears very slowly, usually with a small pain in the base of the neck and/or a stiff neck followed, over a period of time, by rotating or pulling sensations. The hand may have to be used to alleviate the pain and/or control the pulling. This is known as an **antagonistic gesture**. There are three distinct varieties of spasmodic torticollis: tonic (in which the head turns to one side), clonic (which involves shaking of the head) and mixed (which involves both turning and shaking). The turning of the head is generally considered to fall into one of four categories: rotational (in which the head turns to one side or the other), laterocollis (in which the head is pulled toward the shoulder), retrocollis (in which the head is pulled to the back) or anterocollis (in which the head is pulled forward). For most people, spasmodic torticollis involves a combination of turning movements from the four categories. Ramisectomy and rhizotomy are surgical techniques that involve cutting the nerve or nerves supplying overactive muscles, but are now usually used only for spasmodic torticollis patients who have developed resistance to botulinum toxin injections. Myobloc™, a type B toxin, is antigenically distinct from Botox®, a type A toxin. Patients who become non-responsive to one of the toxins can now switch to the other and, in most cases, realize an improvement in their symptoms. *See also* ATLANTO-OCCIPITAL FUSION.

Bibliography
National Spasmodic Torticollis Association. Http://www.torti-collis.org

ST/Dystonia, Inc. Http://www.spasmodictorticollis.org

TOUCH *See under* MECHANORECEPTORS.

TOUGHNESS 'Fracture energy.' 'Work of fracture.' It is a measure of the amount of energy that a material can absorb prior to failure (such as fracture). The greater the energy absorption, the greater is the toughness. **Absorbed strain energy** is the area of the stress-strain curve under the plastic range, between the elastic limit and the breaking point. **Toughness modulus**, usually measured by an impact test, is defined as strain energy absorbed per unit volume of the material prior to failure.

Toughness is closely related to the concepts of ductility and brittleness. **Ductile materials** deform extensively before fracture; the yield point is just beyond the elastic limit and deformation increases without any increase in force at this point. Unlike ductile materials, **brittle materials** are not capable of withstanding large strains. *See also* MENTAL TOUGHNESS.

TOURETTE'S SYNDROME *See under* TIC.

TOXOPLASMOSIS A disease caused by the protozoan parasite *Toxoplasma gondii*, which can produce a variety of syndromes in humans (though most adults have no symptoms). If a woman is exposed to the parasite for the first time during pregnancy, the effects that it will have on her and the baby will depend on how advanced the pregnancy is. During the first three months, it is unlikely that a woman will pass the parasite on to her developing fetus. A woman in the third trimester of pregnancy is most likely to pass on toxoplasmosis to her baby, but the parasite is least likely to cause serious birth defects such as hydrocephalus. The fetus does not have the ability to make antibodies that are carried by infected humans. If a pregnant woman contracts toxoplasmosis, there is a 40% chance that her unborn child will also become infected. In the USA, 1 to 2 out of 1,000 infants are infected. Spores of *Toxoplasma gondii* are passed in the feces of cats infected by mice and can be inhaled or ingested. The parasite reproduces in the cat's intestine, and a form of the parasite ends up in the cat's litter box, sand or soil. This form of parasite become infectious within days and is resistant to most disinfectants. Infected cats usually appear healthy. Women are therefore advised to avoid contact with cats during pregnancy.
See also TERATOGEN.

TRACE ELEMENTS *See under* MINERALS.

TRACHEA Windpipe. It is a broad tube that connects the larynx to the bronchi. The trachea divides into two bronchi, one for each lung.

TRACTION *See* TENSION.

TRAGION An anatomical landmark that is the notch superior to the flap (tragus) of the ear at the superior aspect of the zygomatic bone.

TRAINING A deliberate scheme to assist learning and/or improve physical fitness. Four principles of training are specificity, individual differences, overload and reversibility. The **specificity principle** states that adaptations to training depend on the type of overload imposed; specific exercise elicits specific adaptations to training, thus creating specific training effects. Specificity can be stated as the SAID principle (specific adaptation to imposed demands). The **individual differences principle** states that the benefits to be gained from training are optimized when programs are set to meet the needs and capacities of a particular individual. The **overload principle** states that by exercising at a level above that which the individual has experienced before, a number of training adaptations occur to enable the body to function more efficiently. Overload can be achieved by changing frequency, intensity or duration. Variation is a component of the overload principle and involves manipulating the variables of overload. The **reversibility principle** states that the effects of training are transient and reversible.

See also AEROBIC TRAINING; CROSS TRAINING; FLEXIBILITY; INTERVAL TRAINING; PERIODIZATION; POWER; RESISTANCE TRAINING; SPEED; TAPERING; TRAINING FOR DISTANCE RUNNING.

TRAINING FOR DISTANCE RUNNING Four types of training for endurance performance are described by Hawley et al. (1997): base/foundation; transition, pace/tempo; and speed/power training.
Base/foundation training should be performed for several months during the non-competitive period of an athlete's macro-cycle. The primary emphasis is the establishment of a sound endurance base gained through prolonged (greater than an hour), moderate-intensity (70% of maximal oxygen uptake) workouts. **Transition training** should be performed twice per week for 2 to 4

weeks immediately following the base phase. The aim is to expose the power systems to sustained exercise at an intensity corresponding to the athlete's highest current steady-state pace.

Pace/tempo training is normally undertaken after the athlete has established a solid endurance base, and typically consists of sustained exercise sessions at an intensity of around 85% of maximal oxygen uptake, alternated with short rest intervals of activity at a slower pace. The benefits of pace/tempo training include enhancement of lactate kinetics, stimulation of the specific neurological patterns of muscle fiber recruitment needed during race pace, improved fatigue resistance, and enhanced athletic performance. **Speed/power training** should be performed up to three times per week during the final 14 to 21 days before a major competition. During these sessions, the athlete undertakes 'supra-maximal' efforts at speeds faster than planned race pace. It is a form of interval training. For distance running, it might involve 30 to 90 seconds running at a speed of five seconds per 400 m faster than race pace, with a work-to-recovery ratio of 1 to 5. The goal is to improve running economy and increase running speed.

It seems that maximal oxygen uptake is not compromised when resistance training is added to an endurance program. Improvements in lactate threshold have been observed in untrained individuals as a result of resistance training, but it is unlikely that it would be improved in trained distance runners. Trained distance runners have shown improvements of up to 8% in running economy following a period of resistance training. Concurrent strength and endurance training induces increases in both muscular strength and aerobic power. This type of training, however, interferes with optimal development of muscular strength, but does not affect optimal development of aerobic power. Strength training and endurance should be conducted sequentially, with strength training preceding endurance training. *See also* PERIODIZATION.

Bibliography

Burke, E.R. (1998, ed). *Precision heart rate training*. Champaign, IL: Human Kinetics.

Daniels, J. (1989). Training distance runners: A primer. *Gatorade Sports Science Exchange* 1(11).

Dudley, G.A. and Fleck, S.J. (1987). Strength and endurance training. Are they mutually exclusive? *Sports Medicine* 4, 79-85.

Hawley, J.A. et al. (1997). Training techniques to improve fatigue resistance and enhance endurance performance. *Journal of Sports Sciences* 15, 325-333.

Hawley, J. and Burke, L. (1998). *Peak performance: Training and nutritional strategies for sport*. Sydney: Allen & Unwin.

Janssen, P. (2001). *Lactate threshold training*. Champaign, IL: Human Kinetics.

Jung, A.P. (2003). The impact of resistance training on distance running performance. *Sports Medicine* 33(7), 539-552.

Martin, D. and Coe, P. (1997). *Better training for distance runners*. Champaign, IL: Human Kinetics.

TRAIT Any aspect of appearance, behavior, development, biochemistry, or other feature of an organism. In psychology, it refers more specifically to a person's predisposition to behave in a predictable way. *See under* ANXIETY; PERSONALITY.

TRANQUILIZERS *See under* DEPRESSANTS.

TRANSAMINASE A class of enzymes that transfer amino groups from one compound to another.

TRANSAMINATION *See under* AMINO ACID DEGRADATION.

TRANSCRIPTION *See under* PROTEIN SYNTHESIS.

TRANSDUCER An instrument that transforms energy from one form to another.

TRANSFERASES *See under* ENZYMES.

TRANSFER OF LEARNING *See* MOTOR LEARNING, TRANSFER OF.

TRANSFERRIN *See under* IRON.

TRANSIENT ISCHEMIC ATTACK *See under* STROKE.

TRANSLATION *See under* LINEAR MOTION; PROTEIN SYNTHESIS.

TRANSPORT   See ACTIVE TRANSPORT; PASSIVE TRANSPORT.

TRANSPOSITION   Displacement to the opposite side. In genetics, it is the nonreciprocal insertion of material deleted from one chromosome into another, nonhomologous chromosome.

TRANSPULMONARY PRESSURE   Pressure across the lungs. It is the pressure difference between the airways and the pleural space. It is equal to the difference between intrapulmonary pressure and intrapleural pressure. Intrapleural pressure is an actual or potential space between the visceral pleural membrane covering the lungs and the somatic pleural membrane lining the thoracic wall.

TRANSVERSE PLANE   See under PLANES.

TRANSVERSE TARSAL JOINT   See MID-TARSAL JOINTS.

TRAPEZIOMETACARPAL JOINT   See under CARPOMETACARPAL JOINTS.

TRAPEZIUM   Multangum major. One of the carpal bones in the distal row.

TRAPEZOID   Multangum minor. One of the carpal bones in the distal row.

TRAUMA   See under INJURY.

TRAUMATIC BRAIN INJURY   See under HEAD INJURIES.

TREADMILL   A mechanical device in which a moving belt, driven by a motor, allows walking and running to be performed. The speed and gradient can be varied. Work rate must be estimated from body weight, speed and gradient. Values for maximum oxygen uptake tend to be about 5 to 10% lower when bicycle ergometers are used instead of treadmills. Movement artifacts present more of a problem with treadmills than cycle ergometers. Nevertheless, treadmills are frequently used in exercise testing, especially for people who are unable to cycle. See also BICYCLE ERGOMETER.

TREMOR   An involuntary, rhythmic, shaking movement produced when muscles repeatedly contract and relax. **Physiologic tremor** is the normal tremor found in each person; it is usually too slight to be noticed. **Action tremors** occur when the muscles are active. **Resting tremors** occur when the muscles are resting. **Intention tremors** occur when a person makes a purposeful movement, especially in people who have a disease of the cerebellum or its connections. **Essential tremors** are tremors that usually begin in early adulthood, slowly become more obvious, and have no known cause. **Senile tremors** are essential tremors that begin in older people. **Familial tremors** are essential tremors that occur in families. Essential tremors usually remain mild, but may affect handwriting and make it difficult to use utensils. Essential tremors generally cease when the arms or legs are at rest. Many drugs, especially those for asthma and emphysema, can worsen an essential tremor. Drinking alcohol in moderation may decrease essential tremor in some people, but heavy drinking and alcohol withdrawal can make the tremor worse. Treatment is not usually required for essential tremor, but beta- blockers such as propranolol may be prescribed.

Bibliography
The Merck Manual. Http://www.merck.com

TRIANGULAR FIBROCARTILAGENOUS CARTILAGE COMPLEX   A small meniscus resting on the ulnar side of the wrist. It serves as a site of connection of ligaments as well as a cushion between the carpal bones and the end of the forearm. It is analogous to the meniscus within the knee and can be injured in a similar fashion when the complex is compressed and then a shear force is applied to it.

Tears of the triangular fibrocartilagenous cartilage complex may occur as a result of swinging a bat, throwing a ball of any type, and any sport such as gymnastics that involve loading of the wrist. When this complex is torn or damaged, there is usually pain on the ulnar side of the wrist (especially during pronation and supination of the forearm). Damage to the complex may occur also as a consequence of a distal radius fracture.

TRICARBOXYLIC ACID CYCLE   *See* KREBS CYCLE.

TRICEPS BRACHII REFLEX   The tendon of the *triceps brachii* muscle is tapped with a reflex hammer just above the elbow. This stretches *triceps brachii* muscle and it should respond by reflexively contracting.

TRICEPS SURAE REFLEX   *See* ACHILLES TENDON REFLEX.

TRICYCLIC ANTI-DEPRESSANTS   *See under* DEPRESSION.

TRIGGER FINGER   Locking of the finger or thumb in the flexed position at the interphalangeal joint. The fibrous sheath is thickened at the base of a finger or thumb, usually causing 'triggering,' but sometimes just pain or difficulty in bending the digit.

TRIGGER POINT   An area of tenderness in a tight band of muscle, most typically in the neck, upper back or lower back. Pain is produced by pressure on the trigger point and radiates away from the point of pressure. In athletes, trigger points develop most often because of some mechanical stress to muscle.

TRIGLYCERIDE   *See under* FAT.

TRIIDOTHYRONINE   *See under* THYROID GLAND.

TRIQUETRAL BONE   Os triquetrum. Cuneiform. One of the carpal bones in the proximal row.

TRISOMIC   Of, or relating to, the chromosome state in which each of the various chromosomes, except the sex chromosome, is represented twice.

TRISOMY-X SYNDROME   Triple X syndrome. Females with the karyotype 47, XXX have three X chromosomes instead of the usual two. The mutation occurs in 1 in every 1,000 to 3,000 newborn girls, but it is often not diagnosed until later in life. It is the most common X-chromosome disorder in females. One consistent feature is tall stature. Some females exhibit no or very few symptoms. There are wide individual differences in other signs and symptoms, but these can include small head, speech and language delays, learning disabilities, delayed development of certain motor skills, seizures, delayed puberty and infertility. Mental retardation rarely occurs.

Bibliography
National Association for Rare Diseases. Http://www.rarediseases.org

TROCHANTER   Tuberosity. Tubercle. It is a prominence on a bone where tendons insert.

TROCHANTERIC BURSITIS   *See under* HIP JOINT, BURSITIS.

TROCHANTERION   An anatomical landmark that is the most superior point on the greater trochanter of the femur.

TROPOMYOSIN   *See under* MUSCLE CONTRACTION.

TROPONIN   *See under* MUSCLE CONTRACTION.

TRYPTOPHAN   An essential, eleven-carbon amino acid. It is both glucogenic (glycogenic) and ketogenic, because when degraded for energy some of its carbons are incorporated in alanine and some in acetoacetyl CoA. It is a precursor of a number of significant compounds, e.g. serotonin. *See also under* AMINO ACIDS.

TUBERCLE   *See* TROCHANTER.

TUBEROSITY   *See* TROCHANTER.

TUBEROUS SCLEROSIS Tuberous sclerosis complex. It is a neurologic disorder of infancy and childhood. It is characterized by hard little bumps on the nose and cheeks that resemble acne. These bumps are also scattered through the brain, heart and other organs. It can cause seizures and hemiparesis. Disorders commonly found with tuberous sclerosis include autism, Asperger's syndrome, attention-deficit hyperactivity disorder and mental retardation.

An estimated 1 in 7,000 of the population are affected by tuberous sclerosis. It is inherited as an autosomal dominant trait. Mutations in the TSC1 and TSC2 genes cause tuberous sclerosis. The TSC1 gene makes a protein called hamartin, and TSC2 produces a protein called tuberin. These two proteins function together in cells to regulate and prevent the overgrowth of cells into tumors. When either the TSC1 or TSC2 gene is mutated, nonfunctional versions of hamartin or tuberin are made in the cell. As a result, the hamartin-tuberin protein complex does not form and cells divide too frequently, leading to the formation of noncancerous tumors. Approximately one third of the mutations in the TSC1 or TSC2 genes are inherited from a parent who has the condition. Approximately two thirds of cases arise as new (de novo) mutations. A new mutation means that neither parent has the altered gene, but the affected individual could pass it on to his or her children. Most new mutations involve the TSC2 gene.

Bibliography

Genetics Home Reference. Http://ghr.nlm.nih.gov/ghr
Tuberous Sclerosis Association. Http://www.tuberous-sclerosis.org

TUMOR *See* NEOPLASM.

TUMOR NECROSIS FACTOR A pro-inflammatory cytokine that is produced by monocytes and macrophages. It has an anti-neoplastic effect, but causes inflammation.
See under ARTHRITIS.

TURF TOE A sprain of the plantar-capsular-ligamentous complex of the 1st metatarsophalangeal joint related to two predisposing factors: hard, artificial surfaces and soft-soled, flexible shoes. The plantar-capsular-ligamentous complex is made up of collateral ligaments, the plantar plate, and the *flexor hallucis brevis*, *adductor brevis* and *abductor hallucis* muscles. The plantar plate is a strong, fibrous structure firmly attached to the proximal phalanx and loosely attached to the metatarsal neck through the joint capsule. It blends with the sesamoids and tendons of the *flexor hallucis brevis* muscle to provide structural support. The 1st hallux (great toe) typically bears twice the load of the lesser toes and, during normal gait, it withstands 40% to 60% of the body weight. This load increases several-fold with running or jumping, and it may approach nearly 8-times body weight with a running jump.

Severity of turf toe injury ranges from minor tearing of the capsuloligamentous structure to compression fracture of the metatarsal head or an avulsion fracture with a complete tear of the capsuloligamentous structures. Up to 50% of athletes with turf toe injuries have persistent symptoms after 5 years. In the short term, running and pushing off are compromised, and players frequently miss games and practice.

It occurs commonly in football, especially in linemen, and is caused by hyperextension of the 1st metatarsophalangeal joint during a rapid and explosive push-off. Further hyperextension of the metatarsophalangeal joint can occur when another player lands on the back of the athlete's foot.

Prior to the advent of artificial playing surfaces in the late 1960s, sprains to the 1st metatarsophalangeal joint were relatively uncommon. Artificial grass contains a higher coefficient of friction, which places the forefoot at greater risk to become fixed to the playing surface. Thus, the forefoot becomes more prone to an external force that places the 1st metatarsophalangeal joint in a position of extreme dorsal flexion. A softer, soccer-style shoe replaced the traditional multicleated shoe containing a steel plate in the forefoot that was designed for grass surfaces. This shoe allowed a greater degree of motion in the metatarsophalangeal joints and placed significantly more stress across the forefoot.

Turf toe is not limited to hyperextension of the metatarsophalangeal joint. Several variations have been described that account for damage to specific anatomic structures in the capsular ligamentous-sesamoid complex. These include hyperflexion, and valgus- and varus-type injuries. Hyperflexion occurs when the metatarsophalangeal joint is forced into exaggerated plantar flexion. This injury has been referred to as **sand toe**, as this injury often occurs in beach volleyball. This injury has also been known to occur in football players and dancers. A plantar foot with the metatarsophalangeal joints driven into hyperflexion can result in tearing of the dorsal capsule. Valgus injury is a variant of the dorsal flexion-type injury in which the medial ligamentous structures and, in some cases, the medial sesamoid are damaged. This most often occurs in the setting of push-off, when internal rotation occurs on a fixed forefoot. Untreated, this may lead to bunion formation and contractures on the lateral side of the joint. Varus injury may result from external rotation on a fixed forefoot, with varus instability resulting from a torn lateral capsule as well as rupture of the *adductor hallucis* tendon from the base of the proximal phalanx.

Bibliography

Bowers, K.D. and Martin, R.B. (1976). Turf-toe: A shoe-surface related football injury. *Medicine and Science in Sports and Exercise* 8(2), 81-83.

Ohlson, B. and O'Connor, P.L. (2003). Turf toe. Http://emedicine.com

TURNER'S SYNDROME The clinical features of human females with the karyotype 45, X. It is caused by a division failure that results in only one X instead of the XX or XY chromosome pair in normal cells. Turner's syndrome affects approximately 1 out of every 2,500 female live births. It results in short stature (less than 5 feet), appearance of a short neck because of a lower posterior hairline and/or cervical webbing, a broad chest with widely spaced nipples, and failure to menstruate and mature sexually. The short stature in Turner syndrome is partially due to the loss of SHOX gene on the X chromosome. The SHOX gene is important for long bone growth. The loss of the SHOX gene may also explain some of the skeletal features found in Turner syndrome, such as short fingers and toes, and irregular rotations of the wrist and elbow joints. Girls with Turner syndrome are treated with estrogen to induce breast development and other features of puberty if menses has not occurred by the age of 15 years at the latest. Girls and women should be maintained on estrogen-progesterone treatment to maintain their secondary sexual development and to protect their bones from osteoporosis until at least the usual age of menopause (50 years).

5% to 10% of children with Turner syndrome are found to have a severe constriction ('coarctation') of the aorta. Up to 15% of adults with Turner syndrome are reported to have 'bicuspid aortic valves,' i.e. the aorta with two rather than three components to the valve regulating blood flow. Individuals with Turner syndrome have twice the risk of Type 2 diabetes than the general population. About a third of individuals with Turner syndrome have a thyroid disorder, usually hypothyroidism (the symptoms of which include decreased energy). Girls and women with Turner syndrome may have difficulty with specific visual-spatial coordination tasks, such as mentally rotating objects in space. Some girls and women with Turner syndrome experience difficulty with memory and motor coordination; these problems may be related to estrogen deficiency. *See also* NOONAN SYNDROME.

Bibliography

Turner Syndrome Society of the United States. Http://www.turner-syndrome-us.org

TURNOVER The balance between rate of production and rate of removal of metabolites (such as lactate) from tissues.

TWITCH *See* MUSCLE TWITCH.

TYROSINE A non-essential, nine-carbon amino acid that is a precursor of a number of important molecules including the catecholamines. It is both ketogenic and glucogenic (glycogenic) because when degraded for energy, four of its carbons enter the Krebs cycle as fumarate and four enter via acetoacetyl CoA.

U

UBIQUINONES Lipid-soluble quinone derivatives. The predominant form of ubiquinone in humans is ubiquinone-10 (coenzyme Q_{10}) and it is produced by the liver.

The major sources of ubiquinone-10 in the diet are soybean oil, meats, fish, nuts, wheat germ and vegetables (e.g. spinach). Approximately 14 to 32% of ubiquinone-10 is lost during frying, but the ubiquinone-10 content of vegetables and eggs does not change when boiled. Beef (3 oz, fried) contains 2.6 mg and peanuts (roasted, 1 oz) contain 0.8 mg of ubiquinone-10.

As a nutritional supplement, it has been used in the treatment of cardiovascular disease because of its role in oxidative metabolism. It has been found to increase oxygen uptake and improve exercise performance in cardiac patients.

There is some evidence that ubiquinone levels are lower in trained athletes compared to sedentary individuals, and that ingestion of oral supplements containing ubiquinone increases tissue levels. It has been suggested that ubiquinone may have potential as an ergogenic aid for endurance athletes, but there is no scientific evidence to support this.

Ubiquinones appear to act as antioxidants, and it may protect cardiac tissue from damage associated with inadequate oxygen. Reduced forms of ubiquinones are much better antioxidants. Ubiquinones react with reactive oxygen species to prevent lipid peroxidation in membranes and other lipid structures in the cell. Some ubiquinones play an important role in the recycling of vitamin E during periods of oxidative stress via an NADPH-dependent system. Ubiquinone supplementation, however, may actually be detrimental, because it may induce free radical formation, cell membrane lipid peroxidation and damage to the mitochondria.

Primary ubiquinone deficiency is probably due to mutations in nuclear genes that encode enzymes, which are involved in ubiquinone biosynthesis. It causes exercise intolerance and recurrent myoglobinuria, usually in conjunction with brain symptoms, such as seizures or cerebellar ataxia.

Bibliography

DiMauro, S. (1999). Exercise intolerance and the mitochondrial respiratory chain. *Italian Journal of Neurological Science* 20(6), 387-393.

Oregon State University. The Linus Pauling Institute. Micronutrient Information Center. Http://lpi.oregonstate.edu/infocenter

Powers, S.K. et al. (2004). Dietary antioxidants and exercise. *Journal of Sports Sciences* 22, 81-94.

ULNAR COLLATERAL LIGAMENT i) A ligament that holds the proximal phalanx of the thumb to the metacarpal. ii) *See under* ELBOW JOINT, THROWING INJURIES.

ULNAR NERVE The terminal direct branch of the medial cord, i.e. the 8th cervical to 1st thoracic (C8-T1) roots of the brachial plexus. The nerve travels down the medial aspect of the arm in close proximity to the median nerve. Coursing posteriorly in the distal arm, it passes against the medial head of the triceps and an overlying fascial structure, the **arcade of Struthers**, which is anatomically present in about 70% of people. The nerve passes behind the medial epicondyle of the elbow in the ulnar groove and enters the forearm under the proximal portion of the *flexor carpi ulnaris* muscle. A ligamentous/fibrous arch (the **arcuate ligament**) between the two heads of the *flexor carpi ulnaris* overlies the ulnar nerve, forming the **cubital tunnel**. The nerve travels down the forearm underneath the *flexor carpi ulnaris* lying on top of the *flexor digitorum profundus* muscle. The ulnar nerve innervates both the *flexor carpi ulnaris* and the *flexor digitorum profundus* to the 3rd and 4th fingers proximally in the forearm. The ulnar nerve has two sensory branches: the palmar cutaneous nerve approximately 8 to 10 cm from the wrist and the dorsal cutaneous nerve 5 to 6 cm from the wrist. The ulnar nerve proper then travels through Guyton's canal. The ulnar nerve innervates the musculature of the hypothenar eminence along with both palmar and dorsal interossei and the lumbricals to the third and fourth fingers within the hand. Injury to the ulnar nerve most commonly occurs at the elbow region.

'**Funny bone**' refers to the transient sensation of numbness and tingling that is experienced when the elbow is struck on its posteromedial aspect. The ulnar nerve is violently compressed against the humerus, causing a temporary blockage of the flow of nerve impulses.

See also BOWLER'S THUMB; CUBITAL TUNNEL SYNDROME; GUYTON'S TUNNEL SYNDROME.

ULNAR TUNNEL SYNDROME *See* GUYTON'S TUNNEL SYNDROME.

ULNOCARPAL ABUTMENT SYNDROME *See under* WRIST JOINT, FRACTURES.

ULTRA Beyond a certain limit or more than the normal range.

ULTRAVIOLET LIGHT UV light. It is radiant energy of wavelength smaller or shorter than those at the visible end of the spectrum and longer than 1 nm. UV-A is the wave band comprising radiation between 320 and 400 nm. UV-B is 280 to 320; and UV-C is 100 to 280 nm.

UNCIFORM *See* HAMATE BONE.

UNILATERAL Confined to one side only.

UNITS The base dimensions of the **Système Internationale d'Unités (SI system)** are mass (kg), length (m), time (sec) and temperature (K). The SI system is the internationally accepted system, but many other units continue in regular use. US customary units (more commonly known in the USA as English units) are the non-metric units of measurement that are presently used in the USA.

The seven **base units** of the SI system, with their symbols are (physical quantities in parentheses): meter, m (length); second, s (time); kilogram, kg (mass); ampere, A (electric current), kelvin, K (thermodynamic temperature), candela, cd (luminous intensity); and mole, mol (amount of substance). One of the **supplementary units** of the SI

system is the radian, rad (plane angle). Some of the **derived units** of the SI system are: hertz, Hz (frequency); newton, N (force, weight); joule, J (work, energy, quantity of heat); pascal, Pa (pressure, stress); watt, W (power); and volt, V (electric potential difference). Some of the SI units with **compound names** are: square meter, m^2 (area); cubic meter, m^3 (volume); meter per second, m/s (speed, velocity); meter per second squared, m/s^2 (acceleration); kilogram per cubic meter, kg/m^3 (density); and newton meter, N.m (moment of force). Some of the units that may be used with the SI system are: minute, min (time); hour, h (time); day, d (time); degree, ° (plane angle); metric ton, t (mass); liter, l (volume); kilometer per hour, km/h (speed); degree Celsius, °C (temperature); and revolution per minute, r/min (rotational frequency).

UPPER RESPIRATORY TRACT INFECTIONS Most upper respiratory tract infections are viral nasopharyngeal infections that will improve in 7 to 10 days with symptomatic treatment. The **common cold** is most often caused by one of several hundred rhinoviruses, but coronaviruses or the respiratory synctial virus may also lead to infection. Other viruses, such as influenza, parainfluenza and adenoviruses, may produce respiratory symptoms, but these are often associated with pneumonia, fever or chills. Adenoviruses cause high fever, significant pharyngeal erythema and swelling (associated with conjunctivitis 50% of the time). Significant pharyngeal pain and vesiculation are common with herpes simplex or coxsackievirus.

Group A streptococcus is responsible for up to 20% of acute pharngitis cases during its peak incidence in winter through early spring. Classic symptoms include significant sore throat, fever and tender anterior cervical lymphadenopathy. Nearly half of patients with symptoms will not have Group A streptococcus. For confirmed cases of Group A streptococcus pharyngitis, athletes should be restricted from participation until they are afebrile and have been taking antibiotics for 24 hours.

Classic presenting symptoms of Epstein-Barr virus include sore throat with tonsillar hypertrophy and exudates, significant lymphadenopathy and fatigue. Some athletes also complain of left-sided abdominal discomfort from splenomegaly. If splenic rupture occurs, it usually does so between weeks 2 and 4 of infectious mononucleosis. The reported incidence of splenic rupture is 1 in 1,000 cases. Athletes are generally restricted from training and competition for 3 to 4 weeks. Return to collision sports should be delayed for 4 to 6 weeks.

Colds occur in a seasonal pattern that usually begins in mid-September and concludes in late April to early May. The common cold is quite contagious and the two most likely methods of transmission are hand contact with infectious secretions and inoculation through hand contact with the eyes or nose. Viruses can be spread directly through aerolized droplets. Upper respiratory symptoms usually begin 1 to 2 days after exposure and generally last 1 to 2 weeks, but viral shedding can continue for 2 to 3 more weeks. On average, adults have 2 to 4 colds each year, with most occurring during the winter. Athletes who train in close quarters are susceptible to upper respiratory tract infections. Cleaning shared equipment between users and improving ventilation can help prevent the spread of infection.

Colds can sometimes lead to more serious secondary bacterial infections, such as bacterial sinusitis; or lower respiratory involvement, such as bronchitis or pneumonia. It is not known whether exercise training, per se, increases the risk of acquiring such secondary infections. Some athletes suffering from a cold actually feel better when they exercise. This may be due to an increase in mucous flow. The general consensus among physicians who regularly treat athletes with colds is that it is safe to exercise, as long as the symptoms are located above the neck (runny nose, sneezing, scratchy throat). Exercise should be avoided if there are below-the-neck symptoms such as fever, pharyngeal swelling sufficient to cause airway compromise, and a bad cough with sputum production. It could be argued, however, that any exercise during a cold should be avoided, because the quality of training is compromised and overtraining is possible.

Athletes engaged in moderate regular training appear to have increased resistance to infection, while those engaged in heavy training are more susceptible to infection. During the week following the 1987 Los Angeles marathon race, 12.9% of the marathon competitors reported sickness, compared with only 2.2% of control runners who did participate. Runners training more than 96 km per week doubled their chance for sickness compared with those training less than 32 km per week. *See also* IMMUNITY.

Bibliography

Heath, G.W., Macera, C.A. and Nieman, D.C. (1992). Exercise and upper respiratory tract infections. Is there a relationship? *Sports Medicine* 14(6), 353-365.

Koenig, D. et al. (2000). Upper respiratory tract infection in athletes: Influence of lifestyle, type of sport, training effort, and immunostimulant intake. *Exercise Immunology Review* 6, 102-120.

Nieman, D.C. et al. (1990). Infectious episodes in runners before and after the Los Angeles Marathon. *Journal of Sports Medicine and Physical Fitness* 30, 316-328.

O'Kane, J.W. (2002). Upper respiratory infection. Helpful steps for physicians. *The Physician and Sportsmedicine* 30(9). Http://www.physsportmed.com

Peters, E.M. (1997). Exercise, immunology and upper respiratory tract infections. *International Journal of Sports Medicine* 18(1), S69-S77.

Swain, R.A. and Kaplan, B. (1998). Upper respiratory infections: Treatment selection for active patients. *The Physician and Sportsmedicine* 26(2), 85-96.

Thornton, J.S. (1990). Common concerns about the common cold. *The Physician and Sportsmedicine* 18(6), 120-126.

White, J. (1994). Can colds kill athletes? *The Physician and Sportsmedicine* 22(6), 23.

URACIL A nitrogenous, pyrimidine base found in RNA.

UREA An end product of protein breakdown and the major nitrogenous constituent of urine, representing 60 to 90% of the total nitrogen excreted in a 24-hour period.

See also ENERGY YIELD OF NUTRIENTS; URIC ACID.

UREA CYCLE A cycle of five main reactions taking place in the liver that prepares toxic ammonia for safe travel through the blood and then excretion by the kidney. It leads to the production of urea. It is called a cycle because the amino acid ornithine is continually regenerated to continue the series of reactions.

URIC ACID   A complex nitrogen-containing organic compound that is the major excretory product of the breakdown of amino acids. *See also* GOUT.

URICOSURIA   Excessive amounts of uric acid in the urine.

URINARY INCONTINENCE   Inability to control micturition voluntarily. It affects 5% of the population; 8% of women and 3% of men. Urinary incontinence may be urge, overflow, functional, or stress incontinence.

Urge incontinence (detrusor hyper-reflexia) is caused by detrusor overactivity. It accounts for 40 to 70% of urinary incontinence. Patients with urge incontinence have early, forceful detrusor contractions, well before the bladder is full. Detrusor overactivity may be found in conditions of defective central nervous system inhibition or increased afferent sensory stimulation from the bladder. Disorders that impair the ability of the central nervous system to send inhibitory signals include aneurysm, hemorrhage, multiple sclerosis, Parkinson's disease, stroke and tumors. Urge incontinence may be treated through behavior therapy consisting of bladder retraining. Acetylcholine medication (e.g. oxybutinin hydrochloride) may be used to suppress early contraction of the detrusor muscle.

Overflow incontinence occurs when urine dribbles from the urethra whenever the bladder overfills. **Urinary retention** occurs when the bladder is unable to expel its contained urine. It is generally due to a bladder with contractile dysfunction (hypotonic/atonic bladder) or obstructed urinary outflow. In either case, the large bladder volumes result in the intravesicular pressure exceeding the intra-urethral resistance. It is normal after general anesthesia has been given, because it takes time for the detrusor muscle to regain its activity. Urinary retention in men often reflects hypertrophy of the prostate gland, which narrows the urethra and makes it difficult to void. The goal of treatment in patients with overflow urinary incontinence is to improve bladder drainage. Alpha-adrenergic antagonists such as prazosin decrease internal sphincter tone and can improve urinary flow, but must be used with caution in the elderly due to risk of orthostatic hypotension.

Functional urinary incontinence is due to physical, cognitive or pharmacological factors that prevent the person from reaching toilet facilities in time, e.g. severe arthritis, dementia or the effect of diuretics.

Stress urinary incontinence (outlet incompetence) involves urine loss that results from a decreased tone of the internal and external urinary sphincter. It is the most common type of urinary incontinence. Patients typically lose small volumes of urine with activities such as coughing that result in transiently increased intra-abdominal pressure. It is caused by a derangement of the pelvic supportive structures and may occur as a result of aging, birth trauma or collagen defects. These changes become more pronounced following menopause as estrogen deficiency allows atrophy of the genitourinary tissues. Alpha-adrenergic agonists, such as pseudoephedrine, increase the internal sphincter tone and bladder outflow resistance. Pelvic-floor muscle exercises are effective in 50% to 60% of women with stress urinary incontinence; 10 to 20 pelvic floor contractions for ten seconds each being repeated three times a day. When conservative treatment for stress urinary incontinence fails, surgical intervention is aimed at resupporting the bladder neck.

The risk of incontinence is greater with high-impact activities. It is higher in basketball than volleyball, possibly because the running jumps in basketball result in greater impact than the typical jumping in volleyball. In a survey of all 35 elite trampolinists (mean age 15 years, range 12 to 22 years) in Sweden, 80% reported involuntary urinary leakage, but only during trampoline training. The leakage started after 2.5 (range 1 to 4) years of training. All women above the age of 15 years reported urinary leakage. 18 incontinent women continued the study and their leakage was verified by a pad test. The strength of the pelvic floor muscles was tested with perineometry in ten women and found to be good. A stiff and strong pelvic floor positioned at an optimal level inside the pelvis may be a crucial factor in counteracting the increases in abdominal pressure occurring during high-impact activities. Use of preventive devices such as vaginal tampons or pessaries can prevent leakage during high impact physical activity.

See also MICTURITION.

Chronology

•1948 • Arnold Kegel, a physician, published a paper entitled "Progressive resistance exercise in the functional restoration of the perineal muscles" in the *American Journal of Obstetrics and Gynecology*. Pelvic floor muscle tone is important for good functioning of the bladder, urethra, vagina, uterus and rectum. The idea of using pelvic muscle exercises to cure urinary incontinence was originally developed by Joshua Davies of New York. Kegel invented the world's first biofeedback device, the Kegel perineometer. A vaginal air pressure cone or chamber was connected by an airtube to an air pressure gauge whose dial was calibrated in mmHg. The perineometer gave resistance to the 'vaginal squeeze.' Kegel claimed that 93% of 3000 patients were successful in eliminating incontinence. The device was used 2 or 3 times per day. Modern Kegel exercises involve isometric movement without external resistance (something that Kegel appeared not to believe in).

Bibliography

Bø, K. (2004). Urinary incontinence, pelvic floor dysfunction, exercise and sport. *Sports Medicine* 34(7), 451-464.

Elia, G. (1999). Stress urinary incontinence in women. *The Physician and Sportsmedicine* 27(1), 39-52.

Eliasson, K., Larsson, T. and Mattson, E. (2002). Prevalence of stress incontinence in nulliparous elite trampolinists. *Scandanavian Journal of Medicine and Science in Sports* 12(2), 106-110.

Germann, W.J. and Stanfield, C.L. (2001). *Principles of human physiology*. San Francisco, CA: Benjamin Cummings.

URINARY TRACT   The organs of the body that produce and discharge urine. These include the kidneys, ureters, bladder and urethra.

URTICARIA   Hives. Wheals. Welts. 'Nettle rash.'

Urticaria is pale red swelling (edema) that occurs in groups on any part of the skin. It is formed by blood plasma leaking out of small blood vessels in the skin. This is caused by the release of histamine and other chemical mediators. 10 to 20% of the population will have at least one episode of urticaria in their lifetime. Most cases of urticaria are acute, lasting from a few hours to less than six weeks. Some cases are chronic, lasting more than 6 weeks. Triggers include alcohol, certain foods or food additives, cold, sun exposure, insect stings, exercise and emotional stress. The most common foods that cause hives are nuts, chocolate, fish, tomatoes, eggs, fresh berries and milk. Fresh foods cause hives more often that cooked foods.

A distinction can be made between allergic and non-allergic urticaria. **Allergic urticaria** is the least common form, although it is somewhat more common in children than adults. **Non-allergic urticaria** takes many forms. **Cold-induced urticaria** may occur after a plunge into a swimming pool. **Cholinergic urticaria** is associated with exercise, hot showers and/or anxiety. **Pressure urticaria** develops from the constant pressure of constricting clothing, such as bra straps. **Solar urticaria** arises on parts of the body exposed to the sun. This may occur within a few minutes after exposure. **Dermatographism** is a type of urticaria that forms after firmly stroking or scratching the skin.

See also ANGIOEDEMA.

Bibliography

American College of Allergy, Asthma and Immunology. Http://allergy.mcg.edu/advice/urtic.html.

UTP   Uracil triphosphate. A molecule that consists of the nitrogenous base uracil linked to the sugar ribose. It has a chain of three phosphate groups attached to the ribose. UTP is required during transcription since it is a direct precursor of RNA.

V

VACUOLE   A membrane bound sac found in the cytoplasm of many types of cells that serve to isolate its contents from the general intracellular environment. Prokaryotes do not have vacuoles. A **vesicle** is any small vacuole in an animal cells, which is used for various storage and transport functions. One type of vesicle is a small, circumscribed elevation of the skin containing fluid.

VAGAL   Pertaining to the vagus nerve.

VAGUS NERVES   The tenth cranial nerves. A pair of nerves that originate in the medulla of the brain and pass through the neck, chest and abdomen, where they innervate the heart, lungs, digestive tract and other organs. The vagus nerves are predominantly of the parasympathetic branch of the autonomic nervous system and contain both afferent and efferent neurons.

VALENCE   The power of an element or a radical to combine with (or to replace) other elements or radicals. It has been superseded by the concept of oxidation number. *See* REDOX.

VALGUS   A condition of segments where the longitudinal axis of the segment is angled outwards from its proximal to its distal end. *See* FEMORAL VALGUS; FOREFOOT VALGUS; GENU VALGUS; REAR FOOT VALGUS; TIBIAL VALGUS; VALGUS EXTENSION OVERLOAD SYNDROME.

VALGUS EXTENSION OVERLOAD SYNDROME   An overuse injury related to posterior compartment elbow changes from repetitive valgus stresses. It is most common in throwing athletes. Baseball pitchers suffer valgus extension overload as a result of stress during the late-acceleration and deceleration phases of throwing. Powerful elbow extension and valgus stresses due to throwing lead to medial shear of the posterior compartment. The olecranon tip's medial aspect impinges against the olecranon fossa's medial aspect, causing chondroma-lacia, reactive spurring, flexion contracture and, ultimately, loose body formation.

VALINE   An essential, glucogenic (glycogenic), five-carbon amino acid. It is degraded mainly in skeletal muscle, especially during fasting and uncontrolled diabetes mellitus. It is glucogenic, because three of its carbons form succinyl CoA, an intermediate in the Krebs cycle.

VALSALVA'S MANEUVER   An attempt to exhale air against a closed epiglottis or closed mouth and nostrils. It may result in the 'grunt' that occurs during weightlifting, isometric exercise, or even tennis playing. It stabilizes the abdominal and thoracic cavities, and is nearly reflexive with lifts greater than 50% of one-repetition maximum.

Intra-abdominal pressure is increased, as is intra-thoracic pressure; the muscle contraction can momentarily impede blood flow, venous return to the right atrium of the heart drops sharply, cardiac output decreases, oxygen supply to the brain is decreased, and dizziness or syncope may occur. When the breath is released, the intrathoracic pressure drops and the trapped blood is quickly propelled through the heart, producing an increase in the heart rate (tachycardia) and blood pressure. Immediately after this event, a reflex bradycardia ensues. The increased pressure, immediate tachycardia and reflex bradycardia can bring about cardiac arrest in vulnerable heart patients.

Olympic weightlifters are most vulnerable to blackout when the bar compresses vessels in the neck, just prior to jerking the bar overhead after the clean. Valsalva's maneuver is a useful, but dangerous technique for producing extra force. Prolonged breath holding should be avoided during strenuous weight lifting. Inhalation should occur during the lowering phase and exhalation during the upward, pushing or pulling phase (i.e. 'exhale with effort').

Cerebral blood flow velocity has been shown to significantly increase during dynamic exercise (running) secondary to increases in cardiac output.

Static exercise (weightlifting) induces supraphysiological arterial pressures up to 450/380 mmHg, and thus may alter cerebral blood flow velocity. Studies involving the Valsalva maneuver have demonstrated decreases in cerebral blood flow velocity of 21% to 52%. Intra-ocular pressure, which is an indirect measure of intracranial pressure, elevates to pathophysiologic levels during weightlifting. In a study of nine elite power athletes, including a multi-world record holder in powerlifting, all subjects had resting blood flow velocities within normal ranges. Blood flow velocities were significantly decreased in all subjects during maximal lifting. The drop in cerebral blood flow velocity was significantly less than previous research, which likely reveals the cardiovascular, baroreflex and cerebrovascular system adaptations occurring in these elite power athletes.

Bibliography

Dickerman, R.D. et al. (2000). Middle cerebral artery blood flow velocity in elite power athletes during maximal weight-lifting. *Neurological Research* 22(4), 337-340.

VALUE A code or standard that organizes a system of action and has some persistence through time. Values are concerned with what is considered to be desirable or what 'ought to be' (rather than what is actually) in existence. Williams (1970) identified the following values as characteristic of American society: achievement and success, activity and work, moral orientation, humanitarianism, efficiency and practicality, progress, material comfort, equality, freedom, conformity, science and rationality, nationalism and patriotism, democracy, individualism, racism and group-superiority. Some of these values stand in contrast to others (e.g. individualism vs. conformity).

Democracy is a political system based on the participation of all adults through the process of elections; and an economic system based on providing products and services that meet the needs of a broad range of selective, individual consumers. By **freedom**, is meant pursuit of goals without unreasonable interference from the government or other people, as well as freedom of expression.

Sport films depict sociocultural issues in American society and serve as a purveyor of values.

Altruism, self-sacrificing and character building were themes frequently employed in sport films of the 1930s, whereas tragedies, comedies and biographies were characteristic of the 1940s and 1950s. Sport films reflecting patriotism or nationalism were also in vogue during and shortly after World War II. Sport during the late 1920s through the 1930s, ending with American involvement in World War II in 1941, has been referred to as the "Golden Age of American Sport," a period of immersion in the new sports heroes of the day. The period from the 1920s through 1930s was also the 'golden age' of movies because of attendance and film distribution. Due in part to a changing social and political climate in America, sport films declined during the 1960s. Pearson et al. (2003) selected 590 sports (including 169 films during the 1930s), but only 43 in the 1960s. The 1960s was an anti-hero period, wrought with the social changes of the civil rights and antiwar movements, the women's liberation movement, campus unrest and urban riots. This diverted attention away from sport films in general, and those depicting physical contact in particular, towards social causes and reforms. The post-1960s era has been indicative of major shifts in the depiction of sport figures from diverse social classes and ethnic groups. The 1980s and 1990s appear to reflect the eclectic nature within the sport film genre.

See IDEOLOGY.

Chronology

•1891 • Thomas Edison's rudimentary motion-picture camera, the kinetoscope, was patented. It marked the birth of the movie industry. In 2001, *Sports Illustrated* listed what is considered to be the all-time top fifteen sport movies. The top four were *Bull Durham* (1988), *Raging Bull* (1980), *Rocky* (1976) and *Hoosiers* (1986). Others included *Chariots of Fire* (1981).

•1936 • Leni Riefenstahl's documentary of the Olympic Games in Berlin, which set out to glorify the Nazi party, is regarded as the start of modern film coverage of sports and heavily influenced subsequent television coverage.

Bibliography

Bergan, R. (1982). *Sports in the movies*. New York: Proteus.

Pearson, D.W. et al. (2003). Sport films. Social dimensions over time, 1930-1995. *Journal of Sport and Social Issues* 27(2), 145-161.

Williams, R.M. (1970). *American society: A sociological interpretation*.

3rd ed. New York: Alfred A. Knopf.

Zucker, H.M. and Babich, L.J. (1987). *Sport films: A complete reference*. Jefferson, NC: McFarland.

VARICOSE VEINS A condition in which the valves within a vein become defective and unable to prevent backflow. It usually occurs in the superficial veins of the lower extremities owing to the force of gravity that retards blood flow in an upright position. The veins become excessively distended, impairing circulation from the affected area. **Phlebitis** is a severe case of varicose veins in which the venous wall becomes inflamed and may degenerate; the vein must then be removed surgically. Individuals with varicose veins are generally advised to avoid excessive isometric exercise and the non-rhythmic muscular contractions often used in resistance training, because both the muscle pump and ventilatory pumps are unable to contribute significantly to venous return.

Bibliography
Donaldson, M.C. (1990). Varicose veins in active people. *The Physician and Sportsmedicine* 18(7), 46-52.

VARUS A misalignment in which a segment tends excessively inward (medially) from its proximal its distal end. Tensile stress is placed on the lateral side of the segment's proximal joint and on the medial side of the segment's distal joint. The muscles on the stressed side should be strengthened, while the muscles located on the opposite side should be stretched. Footwear should be worn that either compensates for, or corrects, the misalignment.
See FEMORAL VARUS; FOREFOOT VARUS; GENU VARUS; TIBIAL VARUS; REARFOOT VARUS.

VASCULAR Of, or relating to, vessels(s).

VASCULAR FRAGILITY Vascular problems such as dilation, dissection and rupture can occur as a result of many disorders. See ANEURYSM; EHLERS-DANLOS SYNDROME; MARFAN SYNDROME.

VASOCONSTRICTION Narrowing of blood vessels. It is brought about by adrenergic fibers of the sympathetic branch of the autonomic nervous system. Although there is convincing evidence that vasoconstriction can occur in active muscle, the proposition that the sympathetic nervous system constricts skeletal muscle during exercise poses a paradox, given the robust vasodilation that occurs in muscle during exercise. Ultimately, muscle perfusion is a balance between metabolic vasodilation and sympathetic vasoconstriction.

Bibliography
Buckwalter, J.B. and Clifford, P.S. (2001). The paradox of sympathetic vasoconstriction in exercising skeletal muscle. *Exercise and Sport Sciences Reviews* 29(4), 159-163.

VASODILATION Widening of blood vessels. It is brought about by cholinergic fibers of the sympathetic branch of the autonomic nervous system.

VASODILATORS Drugs that cause vasodilation and thus decrease blood pressure by lowering systemic vascular resistance. See CALCIUM-CHANNEL BLOCKERS; NITRATES.

VASOMOTOR A term which refers to the constriction and dilation of blood vessels, i.e. vasodilation and vasoconstriction. **Vasomotor nerves** are sympathetic nerves that control the smooth muscle of arterioles.

VASOPRESSIN Arginine vasopressin. Anti-diuretic hormone. A peptide hormone secreted by the posterior pituitary gland and controlled by the hypothalamus. The stimulus for the release of vasopressin is increased plasma osmolality. Vasopressin controls the excretion of water by the kidneys. Secretion of vasopressin is increased during exercise and this explains the greater retention of water by the kidneys during and after severe exercise when dehydration occurs. Vasopressin levels also increase greatly after vomiting. Some drugs stimulate the release of vasopressin, but others (e.g. alcohol and caffeine) inhibit it.

VASOVAGAL See under SYNCOPE.

VECTOR i) An invertebrate animal capable of transmitting an infectious agent among vertebrates such as humans. ii) A quantity that has both magnitude and direction, e.g. velocity. A **scalar** has magnitude only, e.g. speed. The direction of an angular motion vector is referred to as the **polarity** of the vector. The polarity of an angular motion vector is determined by a convention known as the 'right hand rule.' The curled fingers of the right hand are placed in the direction of the rotation. The angular motion vector is defined by an appropriate length arrow that coincides with the direction of the extended thumb of the right hand. It is conventional that, in the sagittal plane, all segments moving in a counter-clockwise direction from the right horizontal have a positive polarity and all segments rotating in a clockwise direction have a negative polarity. The angular velocity vector is perpendicular to the plane of rotation. **Vector algebra** is a set of definitions, rules and operations used for computational purposes in the manipulation of vector quantities. The **composition of vectors** is the use of vector algebra to combine vectors that act in the same plane (coplanar) and that have the same point of application (concurrent). **Resolution of vectors** is the reverse process from vector composition.

VEGETARIAN DIET A type of diet that, to some degree, excludes foods originating from animal sources. The major risk of vegetarian diets is nutritional inadequacy. Vegetarians (especially vegans, who exclude all animal products) tend to have low calorie intake. This is partly because much of the food from plant sources is high in bulk and low in calories. There may be a lack of vitamin B_{12} in a diet based mainly on plant foods, while vitamin B_6 iron, riboflavin, calcium and zinc may be less than recommended. Plant foods contain a form of iron called non-heme iron that is not as well absorbed as the heme iron in animal foods. Since vitamin C aids iron absorption in the body, however, the higher vitamin C intakes of vegetarians may offset the lower iron intakes to some degree. A variety of nuts and pulses is necessary in a vegan diet to ensure intake of essential amino acids.

There has been some concern that vegetarian, female athletes are at increased risk for oligomenorrhea, but evidence suggests that low energy intake, not dietary quality, is the major cause.

Chronology

•1839 • Sylvester Graham published his influential book entitled *Lectures on the Science of Human Life*. It promoted rigorous discipline and temperance (abstaining from excess). Graham's philosophy included vigorous exercise. As a teenager, Graham suffered tuberculosis and in his late twenties he suffered a nervous breakdown. In 1830, at the age of 36, after a failed attempt to become a minister, Graham became a professional health reformer. His lectures on proper living, including the Bible's stance on wine and meat, were attended by thousands of people. He believed that sexual desires irritated the body and caused disease, and that the remedy was to get married in order to get the urge out of one's systems. Such beliefs caused much controversy at his lectures. In 1831, New York's temperance leadership invited him to deliver lectures on the relationship between diet and disease. Graham was a vegetarian and he expounded the benefits of homemade bread made with whole-grain wheat, which became known as Graham flour. The recipe for Nabisco's Graham Crackers is basically the same as that created by Sylvester Graham. Graham's version of vegetarianism, "Grahamism" (bran, bread, water and vegetables) did not attract widespread popularity, but was popular for a while among radical communities such as Brook Farm. When the British Vegetarian Society was founded in 1847, he helped found the American Vegetarian Society in 1850 that came out of a meeting called by William Metcalfe who had led a migration of 40 members of the Bible Christian Church from England to Philadelphia in 1817. The *Graham Journal of Health and Longevity* was published from 1837 to 1839, after which time enthusiasm for Grahamism waned. Graham's own health declined steady, until he died in 1851.
•1887 • The Vegetarian Cycling and Athletic Club was founded. Its objective was to provide a means of contact between vegetarian cycling enthusiasts and to show that they could hold their own in athletic competition against their carnivore counterparts.
•1905 • Wilhelm Caspari of Berlin published studies of vegetarianism and physiology. He concluded that there was no dietary advantage to vegetarianism and argued that the apparent remarkable performances of vegetarians in long-distance races could be accounted for by the "struggle for their ideals."
•1923 • John H. Kellog, the 'father of the breakfast cereal industry,' opened Battle Creek College, with a four-year program in physical education and home economics. Kellog practiced and preached vegetarianism. His many publications included a popular health periodical, *Good Health*. The program was soon enlarged to include football. The director hoped that vegetarianism would be an ergogenic aid. The win-loss record of the team in its first season was poor and it was disbanded. The official reason for discontinuing football was that the game was too violent!

Bibliography

Grandjean, A.C. (1987). The vegetarian athlete. *The Physician and Sportsmedicine* 15(5), 191-194.

Green, J. (1986). *Fit for America. Health, fitness, sport and American society.* New York: Pantheon Books.

Grover, K. (1989, ed). *Fitness in American culture. Images of health, sport and the body.* Amhert, MA: University of Massachusetts Press.

Nieman, D.C. (1999). Physical fitness and vegetarian diets: Is there a relation? *American Journal of Clinical Nutrition* 70(3S), S570-S575.

VELOCITY   The rate of change of position (or displacement) with respect to time. **Speed** is the rate of change of distance with respect to time. Velocity is a vector quantity. Speed is the magnitude of velocity, and hence speed is a scalar quantity. The SI unit of velocity is meters per second (m/s). The US customary unit is feet/sec or miles per hour. 1 ft/s = 0.3048 m/s. 1 mph = 0.447 m/s = 1.609 km/h. See also ANGULAR VELOCITY.

VELOCITY RATIO   *See under* MACHINE.

VEIN   A vessel that carries blood to the heart. Veins are **capacitance vessels**, owing to their distensibility, which enables them to pool large volumes of blood and become reservoirs for blood. Veins are formed by the joining together of capillaries. Veins and venules have walls that are not as thick as those of the arteries or arterioles and do not have high elasticity, but do have high compliance. Veins are surrounded by smooth muscle, which, because of the compliance of the venous circulation, functions to regulate the cross-sectional dimensions of the veins and therefore the volume of blood in the venous circulation.

Venous blood volume is also increased by skeletal muscle acting as a pump to propel blood in veins through the one-way valves back to the heart. **Mixed venous blood** is the mixture of venous blood from both the upper and lower body that accumulates in the right side of the heart. It represents an average of venous blood from the whole body.

See also ARTERIAL-VENOUS MIXED OXYGEN CONTENT DIFFERENCE.

VENA CAVA   A large vein through which blood from the body returns to the right atrium of the heart.

VENOMOTOR TONE   Increased contractile activity in venous smooth muscle due to triggering from venoconstrictor neurons of the sympathetic nervous system. Increased venomotor tone leads to: i) constriction of veins, which increases blood pressure within them, forcing blood to return to the heart and briefly increases stroke volume; and ii) increased wall tension decreases venous compliance, raising central venous pressure and producing a sustained increase in stroke volume. Increased venomotor tone therefore promotes an increase in cardiac output and mean arterial pressure. Changes in venomotor tone are an important component of the reflexes that regulate arterial pressure.

VENOUS COMPLIANCE   *See under* COMPLIANCE.

VENOUS POOLING   Accumulation of blood in the veins. When a person stands up, the force of gravity increases the pressure on the blood in the lower veins of the body, causing those veins to expand and enabling the volume of blood within them to increase. Venous pooling is detrimental to the heart's pumping action because it decreases venous return, central venous pressure and arterial pressure. A decrease in mean arterial pressure upon standing (orthostatic hypotension) may cause a person to feel dizzy, but reflex mechanisms normally quickly compensate for it. The presence of aggravating factors, e.g. dehydration or a failing heart, may cause a person to faint upon standing. With fainting, blood that pooled in the veins of the legs moves toward the central veins, thus increasing central venous pressure, venous return and cardiac output. The increase in mean arterial pressure helps restore blood flow to the brain.

See also SYNCOPE; SPINAL PARALYSIS.

VENOUS RETURN   The return of venous blood to the heart. This occurs via the alternate contraction and relaxation of the skeletal muscles that squeezes blood through the veins and towards the heart. The most important influence on venous return is **central venous pressure**, which is the pressure of blood contained in the large veins that lead into the heart. As central venous pressure increases, venous return increases because the increased pressure forces more blood to flow into the atria. Venous return increases during exercise due to vasoconstriction, the muscle pump and the ventilatory pump. Valves prevent backflow.

See also ORTHOSTATIC TOLERANCE.

VENOUS SINUS i) A wide channel containing blood. ii) Air cavities within the facial bones, lined by mucous membranes similar to those in other parts of the airways.

VENOUS THROMBOEMBOLISM *See under* THROMBOSIS.

VENTILATION This is part of respiration. It is the movement of air into and out of the lungs by bulk flow. **Pulmonary (minute) ventilation** is the volume of gas exhaled divided by the time of exhalation in minutes. It is calculated as tidal volume multiplied by respiratory frequency. Pulmonary ventilation is the sum of alveolar ventilation and dead space ventilation.

See also GROWTH; HYPERVENTILATION; HYPOVENTILATION.

VENTILATION-TO-PERFUSION RATIO The matching of blood flow to ventilation. The ideal ventilation-to-perfusion ratio is one, since this ratio implies a perfect match of blood flow to ventilation. **Pulmonary ventilation-perfusion ratio** is the ratio of pulmonary ventilation to cardiac output. It is approximately unity (one) during rest in most individuals, but may increase up to six-fold at maximal exercise. This increase is one reason why pulmonary ventilation is not thought to be a limiting factor of oxygen uptake.

Mismatch of ventilation-to-perfusion ratio is the most common problem with gas exchange. It may occur in any disease that disturbs the distribution of ventilation (e.g. asthma) or the distribution of

pulmonary blood flow (e.g. thrombo-embolism).

VENTILATORY PUMP Respiratory pump. During inhalation, the diaphragm pulls downward and the rib cage expands. This lowers pressure in the thoracic cavity and increases pressure in the abdominal cavity. A pressure gradient is thus created that promotes the movement of blood from the abdominal veins to the central veins in the thoracic cavity. During exhalation, the thoracic pressure increases and abdominal pressure decreases. This creates a pressure gradient that would promote the backward movement of blood from the central veins to the abdominal veins, if such backward flow were not prevented by the closure of valves in the abdominal veins. Instead, the rise in thoracic pressure drives the forward movement of the blood from the central veins to the heart, thereby promoting increased end-diastolic volume and cardiac output.

VENTILATORY RESERVE Breathing reserve. It is the difference between the maximum voluntary ventilation and the maximum ventilation during exercise. Pulmonary ventilation at maximal oxygen uptake is only 60 to 85% of a healthy person's maximal voluntary ventilation, thus ventilatory reserve is a measure of the body's residual potential for further increasing ventilation during exercise of maximal intensity.

VENTILATORY THRESHOLD *See under* LACTIC ACID.

VENTRAL Relating to the front surface of the body.

VENTRICLES i) These are two thick-walled, muscular chambers of the heart. The right ventricle pumps blood to the lungs; the left ventricle pumps blood to the rest of the body. ii) Fluid-filled chambers of the brain that are continuous with the spinal cord.

VENTRICULAR FIBRILLATION *See under* CARDIAC ARRHYTHMIAS

VENULES   Small blood vessels that connect capillaries to veins.

VERRUCAS   Warts that are caused by a virus and can be transferred from one individual to another in floor areas where people walk barefoot. The incubation period is one to six months.

VERTEBRAL COLUMN   *See* SPINE.

VERTEX   i) The intersection of the two lines that form an angle. ii) An anatomical landmark that is the most superior point in the mid-sagittal plane on the skull when the head is held in the **Frankfort plane**, i.e. when the orbitale and tragion are horizontally aligned. *See* STATURE.

VERTICAL JUMP   A complex, multi-joint movement that requires muscle coordination best improved by specific skill development. Traditional strength training, explosive types of weight training, Olympic weightlifting and plyometrics can be effective for increasing the vertical jump. The form of training that is most effect is determined by the relative strengths and weaknesses of the athlete. Traditional weight training strength will only increase jump height in athletes who exhibit low initial strength. Some of the power developed during a vertical jump is derived from the stretch-shortening cycle. Drop jumping, a form of plyometric training, enhances the ability to use the stretch-shortening cycle. It increases the height of jumps preceded by counter movements, but has no significant effect on jumps initiated from a static crouch position. Olympic weightlifters exhibit exceptional vertical jump scores, either because of their training or their genetic endowment. The movement pattern of Olympic style lifting is similar to that of a vertical jump, more so than traditional weight training exercises.

Bibliography
Kraemer, W.J. and Newton, R.U. (1994). Training for improved vertical jump. *Gatorade Sports Science Exchange* 7(6).

VERTIGO   The false sense of motion or spinning. It is the most common symptom of dizziness. Vertigo

may be severe enough to cause nausea and vomiting. Vertigo is usually accompanied by nystagmus.

Benign positional vertigo involves intense, brief episodes of dizziness associated with a change in the position of the head, often when a person turns over in bed or sits up in the morning. It is most often a natural result of aging, and it may also result from head trauma. It seems to be caused by **otoconia**, which are small calcium carbonate crystals, which break loose from their normal attachments in the inner ear and strike against sensitive nerve endings (the **cupula**) within the vestibular apparatus at the end of each semicircular canal (the **ampulla**). This causes a sudden increase in sensory stimulation to the brain. The vestibular nuclei (found within the brainstem) are overexcited, causing dizziness. The otoconia usually dissolve or fall back into the vestibule within several weeks, and no longer cause any symptoms.

Labyrinthitis (vestibular) neuronitis is a presumed viral infection of the vestibular nerve. It causes sudden loss of function in the balance system of one ear. The brain normally compares the two ears. When one ear develops labyrinthitis, the difference between the two ears produces the feeling of spinning.

Menière's disease (endolymphatic hydrops) involves the excessive buildup of fluid in the inner ear. The dizzy episodes are usually linked with vomiting, and the sufferer can often tell an episode is about to start because of a drop in their bearing, a feeling of fullness in the ear, and some tinnitus. It may affect adults at any age and is characterized by sudden episodes of vertigo lasting 30 minutes to an hour or longer.

The cause of vertigo may be a migraine. People who experience a **vestibular migraine** are very sensitive to motion. Another cause of vertigo is **acoustic neuroma**, a benign growth on the acoustic nerve, which connects the inner ear to the brain. Rapid changes in motion, such as riding on a roller coaster, can make a person dizzy.

Treatment of vertigo is symptomatic. Valium and Antivert are vestibular suppressants.

Bibliography

Germann, W.J. and Stanfield, C.L. (2001). *Principles of human physiology*. San Francisco, CA: Benjamin Cummings.

VESICLE   *See under* VACUOLE.

VESICULAR TRANSPORT   *See under* ACTIVE TRANSPORT.

VESTIBULAR REFLEXES   The reflexes for maintaining the position of the eyes and body in relation to changes in orientation of the head.

VESTIBULAR SYSTEM   *See under* BALANCE; EAR.

VIAGRA   *See under* SEX BEHAVIOR.

VIBRATION   *See under* MECHANORECEPTORS.

VIDEO ANALYSIS   *See under* MOTION ANALYSIS.

VIOLENCE   Physical force used to injure, damage or destroy. Collective violence in sport that involves spectators has attracted the attention of sports officials, police, journalists and politicians worldwide. Many theories have been proposed in an attempt to explain collective violence in sport, including Contagion, Convergence, Decision/ Games, Emergent Norm, Rules of Disorder, Value-added and Catharsis.

Contagion theory is based on the premise that the behavior of self-elected leaders in crowds leads to homogenous action as members of a crowd copy each other. This theory fails to explain why some crowds become violent and others remain passive.

Convergence theory is based on the premise that people in a crowd share common values and goals. It is proposed that people exploit the protection of being in a crowd to engage in behavior that is normally repressed. What the theory fails to explain is why persons with similar goals may behave differently in crowds.

Decision/Gaming theory is based on the premise that crowd members engage in a rational decision-making process regarding estimated rewards of action versus potential costs. Field invasion of large groups reduces the risk of an individual being arrested. What the theory fails to explain is spontaneous crowd behavior.

Emergent Norm theory is based on the premise that 'controlling norms' in crowds emerge spontaneously and members of the crowd feed off each other's behavior, especially in moments of ambiguity. It is proposed that conventional norms are overcome by temporary norms, which are deviant and lead to collective violence. The theory fails to explain why violence may be prearranged and ordered, rather than spontaneous.

Rules of Disorder theory is based on the premise that collective violence is a form of social action governed by rules. It was proposed that the hooliganism in mid-1970s English soccer had an inherent orderliness characterized by ritualized violence. This theory de-emphasizes actual violence that may be organized between rival fighting groups.

Value-added theory is based on the premise that crowd behavior is determined by a sequence of incremental steps. It is proposed that precipitating factors at sports events are important determinants of crowd hostility. Unpopular decisions by referees and player violence are two of the strongest and common precipitating factors. A criticism of this theory is that necessary precipitants for violence may not be incremental and may not exist at all.

Catharsis theory is based on the premise that frustration accumulated in daily life can be diffused by behaving aggressively or by observing violent action. It is proposed that sport violence acts as a frustration outlet for both players and fans. There is a belief that violence in sport minimizes other forms of social violence. In fact, there is more evidence that participating in violence promotes further violence.

Fan fighting at North American sports has not expressed itself in terms of routinized rival gang episodes of British and European soccer. The majority of incidents of fan-to-fan aggression occurring at North American games involve individuals or small groups of supporters participating in activities such as common assault, drunken and disorderly behavior, and confrontations with police. The most predictable and widely publicized form of North American fan disorder, according to Young (2002), is the post-event riot. *See also* AGGRESSION.

Chronology

•2000 • At the Staples Center in Los Angeles, after the Lakers won the NBA title in 2000, vandalism, arson and fighting among fans provoked the police into using rubber bullets and batons as players were detained inside the Staples Center for several hours until rioting subsided. Approximately 12 people were injured and the same number of people arrested.

•2004 • Violence erupted during the final minute of a National Basketball Association (NBA) match between the Indiana Pacers and the Detroit Pistons. A fight began when Ron Artest of the Pacers fouled Ben Wallace in the back during a lay-up attempt. Wallace retaliated by shoving Artest's face with both hands and charging at him. Subsequent events included a fan throwing a plastic cup, filled with beverage, at Artest, who then dashed into the stands. During the fight, three Pacers players (Ron Artest, Stephen Jackson and Jermaine O'Neal) punched Pistons fans. The NBA suspended Ron Artest of the Pacers for the entire season. Seven other players received suspensions; four of them, including Reggie Miller of the Pacers, for leaving the bench. Five of the players from the Pacers and five fans faced criminal charges.

Bibliography

Young, K. (1991). Sport and collective violence. *Exercise and Sport Sciences Reviews* 19, 539-86.

Young, K. (2002). Standard deviations: An update on North American crowd disorder. *Sociology of sport Journal* 19(3), 237-275.

VIRAL SHEDDING The expelling of virus particles from the body. Important routes include the respiratory, genital and intestinal tracts. The virus remains in cells of the body after the first infection in a latent or dormant form. At some point, this latency ends and the virus begins to multiply becoming transmittable. Viral shedding may or may not be accompanied by symptoms of a rash. It occurs most often with herpes simplex virus infections.

VIRUSES Infectious agents that consist of DNA or RNA encased in a protein coat. In order to grow or replicate on their own, they invade a host cell and subvert its cellular mechanisms.

See AIDS; CHRONIC FATIGUE SYNDROME; NATURAL KILLER CELLS; UPPER-RESPIRATORY TRACT INFECTION.

VISCERA Organs enclosed within the four great cavities (cranium, thorax, abdomen and pelvis). Most commonly, the term refers to the digestive organs within the abdominal cavity.

See ABDOMINAL OBESITY.

VISCERAL RECEPTORS These receptors are mostly free nerve endings. The specific stimuli for visceral pain are stopping of the blood flow, irritant chemicals, tissue stretch, and spasm of the smooth muscles. Some inner organs are not pain-sensitive, e.g. alveoli of the lungs.

VISCOELASTICITY The property of a material that describes its time-dependent elastic behavior. Viscoelastic materials tend to flow with time, and stress is proportional to the rate of strain. The higher the rate of strain, the smaller the degree to which creep and stress relaxation can occur during deformation. In turn, this increases the stiffness, ultimate stress and toughness of the material. For example, the increased toughness of muscle-tendon units and bones in response to increased strain rates may enable the body to dissipate large amounts of energy as heat. Most biological materials are viscoelastic and will deform slowly in a non-linear manner. In mechanical models of viscoelastic materials such as muscle, the elastic elements are usually represented by springs and the viscous elements by hydraulic pistons ('dashpots').

See RESILIENCE; RHEOLOGY.

VISCOSITY The internal friction of a fluid. It is because of viscosity that a force must be exerted to cause one layer of fluid to slide past another; hence what is meant by viscosity being a fluid frictional property concerned with resistance to shear forces. Viscosity can be defined as shear stress divided by shear strain rate. For a given level of shear stress, the lower the strain rate, the higher the viscosity. Liquids are much more viscous than gases. An ideal fluid is assumed to have zero viscosity.

See HEMOCONCENTRATION; VISCO-ELASTICITY.

Bibliography

El-Sayed, M.S. (1998). Effects of exercise and training on blood rheology. *Sports Medicine* 26(5), 281-292.

VISION The interpretation of what is seen in the external world as a result of stimulation of the retina by light and recognizing differences such as form, color and position. **Near vision** is 25 to 50 cm; **intermediate vision** is 40 cm to 1.5 m; and **distance vision** is 5 or 6 m to infinity.

Refractive vision refers to visual acuity, the product of light rays bending and reaching the receptor cells (rods and cones) of the retina. Visual impulses are transmitted via the optic nerve (2nd cranial nerve) to many parts of the brain for inter-pretation. Refractive problems include myopia (nearsightedness), hyperopia (farsightedness) and astigmatism (blurring and distortion). At around the age of 40 years, the ability of an individual to focus at close distances tends to decline (presbyopia).

Binocular coordination is the ability of the two eyes to work in unison. It is closely linked with balance and postural reflexes. For **bifoveal fixation** to occur, the fovea of the two eyes must be aligned and directed at the same instant toward the object of visual regard. **Fusion** is the process in which the images on the two retinas are combined into a single visual percept. **Stereopsis** is based on the extent of **retinal disparity**, or mismatch, between the two eyes and has been demonstrated in infants of 3 months and upwards. Speed of stereopsis is a measure of the speed of depth perception. If the information is slow or incomplete, the performer will exhibit problems in timing.

Accommodative-vergence facility refers to the ability to quickly and efficiently shift visual atten-tion while maintaining clarity and spatial accuracy.

See also ALBINISM; AMBYLOPIA; BLINKING; CATARACT; COLUBOMA; CONTACT LENSES; CONTRAST SENSITIVITY; DEPTH PERCEP-TION; EYE DOMINANCE; EYE MOVEMENTS; EYE MUSCLE COORDINATION; FIGURE-GROUND PERCEPTION; GLASSES; GLAUCO-MA; KERATOCONUS; MACULAR DISEASE; NYS-TAGMUS; OPTIC NERVE; PERIPHERAL VISION; RETINA; SPORTS VISION; STRABISMUS.

VISUAL ACUITY **Static visual acuity** refers to clarity of eyesight. Standard normal distance mono-cular visual acuity is 20/15; for binocular it is 20/20. If the denominator is larger than 15, the visual acuity is below standard. Static visual acuity is usually evaluated using the Snellen Eye Chart where the smallest feature (usually letters) discernible is evaluated in high contrast conditions. Greater illumi-nation tends to improve acuity, but too much light may create glare that interferes with vision. **Dynamic visual acuity** is the ability to distinguish detail in moving objects. It is measured by flashing check-board targets with varying levels of grid precision on a screen. Static visual acuity is weakly related to dynamic visual acuity at slow speeds, and is not related to dynamic visual acuity at faster speeds. Dynamic visual acuity improves from ages 6 to 20 years and begins to decline after that. Dynamic visual acuity can be improved with training.

VISUAL IMPAIRMENT *See under* BLIND.

VISUAL-MOTOR BEHAVIOR REHEARSAL *See* SYSTEMATIC DESENSITIZATION.

VISUAL RIGHTING REFLEX *See under* LABYRINTHINE REFLEX.

VITAL CAPACITY The maximal volume of gas that can be expelled from the lungs by forceful effort following a maximal inspiration. Vital capacity is the sum of tidal volume, inspiratory reserve volume and expiratory reserve volume.

Forced expired volume is the percentage of vital capacity that is expired in 0.75 minute. It gives an indication of the expiratory power and overall resistance to air movement in the lungs.

VITAMIN A chemical compound required by the body in minute quantity for its essential role in metabolism. Thirteen vitamins have been identified and are classified as either fat-soluble or water-soluble. The **fat-soluble vitamins** are vitamins A, D, E and K. The **water-soluble vitamins** are biotin, the B-complex group (vitamin B_{12}, folacin, niacin, pantothenate, riboflavin, thiamin and vitamin

B_6) and vitamin C. The water-soluble vitamins act as coenzymes. Vitamins can be used repeatedly in metabolic reactions. Intake of water-soluble vitamins should be on a daily basis.

Vitamins must be obtained from the diet. Vitamin A, vitamin D and niacin can be made in the body from other substances, but it is not accurate to say that the body can synthesize them. Vitamin A can be made by cleavage of beta-carotene. Vitamin D can be formed from the action of sunlight on 7-dehydrocholesterol in the skin. Niacin is a normal product from the breakdown of the amino acid tryptophan. Biotin and vitamin K are synthesized by bacteria living in the human gut. Vitamin B_{12} is also synthesized by the action of intestinal bacteria, but insufficient quantity is absorbed via this source to meet human requirements.

Restricting intake of some B-complex vitamins by approximately less than 35 to 45% of the recommended dietary allowance may lead to decreased endurance capacity within a few weeks. It is possible that B-complex vitamin supplementation might be useful in sports with a high-energy expenditure, because of the unavoidable consumption of food products with a low nutrient density in order for energy intake to be high enough.

Dietary deficiencies of most vitamins are not very common among athletes, except in those who restrict their food intake in order to maintain body weight. In addition to dietary deficiency, an increased requirement for vitamins can be caused by increased turnover, decreased absorption by the gastrointestinal tract, and increased excretion in sweat, urine and feces. There is no evidence, however, that vitamin excretion or turnover is increased in athletes.

Surveys have indicated that most elite athletes do take vitamin supplements, often in dosages greater than 50 to 100 times the recommended daily allowance. Although supplementing one's diet with a multi-vitamin tablet may be a reasonable precautionary measure, and even of psychological benefit, there is no justification for taking 'megavitamins' (doses of more than ten times the recommended daily intake). Excess amounts of water-soluble vitamins are simply excreted, though mega-doses of vitamin C have been associated with kidney stones. Fat-soluble vitamins are stored in the fatty tissues of the body and excess amounts can be harmful or even fatal.

Research has shown that a vitamin deficiency impairs physical performance. If this deficiency is corrected, performance usually improves. In general, vitamin supplementation to an athlete on a well-balanced diet has not been shown to improve performance.

Pangamic acid ('vitamin B_{15}') is not a vitamin, because no specific disease state is associated with a deficiency.

Bibliography

Haymes, E.M. (1991). Vitamin and mineral supplementation to athletes. *International Journal of Sport Nutrition* 1(2), 146-169.

Oregon State University. The Linus Pauling Institute. Micronutrient Information Center. Http://lpi.oregonstate.edu/infocenter

Van der Beek, E.J. (1985). Vitamins and endurance training. *Sports Medicine* 2, 175-197.

Van der Beek, E.J. (1991). Vitamin supplementation and physical exercise performance. *Journal of Sports Sciences* 9, 77-90.

VITAMIN A   Retinoids. A fat-soluble vitamin; active forms are retinol, retinal and retinoic acid. **Retinol**, which is required for reproduction and bone health, can be converted to **retinal**, the form required for night and color vision. Retinal can reform retinol or it can irreversibly form **retinoic acid**, which is important for cell growth and differentiation.

Carotenoids are a group of red, orange and yellow pigments normally found in fruit and vegetables. Scientists have identified about 600 carotenoids, 50 of which are typically found in the American diet. The major carotenoids are alpha-carotene, beta-carotene, lutein, zeaxanthin, cryptoxanthin and lycopene. The yellow-orange pigment beta-carotene, which lends it color to cantaloupe, carrots and squash, is the most common carotenoid. The body can convert alpha- caroteine, beta-caroteine and beta-cryptoxanthin to retinal, so they are called **provitamin A carotenoids**. Lycopene, lutein and zeaxanthin have no vitamin A activity, so they are called **nonprovitamin A carotenoids**. Carotenoids are involved in bolstering immune function, enhancing vision and preventing cancer. Carotenoids also scavenge several free radicals, including superoxide radicals and peroxyl radicals. Similar to vitamin C, beta-carotenoid can function both as an antioxidant and a pro-oxidant. Under hyperoxic partial pressures (i.e. greater than 150 mmHg), beta-carotene exerts pro-oxidant properties with a concomitant loss of its antioxidant capacity.

Different dietary sources of vitamin A have different potencies. For example, beta-carotene is less easily absorbed than retinal and must be converted to retinal and retinol by the body. **Retinol activity equivalency** (RAE) is a standard measure of vitamin A and represents vitamin A as retinol. In general, free retinol is not found in foods. Retinyl palmitate, a precursor and storage form of retinol, is found in foods from animals. Cod liver oil (one table spoon) contains 4,080 mcg RAE. Carrot (half a cup, raw, chopped) contains 595 mcg RAE. Whole milk (8 oz) contains 76 mcg RAE.

The recommended daily allowance (RDA) for vitamin A is based on the amount required to ensure adequate stores of vitamin A in the body to support normal reproductive function, immune function, gene expression and vision. The RDA for adults is 900 mcg/day (males) and 700 mcg/day (females). Breastfeeding adult females require 1,300 mcg/day. Vitamin A toxicity has occurred from eating the livers of carnivorous animals or large fish, but most toxicity occurs through supplementation. Vitamin A supplements should not be taken in the first trimester of pregnancy. Large doses of vitamin A may be teratogenic.

Bibliography

Oregon State University. The Linus Pauling Institute. Micronutrient Information Center. Http://lpi.oregonstate.edu/infocenter

VITAMIN B₁ Thiamin. A water-soluble vitamin, the active form of which is the coenzyme thiamin pyrophosphate (thiamin diphosphate), required for a number of metabolic reactions including the oxidative decarboxylation of alpha keto acids, such as pyruvate and alpha ketoglutarate.

Whole grain cereals, beans, lentils, nuts, lean pork and yeast are rich sources of thiamin. Because most of the thiamin is lost during the production of white flour and polished (milled) rice, white rice and foods made from white flour are fortified with thiamin. Long grain white rice that is enriched contains 0.26 mg of thiamin; unenriched, it contains only 0.03 mg. Brazil nuts (1 oz) contain 0.28 mg of thiamin.

The recommended daily allowance (RDA) for thiamin is based on the prevention of deficiency in generally healthy individuals. The RDA for adults is 1.2 mg/day (males) or 1.1 mg/day (females).

Bibliography

Oregon State University. The Linus Pauling Institute. Micronutrient Information Center. Http://lpi.oregonstate.edu/infocenter

VITAMIN B₂ COMPLEX A group of water-soluble vitamins consisting of folic acid, niacin, pantothenic acid and riboflavin. As a co-enzyme, **folic acid** (folacin) is involved in nucleic acid and amino acid metabolism. It is also essential for the synthesis of red blood cells, and it works with vitamin B₁₂ and vitamin B₆ to decrease elevated homocysteine, which is a risk factor for heart attacks. Rich sources of folic acid include green leafy vegetables. Spinach (half a cup, cooked) contains 131 mcg of folate. One cup of fortified breakfast cereal contains 200 to 400 mcg of folate. In order to help prevent neural tube defects, the Food and Drug Administration (FDA) has required since 1998 that 1.4 mg of folic acid per kilogram of grain be added to refined grain products, which are already enriched with niacin, thiamin, riboflavin and iron. The recommended dietary allowance (RDA) is based primarily on the adequacy of red blood cell folate concentrations at different levels of folate intake, which have been shown to correlate with liver folate stores. The RDA for adults is 400 mcg/day. Because pregnancy is associated with a significant increase in cell division and other metabolic processes requiring folate coenzymes, the RDA for pregnant women is higher (600 mcg/day) than for women who are not pregnant (400 mcg/day). Food folate is not as well absorbed as synthetic folic acid. In the USA, the Food and Nutrition Board recommends that women capable of becoming pregnant obtain 400 mcg of synthetic folic acid daily from either fortified foods or a supplement, in addition to consuming food folate from a varied diet.

Niacin (nicotinic acid and nicotinamide) was first isolated as an oxidation product of nicotine. **Nicotinic acid** is converted to **nicotinamide** by the liver in a series of reactions involving ATP, ADP and glutamine. Tryptophan can also be converted into nicotinamide by the liver. Niacin forms part of the large redox coenzymes, nicotinamide adenine dinucleotide (NAD^+) and nicotinamide adenine dinucleotide phosphate (NADP). Good sources of niacin include yeast, meat, poultry, fish, cereals, legumes and seeds. 3 oz of chicken (light meat), cooked without skin, contains 10.6 mg of niacin. One cup of fortified cereal contains 20 to 27 mg of niacin. In plants, especially mature cereal grains like corn and wheat, niacin may be bound to sugar molecules in the form of glycosides, which significantly decreases niacin bioavailability. The RDA for niacin is based on the prevention of deficiency. NE, niacin equivalent, is defined as follows: 1 mg NE = 6 mg of tryptophan = 1 mg niacin. **Pellagra** caused by deficiency of niacin or failure to convert tryptophan to niacin. Most persons with pellagra also suffer from deficiencies of riboflavin and other essential vitamins and minerals. It is characterized by various skin, gastrointestinal and mental disturbances. It can be prevented by about 11 mg of NE per day, but 12 mg to 16 mg per day has been found to normalize the urinary excretion of niacin metabolites in healthy young adults.

Pantothenic acid forms part of coenzyme A, which, in turn, is a component of acetyl CoA. Good sources of pantothenic acid include liver and kidney, yeast, egg yolk and broccoli. Food processing such as freezing and canning of foods may result in a 35% to 75% loss in pantothenic acid. One large egg contains 0.61 mg of pantothenic acid. Half a cup of broccoli (steamed, chopped) contains 0.40 mg. For pantothenic acid, there is an Adequate Intake (AI) based on estimated dietary intakes in healthy population groups. In adults, the AI is 5 mg per day.

Riboflavin is the reactive group for two important coenzymes, flavin mononucleotide (FMN) and flavin adenine dinucleotide (FAD). Most plants and animal-derived foods contain at least small quantities of riboflavin. In the USA, wheat flour and bread have been enriched with riboflavin (as well as thiamin, niacin and iron) since 1943. Riboflavin is easily destroyed by exposure to light. Fortified cereal (one cup) contains 0.59 to 2.27 mg of riboflavin. One egg (large size, cooked) contains 0.27 mg of riboflavin. The RDA for riboflavin is based on the prevention of deficiency, and is 1.3 mg/day and 1.1 mg/day in males and females, respectively.

Bibliography

Food and Nutrition Board, Institute of Medicine (1998). *Dietary Reference Intakes for thiamin, riboflavin, niacin, vitamin B6, folate, vitamin B12, pantothenic acid, biotin and choline.* Washington, DC: National Academy Press.

Oregon State University. The Linus Pauling Institute. Micronutrient Information Center. Http://lpi.oregonstate.edu/infocenter

VITAMIN B$_6$ A vitamin that exists in six forms: pyridoxal, pyridoxine and pyridoxamine; and their phosphate derivatives. For example, the phosphate derivative of pyridoxal, and active coenzyme form, is pyridoxal 5'-phosphate (PLP). As a co-enzyme, it is thought to be important in protein and amino acid metabolism and in the breakdown of glycogen to glucose. Certain plants food contain a unique form of vitamin B$_6$ called pyridoxine glucoside, which appears to be only about half as bioavailable as vitamin B$_6$ from other food sources or supplements. Vitamin B$_6$ in a mixed diet is about 75% bioavailable. Fortified cereal (one cup) contains 0.5 to 2.5 mg of vitamin B$_6$. One banana (medium size) contains 0.68 mg of vitamin B$_6$. Increased dietary protein results in an increased requirement for vitamin B$_6$, probably because PLP is a coenzyme for many enzymes involved in amino acid metabolism.

The recommended daily allowance (RDA) for vitamin B$_6$ is 1.3 mg/day (males, 19-50 years), 1.7 (males, 51 years and older), 1.3 mg/day (females, 19-50 years), 1.5 mg/day (females, 50 years and older), 1.9 mg/day (pregnancy) and 2.0 mg/day (breastfeeding).

Bibliography

Oregon State University. The Linus Pauling Institute. Micronutrient Information Center. Http://lpi.oregonstate.

edu/infocenter

VITAMIN B$_{12}$ Cobalamin. It is a water-soluble vitamin, which is important as a co-enzyme in nucleic acid metabolism. A number of different forms exist. **Cynanocobalamin** is one of the most active forms and the one that is commercially available. Vitamin B$_{12}$ cannot be synthesized by plants or animals, only by micro-organisms. In food, it is bound to proteins and is found almost exclusively in animal products. Therefore strict vegetarians may be at risk of vitamin B$_{12}$ deficiency. **Intrinsic factor**, a glycoprotein produced by the parietal cells of the gastric mucosa, binds with vitamin B$_{12}$. When the intrinsic factor is absent, pernicious anemia results.

Vitamin B$_{12}$ is present in animal products such as meat, poultry, fish and shellfish, and to a lesser extent in milk, but it is not generally present in plant products or yeast. Vegetarians who eat no animal products require supplemental vitamin B$_{12}$. Individuals who are over the age of 50 years should obtain their vitamin B$_{12}$ in supplements or fortified foods like fortified cereals, because of the increased likelihood of food-bound vitamin B$_{12}$ malabsorption. Clams (steamed, 3 oz) contain 84 mcg of vitamin B$_{12}$; mussels (steamed, 3 oz) contain 20.4 mcg of vitamin B$_{12}$; and milk (8 oz, whole) contains 0.9 mcg of vitamin B$_{12}$. The recommended dietary allowance (RDA) for vitamin B$_{12}$ is 2.4 mcg/day in adults (19 to 50 years).

Atrophic gastritis is a condition that decreases the absorption of food-bound vitamin B$_{12}$. Because 10 to 30% of persons older than 50 years have atrophic gastritis, the recommendation for this age group is to obtain vitamin B$_{12}$ from supplements or fortified foods.

Bibliography

Food and Nutrition Board, Institute of Medicine (1998). *Dietary Reference Intakes for thiamin, riboflavin, niacin, vitamin B6, folate, vitamin B12, pantothenic acid, biotin and choline.* Washington, DC: National Academy Press.

Oregon State University. The Linus Pauling Institute. Micronutrient Information Center. Http://lpi.oregonstate.edu/infocenter

VITAMIN C   A water-soluble vitamin that is important for maintaining the structure of cartilage, bone and teeth. Its two active forms, **L-ascorbic acid** (the reduced form) and **dehydroascorbic acid** (the oxidized form), enable it to function both as a receiver and a donor of electrons in redox reactions. In its reduced form, vitamin C is readily oxidized, thus it serves as an antioxidant and reducing agent. It also indirectly activates many enzymes, but it is not a coenzyme. Vitamin C can directly scavenge superoxide, hydroxyl and lipid hydroperoxide radicals. Additionally, vitamin C plays an important role in recycling the vitamin E radical back to it reduced state. In the process of recycling vitamin E, reduced vitamin C is converted to a vitamin C (semiascorbyl) radical. Recycling of vitamin C radical can be achieved by NADH semiascorbyl reductase, or cellular thiols such as glutathione and dihydrolipoic acid. In high concentrations, vitamin C can exert pro-oxidant effects in the presence of transition metal ions such as ferric iron (Fe^{3+}) or copper (Cu^{2+}). The pro-oxidant action of vitamin C stems from its ability to reduce ferric iron (Fe^{3+}) to the ferrous (Fe^{2+}) state. Ferrous iron is known to be a potent catalyst in the production of free radicals. Mega-dose vitamin C supplementation should be avoided due to its pro-oxidant potential.

Unlike most animals, humans lack the necessary enzymes to synthesize vitamin C. **Scurvy** is a disease due to vitamin C deficiency. Symptoms include muscular weakness due to malformation of collagen. Vitamin C is required for hydroxylation of proline to hydroxyproline, without which collagen will not have its necessary strength. Vitamin C is essential for holding iron in its reduced state in many reactions, and is important in facilitating the absorption of non-heme iron from the intestine. There is also some evidence to suggest that vitamin C may increase blood concentration of 2, 3-diphosphoglycerate. There is no convincing evidence that megadoses of vitamin C prevent or cure the common cold. Ingestion of megadoses of vitamin C may result in uricosuria, excessive iron absorption, impaired leukocyte activity, and hypoglycemic-type effects. Abrupt withdrawal of megadoses of vitamin C can result in symptoms resembling scurvy.

Exercise generally causes a transient increase in

circulating vitamin C in the hours following exercise, but a decline below pre-exercise levels occurs in the days after prolonged exercise. These changes could be associated with increased exercise-induced oxidative stress. It is unclear if regular exercise increases the metabolism of vitamin C. The similar dietary intakes and responses to supplementation between athletes and nonathletes suggest that regular exercise does not increase the requirement for vitamin C in athletes.

An orange (medium sized) contains 70 mg of vitamin C. A sweet red bell pepper (half a cup, raw, chopped) contains 141 mg of vitamin C.

The recommended daily allowance (RDA) for vitamin C is based primarily on the prevention of deficiency. For adults it is 90 mg/day (males), 75 mg/day (females), 125 mg/day (male smokers) and 110 mg/day (female smokers). The RDA is higher for smokers because of increased oxidative stress from the toxins in cigarette smoke and the lower blood levels of vitamin C in smokers.

Bibliography

Oregon State University. The Linus Pauling Institute. Micronutrient Information Center. Http://lpi.oregonstate.edu/infocenter

Peake, J.M. (2003). Vitamin C: Effects of exercise and requirements with training. International Journal of Sport Nutrition and Exercise Metabolism 13(2), 125-151.

VITAMIN D A group of ten sterols named vitamin D_1 through D_{10} that exhibit **antirachitic** properties, i.e. they prevent a childhood disease called **rickets**. Vitamin D deficiency affects the mineralization of bones and teeth, causing disease characterized by soft bone that bends under body weight (rickets in children and osteomalacia in adults).

The most important of the ten sterols are D_2 (ergocalciferol) and D_3 (cholecalciferol). Ergocalciferol is found exclusively in plant foods. Cholecalciferol is found in animal foods, such as eggs and fish oils, but most is synthesized in the skin. Although classed as a fat-soluble vitamin, cholecalciferol is not actually a vitamin in the classic sense of dietary need and coenzyme function. Rather, it is a pro-hormone produced in the skin of animals including humans, using ultraviolet radiation in sunlight, from the precursor 7-dehydrocholesterol, which is converted into cholecalciferol. It is also produced in plants using ergosterol as a precursor and is converted to ergocalciferol in the presence of ultraviolet light.

Exposure to sunlight provides most people with their entire vitamin D requirement. Elderly persons have diminished capacity to synthesize vitamin D from sunlight exposure, and frequently use sunscreen or protective clothing in order to prevent skin cancer and sun damage. The application of sunscreen with sun-protection factor (SPF) of 8 decreases production of vitamin D by 95%. In latitudes around 40 degrees north or 40 degrees south, there is insufficient ultraviolet B light available for vitamin D synthesis from November to early March. Ten degrees further north or south this, there is insufficient ultraviolet B light from mid-October to mid-March. About 15 minutes of exposure on the hands, face and forearms 3 times weekly in the morning or late afternoon during the spring, summer and fall should provide adequate vitamin D and allow for storage of any excess in fat for use during the winter with minimal risk of skin damage.

Vitamin D is found naturally in very few foods. Foods containing vitamin D include some fatty fish (such as salmon), fish liver oils and eggs from hens that have been fed vitamin D. In the USA, milk is fortified with 10 mcg of vitamin D per quart. Accurate estimates of dietary intakes of vitamin D are difficult because of the high variability of the vitamin D content of fortified foods. There is no recommended dietary allowance (RDA) for vitamin D, but there is an adequate intake (AI) level that assumes no vitamin D is synthesized in the skin through exposure to sunlight. The AI for adults is 5 mcg/day (19-50 years), 10 mcg/day (51-70 years) and 15 mcg/day (70 years and older). For the elderly, meeting the AI for vitamin D will likely require supplemental sources of vitamin D if they do not drink generous quantities of fortified milk.

Cases of vitamin D toxicity, resulting in hypercalcemia and decreased bone mineral density, have been reported in osteoporosis patients using several nonprescription dietary supplements.

Bibliography

Food and Nutrition Board, Institute of Medicine (1997). *Dietary Reference Intakes for calcium, phosphorus, magnesium, vitamin D and fluoride*. Washington, DC: National Academy Press.

Oregon State University. The Linus Pauling Institute. Micronutrient Information Center. Http://lpi.oregonstate.edu/infocenter

VITAMIN E A fat-soluble vitamin, which, chemically, is one of eight naturally occurring compounds: alpha-tocopherol, which is the most common and biologically active; beta tocopherol; gamma-tocopherol; delta-tocopherol; alpha tocotrienol; beta-tocotrienol; gamma tocotrienol; and delta-tocotrienol.

Due to its high lipid solubility, vitamin E is associated with lipid-rich structures, such as mitochondria, sarcoplasmic reticulum and the plasma membrane. As an antioxidant, vitamin E is particularly important, because of its ability to convert superoxide, hydroxyl and lipid peroxyl radical to less reactive forms. Vitamin E can also break lipid peroxidation chain reactions that occur during free radical reactions in biological membranes. The interaction of vitamin E with a radical results in a decrease in functional vitamin E and the formation of a vitamin E radical. The vitamin E radical can be 'recycled' back to its native state by a variety of other antioxidants. The body excretes some of this altered vitamin E and recycles the rest by adding an electron from another antioxidant, such as vitamin C. This vitamin C radical can regain its antioxidant form by taking an electron from glutathione. The enzyme glutathione reductase restores glutathione to its antioxidant form and depends on selenium. Vitamin E also inhibits platelet activation and monocyte adhesion.

Vegetable oils, nuts, whole grains and green leafy vegetables are rich sources of vitamin E. All eight forms of vitamin E occur naturally in foods, but in varying amounts. Olive oil (one tablespoon) contains 1.6 mg alpha-tocopherol and 0.1 mg of gamma-tocopherol. Soy oil (one tablespoon) contains 1.2 mg of alpha-tocopherol and 10.8 mg of gamma-tocopherol. The recommended dietary allowance (RDA) for vitamin E is based on the prevention of deficiency symptoms. The RDA for adults is 15

mg/day. Most human studies investigating vitamin E supplementation have not demonstrated improvement in exercise performance. High doses of vitamin E can interfere with vitamin K action.

Bibliography

Food and Nutrition Board, Institute of Medicine (2000). *Dietary Reference Intakes for vitamin C, vitamin E, selenium and carotenoids*. Washington, DC: National Academy Press.

Oregon State University. The Linus Pauling Institute. Micronutrient Information Center. Http://lpi.oregonstate.edu/infocenter

VITAMIN K Quinines. Vitamin K is a generic term for derivatives of 2-methyl-1,4-naphthoquinone that have coagulation activity. Vitamin K controls the formation of coagulation factors II (prothrombin), VII (proconvertin), IX (Christmas factor, plasma thromboplastin component) and X (Stuart factor) in the liver. Other coagulation factors dependent on vitamin K are protein C, protein S, and protein Z. Proteins C and S are anticoagulants.

Vitamin K_2 (menaquinones) are synthesized by bacteria in the intestinal microflora and can supply part of the vitamin K requirements. Less than 50% of vitamin K requirement is met by bacterial synthesis. Vitamin K_1 (phylloquinones) is found only in plants and is the major dietary form of Vitamin K.

Green leafy vegetables and some vegetable oils (e.g. olive oil) are rich sources of vitamin K. Soybean oil (one tablespoon) contains 26.1 mcg of vitamin K and broccoli (cooked, one cup, chopped) contains 420 mcg of vitamin K.

Based on consumption levels of healthy individuals, the adequate intake (AI) of vitamin K for adults is 120 mcg (males) and 90 mcg/day (females).

Bibliography

Oregon State University. The Linus Pauling Institute. Micronutrient Information Center. Http://lpi.oregonstate.edu/infocenter

VLDL *See under* CHOLESTEROL.

VOLAR PLATE *See under* METACARPOPHALANGEAL JOINT.

VOLTAGE   The difference in net distribution of charged particles between two locations.

VOMITING   Emesis. The contents of stomach and sometimes the lower portions of the gastro-intestinal tract are forcefully expelled through the mouth. It can be triggered by a variety of stimuli, such as motion sickness, excessive alcohol intake, disease and touching the back of the pharynx. Sensory impulses are sent from the irritated sites to the emetic center of the medulla oblongata, causing the vomiting reflex. The diaphragm and abdominal wall muscles contract, increasing intra-abdominal pressure, the cardiac sphincter relaxes and the soft palate rises to close off the nasal passages. The **cardiac sphincter** is the valve between the distal end of the esophagus and the stomach. Before vomiting a person is typically pale-faced, feels nauseated and salivates. Excessive vomiting can cause dehydration and may lead to severe disturbances in the electrolyte and acid-base balance of the body.

VON HIPPEL-LINDAU DISEASE   A hereditary disease marked by tumors in the retina, brain, other parts of the central nervous system, and various organs throughout the body. The disease is caused by an autosomal dominant mutation in chromosome 3.

VULVA   *See under* GENITO-URINARY INJURIES.

W

WAIST-TO-HIP RATIO *See under* ABDOMINAL OBESITY.

WALKING A form of locomotion that involves placing one foot in front of the other while maintaining contact with the supporting surface. Approximate age of onset of rudimentary upright unaided gait is 13 months.

See also under DEVELOPMENT; GAIT; INFANT WALKERS.

WALKING REFLEX Stepping reflex. A postural reflex that is normal from the first few weeks after birth to about 6 months. It is elicited by holding the infant upright with the feet touching a supporting surface. The pressure on both feet causes the legs to lift and then descend. It resembles a crude form of walking.

WAKE *See under* DRAG.

WARFARIN *See under* THROMBOSIS.

WARM UP Techniques that are used to increase local muscle and total body (core) temperature before vigorous exercise. **Passive warm up**, such as taking a hot bath, involves increasing body temperature without exercising. **Active (general) warm up** involves increasing body temperature by active movements of major muscle groups. **Specific warm up** involves rehearsing the skills involved in a particular sport, but at a decreased intensity level.

Active warm up tends to result in slightly larger improvements in short-term performance (less than 10 seconds) than those achieved by passive heating alone. However, passive warm-up techniques may be important to supplement or maintain temperature increases produced by an active warm up, especially if there is an unavoidable delay between the warm up and the task and/or the weather is cold. Tissue temperature changes brought about by warming up persist for about an hour. The addition of a brief, task-specific burst of activity has been reported to provide further ergogenic effects for some tasks. While active warm up has been reported to improve endurance performance, it may have a detrimental effect on endurance performance if it causes a significant increase in thermoregulatory strain.

It seems that an increase above normal core temperature of two degrees Celsius is sufficient to produce: (i) more rapid and complete dissociation of oxygen from hemoglobin and myoglobin; (ii) acceleration of metabolic rate, leading to more efficient use of energy substrates; iii) decrease of muscle viscosity, leading to an improvement in the mechanical efficiency of muscular contractions; (iv) greater speed and force of muscular contraction; (v) more rapid redirection of blood flow to working skeletal muscle and away from the viscera at the start of exercise, due to vasodilation; (vi) improvement in delivery of energy substrates and removal of metabolic by-products, due to vasodilation; (vii) higher speed of nerve transmission; (viii) decreased risk of injury to muscle, because of higher blood saturation; and (ix) improved flexibility, ability to improve flexibility and decreased risk of injury, due to increased extensibility of tendons, ligaments and other connective tissues.

Vigorous warm-up exercise that normally results in an elevated blood and muscle lactate concentration has the potential to increase the aerobic energy turnover in subsequent high-intensity exercise. The elevation in muscle temperature by prior exercise does not appear to be implicated in the altered metabolic and gas exchange responses observed during subsequent exercise.

The optimal combination of the intensity, duration and mode of warm up exercise is not known, nor is the recovery period allowed before the criterion exercise challenge. It seems, however, that the time between warm-up and the event should be no longer than 15 minutes. For safety and effectiveness, warm up should be done before stretching.

See also ACTIVE RECOVERY; MASSAGE.

Bibliography

Bishop, D. (2003). Warm up I: Potential mechanisms and the effects of passive warm up on exercise performance. *Sports Medicine* 33(6), 439-454.

Bishop, D. (2003). Warm up II: Performance changes following active warm up and how to structure the warm up. *Sports Medicine* 33(7), 483-498.

Safran, M.R., Seaber, A.V. and Garrett, W.E. (1989). Warm-up and muscular injury prevention. An update. *Sports Medicine* 8(4), 239-249.

Shellock, F.G. and Prentice, W.E. (1985). Warming-up and stretching for improved physical performance and prevention of sports-related injuries. *Sports Medicine* 2(4), 267-278.

WARTENBERG'S SYNDROME Neuritis of the radial sensory nerve. It may afflict weight lifters who wear tight wristbands.

WATER The main mechanism in the body for transporting nutrients, internal secretions (such as hormones) and waste products. It is a medium in which chemical reactions take place. Diffusion of gases always occurs across surfaces moistened by water.

Water is also vital for thermoregulation. Water makes up about 60% and 50% of a man's and woman's body, respectively. About 55% of the body's water is found in the cells, about 39% in the interstitial fluid and about 6% in the plasma and lymph.

A normal daily water intake of 2.5 liters is comprised of (approximately) 1.2 liters from ingestion of liquid, 1 liter from food and 0.3 liters from metabolic water produced from energy-producing reactions. Water content in food varies from 95% in succulent fruit and vegetables, to 5% in nuts.

A normal daily water loss of 2.5 liters is comprised of (approximately) 1.5 liters in the urine, 0.6 through the skin as sweat, 0.3 liters as water vapor in expired air and 0.1 liters in feces. Each pound of weight loss corresponds to about 450 milliliters of dehydration.

See also DEHYDRATION; FLUID REPLACEMENT.

WATER INTOXICATION *See under* HYPONATREMIA.

WATER POTENTIAL The potential energy possessed by a mass of water. It is the physical property that determines the direction in which water will flow. This flow is the result of passive transport. In the context of osmosis, water potential determines the ability of water to move. Water always moves from areas of high water potential to low water potential. A hypertonic solution has lower water potential; a hypotonic solution has higher water potential.

WEIGHT The force that results from the action of a gravitational field on a mass. Weight is equal to the ground reaction force when the object is at rest on a horizontal surface. Assuming constant gravitational acceleration, mass can be estimated from weight using Newton's 2nd law. The SI unit is the newton (N). The US Customary unit is pound force (lbf).

WEIGHT CONTROL *See* BODY WEIGHT REDUCTION.

WEIGHTLIFTING BELT *See under* INTRA-ABDOMINAL PRESSURE.

WEIGHT TRAINING *See* RESISTANCE TRAINING.

WELLNESS *See under* HEALTH.

WERDNIG-HOFFMAN DISEASE Infantile spinal muscular atrophy. It is an inherited, degenerative disorder that affects the anterior horn cells of the spinal cord. It involves progressive, symmetrical muscle weakness that usually presents within the first six months of life. It is characterized by hypotonia and wasting of muscles, complete flaccid paralysis, and death (usually within the first 3 years of life). It affects 1 in 20,000 births, and is one of the most common autosomal recessive diseases in childhood.

Bibliography

National Organization for Rare Disorders. Http://www.rarediseases.org

WESTPHAL PHENOMENON The paradoxic contraction of passively shortened muscles. It is seen in dystonia, spasticity and Parkinsonian disorders. It is a typical symptom of deforming muscular dystrophy, reflecting disorders of muscular tone.

WHEEL AND AXLE   A wheel-type device attached to the axle about which it revolves. The radius of the wheel corresponds to the force arm of a lever. When the force is applied to the wheel in order to turn the axle, the mechanical advantage favors force; when the force is applied to the axle in order to turn the wheel, the mechanical advantage favors speed. Most wheel and axle arrangements in the human body favor speed, e.g. the contraction of the oblique abdominal muscles causes rotation of the trunk (wheel) around the spine (axle).

WHEELCHAIR ATHLETICS   About 0.1% of the total population in developed nations are confined to a wheelchair. Body composition of the wheelchair-confined subject is affected by wasting of muscles and osteoporosis in paralyzed limbs. There are fewer skin sores and related hospitalizations for people involved in wheelchair sports programs versus those not involved in regular sports activities.

The mechanical efficiency of a wheelchair is determined by a number of factors, including body mass, physiological efficiency of the user, the mass of the chair and friction in its bearings, the propulsion system, the skill of the athlete, the velocity of movement of the chair and the type of ground surface. Camber tubes or bars, near the center of the large wheels, permit adjustment of the angle of the wheels from 0 degrees (no camber) to 15 degrees (maximum camber). **Camber** is the degree to which the tops of the wheels slant inward. It makes pushing more efficient, decreases the chance that the arm will bump against the wheel, and permits comfortable elbow posture. The effort expended against ground friction and the ascent of any slope is proportional to body mass, but the load imposed by air resistance and a head wind is relatively independent of body mass. In athletes with good trunk control, trunk flexion alternates with trunk extension during the thrust and recovery phases of the arm in all sports, except for track. Having the knees as high as possible and the center of gravity as low as possible

facilitates optimal trunk flexion, which decreases aerodynamic drag, a better driving position for the arms, and increased trunk stability.

Strength of shoulder and elbow muscles is greater in wheelchair-confined subjects compared to the able bodied. Strength in the arm muscles is essential for mounting curbs and ramps in a wheel chair. Strength also facilitates perfusion of the arms during endurance effort. The grip strength of the wheelchair athlete is increased only slightly relative to that of non-disabled athletes, probably because the usual technique of fast wheelchair operation (a 'stroke') does not require gripping of the push rim. There is a negative correlation between speed and the hand time on the rim. Most well-trained sprint athletes adopt a shuttle-type motion, while endurance athletes choose a more circular pattern of arm movements.

Normal wheelchair ambulation demands anywhere from 9 to 55% of maximal oxygen uptake, depending on the age and fitness of the wheelchair user. Stroke volume is increased with training, probably due to a decreased afterload, and is associated with strengthening of the active arm and shoulder muscles. The muscles become stronger and the increase in blood pressure is less at a fixed intensity of isometric contraction. Depending on the extent of training of the arm muscles, arteriovenous oxygen difference during vigorous exercise may be normal or increased.

The principles of training for wheel chair athletics are similar to the able bodied, but there is a smaller margin between an effective training stimulus and overtraining. Overuse can cause stress fractures or cumulative trauma disorders. Upper-extremity injuries are more frequent in athletes who use a wheel chair than other disabled (but ambulatory) athletes. Manual wheelchair users are particularly susceptible to rotator cuff tears, lateral epicondylitis, and cubital tunnel or carpal tunnel neuropathies due to micro-injury caused by the repetitive motions required to propel themselves. Wheelchair track and road racers wear gloves to protect their hands and to make contact with the hand rim more efficient. The impact of the hand hitting the push rim may cause blisters, skin irritation, or fractured bones. When wheelchair use is the primary mode of mobility, it may be difficult to provide sufficient rest to allow complete healing. This can eventually lead to fibrocartilage metaplasia and calcific tendonitis.

Many wheelchair-racing clothes have been made of tight-fitting elastic fabric that presumably serves to improve venous pooling. Excessive constriction about the abdomen and upper thighs should be avoided, however, because this is associated with the development of blood clots in the extremities.

Dynamic arm exercise testing (e.g. arm crank ergometry) can be used to evaluate cardiovascular fitness in people who are unable to perform leg-cycle ergometer exercise owing to neurologic, vascular or orthopedic limitations. Such individuals include those with intermittent claudication, disabling arthritis, or paraplegia. There is a significantly lower physical work capacity and maximal heart rate for wheelchair ergometry compared to arm crank ergometry, but maximal oxygen uptake is similar for both exercise modes. For many people with disabilities, arm exercise is associated with deficient peripheral and central hemodynamic responses, due to inactivity of the skeletal muscle pump. There is evidence that arm work performance, metabolic and cardiopulmonary responses, and aerobic training capability may be improved by decreasing blood pooling and stasis in the legs, thereby enhancing venous return and cardiac output.

Chronology

•1946 • Wheelchair sport started in the USA as a result of World War II veterans surviving catastrophic injuries.
•1948 • In Britain, the first wheelchair games were organized by Sir Ludwig Guttmann at the Stoke Mandeville Paraplegic Unit. It coincided with the Olympic Games in London. The 14 male and 2 female participants were all former military personnel. Guttmann revolutionized treatment of persons with spinal cord injury at Stoke Mandeville Hospital in the late 1940s.
•1949 • The National Wheelchair Basketball Association was founded. It is played under National Collegiate Amateur Association (NCAA) rules with the same court size and basket height, but some differences, e.g. a 'physical advantage foul' is called when a player does not keep firmly seated in the wheelchair at all times.
•1956 • The National Wheelchair Athletic Association was founded in the USA. It is now called Wheelchair Sports, USA and it serves people with spinal cord injuries, spina bifida, poliomyelitis

and postpolio syndrome.
•1972 • The British Paraplegic Sports Society was founded by Sir Ludwig Guttmann. It was later renamed as the British Wheelchair Sports Foundation.
•1976 • Two persons with disabilities held a series of exhibitions and clinics on wheelchair tennis. The National Foundation of Wheelchair Tennis was founded as the governing body of the sport. In the following year, the first tournament was staged in Los Angeles and attracted 30 participants. In wheelchair tennis, a standard tennis racquet is used but the ball may bounce twice before being returned. Wheelchair tennis players are classified according to their skill level, rather than their neurological impairment.
•1988 • The United States Quad Rugby Association was founded. Rugby for persons with quadriplegia ('quad rugby') was developed in the 1970s by two sportsmen with quadriplegia who came from Winnipeg (Manitoba, Canada) and a professor of architecture at Manitoba University. It developed from wheelchair basketball and is a mix of basketball, ice hockey and American football. A basketball court is used for play, with cones placed at either end to identify goal lines. A goal is scored when an offensive player crosses the opponent's goal line while in clear possession of the ball. Ball handlers may take an unrestricted number of pushes, but must bounce or pass the ball within 10 seconds. A volleyball is used instead of a basketball, because it is lighter.

Bibliography

Compton, D.M., Eisenman, P.A. and Henderson, H.L. (1989). Exercise and fitness for persons with disabilities. *Sports Medicine* 7, 150-162.

Ferrera, M.S. et al. (1992). The injury experience of the competitive athlete with a disability: Prevention implications. *Medicine and Science in Sports and Exercise* 24, 184-188.

Ferrara, M.S. and Peterson, C.L. (2000). Injuries to athletes with disabilities: Identifying injury patterns. *Sports Medicine* 30(2), 137-143.

Shephard, R.J. (1988). Sports medicine and the wheelchair athlete. *Sports Medicine* 4, 226-247.

Shephard, R.J. (1990). *Fitness in special populations*. Champaign, IL: Human Kinetics.

Vanlandewijck, Y., Theisen, D. and Daly, D. (2001). Wheelchair propulsion biomechanics: Implications for wheelchair sports. *Sports Medicine* 31(5), 339-367.

WHEEZE An adventitious or abnormal breath sound heard when listening to the chest as a person breathes. Wheezes are continuous and musical sounding, and usually caused by airway obstruction from swelling or secretions. Wheezes can be high or low pitched.

WHIPLASH Trauma due to acceleration and deceleration of the head relative to the trunk in any plane. Many structures can be injured in whiplash, especially cervical structures, but also the brain. Although whiplash can occur in more than one plane, it occurs most commonly as a sagittal plane injury in the victim of a rear-end vehicular collision, where there is sequential acceleration of the vehicle, the victim's trunk and shoulders and, finally, the victim's head. At the instant of impact, the victim's head remains stationary while the vehicle is violently pushed forward. When the victim's trunk and shoulders are accelerated anteriorly, the head is forced into hyperextension. Once its inertia is overcome, the head is thrown forward into flexion ('whiplashed'). A secondary flexion injury may occur if the struck vehicle then strikes another vehicle in front of it and just as suddenly decelerates again, throwing the occupant forward once more. In American football, whiplash may occur when an athlete is tackled or blocked while unprepared.

WHITE BLOOD CELLS See LEUKOCYTES.

WHITE MATTER See under BRAIN; CENTRAL NERVOUS SYSTEM.

WIND Any motion of atmospheric air; it usually refers to the horizontal component of such motion. **Wind chill** is a concept that relates the rate of heat loss from humans under windy conditions to an equivalent air temperature for calm conditions. The **wind chill temperature** is an equivalent air temperature equal to the air temperature needed to produce the same cooling effect under calm conditions. It is not actually a temperature, but rather an index that helps relate the cooling effect of the wind to the air temperature under calm air conditions. Wind will not cause an exposed object to become colder than the ambient air. Higher wind speeds will only cause the object to cool to the ambient temperature more quickly. Wind chill calculations for the public in the USA started in 1973. The old wind chill index has recently been replaced by one in which the difference between the actual and equivalent temperature is only about as half as much. The old index overestimated the wind's cooling effect on human skin. The new index is based on the 5% of the public whose facial skin is the most thermally resistant, i.e.

those whose skin can get cold more quickly, even though the person doesn't necessarily feel cold inside, leaving the skin at greater risk from frostbite. An air temperature of 0 degrees Fahrenheit, with a 15 mph wind gives a wind chill temperature of minus 19 degrees Fahrenheit. At this wind chill temperature, exposed skin can freeze in 30 minutes.

Bibliography
National Weather Service (2001). Http://www.nws.noaa.gov/om/windchill

WINDING See SOLAR PLEXUS CONTUSION.

WINGATE TEST See under ANAEROBIC POWER.

WINGED SCAPULAE See under SCAPULAE.

WITHDRAWAL REFLEX See FLEXOR REFLEX.

WOLFF'S LAW See under BONE.

WORK The result of the utilization of energy to produce a change in a body. **Biologic work** in humans may be mechanical work of muscle contraction, the chemical work that synthesizes cellular molecules, or transport work that concentrates various substances in the intracellular and extracellular fluids. **Mechanical work** is done when a force acts against a resistance to produce motion in a body. If the force is parallel to the ground, mechanical work is the product of force and displacement. Otherwise it is the product of the following: magnitude of force, the cosine of the angle between the force vector and the line of displacement, and the displacement. The Standard International (SI) unit of work is the joule (J). 1 joule is the work done when 1 newton acts to move an object through a distance of 1 meter in the direction in which the force is applied. The US Customary unit is the foot.pound force (ft.lbf). 1 J = 0.737 ft.lbf. 1 J = 0.243 calories. 1 ft.lbf = 1.356 J.

In biomechanics, **external work** is work done by a performer on external objects (environment). **Internal work** is work done by a performer on the body links. In lifting an object of a given weight off the floor, a taller person must exert a force over a long distance and must therefore perform more work than a shorter person. **Positive work** is the work done by a force directed along the displacement. **Negative work (of a force)** is the work done by a force directed opposite to the displacement. In the context of human movement, negative work refers to work performed on, rather than by, a skeletal muscle. Negative work requires 10 to 30% less energy than positive work, possibly because of decreased muscle fiber activation.

Mechanical angular work is the product of the magnitude of the torque applied against an object and the angular distance that the object rotates in the direction of the torque while the torque is being applied. The SI unit is the joule.

The **work-energy principle** for a rigid body is that the total work done by all the forces acting on a rigid body is equal to the change in the body's kinetic energy. It also equals the work of the resultant force and couple.

The **zero-work paradox** is that for movement beginning and ending at rest at the same vertical location, energy is expended, but the work is zero.

See POWER; THERMODYNAMICS.

Bibliography

Zatsiorsky, V.M. (2002). *Kinetics of human motion*. Champaign, IL: Human Kinetics.

WRESTLER'S EAR *See* CAULIFLOWER EAR.

WRIST JOINT   Radio-carpal joint. A condyloid joint where the lower end of the radius articulates with the carpals. The carpal bones form gliding joints with each other. The bony anatomy of the wrist consists of two rows of carpal bones (proximal and distal). The proximal row consists of the scaphoid, lunate and triquetrum. The distal row consists of the trapezium, trapezoid, capitate and hamate. Because there are no musculotendinous structures that insert on either the distal or proximal row of carpals, wrist stability depends entirely upon ligamentous structures and the geometry of the bony configurations.

The movements of flexion, extension, abduction and adduction are permitted at the wrist joint. **Flexion** involves decreasing the angle between the hand and the forearm bones. Muscles that produce flexion are: *flexor carpi radialis, flexor carpi ulnaris* and *palmaris longus*. **Extension** involves increasing the angle between the hand and the forearm bones. Muslces that produce extension are: *extensor carpi radialis longus, extensor carpi radialis brevis, extensor carpi ulnaris* and *extensor digitorum communis*. **Abduction (radial deviation)** involves movement of the hand towards the radius. Muscles that produce abduction are: *extensor carpi radialis longus, extensor carpi radialis brevis, flexor carpi radialis, abductor pollicis longus* and *extensor pollicis brevis*. **Adduction (ulnar deviation)** involves movement of the hand towards the ulna. Muscles that produce adduction are: *flexor carpi ulnaris* and *extensor carpi ulnaris*.

See also HAND MUSCLES.

WRIST JOINT, FRACTURES   The most common mechanism of carpal fractures is an axial load applied to a hyperextended (dorsal flexed) wrist. In sport, this fracture results from falls or contact with another player.

With the wrist in this position, compressive forces are transmitted through the carpals to the distal radioulnar complex. Given a radius-to-ulna load distribution of 4 to 1, the scaphoid and lunate are most likely to be fractured because of their articulations with the radius. In sport, the most common and problematic fracture is the scaphoid fracture. Fracture of the carpal lunate is rare, but Kienböck's disease may occur in athletes. The most common ulnar fracture is a nightstick fracture caused by a direct blow. These fractures are usually seen in hockey, lacrosse or the martial arts. Fractures of the triquetrum are the second or third most common carpal fracture, and are usually avulsions from the dorsum of the bone. Avulsion fractures occur during a fall on the outstretched hand, with the wrist in ulnar deviation and dorsal flexion due to impingement from the hamate or ulnar styloid. **Ulnocarpal abutment syndrome** is impingement of the distal ulna on the ulnar aspect of the carpus, primarily at the ulnar aspect of the lunate and lunotriquetral region. It is common in sports involving repetitive flexion/extension or radial/ulnar deviation when the upper extremity is axially loaded. Isolated pisiform fractures are rare in sport, but may occur secondary to a direct blow to the hypothenar area such as from a pitched ball.

See also under ELBOW JOINT COMPLEX, FRACTURES; HAMATE BONE.

WRIST JOINT INJURIES *See* MEDIAN NERVE; METACARPOPHALANGEAL JOINT; RADIAL NERVE; SCAPHOID IMPACTION SYNDROME; ULNAR NERVE; WRIST JOINT, FRACTURES.

WRY NECK *See* TORTICOLLIS.

XYZ

XANTHINE   A purine base formed in tissues during nucleic acid degradation. It is an intermediate product in the catabolism of adenine and guanine. Xanthine derivatives, e.g. caffeine, are also found in plants.

XANTHOMAS   Tumor-like collections of lipids (triglycerides and cholesteryl esters) that can arise in the tendons, points of continued trauma (e.g. knees and elbows) and palms. They may be a symptom of underlying metabolic disorders that are associated with an increase in blood lipids, such as diabetes and familial hypercholesterolemia. They can appear anywhere on the body, but commonly appear on the elbows, joints, tendons, knees, hands, feet or buttocks.

Xanthelasmas are small deposits of fatty materials under the surface of the skin. They are painless and usually appear in the skin of the eyelids near the nose. They may indicate increased blood cholesterol levels and increased levels of triglycerides.

X-RAY   A form of electromagnetic radiation with wavelengths of between approximately 0.1 nanometers to 200 nanometers. A machine emits the radiation as photons that pass through the body and then get detected by a sensitive film. Structures that are dense (e.g. bone) will block most of the photons and will appear on developed film. Structures containing air will be black on film. Muscle, fat and fluid appear as shades of grey. Metal and contrast media (intravenous or oral contrast) blocks almost all the photons and will appear bright white. X-ray films are useful for detecting fractures, misalignments and abnormal cavities.

Depending on the dose, X-rays can decrease cell division, damage genetic material and harm unborn children. Unborn children are particularly sensitive to X-rays, because their cells are rapidly dividing and developing into different types of tissue. If a pregnant woman is exposed to sufficient doses of X-rays, then birth defects may occur or diseases, such as leukemia, may occur later in life.

YAWNING   Yawning reflex. It is a reflex characterized by a single deep inhalation (with mouth open) and stretching of the muscles of the jaw and trunk. It occurs in many animals. Yawning does not appear to be due to carbon dioxide or oxygen levels in the blood. Yawning and breathing are controlled by different mechanisms. It has been shown that yawning occurs when people are fatigued, when they are awakening and during other times when the state of alertness is changing. It may thus be a means of communicating changing environmental or internal body conditions to others. If so, yawning in humans is most likely vestigial and an evolutionary mechanism that has lost its significance.

Bibliography

Provine, R.R. et al. (1987). Yawning. No effect of 3-5% CO2, 100% O2, and exercise. *Behavioral and Neural Biology* 48(3), 382-393.

YIPS   *See under* STRESS, PSYCHOLOGICAL.

YOGA   *See under* MIND-BODY EXERCISE.

YOHIMBINE   A nitrogen-containing alkaloid extracted from the bark of the yohimbe tree. It functions as an alpha-2 adrenoreceptor blocker, increasing serum levels of norepinephrine. Nutritional supplement adverts have claimed that yohimbine and yohimbe bark increase testosterone levels, but there appears to be no scientific evidence to support this claim.

YOUNG'S MODULUS   *See under* ELASTIC MODULI.

ZEITGEBER   *See under* BIOLOGICAL RHYTHMS.

ZEITGEIST   'The spirit of the time.' It refers to the general set of general beliefs, ideas, etc. of a particular period in history.

ZINC   A metallic element, which, as a 'trace element,' is a co-factor in many different enzymes such as lactate dehydrogenase. Most of the zinc in the human body is located in muscles and bones. In blood, it is found mainly in red blood cells, with much smaller amounts found in plasma. A zinc metalloenzyme in red blood cells, **carbonic anhydrase**, changes the carbon dioxide end product of all energy-producing reactions to a bicarbonate ion that can be safely carried in the blood to the lungs for excretion of its carbon dioxide portion. Another zinc metalloenzyme, alcohol dehydrogenase, catalyses the conversion of ethanol to acetaldehyde, in the first step in one of the pathways for the breakdown of beverage alcohol.

An excessive increase in carbohydrates and low intake of proteins and fat may lead to suboptimal zinc intake in 90% of athletes. Mild zinc deficiency is difficult to detect, because of the lack of definitive indicators of zinc status. In athletes, zinc deficiency can lead to anorexia, significant loss in body weight, latent fatigue with decreased endurance and a risk of osteoporosis.

Shellfish, beef and other red meats are rich sources of zinc. Nuts and legumes are relatively good plant sources. Oysters (6 medium, cooked) contain 43.5 mg of zinc; and beef (3 oz, cooked) contains 5.8 mg of zinc. Zinc bioavailability is relatively high in meat, eggs and seafood, because of the relative absence of compounds that inhibit zinc absorption and the presence of certain amino acids (cysteine and methionine) that improve zinc absorption. The zinc in whole grain products and plant proteins is less bioavailable, due to their relatively high content of phytic acid, a compound that inhibits zinc absorption. The enzymatic action of yeast decreases the level of phytic acid in foods.

The recommended dietary allowance (RDA) for zinc is based on a number of different indicators of zinc nutritional status and represents the daily intake likely to prevent nearly all individuals in a specific age and gender group. In adults, the RDA is 11 mg (males) and 8 mg/day (females). Vegetarians may require up to 50% more zinc, since phytates, as well as calcium, hinder zinc absorption in the body. Children between the ages of 7 months and 12 months should consume zinc-containing foods if they consume human milk, which does not contain enough zinc for them to meet the RDA, or should be given formula containing zinc. A tolerable upper intake level (UL) of 40 mg for adults was based on research showing that zinc adversely affects copper absorption at high levels of intake. Zinc supplementation may decrease copper status, impair immune responses, and decrease plasma HDL cholesterol.

Bibliography

Campbell, W.W. and Anderson, R.A. (1987). Effects of aerobic exercise and training on the trace minerals chromium, zinc and copper. *Sports Medicine* 9, 9-18.

McDonald, R. and Keen, C.L. (1988). Iron, zinc and magnesium nutrition and athletic performance. *Sports Medicine* 5, 171-184.

Micheletti, A., Rossi, R. and Rufini, S. (2001). Zinc status in athletes: Relation to diet and exercise. *Sports Medicine* 31(8), 577-582.

Oregon State University. The Linus Pauling Institute. Micronutrient Information Center. Http://lpi.oregonstate.edu/infocenter

ZOOCHEMICALS   Compounds found in animals with chemical properties or biological effects that suggest health benefits. *See also* PHYTOCHEMICALS.

ZYGOTE   The fusion of a female and a male gamete in sexual reproduction. It is a fertilized egg. *See under* HEREDITY.